Dental Materials

Clinical Applications for Dental Assistants and Dental Hygienists

Dental Materials
Clinical Applications for Dental Assistants and Dental Hygienists

FIFTH EDITION

W. STEPHAN EAKLE, DDS, FADM
Professor of Clinical Dentistry Emeritus
Department of Preventive and Restorative Dental Sciences
School of Dentistry, University of California
San Francisco, California

KIMBERLY G. BASTIN, CDA, EFDA, CRDH, EdD
Associate Professor
Director of Dental Hygiene
Assistant Dean of Health Professions and Wellness
State College of Florida Manatee-Sarasota
Bradenton, Florida

ELSEVIER

Elsevier
3251 Riverport Lane
St. Louis, Missouri 63043

DENTAL MATERIALS: CLINICAL APPLICATIONS FOR DENTAL ASSISTANTS AND DENTAL HYGIENISTS, FIFTH EDITION

ISBN: 978-0-443-11449-6

Copyright © 2026 by Elsevier Inc. All rights are reserved, including those for text and data mining, AI training, and similar technologies.

Publisher's note: Elsevier takes a neutral position with respect to territorial disputes or jurisdictional claims in its published content, including in maps and institutional affiliations.

No part of this publication may be reproduced or transmitted in any form or by any means, electronic or mechanical, including photocopying, recording, or any information storage and retrieval system, without permission in writing from the publisher. Details on how to seek permission, further information about the Publisher's permissions policies and our arrangements with organizations such as the Copyright Clearance Center and the Copyright Licensing Agency, can be found at our website: www.elsevier.com/permissions.

This book and the individual contributions contained in it are protected under copyright by the Publisher (other than as may be noted herein).

> **Notice**
>
> Practitioners and researchers must always rely on their own experience and knowledge in evaluating and using any information, methods, compounds or experiments described herein. Because of rapid advances in the medical sciences, in particular, independent verification of diagnoses and drug dosages should be made. To the fullest extent of the law, no responsibility is assumed by Elsevier, authors, editors or contributors for any injury and/or damage to persons or property as a matter of products liability, negligence or otherwise, or from any use or operation of any methods, products, instructions, or ideas contained in the material herein.

Previous editions copyrighted 2021, 2016, 2011 and 2003.

Senior Content Strategist: Kelly Skelton
Senior Content Development Specialist: Maria L. Broeker
Publishing Services Manager: Deepthi Unni
Senior Project Manager: Beula Christopher
Senior Book Designer: Renee Duenow

Printed in India

Last digit is the print number: 9 8 7 6 5 4 3 2 1

 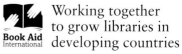

Reviewers

Christy M. Bessette, CDA, EFDA, CRDH, MEd
Dental Assisting Program Director
Cape Coral Technical College
Cape Coral, Florida

Heidi Gottfried-Arvold, MS, CDA
Dental Assistant Program Director/Instructor
Gateway Technical College
Kenosha, Wisconsin

Mandar M. Patole, MDS, BDS
Oral and Maxillofacial Surgeon, Hair Transplant Surgeon and Oral Implantologist
Maharashtra University of Health Sciences (MUHS)
Nashik, Maharashtra, India

Fernanda Perry, DDS, MAEd
Dental Programs Faculty, Dental Assisting Clinical Coordinator
Central Carolina Community College
Sanford, North Carolina

Daniela Taranto, RDH, EdD
Assistant Professor
CTE Teacher at New York City College of Technology
Clara Barton High School
Brooklyn, New York

Therese L. Tippie, EFDA, CDA, CDIPC, BS, MA
Dental Assisting Instructor
South Florida State College
Avon Park, Florida

Preface

LIFELONG LEARNING

The subject of dental materials is rapidly changing as researchers and corporations develop new materials and improve those currently in use. Consequently, dental assistants and dental hygienists are challenged to keep up with the new materials, their physical properties, their handling characteristics, and their clinical applications. As important members of the dental team, dental auxiliary must be adept at placing or assisting in the placement of dental materials, and they play a valuable role in the maintenance of dental materials once they are in the mouth. Dental auxiliary are also instrumental in educating patients in the home maintenance of restorations and prostheses and what to expect with a new prosthesis. Dental auxiliary play major roles in preventive dental education and therapy in most practices.

To stay current, the dental assistant and dental hygienist must be lifelong learners who know how to use available resources to update their knowledge. *Dental Materials: Clinical Applications for Dental Assistants and Dental Hygienists* provides the foundation for that lifelong learning for the new student and serves as an important update on new materials and improvements in materials for the practicing auxiliary. In addition, it provides them with sound criteria for evaluating steps in the restorative process in which they will play a role, such as making accurate alginate and elastomeric impressions, placement of dental sealants, cord retraction, and selection and application of a matrix for composite and amalgam.

KEY GOALS

The goal of *Dental Materials: Clinical Applications for Dental Assistants and Dental Hygienists* is to provide students with the following:
- The principles of dental materials so they can understand the rationale for the use of these materials
- The opportunity to apply newly gained knowledge through clinical and laboratory procedures
- The ability to evaluate their work using accepted criteria
- The opportunity to test their knowledge with review questions and prepare for board examinations
- The opportunity to apply critical thinking through the use of case-based discussion questions

FEATURES

The chapters have the following components:
- **Learning and performance objectives** to guide students in understanding.
- **Key terms** listed and defined in the order of their presentation in the chapters and highlighted in the chapters in colored print.
- **Basic principles and applications, physical properties, and handling characteristics** of the dental materials presented in each chapter.
- **Generous use of color illustrations and photography throughout to aid learning**.
- **Helpful clinical tips or precautions** regarding the use of the materials, highlighted in boxes set apart from the main text for emphasis.
- **Illustrated clinical and laboratory procedures** presented in step-by-step instructions so that students can practice common applications of the materials. Notes at the top of the procedure sheets guide the clinician as to precautions for patients or clinicians and alert the clinician when procedures may not be allowed by all state dental boards.
- **Competency assessment forms** for each procedure to test skills attainment located on the Evolve website.
- **Review questions** to enable students to test their comprehension of the subject matter and prepare for examinations; answers are provided at the end of the book.
- **Case-based discussion topics** that encourage students to relate what they have learned to the actual application in the dental office. Instructors may want to use them as topics for group discussions.
- **Reference lists** at the end of each chapter to help students find additional information about the principles, procedures, and properties of the dental materials discussed.
- **Instructional videos are accessible on EVOLVE website** to enhance and reinforce materials presented.

NEW TO THIS EDITION

- Key Points summarize the important portions of the chapters and highlight important concepts or facts students should know.
- Recall questions are placed throughout each chapter to encourage students to test themselves on comprehension of what they have read.

- Expanded use of information presented in bulleted format to reduce lengthy paragraphs.
- Many chapters are more concise with the reduction or elimination of supplementary information.
- New illustrations and clinical photographs throughout.
- Numerous new instructional videos found on the Evolve website to supplement learning from the text.
- New Clinical tips and Cautions.

EVOLVE

An expanded Evolve website provides a variety of resources for both instructors and students.

FOR INSTRUCTORS

- TEACH Instructor's Resource Manual (includes answer keys, lesson plans, PowerPoints, and student handouts)
- Test Bank
- Image Collection

FOR STUDENTS

- Practice quizzes
- Competency forms
- Instructional video

A NOTE TO EDUCATORS

Dental Materials: Clinical Applications for Dental Assistants and Dental Hygienists is written to be easily comprehended by students with varying amounts of science in their educational backgrounds. Learning and performance **objectives** and key points summaries draw the students' attention to the important concepts and features of the materials. **Key terms** are not only listed but also defined at the start of each chapter. Recall questions throughout the chapters help the student identify if the basic concepts have been comprehended. Helpful **clinical tips** are used throughout the chapters to call attention to clinical points to which the student may not have been exposed, and **cautions** are noted where appropriate for the safety of both the patient and the clinician. Material presented in bulleted form highlights important information and reduce lengthy paragraphs. The book is generously illustrated to help with the comprehension of clinical and **laboratory procedures**, especially for our visual learners. The procedures help the students to see how the materials are actually used, and when students apply their newly gained knowledge, the procedures reinforce learning. **Review questions** help reinforce what the students have learned and help prepare them for board examinations. **Case-based discussion** topics can be used for group discussions and bring the flavor of real-life dentistry to the application of dental materials.

Additional material is included on the Evolve website. **Chapter quizzes** (nearly 300 questions) help students prepare for classroom and board examinations. **Competencies** are included for each procedure so that students can evaluate their own efforts and also receive feedback from their instructors.

YOUR COMMENTS, PLEASE

The authors would appreciate suggestions or comments regarding this book because it is written with your needs in mind. We hope instructors and students will enjoy this book and gain as much from it as we have intended.

W. Stephan Eakle
mouthtools@gmail.com
Kimberly G. Bastin
bastink@scf.edu

Acknowledgments

The authors would like to express their deep appreciation to all those whose invaluable contributions made this edition possible. We extend our heartfelt thanks to the dental researchers and clinicians whose work forms the foundation of this text. Their expertise, along with the clinical illustrations, has greatly enhanced the quality of this edition, offering learners a visual understanding beyond the written word.

We are especially grateful to our colleagues for their insight and suggestions and to the dental manufacturers for providing essential technical information and detailed procedural images. Your support has been integral to the completion of this edition.

A special thank you goes to the editorial team at Elsevier, particularly Kelly Skelton for guiding this edition to completion, and to Maria Broeker, Oviya Balamurugan and Beula Christopher for their unwavering dedication and tireless efforts in bringing this fifth edition to life.

On a personal note, we extend our deepest thanks to our family members—Sheila Eakle, Rachel, Olivia, Sam, and Emi—for your constant energy, inspiration, and understanding. To my friend and colleague, Denny Weir, for the sarcasm that provided motivation; to Jimmy Bastin, for his endless encouragement, feedback, and guidance; and to Toni McLeroy and Mara Beth Womack, both friends and colleagues, for their positivity and enthusiastic support.

Lastly, we are profoundly grateful to our friends and colleagues for their patience and understanding during this demanding process and for their unwavering belief in this project.

To all of you, we extend our deepest gratitude for your dedication and superb efforts on behalf of students and educators. Your contributions have made this journey not only possible but deeply rewarding.

Contents

1 Introduction to Dental Materials, 1
The Role of the Dental Auxiliary in the Use of Dental Materials, 1
Evidence-Based Dentistry, 2
The Historical Development of Dental Materials, 3
The Agencies Responsible for Standards, 3
  American Dental Association, 3
  American National Standards Institute, 5
  US Food and Drug Administration, 5
  International Agencies, 5
Future Developments in Dental Biomaterials, 5
Summary, 5

2 Oral Environment and Patient Considerations, 7
Classification of Dental Materials, 9
  Preventive/Therapeutic Materials, 9
  Restorative Materials, 9
  Auxiliary Materials, 9
Biocompatibility, 9
  Adverse Response, 10
Biomechanics, 10
Oral Factors Affecting Dental Materials, 10
  Force, Stress, and Strain, 10
Moisture and Acid Levels, 12
  Effect of pH, 12
Galvanism, 13
Temperature, 13
  Expansion and Contraction, 13
  Thermal Conductivity, 14
Retention, 14
  Mechanical and Chemical Retention, 14
  Bonding, 15
Microleakage, 16
Esthetics and Color, 16
  How We Sense Color, 16
  Components of Color, 16
  Optical Properties, 17
  Viewing Color, 17
Oral Biofilm and Dental Materials, 17
  Community of Microorganisms, 17
  Formation of Oral Biofilm, 17
  Biofilm and Oral Disease, 18
  Probiotics, 18
  Biofilm and Systemic Diseases, 18
  Biofilm on Dental Materials, 18
  Managing the Oral Biofilm, 18
Detection of Restorative Materials, 19
  Methods of Identification, 19
Summary, 21

3 Physical and Mechanical Properties of Dental Materials, 24
Physical Structure, 25
  Atoms, 25
  Types of Bonds, 25
  The Three States of Matter, 26
Properties of Dental Materials, 26
  Physical Properties, 26
  Mechanical Properties, 27
Classification of Materials, 28
Composition, 29
Reaction Activated by Mixing, 30
Manipulation of Materials, 31
  Ratios of Components, 31
  Effect of Temperature and Humidity, 31
  Mixing of Components, 31
Shelf Life, 31
Summary, 32

4 General Handling and Safety of Dental Materials in the Dental Office, 34
Material Hazards in the Dental Environment, 34
  Exposure to Particulate Matter, 34
  Exposure to Biological Contaminants, 35
Bioaerosols in the Dental Setting, 35
  Dental Bioaerosols, 35
Chemical Safety in the Dental Office, 36
  Hazardous Chemicals, 36
  Skin and Eyes, 38
  Inhalation, 38
  Ingestion, 38
  Exposure to Bisphenol A, 38
  Exposure to Mercury, 38
Acute and Chronic Chemical Toxicity, 38
  Acute Chemical Toxicity, 38
  Chronic Chemical Toxicity, 38
Personal and Chemical Protection, 39
  Hand Protection, 39
  Eye Protection, 39
  Protective Clothing, 39
  Inhalation Protection, 39
Control of Chemical Spills, 40
  Mercury Spill, 40
  Flammable Liquids, 40

Acids, 40
Eyewash, 40
Ventilation, 40
General Precautions for Storing and Disposing of Chemicals, 41
Storage, 41
Disposal of Chemicals, 41
Empty Containers, 41
Regulations for Hazardous Waste Disposal, 42
Dental Laboratory Infection Control, 42
Hazard Communications, 43
Occupational Safety and Health Administration Hazard Communication Standard, 43
Hazard Communication Program, 43
Labeling of Chemical Containers and Safety Data Sheets, 44
Labeling Exemptions, 44
Eco-Conscience Green Practices, 46
Patient Safety, 47
Summary, 48

5 Impression Materials, 51

Overview of Impressions, 52
Types of Impressions, 53
Impression Material Types, 53
Impression Trays, 54
Stock Trays, 54
Triple Trays (Closed-Bite Trays), 54
Bite Registration Trays, 54
Custom Trays, 54
Hydrocolloids, 54
Reversible Hydrocolloid (Agar), 55
Irreversible Hydrocolloid (Alginate), 56
Making Alginate Impressions, 57
Criteria for Clinically Acceptable Impressions, 61
Two-Consistency Alginate System, 61
Elastomers, 62
Use of Adhesive, 62
Elastic Recovery, 63
Wettability, 63
Polysulfides, 63
Silicone Rubber Impression Materials, 63
Polyvinyl Siloxane (Vinyl Polysiloxane), 64
Vinyl Polyether Silicone Hybrid, 68
Components of Impression Making for Crown and Bridge Procedures, 69
Gingival Retraction, 69
Making the Impression, 72
Digital Impressions, 73
Learning Curve, 73
Scanning Devices, 74
Advantages and Disadvantages of Digital Impressions, 76
Soft Tissue Management, 76
Expanded Use of Digital Impressions, 77
Inelastic Impression Materials, 77
Dental Impression Compound, 77
Impression Plaster, 78
Zinc Oxide Eugenol Impression Material, 78
Impression Wax, 78
Infection Control Procedures, 78
Disinfecting Impressions, 78
Disinfecting Casts, 79
Sterilizing Impression Trays, 79
Summary, 79

6 Gypsum and Wax Products, 93

Gypsum Materials, 94
Uses of Gypsum Materials, 94
Desirable Qualities, 94
Behaviors of Gypsum Products, 95
Formation of Gypsum, 95
Production of Gypsum Products, 95
Physical Properties, 96
Classification of Gypsum Products, 98
Impression Plaster (Type I), 98
Model Plaster (Type II), 98
Dental Stone (Type III), 99
Dental Stone, High Strength/Low Expansion (Type IV), 99
Dental Stone High Strength/High Expansion (Type V), 99
Metal-Plated and Epoxy Dies and Resin-Reinforced Die Stone, 99
Investment Materials, 99
Manipulation of Gypsum Products, 100
Material Selection, 100
Proportioning (Water-to-Powder Ratio), 100
Mixing: Spatulation, 100
Setting Times, 101
Control of Setting Times, 102
Fabricating Diagnostic/Working Casts, 103
Storage, 104
Cleanup, 105
Infection Control and Safety Issues, 105
Separating the Impression from the Cast, 105
Trimming the Casts, 105
Composition and Properties of Dental Waxes, 106
Composition of Waxes, 106
Properties of Waxes, 106
Melting Range, 106
Flow, 107
Excess Residue, 107
Thermal Expansion, 107
Classification of Waxes, 107
Waxes are Grouped as Follows, 107
Pattern Waxes, 107
Processing Waxes, 108
Impression Waxes, 109
Other Waxes Utilized in the Dental Office, 109
Manipulation of Waxes, 109
Lost Wax Technique, 109
Summary, 111

7 Principles of Bonding, 120

Basic Principles of Bonding, 121
    Surface Wetting, 121
Etching Enamel and Dentin, 121
    Enamel Etching, 121
    Dentin Etching, 123
    Bond Strength, 125
Bonding Systems, 126
    Components of Bonding Systems, 126
    History of the Development of Bonding Systems, 127
    Modes of Cure of Adhesives, 128
    Oxygen-Inhibited Resin Layer, 129
Classification of Bonding Systems, 129
    Etch-and-Rinse Bonding Systems, 129
    Self-Etch Bonding Systems, 130
    Clinical Application of Universal Bonding Adhesive, 132
    Biocompatibility, 134
    Compatibility with Other Resins, 134
    Contamination of Bonding Site, 135
Bonding of Restorations, 135
Summary, 136

8 Composites, 139

History of the Development of Composite Resin for Dentistry, 140
Direct-Placement Esthetic Restorative Materials, 140
Composite Resin, 141
    Components, 141
    Polymerization, 141
    Physical and Mechanical Properties of Composite Resins, 142
Classification of Composites by Filler Size, 145
    Macrofilled Composites, 145
    Microfilled Composites, 145
    Hybrid Composites, 145
    Microhybrids, 146
    Nanohybrids, 146
    Nanocomposites, 146
    Other Composite Types, 147
Clinical Handling of Composites, 150
    Uses of Composite Resins, 150
    Selection of Materials, 150
    How to Match the Shade, 150
    Color Characteristics: Hue, Chroma, and Value, 150
    Placing the Composite, 153
    Resin-to-Resin Bonding, 153
    Contaminants, 155
    Layering (Stratification) of Composite, 154
    Shelf Life, 155
    Dispensing and Cross-Contamination, 155
    Matrix Systems, 156
    Light-Curing, 160
    Finishing and Polishing Composites, 163
Why Composites Fail, 163
    Composite Repair, 163
Indirect-Placement Composite Resins, 163
Summary, 164

9 Glass Ionomers, Compomers, and Bioactive Materials, 170

Glass Ionomer Cements, 170
Conventional Glass Ionomer Cements, 170
    Physical and Mechanical Properties of Glass Ionomer Cement, 171
    Uses for Glass Ionomer Cements, 171
Resin-Modified (Hybrid) Ionomers, 173
    Properties, 173
    Curing Modes, 174
    Use for Pediatric Dentistry, 174
    Other Uses, 174
    Nano-Ionomers, 174
    Clinical Application of Glass Ionomer Cements, 174
Compomers, 176
    Fluoride Release, 176
    Packaging, 176
    Setting Reaction, 176
    Bonding, 176
    Uses, 176
    Placement and Finishing, 176
    Properties, 176
    Giomers, 176
Bioactive Dental Materials, 177
    Physical Properties, 177
    Uses, 177
Summary, 177

10 Dental Ceramics, 180

Dental Ceramics, 181
    A Brief History of Dental Ceramics, 181
    Advantages and Disadvantages of Ceramic Restorations, 181
    Classification of Dental Ceramics, 181
    Glass and Nonglass Ceramics, 181
Glass-Based Ceramics, 182
    Porcelain, 182
Nonglass-Based Ceramics, 183
    Alumina, 183
    Zirconia, 183
Physical and Mechanical Properties, 183
    Flexural Strength, 183
    Thermal Properties, 184
    Optical Properties, 184
    Biocompatibility, 184
Ceramic Processing Techniques, 185
CAD/CAM Technology, 185
    Basic Components of CAD/CAM Systems, 185
CAD/CAM Restorations, 185
    Ceramic CAD/CAM Materials, 185
Summary of CAD/CAM Steps for Producing a Restoration, 188

Clinical Applications for Ceramic Materials, 189
   Rationale for the Selection of Ceramic Materials, 189
   Ceramic Veneers, 189
   Ceramic Inlays, Onlays, Fixed Bridges, 191
   Finishing and Polishing Ceramic Restorations, 191
   Cementation of All-Ceramic Restorations, 191
   Maintenance of All-Ceramic Restorations, 192
   Porcelain-Fused-to-Metal Restorations, 193
Shade Taking, 195
   Involving the Dental Auxiliary and the Patient, 195
   Steps for Ceramic Shade Taking, 195
   Devices for Taking the Shade, 197
Summary, 198

11 Dental Amalgam, 203

Dental Amalgam, 204
   Alloys Used in Dental Amalgam, 204
   Silver-Based Amalgam Alloy Particles, 204
   Setting Transformation (Amalgamation), 204
   Properties of Amalgam, 205
   Applications for Dental Amalgam, 207
Matrix Systems, 207
   Use of Matrix Bands, 207
   Sectional Matrix Systems, 213
   Manipulation of Amalgam (See Procedure 11.1), 213
   Dispensing of Alloy and Mercury, 213
   Trituration, 213
   Consequences of Improper Handling, 214
   Working and Setting Times, 214
   Placement and Condensation, 215
   Finishing and Polishing, 215
   Use of a Cavity Sealer, 215
Longevity of Amalgams, 216
   Repair of Amalgam, 217
   Bonding Amalgam, 217
   Allergy to Amalgam, 217
The Safety of Dental Amalgam, 217
   ADA Stance on Dental Amalgam Safety, 217
   Concerns About Mercury Exposure, 217
   Restrictions on Amalgam Use, 218
Summary, 219

12 Metals and Alloys, 226

Structure of Metals and Their Alloys, 227
   Pure Metals, 227
   Lattice Structure, 227
   Alloys, 227
   Properties of Casting Alloys, 229
Porcelain Bonding Alloys, 232
   Porcelain-Bonded-to-Metal Restorations, 233
Identalloy Program, 234
Solders, 234
   Gold Solders, 234
   Flux, 235
   Silver Solders, 235
Wrought Metal Alloys, 235
   Stainless-Steel Alloys, 235
   Preformed Provisional Crowns, 236
Metals Used in Orthodontics, 236
   Archwires, 236
   Brackets and Bands, 237
   Retainers and Removable Orthodontic Appliances, 237
   Space Maintainers, 238
Metals Used in Endodontics, 239
   Endodontic Files and Reamers, 239
Endodontic Posts, 239
   Purpose of the Post, 239
   Classification of Posts, 239
Summary, 242

13 Dental Implants, 246

Dental Implants, 247
   Subperiosteal Implants, 247
   Transosteal Implant, 247
Endosseous Implants, 247
   Indications for Implants, 247
   Contraindications for Implants, 248
   Benefits of Implants, 248
   Implant Components, 248
   Implant Materials, 249
   Implant Fixture Designs, 250
Image-Guided Implant Planning, 251
   Implant Planning Software, 251
   Advantages of Guided Implant Surgery, 251
   Computer-Aided Design/Computer-Aided Machining Technology, 252
Implant Placement, 252
   Informed Consent, 252
   Surgical Risks, 252
   Preparation of the Patient for Surgery, 253
   Postsurgical Instructions, 253
   Implant Placement Surgeries, 253
   Two-Stage Surgical Procedure, 253
   One-Stage Surgical Procedure, 253
   Immediate-Placement Surgical Procedure, 254
   Immediate Loading, 254
Restorative Phase, 255
   Implant Impression and Laboratory Components, 255
   Impression Procedures, 255
   Retention of the Implant Crown, 255
   Retention of the Removable Prosthesis, 258
Mini-Implants, 258
   Uses for Mini-Implants, 259
Bone Grafting, 259
   Purpose of Bone Grafting, 259
   Types of Bone Grafts, 259

Implant Longevity, 261
   Long-Term Success, 261
   Implant Failure, 262
Implant Maintenance, 263
   Biological Seal, 263
   Peri-Implantitis, 263
   Tissue Management, 263
   Home Care, 263
   Hygiene Visit, 266
Sutures, 269
   Types of Sutures, 269
   Suturing Techniques, 270
Summary, 270

14 Polymers for Prosthetic Dentistry, 275

Review of Polymer Formation, 276
   Copolymers, 276
   Polymerization, 276
   Cross-Linked Polymers, 276
   Polymerization Reactions, 276
Acrylic Resins (Plastics), 276
   Uses of Acrylics, 276
   Modifiers, 277
   Properties, 277
   Curing, 277
   Allergic Reaction, 278
   Acrylic Resins for Denture Bases, 278
   Polymerization Reaction, 278
   Processing Methods for Complete Dentures, 280
   Processing of a Removable Partial Denture, 283
Digital Dentures, 284
Denture Reline Materials (Liners), 285
   Soft Relining Materials, 286
   Home Care for Soft Liners, 287
   Hard Relining Materials, 287
   Laboratory Reline, 289
   Over-the-Counter Liners, 289
Detection and Management of Denture Sores, 289
   Signs and Symptoms, 289
   Causes of Denture Sores, 289
   Treatment of Denture Sores, 289
   Home Care for Denture Sores, 290
Denture Teeth, 290
   Acrylic Resin Teeth, 290
   Composite Resin Teeth, 292
   Porcelain Teeth, 292
Characterization of Dentures, 292
Plastics for Maxillofacial Prosthetics, 293
Denture Repair, 294
   Chemical-Cured Acrylic Repair Material, 294
   Light-Cured Repair Material, 295
Custom Impression Trays and Record Bases, 295
   Chemical-Cured Tray Material, 295
   Light-Cured Tray and Record Base Material, 297
   Infection Control Procedures, 297
Instructions for New Denture Wearers, 298
   What to Expect With Your New Dentures, 298
Care of Acrylic Resin Dentures, 298
   Home Care, 299
   In-Office Care, 299
   Storage of Dentures, 300
Summary, 300

15 Provisional Restorations, 306

Dental Procedures That May Require Provisional Coverage, 307
Criteria for Provisional Coverage, 307
Maintain Prepared Tooth Position Relative to Adjacent and Opposing Teeth, 307
Protect the Exposed Tooth Surfaces and Margins, 307
   Protect the Gingival Tissues, 308
   Provide Function, 308
   Esthetics and Speech, 309
   Retention, 309
Properties of Provisional Materials, 309
   Strength, 309
   Hardness, 309
   Tissue Compatibility, 309
   Esthetics, 309
   Provisional Crown Materials, 310
   Preformed Crowns, 310
   Stainless-Steel Crowns, 311
   Aluminum Shell and Tin-Silver Alloy Crowns, 311
   Fitting the Crown, 311
   Polycarbonate Crown Forms, 312
   Customized Provisional Crowns, 313
Materials for Custom Provisional Restorations, 314
   Methacrylate Provisional Materials (Acrylics), 314
   Composite Resin Provisional Materials, 315
   Methods of Fabrication of Custom Provisionals, 316
   Direct Technique, 316
   Indirect-Direct Technique, 319
   Advanced Techniques, 319
Handling the Provisional Restoration, 320
   Cementing the Provisional Restoration, 320
   Removing the Provisional Restoration, 320
   Cleanup, 321
Patient Education, 321
   Home Care Instructions, 322
Summary, 322

16 Dental Cement, 333

Dental Cements, 334
   Classification, 334
   Uses of Dental Cements, 334
Type I Cements: Luting Agents, 339
   Properties of Luting Cements, 339
   Selecting A Luting Cement, 342
Classification of Luting Cements, 342
   Water-Based Luting Cements, 343
   Resin-Based Luting Cements, 347
   Oil-Based Luting Cements, 351

    Bioactive Cements, 353
    Handling of Cements, 353
        Storage, 353
        Pre-cementation Check, 353
        Mixing, 353
        Working and Setting Times, 354
        Loading the Restoration, 355
        Removal of Excess Cement, 355
        Cement-Associated Peri-Implant Disease, 356
        Cleanup, Disinfection, and Sterilization, 356
        Care Around Margins, 356
    Summary, 357

17 Abrasion, Finishing, Polishing, and Cleaning, 369

    Finishing, Polishing, and Cleaning, 370
        Factors Affecting Abrasion, 371
        Mode of Delivery of Abrasives, 373
        Microparticle Abrasives, 374
        Materials Used in Abrasion, 374
    Finishing and Polishing Procedures, 379
        Margination and Removal of Flash, 380
        Finishing and Polishing Amalgam, 381
        Procedures for Finishing and Polishing Amalgam Restorations, 381
        Finishing and Polishing Composite, 381
        Finishing and Polishing Gold Alloy, 382
        Finishing and Polishing Ceramics (Porcelain), 382
    Polishing During Oral Prophylaxis (Coronal Polish), 383
        Amalgam, 383
        Composite, 383
        Gold Alloys and Ceramics, 383
        Resin/Cement Interface, 384
        Implants, 384
        Air Polishing and Air Abrasion, 384
    Laboratory Finishing and Polishing, 386
    Rag Wheel, 386
    Felt Cones and Wheels, 386
    Safety/Infection Control, 387
    Patient Education, 387
    Summary, 387

18 Preventive and Desensitizing Materials, 394

    Fluoride, 395
        Topical and Systemic Effects, 395
        Protection Against Erosion, 396
        Bacterial Inhibition, 396
        Fluoride and Antibacterial Rinses for the Control of Dental Caries, 396
        Methods of Delivery, 398
        Safety, 402
    Pit and Fissure Sealants, 403
        Purpose, 403
        Indications, 404
        Susceptibility of Teeth to Fissure Caries, 405
        Composition, 405
        Working Time, 405
        Color and Wear, 406
        Placement, 406
        Patient Record Entries, 407
        Effectiveness, 407
        Troubleshooting Problems With Sealants, 408
        Glass Ionomer Cement as a Sealant, 408
    Desensitizing Agents, 408
        Mechanism of Tooth Sensitivity, 409
        Treatment, 410
        Categories and Components of Desensitizing Agents, 410
    Remineralization, 411
        Products, 411
        Resin Infiltration, 412
    Summary, 412

19 Teeth Whitening Materials and Procedures, 421

    Teeth Whitening (Bleaching), 421
        Types of Stains, 422
        History of Peroxide Whitening, 423
        How Whitening Works, 423
    Whitening, 424
        Pretreatment Evaluation, 424
        Treatment Methods, 424
        Types of In-Office Treatments, 425
        Whitening of Nonvital Teeth, 427
        Home Whitening (Prescribed by the Dentist), 427
        Over-the-Counter Products, 429
        Nondental Options, 430
        Role of the Dental Auxiliary, 430
        Potential Side Effects of Teeth Whitening, 430
        Restorative Considerations, 431
        Retreatment, 432
    Enamel Microabrasion, 432
        Adverse Outcomes, 432
    Summary, 432

20 Preventive and Corrective Oral Appliances, 440

    Preventive and Corrective Oral Appliances, 440
        Sports Mouth Guards, 440
        Night Guards (Bruxism Mouth Guards), 442
        Oral Appliances to Treat Snoring and Obstructive Sleep Apnea, 445
        Preventive Orthodontics, 446
        Space Maintainers, 446
        Interceptive Orthodontics, 446
        Thumb Sucking Appliance, 446
        Palatal Expansion Appliances, 446
        Crossbite Corrector, 447
        Orthodontic Tooth Aligners, 447
        3D Printing, 447
    Summary, 449

Appendix

Answers to Review Questions, 454

Glossary, 456

Index, 464

List of Procedures

- 4.1 Safety Data Sheet and Label Exercise, 48
- 5.1 Making an Alginate Impression, 80
- 5.2 Making a Double-Bite Impression for a Crown, 83
- 5.3 Bite Registration With Elastomeric Material, 85
- 5.4 Wax Bite Registration, 87
- 5.5 Disinfection of Impression Material or Bite Registration, 89
- 6.1 Mixing Gypsum Products, 111
- 6.2 Pouring the Cast: Anatomic Portion, 112
- 6.3 Pouring the Cast: Art (or Base) Portion, 114
- 6.4 Separating the Impression From the Cast, 115
- 6.5 Trimming Diagnostic Casts, 115
- 7.1 Enamel and Dentin Bonding Using the Etch-and-Rinse Technique, 136
- 8.1 Placement of Class II Composite Resin Restoration, 165
- 10.1 Surface Treatment for Bonding Glass-Based Ceramic Restorations, 198
- 11.1 Placing and Carving Class II Amalgam, 220
- 13.1 Suture Removal, 271
- 14.1 Fabrication of Custom Acrylic Impression Trays, 301
- 15.1 Metal Provisional Crown, 322
- 15.2 Polycarbonate Provisional Crown, 324
- 15.3 Custom Provisional Coverage: Direct Technique, 327
- 15.4 Intracoronal Provisional Cement Restoration, 328
- 16.1 Bonding Orthodontic Brackets, 357
- 16.2 Zinc Oxide Eugenol Cement (ZOE): Primary and Secondary Consistency, 359
- 16.3 Zinc Phosphate Cement: Primary Consistency, 360
- 16.4 Zinc Polycarboxylate Cement: Primary Consistency, 361
- 16.5 Glass Ionomer Cement: Pre-Dosed Capsule, 362
- 16.6 Resin-Based Cement for Indirect Restorations: Ceramic, Porcelain, Composite, 363
- 16.7 Self-Adhesive Technique for Indirect Restorations: Ceramic, Porcelain, Composite, 365
- 17.1 Finishing and Polishing a Preexisting Amalgam Restoration, 388
- 17.2 Polishing a Preexisting Composite Restoration, 389
- 18.1 Applying Sodium Fluoride Varnish, 413
- 18.2 Applying Topical Fluoride, 413
- 18.3 Applying Silver Diamine Fluoride (SDF), 415
- 18.4 Applying Dental Sealants, 415
- 19.1 In-Office Whitening, 433
- 19.2 Clinical Procedures for Home Whitening, 435
- 19.3 Fabrication of Custom Whitening Trays, 436
- 20.1 Fabrication of a Sports Mouth Guard (Protector), 450

Introduction to Dental Materials

Chapter Objectives

On completion of this chapter, the student should be able to:

1. Explain the importance of the study of dental materials for the allied oral health practitioner.
2. Examine why it is necessary that the allied oral health practitioner have an understanding of dental materials in the delivery of dental care.
3. Discuss evidence-based decision-making as it relates to dental materials. What questions might you ask yourself or your practice to ensure you are increasing the potential for successful patient care outcomes?
4. Review the historical development of dental materials.
5. List and compare the agencies responsible for setting standards and specifications for dental materials.
6. Discuss the requirements necessary for a consumer product to qualify for the American Dental Association Seal of Acceptance.

The study of dental materials (biomaterials) is the science covering the evolution, development, properties, manipulation, care, and evaluation of materials used in the treatment and prevention of dental diseases and the interactions of these materials with the tissues of the face and mouth. Specifically, it includes principles of engineering, chemistry, physics, and biology. Dental biomaterials science is continually evolving as dentistry keeps up with the requirements for delivering optimal health care while delivering minimally invasive dentistry.

The tooth and the tooth's supporting structure, esthetics, and function are important considerations for the patient's overall well-being. The dentist, dental assistant, and dental hygienist should have a working knowledge of why materials behave as they do and how we can help to maximize their performance. Through an understanding of how the basic principles of biomaterials affect the choice, manipulation, patient education, and care of all materials used to assist in rendering dental services, the dental team can help to ensure the ultimate success of a patient's dental work and contribute to their quality of life.

THE ROLE OF THE DENTAL AUXILIARY IN THE USE OF DENTAL MATERIALS

Over the years, efforts have been made to employ allied oral health practitioners (also referred to in the text as dental auxiliaries), dental assistants, and dental hygienists in performing intraoral tasks to efficiently deliver health care and enhance the productivity of the dental practice. Until 1970 only dental hygienists were permitted to perform intraoral functions in all states. Although laws vary from state to state, virtually every state has modified, updated, and changed its state restrictions to allow for the performance of intraoral procedures by all allied oral health practitioners. At present, several states allow for the placement as well as care of restorative and other therapeutic agents in the patient's mouth by dental auxiliaries, which includes the new category of advanced practice dental therapists.

In the traditional role, the dental assistant is directly responsible for the manipulation and delivery of dental materials within specific guidelines outlined by the dental manufacturer, while the dental hygienist's responsibilities more frequently include the care of the restorative material once it has been placed and the application of therapeutic and preventive agents. Expanded function auxiliaries provide restorative services after the dentist has prepared the tooth for restoration. These services may include placement and carving or finishing of the restorative material, placement of the retraction cord, and taking a preliminary impression for crown and bridge restorations and/or endodontic procedures. The dental therapist may provide basic preventive and restorative treatment to children and adults in affiliation with, or under the general supervision of, a dentist. Typically, dental therapists work primarily in settings that serve low socioeconomic populations or in a dental health professional shortage area. State regulations determine the educational requirements and scope of practice for the expanded function auxiliary and the dental therapist.

All oral health practitioners must have a complete understanding of the potential hazards in the manipulation and disposal of materials and be educated to handle them safely. Background knowledge of the basic principles of dental materials is also essential to appreciate the selection of a particular restoration or treatment procedure for individual patient application. In many circumstances, it becomes the auxiliary's role to educate the patient on the reasons the dentist has recommended a particular material or the choices the patient may have for a particular circumstance.

Dental materials are classified as preventive, restorative, or therapeutic. The search for the ideal material, designed to prevent and treat disease or restore tooth structures, continues to elude the profession. Many significant improvements have happened in dental materials in recent years; however, despite these improvements, the perfect material does not yet exist. The ideal material would be biocompatible and esthetic, bond permanently to tooth structures, and be useful in repairing or regenerating missing tissues.

This may seem overwhelming, given the ever-growing variety and changes of materials available, recommendations for their use or disuse, and rapidly developing techniques in their manipulation, placement, and care. Professional journals, weblinks, dental material manufacturers or manufacturer's representatives, and other resources can provide invaluable information. The knowledgeable dental assistant continually reviews products recommended and used by their dental practice to provide a reliable resource for patients and dentists.

> **Why Study Dental Materials?**
>
> *To enhance safety:* Appropriate handling and disposal of dental materials.
> *To promote awareness:* Awareness of the overall success of a particular material's properties in dental applications.
> *To maintain materials properly:* Recognition of dental materials present in the oral cavity; effective cleaning, polishing, and instrumentation.
> *To deliver correctly:* Accurate knowledge of the behavior of a dental material on application, correct manipulation of the material, and effective delivery or assistance in delivery of the material.
> *To educate patients:* Ability to present options concerning dental material choices, maintenance of materials present, and reasons for possible failure.

EVIDENCE-BASED DENTISTRY

The American Dental Association (ADA) defines *evidence-based dentistry* as an approach to oral health care that requires the judicious integration of systematic assessments of clinically relevant scientific evidence relating to the patient's oral medical history with the dentist's clinical expertise and the patient's treatment needs and preferences. Searches through scientific literature identify thousands of citations for materials and techniques in restoring and treating oral structures. With this wealth of scientific information, evidence-based decision-making (EBDM) aids the clinician in making decisions about what is relevant to incorporate into practice. The following questions should be asked to appropriately incorporate EBDM into your practice:

- How does your practice make decisions regarding the techniques, technology, and products used?
- How do you analyze the published scientific literature to make sure a product provides a clinical benefit to the patient?
- Do you try product samples before giving them to your patients?
- How does your office stay informed about the newest advances in dentistry?
- How do you incorporate the patient's needs and choices into your decision-making process?

Evidence alone does not replace clinical expertise or input from the patient. EBDM requires an understanding of new concepts and the development of new skills. The clinician must be able to incorporate the best research evidence along with clinical expertise and patient preferences. Developing an evidence-based approach to addressing patient problems will greatly increase the potential for successful patient care outcomes by understanding the cause-and-effect relationship between the biomaterials selected and the success of the treatment rendered. The ADA offers a website (https://www.ada.org/resources/ada-library/evidence-based-databases) for dental professionals and their patients to access the most current, clinically relevant information. The EBDM approach is based on scientific research and clinician expertise and is tailored to the patient's needs (Fig. 1.1).

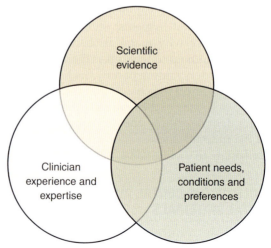

FIG. 1.1 The elements of evidence-based dentistry. (From Sakaguchi RL, Powers JM. *Craig's Restorative Dental Materials.* 13th ed. Mosby; 2012.)

> **? Do You Recall?**
>
> Why should evidence-based decision-making be an integral part of the dental practice?

THE HISTORICAL DEVELOPMENT OF DENTAL MATERIALS

The concept of using materials to alter the appearance and/or function of the natural dentition occurred prior to the first century. Just as today, the diet of our cave-dwelling ancestors was a chief contributor to dental disease. Preventive dentistry had an early beginning as well, with fluoride first mentioned in 1874. The first community water fluoridation program was introduced in 1945.

Whether through the desire for a natural look or more ornamentation, history shows that the appearance of teeth was important to our early ancestors.

The history of dental materials and techniques in the restoration, replacement, and beautification of our teeth is full of ingenuity (Table 1.1). Even early humans knew the importance of maintaining these important structures and, more often than not, suffered the pain associated with their neglect. Through centuries of dental practice, dental professionals have been challenged with the restoration of tooth and oral structures lost to disease and trauma.

THE AGENCIES RESPONSIBLE FOR STANDARDS

Most of the triumphs and atrocities of dentistry were discovered by trial and error, mainly at the expense of the patient. It is only in more recent times that the study of dental materials includes standards set forth to evaluate a material or technique before it is tried in the patient's mouth.

AMERICAN DENTAL ASSOCIATION

Dentistry continued to try to elevate and regulate the practice of the profession with the establishment of the ADA in 1859.

Seal of Acceptance

By 1930 the ADA had established guidelines for testing products and awarded the first Seal of Acceptance in 1931 (Fig. 1.6). Members of the ADA's Council on

Table 1.1 Historical Development of Dental Materials

ERA	DEVELOPMENTS
Ancient times	600–300 BCE—Etruscans practice dentistry with artificial teeth and gold work.
Middle Ages	700—Chinese medical text mentions "silver paste" for tooth structure replacement.
Sixteenth century	1530—*The Little Medicinal Book for All Kinds of Diseases and Infirmities of the Teeth*, the first book devoted entirely to dentistry, is published in Germany. Written for barbers and surgeons who treat the mouth, it covers practical topics such as oral hygiene, tooth extraction, drilling teeth, and placement of gold fillings.
Eighteenth century	1874—Fluoride first mentioned. Pierre Fauchard introduces the technique of joining maxillary and mandibular dentures with springs and hinges (Fig. 1.2). This was done to compensate for the weight of the dentures, which made retention of the maxillary denture virtually impossible. Casts constructed of plaster and wax are used for the construction of dentures with finely carved ivory teeth (Fig. 1.3) and animal and cadaver teeth. Denture teeth fired from porcelain in France. First dental assistant employed by C. Edmund Kells of New Orleans.
Nineteenth century	1901—Fredrick McKay credited with noting dental fluorosis in Colorado Springs (Fig. 1.4). 1945—First community water fluoridation system. Denture bases made of rubber by the Goodyear brothers. Silver coins mixed with mercury as the first dental amalgam. "Amalgam War"—American Society of Dental Surgeons passes a resolution not to use amalgam. G.V. Black develops an acceptable amalgam formula. Silicate cements developed for esthetic restorations. Cohesive gold foil introduced (Fig. 1.5).
Twentieth century	Dr. William Taggart develops the method to cast gold inlays. Dr. Alfred Fones opens the first school for dental hygienists. Development of acrylic resin for fillings and dentures. Fluoride placed in community drinking water. Development of the acid-etch technique for bonding. Composites replace silicate cements for esthetic restorations. Light-activated composites. Modern ceramics are developed for esthetic and restorative alternatives. First commercial home tooth-whitening product to be marketed.

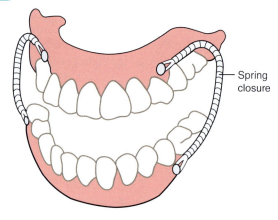

FIG. 1.2 A denture with spring closure, much like those worn by George Washington.

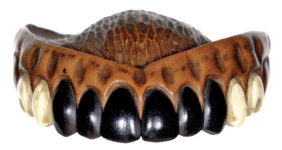

FIG. 1.3 A denture of carved black and white ivory teeth.

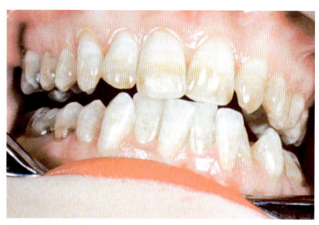

FIG. 1.4 Severe dental fluorosis.

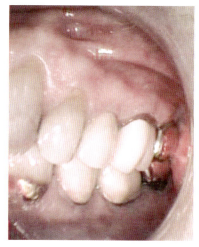

FIG. 1.5 Class V gold foil restoration on the facial surface of the mandibular first premolar.

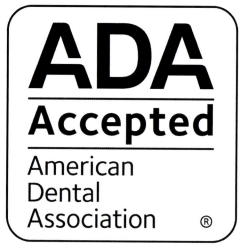

FIG. 1.6 The American Dental Association (ADA) Seal of Acceptance.

Consumers and dentists alike recognize this important symbol of a dental product's safety and effectiveness. The ADA Seal of Acceptance is designed to help consumers make informed decisions about the safety and efficacy of products. Consumers can be confident in products bearing the ADA seal as these products have undergone voluntary yet strict testing. The ADA review process outlines a broad spectrum of requirements that must be met to qualify for the ADA seal. A list of products and guidelines for qualification for the ADA Seal of Acceptance are available online at https://www.ada.org/resources/research/science-and-research-institute/ada-seal-of-acceptance.

? Do You Recall?

Why is the American Dental Association Seal of Acceptance important to the dental consumer?

Scientific Affairs and ADA staff scientists reviewed dental drugs, materials, instruments, and equipment for safety and effectiveness before awarding the ADA seal. The ADA seal has evolved since its inception; in 2005 the ADA decided to phase out the seal for professional products and award it only to consumer products. Although the ADA review process is strictly voluntary, more than 300 consumer dental products carry the ADA Seal of Acceptance. Most common among these are toothpaste, toothbrushes, mouth rinses, floss and other interdental cleaners, sugar-free chewing gum, and denture adherents and cleansers.

AMERICAN NATIONAL STANDARDS INSTITUTE

The American National Standards Institute (ANSI) was founded in 1918. The mission of this not-for-profit organization is to enhance the global competitiveness of US businesses while helping to ensure the safety and health of consumers and the protection of the environment. The development of ANSI/ADA Specification Number 41, Recommended Standard Practices for Biological Evaluation of Dental Materials, represents the establishment of biological tests for dental materials.

US FOOD AND DRUG ADMINISTRATION

The US Food and Drug Administration (FDA) is one of the oldest consumer protection agencies and is charged with protecting the public by ensuring products meet certain standards of safety and efficacy. The original Pure Food and Drug Act of 1906 did not include provisions to ensure medical and dental device safety or claims. In 1976 the Medical Device Amendments were signed to give the FDA regulatory authority over medical and dental devices that are now classified and regulated according to their degree of risk to the public. Dental materials, considered devices by the FDA, as well as over-the-counter products sold to the public, are subject to control and regulation by the FDA Center for Devices and Radiological Health. There are three classifications of medical (including dental) devices, grouped according to the amount of control needed to ensure their safety and efficacy:

- *Class I:* Lowest risk, good manufacturing standards and record-keeping practices, materials such as examination gloves and prophylaxis (prophy) paste, and some over-the-counter products.
- *Class II:* Products required to meet performance standards set by the FDA or ADA, such as amalgam and composite materials.
- *Class III:* The most regulated devices that support or sustain human life, including products such as endosseous implants and bone-grafting materials. These require premarket approval of the FDA, involving scientific review to ensure their safety and effectiveness.

INTERNATIONAL AGENCIES

Two international agencies, the FDI World Dental Federation and the International Organization for Standardization (ISO), represent the standards used to develop specifications and testing at the international level. These standards are developed through the ISO's technical committee for dentistry (ISO/TC 106).

Under Canada's Medical Devices Regulations, dental manufacturers that apply for a license to distribute materials used in dentistry within Canada must provide a valid certificate showing that their quality management system complies with the ISO standard for quality systems (ISO 13485:2003). To receive such a certificate, manufacturing companies are audited to ensure their procedures comply with requirements set out in the standard. These international standards are invaluable in meeting today's high demand for dental materials and devices.

FUTURE DEVELOPMENTS IN DENTAL BIOMATERIALS

The dental materials used today are much better than those used in the past, but they are still far from being perfect. Materials continue to be developed, and techniques for their manipulation have improved. Despite much more effort in health promotion and disease prevention, dental caries remains a major global public health problem. Dental restorations are still needed.

The ADA, FDA, and ISO are committed to continuing to evaluate, test, monitor, and assess risks and review claims and labels of all materials used in dentistry (see Chapter 4). Current research concentrates on bringing technology to the dental office, reducing the number of dental visits, and making dental appointments faster, minimally invasive, and more comfortable for the patient, resulting in optimum patient-centered care.

SUMMARY

There have been many advances in the quality and efficacy of dental materials; the challenge to dental professionals is to use evidence-based practice to critically review the claims, performance, and long-term end-product results of the materials and devices chosen. The input of the allied oral health practitioner is imperative in the successful choice of these materials to deliver quality service to the patient.

The allied oral health practitioner will continue to play an important role in the successful delivery, manipulation, and maintenance of dental-related technologies and materials. Embrace the study of dental materials, for it is the advancement of this science that will ultimately change the way we look at the replacement of oral structures.

Case-Based Discussion Questions

1. Compile a list of 5 to 10 dental products that display the ADA Seal of Acceptance and are found in your local drugstore or supermarket.
2. *How is the seal displayed on the items identified in case study question 1? Ask family and friends if the seal is important in their selection of a dental product. How does the presence of the seal affect your recommendation of a particular product?*
3. Research a dental product by using the Internet or by contacting a manufacturer's representative.
4. *What information is available on the dental product? What type of research has been done? How is the product marketed? What assistance is available to the consumer or dental office?*

BIBLIOGRAPHY

American Dental Association (ADA): Home page. Available from http://www.ada.org.

ADA: ADA: history of dentistry timeline. Available from https://www.ada.org/resources/ada-library/dental-history

ADA: Policy on evidence-based dentistry. Available from https://www.ada.org/resources/research/science-and-research-institute/evidence-based-dental-research.

ADA: ADA Seal of Acceptance. Available from https://www.ada.org/resources/research/science-and-research-institute/ada-seal-of-acceptance.

ADA: ADA Seal Products. Available from https://www.ada.org/resources/research/science-and-research-institute/ada-seal-of-acceptance/product-search#sort=%40productname%20ascending.

Forrest JL, Miller SA, Overman PR, et al: *Evidence-based decision-making: a translational guide for dental professionals,* Philadelphia, 2009, Lippincott Williams & Wilkins.

International Standards Organization (ISO)/TC 106: Dentistry. Available from https://www.iso.org/caring-about-health-and-safety.html

Ring ME: *Dentistry: an illustrated history,* New York, 1993, Harry N. Abrams.

U.S. Food and Drug Administration: Home page. Available from http://www.fda.gov.

Wynbrandt J: *The excruciating history of dentistry: toothsome tales & oral oddities from Babylon to braces,* New York, 2000, Martin's Press.

Oral Environment and Patient Considerations

2

http://evolve.elsevier.com/Eakle/materials/

Chapter Objectives

On completion of this chapter, the student should be able to:
1. Identify the qualities of the oral environment that make it challenging for long-term clinical performance of dental materials.
2. Describe the long-term clinical requirements of therapeutic and restorative materials.
3. List and give examples of four types of biting forces and the tooth structures most ideally suited to them.
4. Define stress, strain, and ultimate strength and compare the ultimate strength of restorative materials during each type of stress to tooth structures.
5. Summarize how moisture and acidity in the mouth can affect dental materials.
6. Explain how galvanism can occur in the mouth and how it can be prevented.
7. Discuss thermal conductivity and thermal expansion and contraction, and compare the values of thermal expansion and conductivity of restorative materials with those of tooth structures.
8. Determine how mechanical and chemical adhesion, or bonding, work to retain restorations.
9. Describe the factors that determine successful adhesion, including wettability, viscosity, film thickness, and surface characteristics.
10. Describe microleakage and how it can lead to recurrent decay and postoperative sensitivity.
11. Define biocompatibility and discuss why requirements for biocompatibility may fluctuate.
12. Describe tooth color in terms of hue, value, and chroma.
13. Discuss the characteristics of oral biofilm and its role in the etiology of dental caries and periodontal disease.
14. Explain the importance of detection of restorations and methods for detection.

KEY TERMS

Adhesion the act of sticking two things together. In dentistry, the term adhesion is used to describe the bonding or cementation process. Chemical adhesion occurs when atoms or molecules of dissimilar substances bond together and differs from cohesion in which attraction among atoms and molecules of like (similar) materials holds them together

Adverse Response an unintended, unexpected, and harmful or unwelcomed response of an individual to dental treatment or biomaterial

Auxiliary Materials materials used to fabricate and maintain restorations, directly or indirectly

Biocompatible the property of a material that allows it not to impede or adversely affect living tissue

Biofilm a complex community of oral microorganisms living on surfaces within the mouth. When these colonies are found on teeth or restorations, they are commonly called dental plaque

Bonding to connect or fasten; to bind

Chroma the intensity or strength of a color (e.g., a bold yellow has more chroma than a pastel yellow)

Coefficient of Thermal Expansion the measurement of change in volume or length in relation to change in temperature

Compressive Force force applied to compress an object

Corrosion deterioration of a metal caused by a chemical attack or electrochemical reaction with dissimilar metals in the presence of a solution containing electrolytes (such as saliva)

Dimensional Change a change in the size of matter. For dental materials, this usually manifests as expansion caused by heating and contraction caused by cooling

Exothermic Reaction the production of heat resulting from the reaction of the components of some materials when they are mixed

Fatigue Failure a fracture resulting from repeated stresses that produce microscopic flaws that grow

Film Thickness the minimal attainable thickness of a layer of a material. It is particularly important in the context of dental cements

Flexural Stress bending caused by a combination of tension and compression

Fracture Toughness a measure of the energy needed to fracture a material

Galvanism an electrical current transmitted between two dissimilar metals in a solution of electrolytes

Hue the color of a tooth or restoration. It may include a mixture of colors, such as yellow-brown

Insulators materials having low thermal conductivity

Interface the surface between the walls of the preparation and the restoration or between two dental materials

Microleakage leakage of fluid and bacteria caused by microscopic gaps that occur at the interface of the tooth and the restoration margins

Opaque optical property in which light is completely absorbed by an object

Percolation movement of fluid in the microscopic gap of a restoration margin as a result of differences in the expansion and contraction rates of the tooth and the restoration with temperature changes associated with ingestion of cold or hot fluids or foods

Resilience a measure of the energy needed to permanently deform a material

Restorative Materials materials used to reconstruct the tooth structure

Retention a material's ability to maintain its position without displacement under stress

Shearing Force force applied when two surfaces slide against each other

Solubility susceptible to being dissolved

Strain distortion or deformation that occurs when an object cannot resist a force

Stress the internal force, which resists the applied force

Surface Energy the electrical charge that attracts atoms to a surface

Tarnish discoloration resulting from the oxidation of a thin layer of a metal at its surface. It is not as destructive as corrosion

Tensile Force force applied in opposite directions to stretch an object

Therapeutic Materials materials used to treat disease

Thermal Conductivity the rate at which heat flows through a material

Torsion or Torque a twisting force that combines tensile and compressive forces

Translucency optical property in which varying degrees of light pass through or are absorbed by an object

Transparent optical property in which light passes directly through an object

Ultimate Strength the maximum amount of stress a material can withstand without breaking

Value how light or dark a color is. A low value indicates a darker color and a high value indicates a brighter color

Viscosity the ability of a liquid material to resist flow, e.g., ketchup is more viscous than water

Vitality a lifelike quality

Water Sorption the ability to absorb moisture

Wetting the ability of a liquid to wet or intimately contact a solid surface. Water beading on a waxed car is an example of poor wetting

---

To become effective in the selection, manipulation, and handling of dental materials, it is important that the dental auxiliary has an appreciation for the complexity and challenges of the oral environment. Dental biomaterials placed and used within the oral cavity must be biocompatible, durable, nonreactive under acid or alkaline conditions, compatible with other materials, and esthetically acceptable. Numerous factors in the mouth can adversely affect restorative dental materials. The influencing factors include but are not limited to the following: hot or cold foods and beverages acidic or alkaline foods and beverages hard or sticky foods heavy biting forces or parafunctional habits such as clenching or grinding of the teeth. These factors can cause: breakdown of the dental materials over time, chipping of restoration margins, fracture of the dental materials, and roughening of the restoration surface. Materials must be selected that have physical and mechanical properties that can hold up in harsh oral conditions. The severity of the conditions in the oral environment may vary somewhat from patient to patient and in specific circumstances.

The degree of compatibility may depend on how and/or how long the material is expected to survive in the oral environment. **Therapeutic materials**, those used to treat disease, are generally used for short periods of time, whereas **restorative materials**, those used to reconstruct the tooth structure, are expected to remain in contact with tissues for indefinite lengths of time. Consider the following cases. If a therapeutic agent were to be used to treat a specific condition, such as a denture sore, it would need to be biocompatible with the tissues but would not need to last long. If a material were being used as a permanent restoration, such as a gold crown, biocompatibility and longevity would both be required.

Patient concerns, questions, and demands must also play a part in the decision process. The patient should be brought into the decision-making process very early. Tooth-colored materials are frequently requested by patients, but they may not be aware of the limitation of that choice. The patient may desire porcelain or composite veneers to cover discolored anterior teeth or to close spacing (Fig. 2.1). If the patient grinds their teeth, porcelain may chip or wear the opposing teeth or the restorations themselves. On the other hand, composite veneers may wear down excessively under the same conditions. The patient needs to be educated as to the limitations imposed by the particular oral condition(s) and the appropriate restorative choices to produce long-lasting results. The auxiliary is frequently involved in this education and must have a good understanding of how materials function in the oral environment.

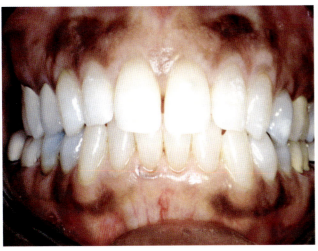 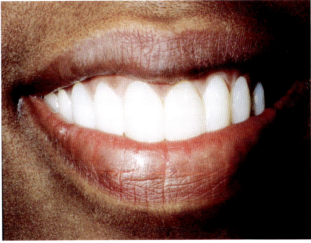

FIG. 2.1 Closing a diastema (i.e., a space) between teeth 8 and 9 with composite restorative material. (Courtesy Dr. Stephan Eakle.)

CLASSIFICATION OF DENTAL MATERIALS

Dental materials may be classified by their use: preventive/therapeutic materials, restorative materials, and auxiliary materials.

PREVENTIVE/THERAPEUTIC MATERIALS

Preventive/therapeutic materials are used to prevent dental related disease or trauma or for their therapeutic action on the teeth or oral tissues. Materials in this category include:
- Pit and fissure sealants to help prevent caries
- Mouth guards to prevent damage to teeth from grinding and injury from athletic activities
- Materials with an antibacterial effect found in some restorative and base materials
- Fluoride and fluoride-containing materials to prevent or reduce the progression of caries

RESTORATIVE MATERIALS

Restorative materials include materials used to repair or replace a tooth structure lost to oral disease or trauma or to change the appearance of the teeth. Restorations are classified as direct and indirect.

Direct Restorations
Direct restorations are placed immediately and directly into a prepared tooth in a pliable state that then sets to harden. This procedure can be done in a single office visit.

Indirect Restorations
Indirect restorations involve customized tooth replacements that require fabrication outside the mouth, usually in a lab. These restorations typically require a second appointment to fit and cement the restoration; however, some newer procedures allow for fabrication and placement in one appointment.

AUXILIARY MATERIALS

Auxiliary materials are those materials used to help fabricate and maintain restorations, directly or indirectly. Auxiliary materials include:
- Impression materials
- Gypsum
- Dental waxes
- Finishing and polishing materials

 Do You Recall

What is the difference between an indirect restoration and a direct restoration?

BIOCOMPATIBILITY

To be **biocompatible**, materials must not impede or adversely affect living tissue and should interact to the benefit of the patient. The study of dental biomaterials must include a thorough understanding of each material's biological properties. All materials contain potentially irritating ingredients. Adverse responses may include postoperative sensitivity, toxicity, and hypersensitivity. Postoperative sensitivity is often associated with dental operative procedures. This may be due to the toxicity of the restorative, preventive, or therapeutic material or bacterial invasion into or near the pulpal tissues.

A material may be acceptable for use on hard tissues (tooth structure), whereas it may not be acceptable for use on soft tissues (gingiva or mucosa). Some materials may be therapeutic when used in small quantities or for short periods of time but may be irritating or toxic when used for longer periods of time or in increased quantities or higher concentrations. Topical fluoride is of great benefit when used according to the manufacturer's directions; however, acidulated versions can be irritating to soft tissues and even excessively etch enamel or some restorations.

Dentistry is not alone in its attention to the development of biocompatible materials. Orthopedic surgeons must consider biocompatibility when placing artificial hips and knees, as does the cardiologist when placing heart catheters and prosthetic heart valves. All dental team members must consider the short-term and long-term functional and biocompatible responses of any material.

ADVERSE RESPONSE

A patient may have an **adverse response** to dental material. The response may be due to the material itself or may be due to breakdown of the components of the material in the oral environment. An example of an adverse response is seen with patients allergic to some metals, particularly nickel. Some nickel-containing alloys are used in dentistry for fabrication of crowns, bridges, partial denture frameworks, or in orthodontic wires. Inflammation of tissues from an allergic reaction to nickel may be seen at crown margins of metal-based crowns (Fig. 2.2), on a patient's lips when wearing some orthodontic appliances, and on a patient's attached gingiva in contact with the metal framework of a removable prosthesis. A complete health history, including an interview with the patient and a thorough examination of oral tissues, can help to identify hypersensitive individuals. Frequently, several different materials are used in combination to produce a restoration, such as a porcelain-fused-to-metal crown cemented with glass ionomer cement. The use of multiple materials makes it more difficult to determine which material is responsible for the adverse response. In general, materials intended for permanent replacement of tooth structures should exhibit no adverse biological responses.

Textbook chapters five through 20 will clearly outline the limitations as well as precautions for the use of each dental material.

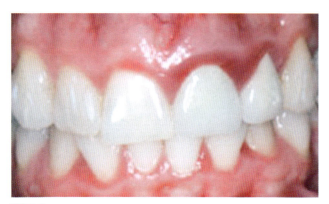

FIG. 2.2 Allergic reaction to nickel. Porcelain-fused-to-metal crowns have been placed on teeth 9 and 10. The tissue is red and inflamed and bleeds easily because of chronic inflammation from allergy to the metal in the crown.

BIOMECHANICS

The function of a material depends on the physical and mechanical properties (see Chapter 3) of that material as well as how the material is being used. Designs for restorations require an understanding of the biomechanical properties of the material. Much like an engineer, the dentist must design a dental bridge by taking into consideration the load that will be placed on the bridge, the length of the span, and the stability of the supporting structures. For example, a material may be used successfully to restore anterior teeth, where biting forces are not as strong, whereas this same material may be undesirable to restore the occlusal surfaces of posterior teeth, where biting forces are heavier. Excessive wear of a material may occur when a stronger material applies force against a weaker material, such as porcelain against composite resin, and may be intensified by surface roughness on the porcelain and by parafunctional habits such as clenching or grinding. Dentists must consider the performance of a material based on a thorough knowledge of the material's properties, the intended application of the material, and the impacting factors in each patient's oral environment.

ORAL FACTORS AFFECTING DENTAL MATERIALS

A number of factors in the oral environment will have an effect on the functionality and durability of the dental materials used in the oral cavity and thus will have an influence on which material the clinician will select.

FORCE, STRESS, AND STRAIN

Force

A force is a push, pull, or twist (or combination of these) applied to a material. When a weight is placed on an object, the weight applies force to that object. The force applied at the surface creates **stress** within the object that tries to resist the weight. If there was no resistance to the weight, then the material would be flattened or displaced.

Materials used to restore teeth must withstand varying degrees of force, or *load*, applied through muscular action, resulting in the pushing or pulling of a restoration by the teeth or food bolus during mastication. For some patients, the forces come from parafunctional habits such as clenching or grinding (called *bruxism*). Normal biting force varies among individuals and from one area of the mouth to another. Biting force is largely a measurement of the strength of the muscles of mastication and the surface area over which the force is applied during the normal chewing of foods. When clenching or grinding, this force is increased due to the lack of a food cushion and the resultant direct contact of tooth surfaces. Normal masticatory forces on the occlusal surface of molar teeth average 90 to 200 pounds per square inch and can increase to as much as 28,000 pounds per square inch on a cusp tip. Masticatory forces are greatest in the molar region and gradually decrease, moving toward the anterior part of the mouth from the premolars to the incisors. Denture wearers apply 40% less force than patients with intact dentitions, but denture wearers whose dentures are supported by implants or roots regain much of the biting force.

A study of the anatomy of teeth reveals that each kind of tooth shape (i.e., incisor, premolar, molar) is designed to apply specific types of force. The three basic types of force are as follows:

- **Compressive Force**—force applied to compress or squeeze an object; crushing, biting forces. Posterior teeth are ideally suited for this type of force. Their large occlusal surface and multirooted base are well suited to resist a crushing force.
- **Tensile Force**—force applied at each end of a material in opposite directions to stretch an object or pull it apart. When tensile force is applied to a rubber band, it is stretched.
- **Shearing Force**—force applied when two surfaces slide against each other in opposite directions. When the maxillary and mandibular incisors are used for cutting, shearing forces are applied. When we use the anterior teeth to bite into food, we slide the mandibular teeth forward or to the side across the maxillary teeth to shear it off.

Torsion

Another type of force is **torsion or torque**. It is a twisting force that has tensile and compressive forces. This force is more descriptive of events during normal chewing. When chewing a combination of compressive, tensile, and shear forces occur, resulting in torsion. When a patient wears full dentures, they may complain that the dentures become dislodged when chewing certain foods. This results from torque on the dentures, which are not well suited to withstand the combination of compressive, tensile, and shear forces while eating (Fig. 2.3).

> **Clinical Tip**
>
> Dislodging of dentures is often due to the tipping forces and possibly torque that break the peripheral seal, causing the loss of suction and resulting in the movement of the denture away from the ridge.

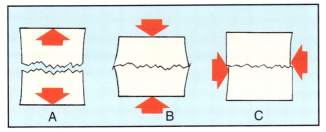

FIG. 2.3 Types of stress and strain: **(A)** Tensile stress pulls and stretches a material. **(B)** Compressive stress pushes it together. **(C)** Shearing stress tries to slice it apart. (From Bird DL, Robinson DS. *Torres and Ehrlich Modern Dental Assisting*. 11 ed. Saunders; 2015.)

The forces used in chewing a sticky caramel candy are different from those used in chewing a peanut. The caramel is compressed as the person bites down and it sticks to the teeth. Then it is torn apart by tensile forces as the jaws separate. The peanut is crushed by compressive forces and ground with shearing forces as the posterior teeth slide across each other in the chewing cycle.

Flexure

Flexure or bending force is a combination of compressive, tensile, and shear forces. When a long plastic rod is flexed into an arch shape, compression occurs on the inside surface of the arch and tension occurs on the outside of the arch, while shear occurs inside of the rod itself. **Flexural stress** is the materials resistance to the combined bending forces.

Stress and Strain

When a force is exerted on a tooth or restorative material, the tooth or material creates stress to resist the force. Stress is expressed as pounds per square inch (psi) or megapascals (MPa) in the metric system. If an object is fixed in position, it may be deformed by force if the magnitude is great enough, and the object is considered strained. Stress, then, is the amount of force exerted from within an object to resist an external force, and **strain** is the amount of change that the force has produced in the object. When the strain is caused by a compressive force, the object is shortened while a tensile force causes the object to lengthen. If the object does not return to its original shape after the stress is removed, it has undergone permanent deformation. Elastic deformation occurs when a stressed material returns to its original shape after the stress is removed (like a rubber band).

Fracture Toughness Strength

Fracture toughness is a mechanical property of materials that measures the energy needed to fracture a material. When increasingly higher forces are applied to a material, it will eventually fracture and the point of fracture is called the **ultimate strength**.

Resilience

Resilience indicates the energy needed to permanently deform a material. Brittle materials such as composites, amalgam, or ceramics are not resilient and do not deform readily and will fracture if loaded too heavily. Any flaws in the materials will cause stress to concentrate in those areas and ultimately reduce the strength of the material, leading to fracture.

Values of compressive and tensile forces applied to the tooth structure and restorative materials are expressed in Table 2.1. Use the table to compare the ultimate compressive and tensile strengths of tooth structure types to the various restorative materials to understand why a certain material may function better in one application than another.

TABLE 2.1	Ultimate Compressive and Tensile Strengths of Tooth and Restorative Structures	
STRUCTURE	ULTIMATE COMPRESSIVE STRENGTH (LB/IN^2)	ULTIMATE TENSILE STRENGTH (LB/IN^2)
Enamel	56,000	1500
Dentin	43,000	4500
Amalgam	45,000–64,000	7000–9000
Porcelain	21,000	5400
Composite resin	30,000–60,000	6000–9000
Acrylic	11,000	8000

Fatigue Failure

During mastication, stress occurs repetitively over time. Failures rarely occur in a single-force application; rather, they occur when stress is frequently repeated. These repeated stresses may produce microscopic flaws that grow over time, resulting in fracture; this is known as **fatigue failure**. A metal wire bent repeatedly will eventually break; this is another example of fatigue failure. Teeth and restorative materials under chewing or grinding forces are subjected to repeated stresses by a mixture of forces applied in a variety of directions and intensities. As a result, the teeth or restorations may crack or fracture. Additionally, conditions of the oral cavity such as moisture, temperature, and pH fluctuations may also contribute to fatigue failure.

MOISTURE AND ACID LEVELS

The oral cavity is always in contact with moisture in the form of foods, saliva, and blood. This moisture can vary from acidic to alkaline depending on foods, beverages, medications, and the amount of acid-producing bacteria present (**biofilm**).

EFFECT OF pH

The normal resting pH of saliva ranges from 6.2 to 7.0 (neutral), but it can fluctuate higher or lower by several points during the course of a day. Many materials that would be compatible in a neutral environment will not be compatible in an acidic one. Some beverages have varying levels of acidity ranging from slightly to very acidic. Citrus fruits and sports drinks contain citric acid and can attack enamel and some restorative materials. Bottled and purified waters may have a lower pH when natural minerals are removed during the purification processes. Acidulated topical fluorides can also attack some materials, such as glass ionomer cements, composite resins, and ceramics.

Most materials are adversely affected by moisture, either during placement or in the long-term clinical behavior of the material. The breakdown of many restorative materials is directly related to the effects of moisture, acid, and stress. Materials designed for long-term retention in the mouth must not rapidly deteriorate under these conditions.

Solubility

Desirable materials should have low **solubility**; that is, not susceptible to being dissolved in a solvent, and, in the case of the oral environment, saliva is the main solvent. Gold and porcelain are retained in the oral environment for many years because of their insoluble nature. Glass ionomer cement materials, frequently used as tooth-colored restorations, are much more soluble. They tend to "wash out" or change in mass over time, requiring replacement (Fig. 2.4).

Water Sorption

Some materials also have the undesirable characteristic of **water sorption** or the ability to absorb moisture; this may result in staining or a slight swelling of the material. Staining of resins and acrylics from repeated exposure to coffee, tea, and other dyed beverages is due to water sorption. Dentures placed in a glass of water will take up the liquid and become slightly larger. Some acrylics will absorb both odors and tastes from foods due to the microscopic porosity of the material. Directions on routine home care can help alleviate this problem for the patient (see Chapter 14).

 Do You Recall

What types of materials cause the pH of the oral cavity to increase or decrease?

Corrosion

Metals suffer from the effects of moisture and acidity, with the exception of noble metals such as gold and platinum. The deterioration or dissolution of the metal in response to a chemical attack (acid), or in an electrochemical reaction with other metals because of the moisture and acid present in the oral environment, is

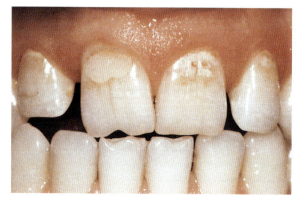

FIG. 2.4 "Washed-out" glass ionomer restoration on tooth 8 is stained, owing to porosities and the solubility of this restorative material.

called **corrosion**. Metals such as steel cannot be used in the oral cavity because the metal breaks down in the wet environment, becoming iron oxide (commonly known as *rust*). When steel is coated first with a barrier to corrosive components, the barrier gives steel its stainless quality. Dental amalgams are particularly susceptible to corrosion, causing marginal breakdown and discoloration of tooth structures (see Chapter 11). The result of corrosion is also seen on dental instruments that are processed in autoclaves due to the oxidation of the metal's surface. Corrosion begins at the surface of the metal and migrates deeper into the metal than **tarnish**, which is limited to the surface and can be seen as discoloration. Corrosion can accelerate in crevices between the tooth and restoration and on rough surfaces. Polishing of amalgams to produce a smooth surface has been recommended to help delay this process. In high-copper amalgams, this may not be as critical to their longevity since they are more corrosion resistant than low-copper amalgams (Fig. 2.5).

GALVANISM

An environment containing moisture, electrolytes, and dissimilar metals makes the generation of an electric current possible. The ions in the saliva facilitate the movement of electrical current from one type of metal to another. The phenomenon of electric current being transmitted between two dissimilar metals is called **galvanism**. The current may result in stimulation of the pulp, called *galvanic shock*. The classic example of a metal fork touching a metal restoration or biting on aluminum foil will be familiar to anyone with metal restorations, and unfamiliar to those who have no metal restorations. Some patients may even feel a galvanic shock or report a metal taste when instruments are used against the surface of a dissimilar metal restoration. When it becomes necessary to place differing types of metal restorations, such as a gold crown in contact with an amalgam restoration, insulation under the restorations in the form of bases or liners can help to lessen the stimulation. Provisional (temporary) aluminum crowns placed opposite or adjacent to amalgam or metal crowns can also cause this phenomenon (Fig. 2.6). In this situation, the selection of a polycarbonate or acrylic provisional crown would be a better choice. In time, the galvanic stimulation will fade as oxides form on the surface of the metal, acting as a barrier against the galvanic current.

> **? Do You Recall**
>
> Why does galvanism occur between two dissimilar metals?

TEMPERATURE

EXPANSION AND CONTRACTION

The ingestion of hot and cold foods and beverages or smoking may alter the temperature of the oral environment. With few exceptions, all forms of matter expand when they are heated and contract when cooled, resulting in **dimensional change**. Atoms or molecules in a material vibrate over a greater range when the material is heated, causing it to expand. Acceptable materials used as restorations and replacements of a tooth structure should have characteristics of expansion and contraction similar to those of tooth structures. Excessive expansion of a restoration within a tooth may result in the fracture of the remaining tooth structure; excessive contraction may result in leakage of fluids and bacteria into the open gaps between the tooth and restoration, resulting in sensitivity. Expansion and contraction are measured as the **coefficient of thermal expansion (CTE)**, the measurement of change in volume or length in relation to change in temperature. (Refer to Table 2.2 to review the values of thermal expansion.)

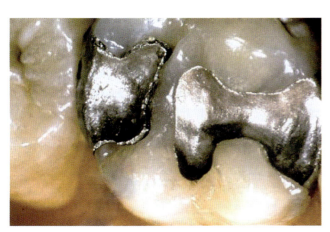

FIG. 2.5 Two amalgam restorations. *Left:* A low-copper amalgam with severe marginal breakdown. *Right:* A high-copper amalgam restoration with minimal marginal discrepancy. Both restorations were placed at the same time. (From Anusavice KJ. *Quality Evaluation of Dental Restorations: Criteria for Placement and Replacement.* Quintessence Publishing; 1989.)

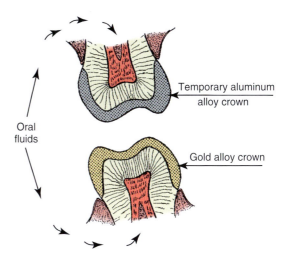

FIG. 2.6 Galvanism illustration of how dissimilar metals in opposing teeth can create a galvanic current, with saliva providing a solution of electrolytes.

TABLE 2.2	Thermal Properties of Tooth and Restorative Structures	
STRUCTURE	COEFFICIENT OF THERMAL EXPANSION ($\times 10^{-6}$/°C)	THERMAL CONDUCTIVITY (K [MCAL CM]/CM^{2}SEC°C)
Enamel	11	2.0
Dentin	8	1.30
Amalgam	20–28	54
Gold	15	350
Porcelain	15	2.50
Composite resin	26–40	2.60

Amalgam readily heats up and expands or cools and contracts with a small temperature change, whereas composite resin is not a good conductor of temperature and requires a greater temperature change to expand or contract. Both of these materials have rates of expansion and contraction that differ significantly enough from enamel and dentin that the marginal integrity of the restoration may be compromised. The difference in CTE value of unfilled acrylic and sealants with tooth structure is the highest, and the value of gold is the closest to human teeth.

Repeated shrinkage and expansion of a restoration during ingestion of cold and hot fluids and foods produces the opening and closing of a gap with movement of oral fluids between the restoration and the tooth surface, a phenomenon called **percolation**. Percolation allows the ingress of bacteria and oral fluids and may lead to recurrent caries, staining, and pulpal irritation.

THERMAL CONDUCTIVITY

Thermal conductivity is the rate at which heat flows through a material over time. Enamel and dentin are poor thermal conductors, whereas metals are excellent conductors. Gold is one of the best thermal conductors, even better than amalgam. Nonmetals such as ceramics, composites, acrylics, and cements are very poor conductors. Poor conductors can be used as restorations or as **insulators**. For instance, a patient wearing a denture may not sense the temperature of a liquid because of the insulation produced by the acrylic denture base.

When a metal restoration conducts temperature changes into the tooth from foods and beverages taken into the oral cavity, the pulp of the tooth may feel the resultant stimulation as sensitivity, particularly if the overlying dentin is thin. Dentin acts as a natural insulator, but when it is too thin, temperature changes may be felt by the pulp. When metal restorations are placed close to the pulp of the tooth, material such as cement is often placed between the tooth structure and the restoration to act as an insulating base to delay and absorb the transfer of temperature. Metals placed against tissue, such as a partial denture framework and some orthodontic appliances, can also conduct temperature to the soft tissues.

Table 2.2 gives values of thermal expansion and thermal conductivity. Compare the values of restorative materials with those of tooth structures to determine the potential for marginal leakage through percolation and/or the need for insulation. When there is a large difference between the CTE for the restorative material, such as amalgam, and that for the tooth structure, the percolation will be greater. Note that, whereas composite has a higher CTE compared with a tooth structure, bonding it to the tooth structure helps to prevent percolation.

In addition to temperature considerations for materials already present in the mouth, it is important to consider the temperature of materials as they are placed into the mouth. Ice-cold water used when mixing alginate may cause the patient pain when the very cold alginate contacts metal restorations. The components of some materials, when mixed, may result in a chemical reaction that produces heat. For example, when the powder and liquid of a chairside denture reline material are mixed, the reaction produces heat (an **exothermic reaction**). If the material is left in the mouth while this reaction is occurring, it is possible that the tissues could receive a thermal burn.

> **Clinical Tip**
>
> An exothermic reaction must be minimized by proper mixing and handling to prevent the excess heat from coming into contact with a susceptible tooth surface. Acrylic used to make temporary crowns and bridges in the mouth will release heat as it polymerizes and sets. If the acrylic is left in the mouth too long, the heat can damage the pulp or burn any soft tissues it contacts.

RETENTION

An important factor in the selection of a material is how it will be retained within or on the tooth. The **retention** of a material is its ability to maintain its position without displacement under stress. Retention may be secured through mechanical, chemical **adhesion**, or **bonding** mechanisms between materials.

MECHANICAL AND CHEMICAL RETENTION

Mechanical retention involves the use of undercuts or other projections into which the material is locked in place. The undercuts used in a typical amalgam preparation are an illustration of mechanical retention (Fig. 2.7). Note that the opening of the cavity preparation is smaller than the internal floor of the preparation. Once the material is hardened in place, it is retained through this undercut design.

When a significant amount of the tooth structure has been removed, undercuts can no longer be successfully used because the cusps or other parts of the tooth will be undermined and weakened. At this time, the clinician may wish to place a restoration covering

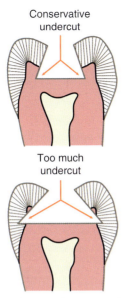

FIG. 2.7 The retentive undercuts of a conservative preparation *(top)* and an excessively undercut reparation that compromises the remaining tooth structure *(bottom)*.

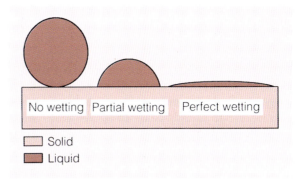

FIG. 2.8 Wetting characteristics of a liquid on a solid surface. (From Van Noort R. *Introduction to Dental Materials*. 14th ed. Mosby; 2013:53.)

the remaining tooth structure (a crown) and hold it in place with a dental cement. Dental cement retains the restoration by chemically and/or mechanically connecting the two surfaces.

BONDING

Bonding is a term commonly used when describing the retention of materials. Bonding of materials occurs when the tooth surface is prepared with an acid-etch technique to create microscopic roughness and pores in enamel and dentin. A fluid bonding material is then allowed to flow into the roughened surfaces and pores and, when hardened, it mechanically locks into the tooth structure. Restorative materials that adhere chemically to the bonding material are then placed. This technique offers several advantages in producing retention. It requires less removal of a healthy tooth structure because no undercuts are necessary, it produces a stronger retentive force between tooth and restoration, and it can seal the margin of the restoration to prevent the leakage of bacteria and fluids through percolation (see Chapter 7).

Many of today's restorative materials use a combination of mechanical and chemical or bonding adhesion for optimal retention. Retention by mechanical undercuts alone will not adequately seal the margins of a restoration and will frequently place the tooth structure in jeopardy of fracture when undercuts leave vulnerable areas of the tooth structure unsupported. Bonding requires the intimate contact of surfaces to produce the best bond strength.

Factors Affecting Bond Strength

Several factors can affect this bond strength and the success of a material as an adhesive. These factors include wetting, viscosity, film thickness, and surface characteristics of the tooth, restoration, and adhesive.

Wetting. **Wetting** is the degree to which a liquid adhesive is able to spread over the surface of a tooth and restorative material. When a liquid wets a surface well, it has a low angle of contact (Fig. 2.8 see also Chapter 7). The better the adhesive is able to spread on the surface of the tooth and restoration, the more retentive it is.

Viscosity. **Viscosity** is the resistance of a liquid material to flow. It can hinder the ability of a liquid to wet a material. Materials with high viscosity are thicker and do not flow well, and therefore may not be effective in wetting an area. Water has low viscosity and flows well, while tar is very thick and viscous. Some dental materials, such as impression materials and cements, are initially in a fluid state, but become more viscous as they start to set.

Film Thickness. **Film thickness** is the minimal thickness obtainable by a layer of a liquid material after it sets under pressure. It is particularly important when working with dental cements. When cementing a crown, if the film thickness of the cement is too great, it may prevent the crown from seating completely. A thin film of cement is desirable to allow the cement to completely wet the surfaces and for excess material to flow from under the crown when it is seated under pressure during cementation.

Surface Characteristics. Surface characteristics that can affect the adhesive retention of a material include:
1. The cleanliness of a surface
2. Moisture contamination
3. Surface texture
4. Surface energy

Even slight contamination of debris from tooth preparation, microorganisms in biofilm, and products of saliva can prevent close contact of the adhesive with the surface. Also, microscopic surface irregularities can trap air as the adhesive flows over them, resulting in incomplete wetting of the surface.

Surface Energy. The surface energy of liquids is also called *surface tension*. Molecules within a drop of liquid are attracted to molecules at the center of the drop, creating tension at the surface. With liquids, if the surface energy is high, the liquid can flow readily over a solid substrate. When liquids bead up on a surface, such as on wax or many plastics, the surface has low surface energy.

Solids also develop surface energy. When enamel is etched, a high surface energy is created that can attract liquids across the surface. Liquids generally wet or spread over high surface energy surfaces better. Metals, ceramics, and enamel have high surface energies.

Many factors in the oral environment are not favorable for retention of materials. The dentist is responsible for the mechanical design of the tooth preparation, but is not solely responsible for controlling all factors that impact retention. The dental auxiliaries play an essential role in delivering materials and controlling the conditions of the oral environment during their delivery. In many states, dental auxiliaries routinely place therapeutic and restorative materials. An understanding of the factors that influence retention is essential to achieving a successful restoration.

MICROLEAKAGE

The need for replacement of restorative materials can be significantly influenced by microleakage. The surface between the walls of the tooth structure (preparation) and the restoration is called the **interface**. If this tooth/restoration interface is not sealed, there may be a space into which fluids and microorganisms can penetrate. This seepage of harmful materials is called **microleakage** and is responsible in part for recurrent decay, marginal staining, and postoperative sensitivity. Microleakage may be due to the deterioration of the dental material, percolation due to differences in CTE, or lack of adhesion of the material to the tooth. It is easy to understand why the leakage of bacteria and other fluids between preparation and restoration sets up an environment for recurrent decay and staining. Postoperative sensitivity may be due to microleakage as well (Fig. 2.9). Tubules found within the hard material of the dentin are filled with fluids under pressure from the pulp. When the enamel of the tooth is removed, fluids can flow out of the much larger dentinal tubules and chemicals and bacteria can flow in, causing irritation of the pulp and sensitivity. Procedures for ensuring the proper seal of the dentinal tubules are described in Chapter 7.

 Do You Recall

What methods can be utilized to prevent microleakage around a restoration?

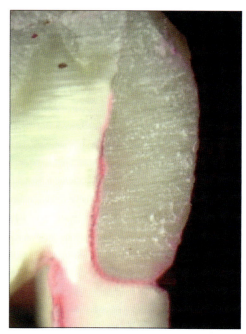

FIG. 2.9 Microleakage allows the seepage of fluids and microorganisms into the restoration-tooth structure interface. Microleakage can be seen as a pink dye penetrating along the internal surface of the class II composite restoration. (From Sakri MR, Kippal P, Patil BC, Haralur SB. Evaluation of microleakage in hybrid composite restoration with different intermediate layers and curing cycles. *J Dent Allied Sci.* 2016;5(1):14–20.)

ESTHETICS AND COLOR

Esthetic dentistry is a rapidly growing elective procedure that is in high demand and may be of equal, if not greater, concern to the patient than function.

HOW WE SENSE COLOR

Our eyes sense light through the cone cells in the retina in three different ranges of wavelength: red, green, and blue. Having three types of color-sensing cells does not limit us to just three colors. The stimulation of two or more types of cone cells, the amount of light they detect, and the interpretation of that light by our brain determine the overall response to a particular color. Mixtures of red, green, and blue light allow you to see many colors. The television mixes these primary colors of light to produce full-color pictures.

COMPONENTS OF COLOR

Three components—hue, chroma, and value—describe the color resulting from the mixing of primary colors:

Hue is the dominant color of the wavelength detected. Tooth colors are predominantly seen in the yellow and brown range.

Chroma refers to the intensity or strength of the color; teeth are rather pale in color.

Value describes how light or dark the color is. Teeth have value ranges at the light end of the value scale. As we age, the tooth value gets darker.

OPTICAL PROPERTIES

The perceived color of ceramic and composite restorations and teeth is influenced by their optical properties. Light that reaches the surface of the tooth or restoration can be transmitted through, absorbed by, and scattered or reflected by it. If light passes directly through an object (like window glass), it is **transparent**. If light is completely absorbed, scattered, and/or reflected by the object, it is **opaque**. Light is reflected off the surface (called *reflectance*), depending on the surface texture and amount of polish. Usually, teeth and esthetic restorations will reflect and transmit light to various degrees; this is called **translucency**. It gives tooth or restoration a lifelike quality called **vitality**. Manufacturers over time have adjusted the components of composite resins so they can absorb, transmit, scatter, and reflect light to mimic a natural tooth structure. The same can be said for modern ceramics.

VIEWING COLOR

Individuals see the many colors, components, and reflections of color somewhat differently in varying situations. This phenomenon, known as **metamerism,** means that colors look different under different light sources (Fig. 2.10). It is important that we have a standardized measure of color, such as a shade guide, to give us an objective measure (Fig. 2.11). It is also important that we produce an environment that reduces the possibility of extraneous color reflection, producing an inaccurate color match for the restoration. A detailed discussion on shade selection is presented in Chapter 10.

ORAL BIOFILM AND DENTAL MATERIALS

It is important to have a basic understanding of **oral biofilm**, what it is, how it functions in health and disease, and how to manage it to maintain a healthy mouth.

COMMUNITY OF MICROORGANISMS

The oral biofilm is a three-dimensional, complex, structured community of microorganisms that can be found on mucous membranes, teeth, intraoral restorations, dental implants, and removable prostheses. Over 700 species of microorganisms can colonize the mouth. These microorganisms include bacteria, viruses, and fungi. In any one individual, approximately 200 of these species may exist as part of the normal oral microbiota. Of these, bacteria are found in the greatest numbers and species.

The oral biofilm exists in a dynamic symbiotic (beneficial to host and microorganisms) relationship with the host. The biofilm provides some level of protection for the structured community of microorganisms from invading bacteria, fungi, and viruses, and toxic substances such as antibiotics or chemicals. The biofilm also provides a type of circulatory system for the uptake of nutrients (derived from adjacent tissues, from salivary secretions, from other microorganisms, and from the host diet) and for elimination of metabolic by-products through water-filled spaces between colonies.

FORMATION OF ORAL BIOFILM

Biofilm (or dental plaque) forms on teeth soon after eruption. Likewise, it quickly re-forms after a professional cleaning and forms on newly placed restorations. The initial layer on the surfaces of the teeth or restorations comes from salivary and gingival crevicular fluid components such as proteins, glycoproteins, lipids, albumin, and mucin and is called the acquired pellicle. That layer acts as a base for bacterial attachment. The majority of the first colonizers are from the *Streptococcus* genus (e.g., *S. mutans, S. salivarius*) and occupy up to 90% of the surface, while other early colonizers occupy the remainder. The early colonizers are

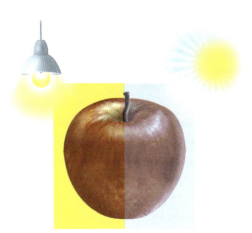

FIG. 2.10 Example of metamerism: the apple changes color depending on the light source used to illuminate it. (From Sakaguchi RL, Powers JM. *Craig's Restorative Dental Materials.* 13th ed. Saunders; 2012:58.)

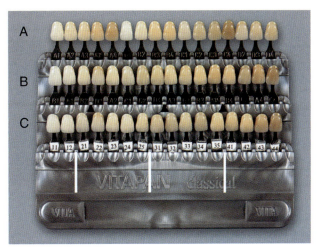

FIG. 2.11 Tab arrangements of the Vitapan classical shade guide. Manufacturer's arrangement according to **(A)** hue, **(B)** value scale, and **(C)** lightest to darkest. (From Paravina RD, Powers JM. *Esthetic Color Training in Dentistry.* Mosby; 2004.)

mostly gram-positive bacteria (they have a thick cell wall that retains a stain used in the laboratory). Within a couple weeks, gram-negative bacteria (which have a thin cell wall that does not retain the stain) begin to proliferate. Later colonizers are mostly anaerobes (they thrive where there is little or no oxygen) that can contribute to periodontal disease, and they attach to the growing plaque. As the bacterial community grows, the adherent bacteria form a protective matrix from extracellular polysaccharides they secrete. The matrix can help protect them from competing microorganisms, antibiotics, and antibacterial mouth rinses.

Factors That Affect the Biofilm

A state of microbial homeostasis (a stable state of equilibrium) forms until it is thrown out of balance by factors affecting the oral environment, such as change in the host immune system, dietary changes, or other systemic changes. Oral factors such as the temperature of the oral cavity, the pH of the saliva, and available nutrients affect the rate of growth of the biofilm. The temperature can change rapidly with the introduction of hot or cold foods and beverages. The pH can vary from its normal range of 6.5 to 7.5 due to the introduction of sugars that are metabolized by certain bacteria, resulting in acid production. Acidic and alkaline foods can also alter the pH, but the saliva dilutes and buffers the foods so that gradually the saliva returns to its normal range. This pH balancing may not happen in patients with dry mouth or saliva with low buffering capacity.

BIOFILM AND ORAL DISEASE

Most of the bacteria in the biofilm are harmless, but pathogens are present in small numbers. If systemic or oral conditions change, the potential exists for certain pathogens for both tooth decay and/or periodontal disease to proliferate and cause disease.

Changes in diet and consumption of foods high in sugars and fermentable carbohydrates can cause the proliferation of acid-producing and acid-tolerant bacteria, such as mutans-type *Streptococci* and *Lactobacilli*. These bacteria can cause dental caries. Changes in other oral factors can cause the growth of periodontal pathogens, leading to gingivitis, periodontitis, and peri-implantitis.

PROBIOTICS

Prescribed antibiotics can kill beneficial bacteria as well as pathogens. As a result it can be a challenge to maintain a healthy level of beneficial bacteria in the mouth and gut. Numerous studies have shown that the introduction of helpful bacteria, called *probiotics*, can help. Probiotics are live microorganisms that are consumed by an individual to promote health. The bacteria can be added to milk, yogurt, or sour cream or are available as tablets, capsules, or drops. Probiotics are becoming more popular as a way to increase the numbers of helpful bacteria to the gastrointestinal (GI) tract and even the mouth. By increasing the numbers of beneficial bacteria, they can help suppress the harmful bacteria. They also help promote a healthy digestive tract and immune system.

BIOFILM AND SYSTEMIC DISEASES

Increasing research studies are showing a correlation between periodontal disease and certain systemic diseases, such as heart disease, diabetes, some respiratory ailments, Alzheimer, and certain complications with pregnancy. It is believed that the ulceration of the gingival sulcus caused by the bacteria in subgingival plaque allows pathogenic bacteria to enter the bloodstream and affect distant organ systems (Fig. 2.12).

BIOFILM ON DENTAL MATERIALS

Biofilm (dental plaque) in the oral cavity is well documented as having a primary role in the formation of dental caries and periodontal diseases. The role of biofilm adhesion on dental material is less well known. Surface roughness has a direct correlation with biofilm accumulation. Roughness from abrasion, coronal polishing agents, hand and ultrasonic scaling, and lack of finishing (smoothing and shaping) and polishing after fabrication or initial placement of a restoration are all associated with increased biofilm accumulation. Biofilm accumulation at the margins of rough or faulty restorations may, in part, contribute to the development of recurrent caries. Biofilms do not accumulate as readily on polished cast alloys and ceramic restorations, possibly because of their smooth surfaces. Amalgam tends to have a biofilm that is less active, likely because of the effect of mercury on the bacterial population. Control of biofilm accumulation on dental implants has been shown to play a significant role in the ultimate success of the implant. Fluoride-releasing materials found in some restorations can counteract the acids produced by biofilms. Dentures tend to develop a biofilm that is high in *Candida* (a yeast) and is associated with chronic irritation of the underlying oral mucosa known as denture stomatitis. Occasionally, denture stomatitis requires treatment with an antifungal medication to clear it up. So, prevention is the best treatment.

MANAGING THE ORAL BIOFILM

Currently, we do not have a way to totally eliminate pathogens in the oral biofilm, but we can manage the biofilm so that a healthy mouth can be maintained. The American Dental Association (ADA) recommends twice-daily brushing for a minimum of two minutes and daily flossing as a basic minimum oral hygiene routine. Tooth brushing with a fluoride-containing paste can be accomplished with manual or power brushing. Interdental cleaning is commonly done with dental floss, but a variety of other aids are available, such as toothpicks, balsa sticks, interproximal plastic

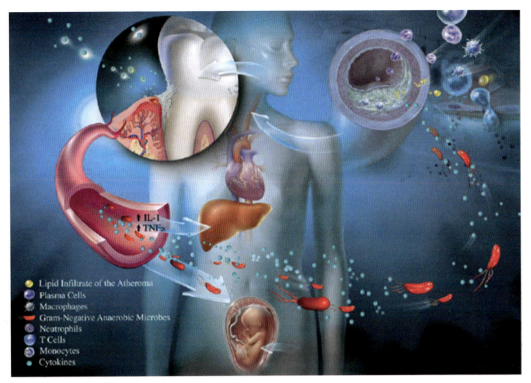

FIG. 2.12 Subgingival plaque bacteria and/or their by-products may gain access to distant sites in the body through the circulatory system and may potentially contribute to systemic inflammation. In this way, a dental biofilm infection may contribute to various systemic diseases and conditions. (From Gurenlian JR: The Role of Dental Plaque Biofilm in Health. *J Dent Hygiene*, vol 81, No. supplement 1, Oct 2007, Fig 4; with permission of MCNEIL-PPC, Inc.)

cleaners, and oral irrigators. Additional oral hygiene measures may include tongue brushing or scraping. ADA-accepted antimicrobial mouth rinses, especially those with a combination of essential oils or chlorhexidine, can be helpful in managing gingivitis and supragingival plaque.

It is important for denture wearers to clean their dentures daily with a denture brush and nonabrasive paste and use a denture effervescent soak to remove the adherent biofilm.

Do You Recall

In what ways does oral biofilm contribute to the failure of restorative materials?

Caution

It is important that the oral health practitioner carefully identify the locations and types of restorations present in the patient's mouth and take precautions to avoid altering their surfaces while instrumenting teeth or adjacent restorations.

DETECTION OF RESTORATIVE MATERIALS

Oral health care professionals must be able to identify restorative materials within the oral environment to treat them appropriately. Identification of restorative materials, which may be obvious with amalgam materials, may also be difficult when identifying tooth-colored materials such as composite resin or ceramics. In addition, restorations may be composed of different materials, such as a ceramic inlay cemented with resin-based cement.

METHODS OF IDENTIFICATION

Identification of restorative materials may be done by:
- Appearance
- Location
- Tactile sensitivity
- Radiography

A restoration that matches the color of the tooth well may be difficult to distinguish from the surrounding tooth structure (Fig. 2.13). Well-developed tactile sensitivity skills with a dental explorer, adequate illumination, liberal use of air to dry the teeth and restorations, and even magnification may be needed to detect some esthetic restorations. The location of margins, especially those placed subgingivally, makes visual inspection of many materials impossible. Drying the teeth well often makes detection of composites easier. Saliva tends to hide the distinction between the tooth surface and the margins of the restoration, as well as the differences in the texture and luster (shininess) of the restoration surfaces.

Tactile Evaluation

Tactile evaluation of the tooth surface can be a helpful means of clinical assessment. The surface of some

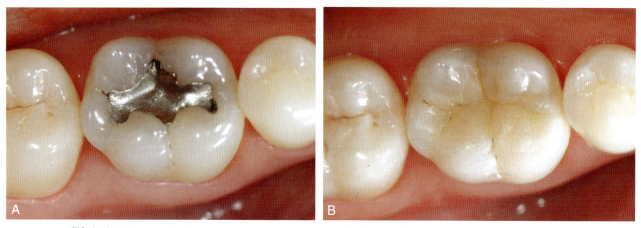

FIG. 2.13 Detection of tooth-colored restorations can be visually difficult. **(A)** Amalgam on the occlusal surface of the lower first molar is obvious. **(B)** The amalgam has been replaced with a composite restoration that matches the tooth color very well and is hard to see. (From Ritter AV, Boushell LW, Walter R. *Sturdevant's Art and Science of Operative Dentistry*. 7th ed. Elsevier; 2019.)

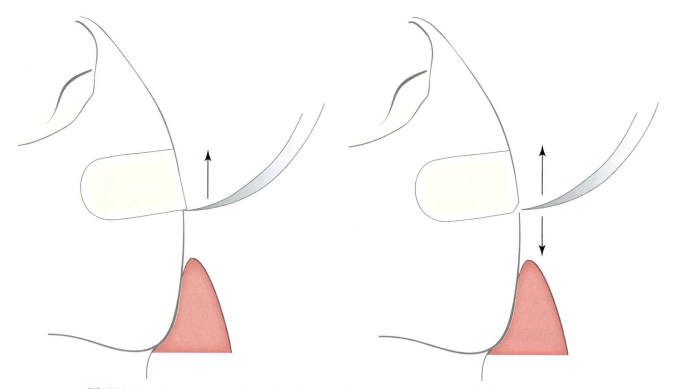

FIG. 2.14 The restoration margin in the first drawing extends over the cavosurface margin of the preparation (an overhanging margin), causing a trap for food and biofilm, and if located on the proximal surface will make flossing difficult. The restoration margin in the second drawing does not meet the cavosurface margin of the preparation (a deficient margin), causing a trap for biofilm and possibly leading to recurrent caries.

composite and glass ionomer restorations may feel rougher than enamel. Tracing the enamel surface onto the restoration with the sharp tip of an explorer is the best way to distinguish this difference. The clinician may detect a smooth surface on the enamel and a "scratchy" surface on the restoration. This difference may be noticed at the cavosurface margin (the margin of the cavity preparation that meets the tooth surface) (Fig. 2.14). Once the presence of a restoration is identified, the entire cavosurface margin should be evaluated. The cavosurface margin should be almost undetectable as the tip of the explorer passes from the restoration to the tooth. Sealants have a smooth, glassy surface covering the anatomical pits and fissures of the tooth surfaces; the explorer feels like it is skating on ice. Porcelain has a very smooth, glassy surface, and the explorer glides easily over the surface. Note the tip of the explorer as it glides against the margin of the restoration.

Illumination and Transillumination

Adequate direct illumination and transillumination are helpful for the detection of many anterior restorations. With transillumination, light can pass through teeth to varying degrees based on the intensity of the light and the thickness of the teeth. A mouth mirror placed lingual to the incisors can reflect the operatory or loupe light through these thin teeth. The light will not pass through the restoration as well as enamel, so it will stand out. This, along with the knowledge that most anterior restorations are prepared from the lingual surface to preserve as much natural enamel on the facial surface as possible, will help in the identification of many class III and IV restorations.

Magnification and Air

Magnification and the liberal use of air will help to distinguish the glossy surface of enamel versus the more opaque surface of composite and resin restorations. (However, newer generations of composites allow them to be polished to a very smooth, lustrous surface similar to enamel.)

Radiographs

Radiographs are a valuable tool for the detection of restorations and the assessment of restorative components. Most modern composites are radiopaque, but some older ones are radiolucent. Glass ionomers are radiopaque, as are many resin-based cements and ceramics (Fig. 2.15 illustrates various types of restorative materials as seen intraorally as well as their corresponding radiographic appearance). Note that the restoration on tooth 20 is an older radiolucent type of composite material, whereas the composite on tooth 13 is a radiopaque type. The other radiopaque restorative materials include the amalgam restorations seen on teeth 14, 15, and 17, as well as the gold crown on implant 18 and a porcelain fused to a metal crown on 19.

For most difficult-to-detect restorations, it is necessary to use a combination of the above-described methods to determine the presence and type of material before clinical procedures are performed.

Ideal Conditions for Assessing Restoration

- Dry field
- Good lighting
- Sharp explorer
- Radiographs
- Magnification
- Good knowledge of the material

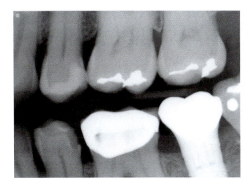

FIG. 2.15 Radiograph of the restorations. Note the radiopacities: composite 13 DO; amalgam 14, 15, and 17; gold crown 18 implant; and PFM. crown 19. Radiolucency of an older type of composite is seen in 20 DO.

SUMMARY

The oral environment presents unique challenges to the successful use of dental materials as restorative and therapeutic agents. An understanding of the limiting factors in the oral environment and an appreciation for how these limitations affect the selection of materials are essential to the successful use of dental materials. Materials used must be biocompatible, exhibit long-term clinical durability, and be esthetically acceptable. No one material is superior in all of these areas.

The dental auxiliary must have an understanding of the limitations as well as the criteria for selection of therapeutic and restorative materials. With this knowledge, the practitioner can educate the patient about the materials used in their mouths as well as select, properly manipulate, and maintain materials to ensure their ultimate success.

INSTRUCTIONAL VIDEOS

See the Evolve Resources site for a variety of educational videos that reinforce the material covered in this chapter.

CHAPTER 2 Oral Environment and Patient Considerations

Get Ready for Exams!

Review Questions

Select the one correct response for each of the following multiple-choice questions.

1. The safe interaction of a dental material with the rest of the body is defined as the material's:
   a. Radioactivity
   b. Carcinogenicity
   c. Biocompatibility
   d. Therapeutic reaction
2. What does the study of dental materials include knowledge of?
   a. The chemical reactions of the material
   b. The physical reactions of the material
   c. The ways to manipulate the material
   d. Causes for the failure of the material
   e. All of the above
3. What is the internal reaction to an externally applied force called?
   a. Strain
   b. Stress
   c. Hardness
   d. Elasticity
4. When increasingly higher forces are applied to a material, it will eventually fracture and the point of fracture is called:
   a. A fatigue fracture
   b. Tensile strength
   c. Ultimate strength
   d. A compressive fracture
5. Material subject to repeated stresses, such as in mastication, may be subject to a fracture due to:
   a. Flexural stress
   b. Force exerted over a large area
   c. Forces stretching an object
   d. Fatigue failure
6. Which of the following restorative materials is the most soluble?
   a. Amalgam
   b. Glass ionomer
   c. Porcelain
   d. Acrylic
7. Corrosion is of greatest concern for which of the following restorative materials?
   a. Gold
   b. Composite resin
   c. Amalgam
   d. Porcelain
8. What is the surface discoloration of a metal restoration called?
   a. Corrosion
   b. Tarnish
   c. Crystallization
   d. Metallurgy
9. Restorative materials with values of thermal conductivity similar to enamel include:
   a. Gold
   b. Composite resin
   c. Amalgam
   d. Silver
10. Susan has just had an MOD amalgam placed on tooth 30. When biting, this tooth is in contact with a gold crown on tooth 3. Susan complains of an electric shock sensation and metal taste. This is most likely due to:
    a. Galvanism
    b. Corrosion
    c. Tarnish
    d. Metamerism
11. Microleakage may be responsible for:
    a. Recurrent decay
    b. Marginal staining
    c. Postoperative sensitivity
    d. All of the above
12. What may the excessive film thickness of cements cause?
    a. An increase in retention
    b. A decrease in marginal leakage
    c. Improper seating of the restoration
    d. Fracture of the restoration
13. What is the seepage of fluids and debris extending along the tooth-restoration interface called?
    a. Metamerism
    b. Trituration
    c. Microleakage
    d. Deformation
14. What are colonies of bacteria growing on the teeth called?
    a. Principle invaders
    b. Parasites
    c. Dental plaque
    d. Primary intruders
15. Color shades can vary depending on the incident light or source of light. What is this effect called?
    a. Spectrum
    b. Chroma
    c. Meniscus
    d. Metamerism
16. What is the term used to describe the intensity of color?
    a. Hue
    b. Value
    c. Chroma
    d. Opacity
17. What is an oral biofilm?
    a. A slick film of mucus that develops on surfaces within the mouth
    b. Composed of bacteria only
    c. Never in balance since the types of microorganisms are constantly changing and there is a complex organization of microorganisms on oral surfaces and restorations
    d. Is a complex organization of microorganisms on oral surfaces and restorations
18. pH in the oral cavity can fluctuate higher or lower during the course of the day.
    a. True
    b. False

Get Ready for Exams!—cont'd

19. An adhesive that spreads on the surface of the tooth and restoration will be more _____.
    a. Viscous
    b. Retentive
    c. Soluble
    d. Corrosive
20. Evidence-based research is showing a correlation between periodontal disease and certain systemic diseases, such as:
    a. Heart disease
    b. Diabetes
    c. Respiratory ailments
    d. Low-term birth weight and other pregnancy complications
    e. All of the above

For answers to the Review Questions, see the Appendix.

Case-Based Discussion Topics

1. A 45-year-old patient comes to the dental office with the chief complaint of having to wear a maxillary removable partial denture. The patient wishes to have this removable prosthesis replaced with a fixed bridge. Examination reveals that the partial denture replaces teeth 6 through 11.
Discuss the stresses that would be placed on a bridge of this span.

2. A 25-year-old teacher comes to your office with the chief complaint of losing a distal-incisal class IV composite from tooth 9. The patient explains that this restoration has been in place for only a few days.
Discuss the factors that might affect the bond strength of this restoration and what can be done to help prevent this from happening again.

3. Look into a mirror or position yourself to examine someone else's mouth, and check the following:
    a. Check how tooth surfaces contact in the posterior, middle, and anterior teeth when in normal occlusion, biting edge to edge on anterior teeth, and moving the jaw laterally (side to side) and front to back.
Which forces are being exerted by these teeth, and when?
    b. Check for metal and resin restorations. Place a piece of ice on the enamel of a tooth, on a metal restoration, and on a resin restoration.
How long does it take to feel sensation in the pulp for each? What is this property called?
    c. Look at the gingival, middle, and incisal/occlusal third of the anterior and posterior teeth.
How does the color of the area change? Is there a change in translucency or opacity? Place something bright red close to the teeth, and direct the dental lamp or other bright light onto the teeth. How do these factors affect the color?

BIBLIOGRAPHY

Gurenlian JR: The role of dental plaque biofilm in oral health, *J Dent Hyg* 81(5):116, 2007.

Marsh PD: Ecological events in oral health and disease: new opportunities for prevention and disease control? *J Calif Dent Assoc* 45(10):525–537, 2017.

Powers JM, Wataha JC: *Dental materials: foundations and applications,* St. Louis, 2016, Elsevier.

Bird DL, Robinson DS: *Modern dental assisting,* ed 13, St. Louis, 2021, Elsevier.

Sakaguchi RL, Ferracane J, Powers JM: *Craig's restorative dental materials,* St. Louis, 2018, Mosby.

Shen C, Rawls HR, Esquivel-Upshaw JF: *Phillips' science of dental materials,* Philadelphia, 2021, Saunders.

Twetman S, Jørgensen MR, Keller MK: Fifteen years of probiotic therapy in the dental context: what has been achieved? *J Calif Dent Assoc* 45(10):539–545, 2017.

Van Noort R: *Introduction to dental materials,* London, 2014, Mosby.

3 Physical and Mechanical Properties of Dental Materials

http://evolve.elsevier.com/Eakle/materials/

Chapter Objectives

On completion of this chapter, the student should be able to:
1. Describe primary and secondary bonds and give an example of how each determines the properties of the material.
2. List the three forms of matter and give a defining characteristic of each.
3. Define density and explain the relationship between density, volume, and crystalline structure.
4. Define hardness and describe how hardness contributes to abrasion resistance.
5. Define elasticity and give an example of when elasticity is desirable in dental procedures.
6. Relate stiffness and proportional limit, and describe how these properties apply to restorative dental materials.
7. Define ductility and malleability, and explain how these characteristics contribute to the edge strength of a gold crown.
8. Explain the difference between toughness and resilience.
9. Describe brittleness and discuss how this property applies to restorative dental materials.
10. Define viscosity and **thixotropy** and describe the clinical significance of each.
11. Differentiate between therapeutic, preventive, and restorative materials.
12. List and describe the three main types of restorative dental materials.
13. Describe the reaction stages a material undergoes to acquire its final state.
14. Identify the variables in the manipulation of a material.

KEY TERMS

Primary Bonds strong bonds with electronic attractions; ionic bonds, covalent bonds, metallic bonds

Secondary Bonds weaker bonds than primary bonds; hydrogen bonds, van der Waals forces, London dispersion forces

Brittle hard materials that break easily when stress is applied. They break suddenly with little plastic deformation, e.g., glass

Density the measure of the c weight of a material compared with its volume

Hardness the resistance of a solid to penetration

Ultimate Strength the maximum amount of stress a material can withstand without breaking

Elasticity the ability of a material to recover its shape completely after deformation from an applied force

Elastic Deformation deformation of a material that recovers its original shape and size when the force is removed

Elastic Limit the greatest stress a structure can withstand without permanent deformation

Plastic Deformation deformation of a material causing permanent changes in size or shape due to an applied force

Yield Stress the stress at which plastic deformation begins; also called yield point on a stress-strain curve

Stiffness a material's resistance to deformation

Young's Modulus or Elastic Modulus measures the resistance of a material to being deformed

Resilience the ability of a material to absorb energy without permanent deformation

Toughness the ability of a material to resist fracture

Ductility the ability of an object to be pulled or stretched under tension without rupture

Malleability the ability to be compressed and formed into a thin sheet without rupture

Edge Strength the ability of a material to withstand fracture at a thin edge, such as at margins of a restoration

Durability the ability of a material to withstand damage due to pressure or wear

Viscosity the ability of a liquid material to resist flow

Thixotropy a characteristic of some gels and liquids to flow more readily under mechanical force such as mixing, stirring, or shaking

Direct Restorative Materials restorations placed directly into a cavity preparation

Indirect Restorative Materials materials used to fabricate restorations outside the mouth that are subsequently placed into the mouth

Permanent Restorations restorations expected to be long lasting

Temporary Restorations restorations expected to last several days or weeks

Intermediate Restorations restorations expected to last several weeks to months

Mixing Time the amount of time allotted to bring the components of a material together into a homogeneous mix

Working Time the lapse of time from the start of mixing the material until it begins to harden and is no longer workable because it has reached its initial set

Initial Set Time coincides with the end of working time and is the time at which the material can no longer be manipulated in the mouth

Final Set Time the time needed for the reaction that begins when the material is mixed to go to completion, and the material hardens to its permanent state

Chemical Set Materials materials that set through a timed chemical reaction with the combination of a catalyst and base

Light-Activated Materials materials that require light in the blue wave range to initiate a reaction

Dual Set Materials materials that polymerize either from exposure to light in the blue wave range or from a chemical reaction

Shelf Life the useful life of a material before it deteriorates or changes in quality

---

To predict how a material will react under oral conditions, it is necessary to have an understanding of its physical properties. Chapter 2 discussed how the oral environment could affect and challenge the properties of dental materials. This chapter discusses how those properties are achieved, how they influence the clinician's selection of a material, and how and when properties can be manipulated. Both physical and mechanical properties must be considered when choosing the best restorative dental material. Physical properties are those properties of materials that can be measured and observed without having to change the composition of the material, and they help describe it. Physical properties include properties such as color, thermal conductivity, and solubility. Mechanical properties are properties that define the material's ability to perform in the oral environment and resist stresses and strains. Mechanical properties are considered a subset of physical properties and include properties such as elasticity, ductility, durability, and ultimate strength.

Electrochemical properties are seen in the reactions of materials as they set or their reactions to corrosive elements in the oral environment and their chemical stability and durability in the mouth.

To begin a discussion of the properties of dental materials, it is important to begin with a review of the physical structure of matter.

PHYSICAL STRUCTURE

ATOMS

Atoms are the basic building blocks of matter. They are composed of particles called neutrons, protons, and electrons (Fig. 3.1). Protons have positive electrical charges, electrons have negative charges, and neutrons have no electrical charges. Electrons are found in orbits (also called shells) around the nucleus. It is the outermost orbit in which electrons (called valence electrons) will interact with other atoms. The number and configuration of electrons in their orbits affect how reactive they are with other atoms. Atoms attempt to form the most stable configurations possible by filling their outermost orbits with electrons when bonding with other atoms. To do this, they will transfer or share electrons.

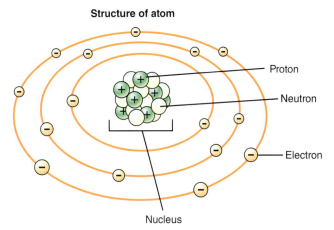

FIG. 3.1 The atomic structure. Heavy neutrons and protons form the nucleus of the atom, and electrons circle around the nucleus in shells or orbits.

TYPES OF BONDS

Two categories of bonds are formed between two atoms; strong bonds are called **primary bonds** and weaker bonds are called **secondary bonds**.

Primary Bonds

Strong bonds that bind the atoms of a molecule:
1. Ionic bonds—one atom gives up electrons and another atom gains electrons in the outer shell.
2. Covalent bonds—two nonmetal atoms share electrons in their outer shell.
3. Metallic bonds—multiple atoms in a lattice configuration share a sea of electrons that move throughout the lattice.

Secondary Bonds

Weak bonds that are adhesive forces acting between molecules (broadly called van der Waals forces):
1. Permanent dipole interactions—negatively charged pole in one atom attracts positively charged pole in an adjacent atom to form weak bonds.

2. Temporary dipole interactions—constantly circulating electrons in one molecule cluster briefly causing a negative charge that attracts a positive charge from a nearby molecule, called London dispersion force. These are the weakest of the secondary bonds.
3. Hydrogen bonds—dipole-dipole interaction involving hydrogen atoms, where a positive electromagnetically charged atom (commonly hydrogen) attracts a strong negatively charged atom (adjacent dipole) to bind hydrogen to a larger atom (i.e., oxygen). These are the strongest of the secondary bonds.

> **KEY POINTS: Physical Structure**
>
> 1. Atoms are the basic building blocks of matter, composed of particles called:
>   - Neutrons
>   - No electrical charge
>   - Protons
>   - Positive electrical charge
>   - Electrons
>   - Negative electrical charge
> 2. Atoms form bonds with other atoms:
>   - Primary bonds
>   - Strong bond
>   - Secondary bonds
>   - Weak bond

THE THREE STATES OF MATTER

Matter exists in three states or phases:
- Solid—it has the strongest attraction between atoms and molecules and has both shape and volume.
- Liquid—it has volume but no definitive shape.
- Gas—it has neither shape nor volume.

Most materials are mixtures of more than one state of matter. Gases are used mostly as propellants in dispensing or mixing dental materials. Therefore this chapter will limit the discussion to the general properties common to solids and liquids.

Solids

Atoms in solids are packed tightly together, and this restricts their movement, providing them with a fixed shape. Primary bonds hold the atoms of solids together, giving them strength and stability. Solids maintain their shape and resist forces that try to deform them. Solids are found in two main forms: crystalline or amorphous. Crystalline solids have an ordered three-dimensional symmetrical pattern or lattice network that repeats throughout the crystal (Fig. 3.2).

Noncrystalline solids, called **amorphous** solids, have atoms in nonrepeating arrangements similar to liquids. They do not have a definite melting point but soften gradually as heat is applied. Examples of amorphous solids include many dental waxes and glass-type ceramics.

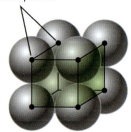

FIG. 3.2 Lattice network in a crystalline solid. Depicted is a simple cubic lattice cell. (From Lattice Structures in Crystalline Solids by Rice University.)

Liquids

Molecules in a liquid state are not confined to patterns, allowing them to change shape and flow. The study of flow is the science of rheology. Fluid flow can be steady or unsteady, and flow has a major influence on the handling or delivery of dental materials. The movement of a liquid will depend on the characteristics of the liquid and the surface on which it is placed.

Viscosity is the resistance of a liquid to flow. Values of viscosity depend on the nature of the fluid; thin liquids have low viscosity, and thicker liquids have high viscosity. Water flows readily and therefore has very low viscosity, whereas higher viscosity liquids (honey, for example) have a greater ability to resist flow. The viscosity of liquids usually decreases as the temperature increases. Some viscous liquids will flow more readily under stress (a property called **thixotrophy**), for example, when they are mixed, shaken, stirred, or manipulated.

Liquids when heated eventually vaporize or boil. Water transforms from a liquid state to a gas state (steam) at its boiling point of 100°C at standard atmospheric pressure. The lower the atmospheric pressure, the lower the boiling point.

> ** Do You Recall?**
>
> What property does a material have when it flows better under stress or pressure?

PROPERTIES OF DENTAL MATERIALS

Properties of dental materials are of three basic types: physical, mechanical, and chemical (or electrochemical).

PHYSICAL PROPERTIES

Physical properties are those properties that can be observed and measured without changing the composition of the material. Physical properties include:
- Melting and boiling points

- Density
- Viscosity
- Thermal conductivity
- Thermal expansion

Density is a measure of the weight of a material compared with its volume. It is a measure of the compactness of matter or how much mass is squeezed into a given space. A brick and a sponge of the same dimensions have the same volume, but the brick is much denser (Fig. 3.3). Enamel is the densest of the tooth structures, and gold is a dense restorative material.

MECHANICAL PROPERTIES

Mechanical properties are a subset of physical properties. They are physical properties that are seen when a load or force is applied to a material. They include properties such as:
- Hardness
- Stress
- Strain
- Fatigue
- Strength
- Elasticity
- Stiffness
- Resilience
- Toughness
- Ductility
- Malleability
- Durability

Hardness is the resistance of a solid to penetration. Hardness is also used to define a material's resistance to wear and abrasion. The hardness of a dental structure or material determines the extent to which it is scratched by an abrasive material. Enamel and porcelain, two of the hardest materials, are more resistant to being scratched in comparison to cementum and dentin, or composite resins and gold crowns. For this reason, it is very important that the type of restorative material or tooth surface be determined first before beginning procedures with abrasive agents.

Stress develops within a material when a force is applied (see Chapter 2). The larger the area over which the force is distributed, the lower the stress. Stress can occur singularly or in various combinations, depending on the directions of the applied forces.

When a solid is subjected to an external force of sufficient magnitude, it undergoes a change in size and shape and is considered strained. The amount of stress placed on a material at the time it breaks is known as its **ultimate strength**. A material does not necessarily have to break when subjected to an external compressive, shearing, or tensile force; it may deform. If this deformation is not permanent and the material recovers from the force completely, it has good **elasticity** and has undergone **elastic deformation**. Plastic deformation, on the other hand, occurs when a force or stress produces an irreversible change in a solid material's shape or size.

Not all materials return to their original shape when the deforming force is removed. Materials that do not return to their original shape have exceeded their **elastic limit** and start to permanently (or plastically) deform. The stress at which **plastic deformation** begins is called **yield stress**.

Young's modulus measures the resistance of a material to being deformed. The **stiffness** of a material, that is, the lack of elasticity, means that it resists being deformed, and it is measured by Young's modulus (also called elastic modulus). Stiffer materials have a higher modulus; enamel has a high modulus. Restorative materials should have a modulus that is compatible with tooth structure. We usually do not want dental restorations to bend or compress when a force is applied, so materials such as amalgam, composite resin, and ceramics should be stiff.

Resilience is the amount of energy a material can absorb without permanent deformation. Impression materials and orthodontic wire must be resilient to be successful.

Toughness is the ability of a material to absorb energy without fracture; restorative materials must exhibit toughness. Brittle materials have limited toughness because small amounts of deformation will cause fracture.

Pulling or stretching of orthodontic wire under tensile stress is a measure of its **ductility** (Fig. 3.4); that is, the

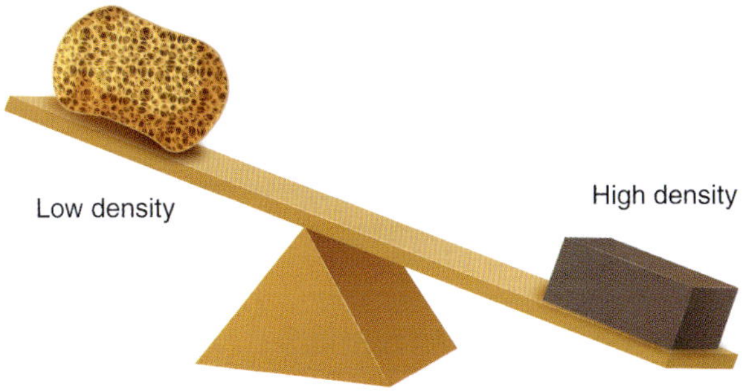

FIG. 3.3 The sponge on the left is porous and low in density, while the brick on the right lacks porosity and is very dense. So the brick weighs more even though the two are about the same in volume.

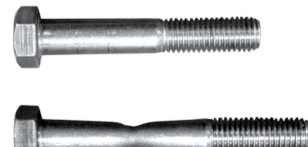

FIG. 3.4 Ductility. Stainless steel is an example of a very ductile metal. When placed under enough stress, it will elongate significantly before it fractures. (Courtesy Fastenal Company, Winona, Minnesota.)

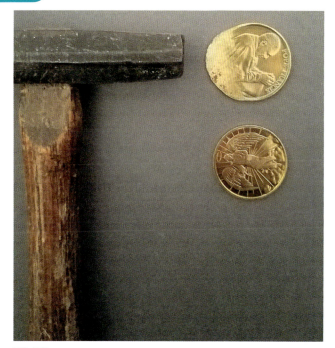

FIG. 3.5 Malleability. The two coins are made from malleable metal and were originally the same size. The left side of the top coin has been pounded with a hammer to a thin edge without breaking. This property is an indication of malleability. (Courtesy Dr. Steve Eakle.)

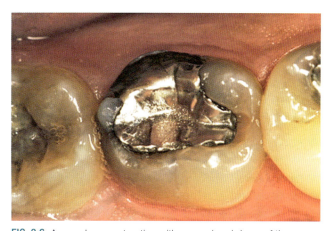

FIG. 3.6 An amalgam restoration with severe breakdown of the margins, creating a space or ditch between the amalgam and the cavity preparation. (Courtesy S. Geraldeli; From Anusavice KJ, Shen C, Rawls H. *Phillips' Science of Dental Materials.* 12th ed. Saunders; 2013:357.)

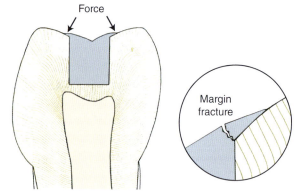

FIG. 3.7 Brittle material. Amalgam is a brittle material. If a thin edge of amalgam is left overlapping the enamel at the margin after carving, this excess amalgam may fracture away under chewing forces, creating ragged margins or a gap that collects plaque. (From Anusavice KJ, Shen C, Rawls H. *Phillips' Science of Dental Materials.* 12th ed. Saunders; 2013:57.)

amount of dimensional change it can withstand without breaking. Materials with poor ductility are classified as **brittle**. These materials are much weaker when subjected to tensile forces than to compressive forces. **Malleability** means that the material responds easily to compressive stress and can be hammered into a thin sheet without fracture (Fig. 3.5). The combination of malleability and ductility gives gold the ability to resist fracture even at fine margins, giving this metal **edge strength**. Amalgam does not have good edge strength. If an insufficient amount of amalgam is present at the edge of a restoration, the forces of mastication will likely cause a fracture of the material around the margin (Figs. 3.6 and 3.7).

In most cases, noble metals tend to be ductile and malleable, whereas ceramics are brittle. Ceramics and composites are described as brittle because they will sustain little strain before fracture occurs.

Fatigue occurs within a material when it is subjected to repeated stresses and can result in a sudden failure or fracture of the material. Microscopic flaws or cracks develop within the material that progress with repeated loading. Weak cusps of a tooth may fracture over time from repeated chewing forces placed on them (Fig. 3.8).

Durability refers to the ability of a material to withstand damage due to pressure or wear.

Chemical Properties

Chemical properties are those that involve a chemical reaction where atoms are rearranged, resulting in the material becoming one or more different materials. Some of the chemical reactions in the mouth involve an electrical current, and these are called electrochemical reactions. **Corrosion** is the most common electrochemical property seen in the oral cavity and is seen most often with metals (see Chapter 2). A very common example of corrosion outside the mouth is a rusting iron gate or nail. Oxygen in the air oxidizes the iron, chemically changing it and forming iron oxide, otherwise known as rust.

Galvinism, as described in Chapter 2, is an electrochemical reaction that occurs when two dissimilar metals contact each other in the presence of a solution containing electrolytes (such as saliva). It acts like a battery and produces an electric current, causing the patient to experience electric shocks and/or a metallic taste.

CLASSIFICATION OF MATERIALS

Restorative dental materials can be classified by their composition and divided into the categories of:
- Metals and alloys

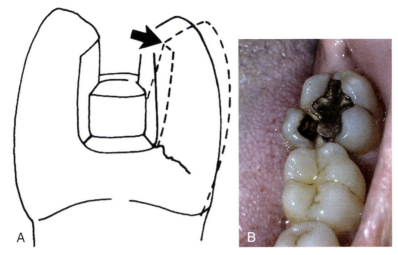

FIG. 3.8 Material fatigue. **(A)** Crack develops and propagates under cusp as it flexes under repeated chewing pressure. **(B)** Fatigue fracture of ML cusp of the lower second molar. (Courtesy Dr. Steve Eakle.)

- Ceramics
- Polymers

Metals have properties such as strength, the ability to conduct electricity and heat, malleability, ductility, and luster. Metals and their alloys are used for amalgam restorations, implants, partial denture frameworks, orthodontic brackets and bands, and crowns and bridges.

Ceramics are strong but generally rigid and brittle and melt at high temperatures. They are poor conductors of heat and electricity. Ceramics are popular for esthetic crowns and veneers.

Polymers can occur in long chains that have certain properties depending on how the chains are linked to each other. Some polymers can be flexible, easily shaped, and rubbery, while others can be hard, rigid, and difficult to mold into shapes. They can be used for denture bases and denture teeth, for example.

Materials can also be classified by their application, how they will be used and fabricated, and their expected longevity. As stated in Chapter 2, they may be preventive, therapeutic, or restorative. Restorations may be further classified as **direct restorative materials** or **indirect restorative materials**.

- Direct restorative materials are fabricated directly in the mouth.
- Indirect restorative materials are fabricated outside the mouth (often in dental laboratories, using replicas of the patient's dentition) and then placed in the patient's mouth.

Materials are classified by longevity, that is, how long they are expected to hold up in the oral cavity. Although all materials will degrade, wear, or fracture over time:

- **Permanent restorations** are expected to be a long-lasting replacement for missing, damaged, or discolored teeth.
- **Temporary restorations**, also called provisional restorations, are used for short periods of time, for example, several days to weeks. They function in place of permanent restoration to protect the teeth, prevent sensitivity and unwanted tooth movement, maintain the health and contours of the periodontal tissues, enable the patient to function normally, and provide temporary esthetics in the prepared area.
- **Intermediate restorations**, like provisional restorations, are placed for a limited time; however, the time may extend from several weeks to months. These restorations are not expected to replace the tooth structure permanently and are generally used when there is other ongoing treatment, such as orthodontics or implant therapy that is needed before a permanent restoration is required.

KEY POINTS: Classification of Dental Materials

1. By composition:
   - Metals and alloys
   - Ceramics
   - Polymers
2. By application:
   - Direct restorative materials
     - Fabricated directly in the mouth
   - Indirect restorative materials
     - Fabricated outside the mouth
3. By longevity:
   - Permanent
   - Temporary
   - Intermediate

COMPOSITION

Materials may be classified by their composition. Components and the reactions of those components may aid in the classification of materials. Many types of dental materials require the combination of two components to form the resulting final material. These initial two components may begin as:

- Water and powder
- Liquid and powder
- Paste and liquid

- Paste and paste
- Paste and initiator (blue light)

Many of these components are classified as catalyst and base; the catalyst is responsible for the speed at which the reaction occurs and is often the liquid component. Components may be measured and dispensed as a catalyst and base or packaged in predosed amounts.

> **Clinical Tip**
>
> Standardization of measurements in predose packages eliminates the errors produced in measuring.

REACTION ACTIVATED BY MIXING

When components are mixed together, a reaction occurs. This reaction may be:
- Physical—involving the evaporation or cooling of liquid
- Chemical—creating new primary bonds

Most reactions of the two components result in a solid structure. Before the material reaches its ultimate solid state, the process goes through stages:
- The manipulation stage—includes mixing and working time
- The reaction stage—includes initial and final set times

Both stages are defined in units of time as follows:
- **Mixing time** is the time the dental auxiliary has to bring the components together into a homogeneous mix. To allow the clinician the full working time, mixing times must be strictly observed.
- **Working time** is the time from mixing the material until it begins to harden and is no longer workable because it has reached its initial set.
- **Initial set time** coincides with the end of working time, and it occurs when the material can no longer be manipulated in the mouth.
- **Final set time** is the time needed for the reaction that begins when the material is mixed to go to completion, and the material hardens in its permanent state (Fig. 3.9).

Mixing and working times often offer some control variables. Mixing slowly and cooling the components may increase the working time; the addition of more catalysts may decrease the working time. Control of these variables is important in some situations. The amount of working time may also be controlled by how the reaction stage is initiated:

1. **Chemical set materials** are those that are set through the timed chemical reaction of a catalyst and base. Once the two components come into contact with each other, the chemical reaction begins and continues through the reaction stage. The clinician has little or no control over the time, except for cooling or warming the material before mixing. For this reason, many clinicians have selected light-activated systems.
2. **Light-activated materials** use a light source in the blue light range to initiate the reaction stage (Fig. 3.10; see Chapter 8). Chemicals that cause the setting reaction are present in the material but do not react until the material is exposed to the blue light source, thus giving the clinician unlimited working time.
3. **Dual set materials** have a slow chemical set that is activated when components are mixed, but the set can be accelerated by light curing. This gives the clinician much more control over the working time and gives assurance of complete setting in areas of the mouth or preparations that are deeper or more difficult to gain access to the curing light.

The setting times, initial and final, are important to the auxiliary as well as the clinician. The material must not be disturbed after the initial set has occurred. Moisture and pressure controls are frequently important during the initial set. Moisture contamination, from saliva or blood, during the initial set time may have an adverse effect on many dental materials, leading to failure. For materials needing intimate contact with the tooth, such as cement, continued firm pressure from biting force or from holding the material firmly in the mouth is essential. The final set of materials may occur while the patient is still in the office or several hours later.

> **Do You Recall?**
>
> What variables can increase the mixing time of a dental material?

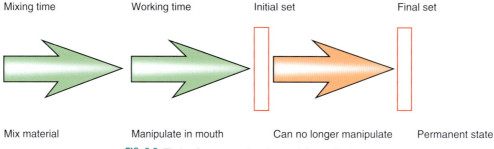

FIG. 3.9 Timing for a procedure from mixing to final set.

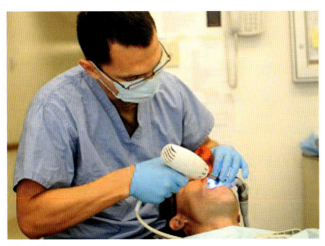

FIG. 3.10 Light curing unit that emits light in the blue wave range is used to cure light-activated material in the mouth.

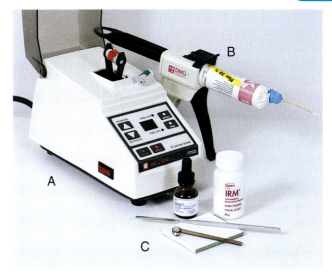

FIG. 3.11 Types of material mixing. (A) Device called a triturator is used to mix encapsulated, premeasured materials. (B) A gun-type automixing dispenser mixes materials contained in a two-barrel cartridge (one barrel with base and one with catalyst) by expressing them through a mixing tip. (C) Powder and liquid hand-mixed material that will be mixed on a paper pad (or a slab) with a metal spatula. A scoop for the powder is seen on the pad of paper.

Appropriate patient postoperative instructions related to when and what to eat, what to avoid, or how to place pressure on the restoration are essential to avoid a fracture of these materials.

MANIPULATION OF MATERIALS

Manipulation of a material's components is an important consideration for the dental auxiliary. It is through this manipulation that the final characteristics of the material are achieved. Some materials offer variation in their manipulation; others are very technique sensitive, and even the slightest variation will have a detrimental effect on the final product.

RATIOS OF COMPONENTS

The manufacturer, using the weight or volume of the components, recommends specific ratios. Many materials are produced as separate components that need to be measured and dispensed according to manufacturers' recommendations. Additionally, manufacturers produce materials in premeasured units, eliminating the need to measure and dispense the components, and thus standardizing the ratios.

Changing the ratios of the materials by adding more of a catalyst may result in a faster reaction; increasing the amount of water or liquid component may also result in a less dense, weaker material. These ratio changes are variables that permit the clinician to alter manipulation and reaction times for some materials but are contraindicated with other materials because of adverse effects. Manufacturers give directions for when variation is needed and how much variation in ratio the material can withstand without adverse results. The auxiliary is most often responsible for measuring and dispensing the components; strict adherence to ratios is required for some materials, whereas others allow some flexibility.

EFFECT OF TEMPERATURE AND HUMIDITY

External variables, such as the material and room temperature and humidity, can also play an important part in the manipulation of materials. In general, high temperatures and humidity will accelerate the reaction of a material's components, and low temperatures and humidity will retard or slow the reaction.

MIXING OF COMPONENTS

How the components of a material are mixed, that is, quickly or slowly, on a paper or wax pad or a glass slab, or by hand-mixing or using automix dispensers, will affect the final material and its consistency (Fig. 3.11). Materials mixed slowly on a chilled glass slab will usually produce a slower reaction. Automixed materials will give a more consistent result because the materials are mixed by equipment in a standardized manner with controlled proportions, eliminating the variables of human error.

SHELF LIFE

The **shelf life** of a material refers to the time a material can be stored before it becomes unsuitable for use. The shelf life varies from material to material and will be impacted by how it is stored. Temperature extremes and high humidity should be avoided. Plaster and other gypsum products should be stored in sealed containers to prevent deterioration from exposure to high humidity. Some materials require refrigeration to prolong their shelf life, and others need to be protected from direct light and may be packaged in light-blocking containers.

Always refer to manufacturers' directions to determine the conditions of storage and expiration. The expiration date for all materials stored in the office should be monitored carefully. Materials should be organized to allow for the use of older materials before new shipments to prevent them from expiring. Many materials will lose their potency or fail to set properly if they have passed their expiration date. Materials past expiration should not be utilized because they may lack their optimum performance and the treatments they were used with may fail. The American Dental Association requires materials that meet its specifications to stamp a date of production on the packaging of the material.

 Do You Recall?

Why is it important to store materials according to the manufacturer's instructions to prolong shelf life?

the dental auxiliary or clinician makes in selecting and manipulating the components while keeping in mind those variables that cannot be altered. Controlling variables of manipulation and reaction stages has become increasingly important with more sophisticated materials and more challenging clinical situations. Hand-mixing of materials allows for some control of manipulation and reaction stages. However, inconsistencies in mixing and time demands have become problematic in many clinical situations. Manufacturers are producing materials in various forms to address these concerns. Premeasured materials are manufactured to standardize the amount of catalyst and base included in the mix, thus preventing inconsistencies in resultant physical properties. Automix materials standardize the amount of catalyst and base and produce a consistent, homogeneous mix. It is important to refer to manufacturers' directions for instructions on storage, proportioning, mixing, and variables that may be altered to produce the best final results for a given clinical scenario.

SUMMARY

The physical structure of a material helps define the characteristics expected from that material. The success of dental materials is directly related to the choices

INSTRUCTIONAL VIDEOS

See the Evolve Resources site for a variety of educational videos that reinforce the material covered in this chapter.

Get Ready for Exams!

Review Questions

Select the one correct response for each of the following multiple-choice questions.

1. What is a defining characteristic of a solid?
   a. Shape and volume
   b. Shape only
   c. Neither shape nor volume
   d. Volume but no shape
2. What is the type of primary bond where atoms share electrons in their outer shells?
   a. Atomic bond
   b. Covalent bond
   c. Ionic bond
   d. Metallic bond
3. What is the correct term for describing the maximum amount of stress a material can withstand without breaking?
   a. Toughness
   b. Elasticity
   c. Ultimate strength
   d. Ductility
4. When the weight of a material increases in relationship to its volume, this is described as:
   a. Elastic
   b. Resilient
   c. Density
   d. Hard
5. Hardness determines the material's ability to:
   a. Deform an object
   b. Break an object
   c. Be easily compressed
   d. Resist scratching
6. A material is thought to have _____, when deformation is not permanent and a material recovers.
   a. Toughness
   b. Elasticity
   c. Malleability
   d. Ductility
7. Resistance to flow is known as:
   a. Viscosity
   b. Film thickness
   c. Density
   d. Curing
8. Thixotropic materials are those that:
   a. Have poor viscosity
   b. Flow under mechanical forces
   c. Flow at higher temperatures
   d. Flow at lower temperatures
9. Mixing time is the length of time from:
   a. The beginning of mixing to the end of setting time
   b. The beginning of mixing to the initial set time
   c. The beginning of mixing to the beginning of working time
   d. The beginning of mixing to the end of working time

Get Ready for Exams!—cont'd

10. A material mixed slowly on a cooled glass surface will:
    a. Have a shorter setting time
    b. Have a setting time that is unchanged
    c. Have a longer setting time

For answers to Review Questions, see the Appendix.

Case-Based Discussion Topics

1. While attending your state dental convention, you find a great deal on dental plaster. To take advantage of this offer, you must buy five 25-pound containers. When the plaster is delivered to the office, you find that there is not enough space to store the material, so it is decided to store it in the dentist's garage. Although the material in the first container has normal setting reactions, the material in containers opened later is inconsistent in working and setting times.
What may account for these inconsistencies?

BIBLIOGRAPHY

Bird DL, Robinson DS: *Modern dental assisting,* 13 ed, St. Louis, 2021, Elsevier.

Darby ML, Walsh MM: *Dental hygiene: theory and practice,* 4 ed, St. Louis, 2015, Saunders.

Powers JM, Wataha JC: *Dental materials: foundations and applications,* 11 ed, St. Louis, 2016, Elsevier.

Sakaguchi RL, Ferracane J, Powers JM: *Craig's restorative dental materials,* 14 ed, St. Louis, 2019, Elsevier.

Shen C, Rawls H, Esquivel-Upshaw JF: *Phillips' science of dental materials,* 13 ed, Philadelphia, 2022, Elsevier.

Van Noort R: *Introduction to dental materials,* 4 ed, London, 2013, Mosby.

4 General Handling and Safety of Dental Materials in the Dental Office

http://evolve.elsevier.com/Eakle/materials/

Chapter Objectives

On completion of this chapter, the student should be able to:

1. Identify five job-related health and safety hazards for employees in dental offices, and explain the methods of prevention for each one.
2. Explain the components of the Occupational Safety and Health Administration Hazard Communication Standard.
3. Describe the ways that chemicals can enter the body.
4. Define the employee and employer responsibility for safety training.
5. Describe the basic infection control methods for the handling of dental materials in the treatment area.
6. Identify the concepts and benefits of *going green* in the dental practice.
7. Discuss how the American Dental Association's Top 10 Initiatives of Sustainability can be incorporated into a general dental practice.

Key Terms

Particulate Matter extremely small particles (e.g., dust from dental plaster or stone)

Personal Protective Equipment (PPE) gloves, masks, gowns, eyewear, and other protective equipment for the employee

Bioaerosol a cloudlike mist containing droplets, tooth dust, dental material dust, and bacteria of a particle size less than 5 μm in diameter

Splatter small particles that may contain blood, saliva, oral particulate matter, water, and microbes

Hazardous Chemical a chemical that can cause burns to the skin, eyes, lungs, and so on, is poisonous, or can cause fire

Toxicity adverse reaction to a product or a chemical that can cause damage to the body

Flash Point the lowest temperature at which the vapor of a volatile substance will ignite with a flash; a low flash point means that a substance can catch fire easily

Ignitable a material or chemical that can erupt into fire easily

Corrosive usually an acid or strong base that can cause damage to metals and equipment, a gradual chemical destruction of metallic materials, as the rusting of metal instruments

Reactive how likely one substance is to react with another substance and change its chemical makeup in the process. Some reactions may give off heat, energy, or toxic gases

Safety Data Sheet (SDS) product reports from the manufacturer containing important information about the chemicals, hazards, handling, cleanup, and special PPE related to a product

---

Dental health care personnel use a wide variety of chemical-containing dental materials for patient treatment and laboratory procedures. All chemicals are capable of causing harmful effects if they are absorbed into the human body. The safety of the patient and the dental professional handling dental materials is of paramount concern. Safety for the work environment is a shared commitment of the dental team and the patient. Clinicians should be very familiar with the regulations for safe practice in the prevention of transmission of potentially pathogenic microbes to both patients and dental personnel. This chapter concentrates on how to prevent exposure to potentially hazardous materials. All dental personnel must understand the safe use, cleanup, and disposal methods for all the materials used in the dental office. This chapter also discusses compliance with governmental regulations and explains health and safety procedures.

MATERIAL HAZARDS IN THE DENTAL ENVIRONMENT

EXPOSURE TO PARTICULATE MATTER

During the manipulation of many dental materials, **particulate matter** can be generated. Items such as gypsum products, alginate, microblasting (sandblasting with very fine particles) materials, and pumice may generate dust during handling. Gypsum models, processed acrylic, porcelain, and various restorative materials may generate dust during the grinding and polishing processes. Pneumoconiosis is a fibrotic lung disease that can be caused by chronic exposure to these dusts. Black lung disease is the diagnosis for coal miners who inhale coal dust over a period of time. It is important for each person handling and manipulating these materials to have and use the proper **personal protective equipment (PPE),** such as dust or surgical masks, eyewear, gowns, and (when appropriate) hair coverings or tiebacks. Appropriate exhaust ventilation in dental laboratories where grinding or trimming of materials is performed is equally important.

Material Hazards in the Dental Office

- Exposure to particulate matter
- Exposure to biological contaminants
- Exposure to airborne contaminants
- Exposure to toxic effects of chemicals
- Exposure to mercury

EXPOSURE TO BIOLOGICAL CONTAMINANTS

Dental personnel come in contact with a variety of microorganisms via exposure to blood, body fluids, or oral and respiratory secretions. These microorganisms may include viruses such as hepatitis B, hepatitis C, human immunodeficiency, and herpes simplex and various bacteria. Dental personnel can be protected from the occupational transmission of infectious diseases through strict adherence to the requirements of the Occupational Safety and Health Administration (OSHA), the Canadian Centre for Occupational Health Bloodborne Pathogens Standard, and to the infection control guidelines issued by the Centers for Disease Control and Prevention. Another excellent resource for the dental team is the Organization for Safety, Asepsis, and Prevention. Most US states have regulations specific to infection control for dentistry. It is imperative the dental auxiliary is familiar with both state and federal regulations and guidelines.

Dental personnel must consider the possibility that equipment, storage containers, and dental materials may become contaminated during handling. Therefore it is important to use proper barrier protection such as overgloves or plastic covers when handling bottles, cans, syringes, or tubes that contain many of the dental materials used in a modern dental practice (Fig. 4.1).

Areas and equipment in each operatory must be clearly marked so dental personnel know which area or item is potentially contaminated thus allowing the necessary precautions be taken in handling that item. When unsure, use a protective covering or disinfect the item with the appropriate germicide.

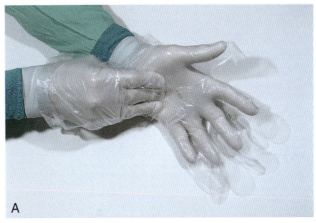

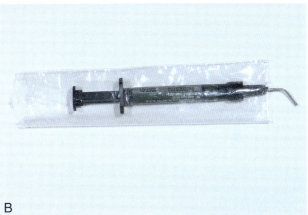

FIG. 4.1 (A) Overgloves are used to prevent cross-contamination when multiple-use dental material containers and dispensers are handled. **(B)** Syringe is barrier protected with a disposable plastic cover.

BIOAEROSOLS IN THE DENTAL SETTING

A **bio-aerosol** (*bio*, living; *aerosol*, mist) is a cloudlike mist containing microbes such as bacteria, viruses, molds, fungi, and yeast. Airborne microorganisms can be found in any building. Air-conditioning systems, humidifiers, carpets, wall coverings, and plants can easily become microbial breeding grounds.

DENTAL BIOAEROSOLS

In addition to the usual sources of airborne microorganisms, bioaerosols and **splatter** in the dental office are even more complex. This is because the aerosols and splatter created during many dental procedures contain oral fluids, blood, dental materials, powder, latex particles, and dust from metal, composites, amalgams, and oral hygiene products (Fig. 4.2). Particles that exit the patient's mouth during dental procedures can be separated into two categories:
1. Particulates that are greater in diameter than 50 μm (considered splatter)
2. Smaller particles less than 50 μm (considered aerosols)

Splatter. The larger splatter particulates can land on the provider's eyewear, skin, and PPE; or on other

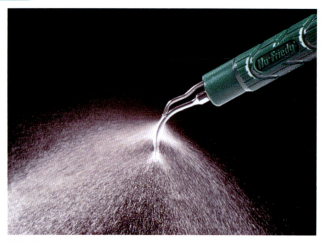

FIG. 4.2 Aerosol and droplets generated by ultrasonic scaler procedures. (Photo © Hu-Friedy Mfg. Co., Inc., Chicago, Illinois, used with permission.)

spaces and equipment and on the floor in the treatment area as far away as 3 feet.

Aerosols. The smaller particulates remain airborne from minutes to hours and can be the source of respiratory infection if inhaled.

The bioaerosols and splatter created by the dental handpiece, ultrasonic scaler, and by air abrasion procedures can contain particles of human teeth, oral fluids, bacteria and viruses, old restorations, lubricating oil, and abrasive powder.

Aerosols can be created by the following procedures:
- The use of a slurry of certain air-water powder products during hygiene procedures (use of the ultrasonic scaler and air polishing)
- Soft tissue treatments with lasers and electrosurgical units and may contain gases, tissue debris, and other infectious materials
- Grinding and polishing procedures in the laboratory

Recommendations for the reduction of bioaerosols during dental procedures include:
- Use of antiseptic rinses before treatment
- Use of high-volume evacuation
- Use of rubber dam when possible
- Reduction of biofilm prior to procedures by coronal polishing or by brushing and flossing

Allergens, toxins, irritants, and infectious agents will continue to build up when the amount of bioaerosol in the environment exceeds the capacity of the air filtration system. Dental personnel can suffer from allergic responses, infectious diseases, and respiratory problems as a result of prolonged exposure to bioaerosols and chemical irritants.

 Do You Recall?

What personal protective equipment should be worn by the dental professional to protect them from particulate matter and aerosols?

 Clinical Tip

Make sure the clinical or laboratory environment where aerosols are generated is well ventilated and the air is not recycled in the system. Use PPE appropriate for the type of aerosol exposure, that is, special high-filtration masks may be needed.

Management of Bioaerosols in the Dental Environment

The effects of bioaerosols can be minimized in dental offices through the following procedures:
- Monitor HVAC (heating, ventilation, and air-conditioning) systems to ensure optimal performance for the removal of particulates and to eliminate excess moisture
- Clean the air filtration system frequently
- Use proper oral and laboratory evacuation and ventilation techniques during bioaerosol-producing procedures
- Use a vacuum dust collection system during dust-producing laboratory procedures
- Use high-volume evacuation during all intraoral procedures that produce aerosol
- Use rubber dams (to minimize exposure to oral fluids)
- Use preprocedural mouth rinses
- Conduct preprocedural removal of biofilm through coronal polishing, brushing, and flossing
- Wear appropriate PPE:
  - Masks
  - Protective clothing such as an overgown or lab jacket
  - Proper eyewear and face shields
  - Gloves; minimize the use of latex products and use powder-free gloves
- Keep all containers tightly covered
- Pour chemicals rather than spraying
- Use lids on ultrasonic cleaners and other chemical containers

CHEMICAL SAFETY IN THE DENTAL OFFICE

HAZARDOUS CHEMICALS

A **hazardous chemical** is defined as any chemical that has been shown to cause a physical or health hazard. It can be any substance that can catch fire, react, or explode when mixed with other substances, or is corrosive or toxic. It is the chemical manufacturers' and importers' responsibility to assess the hazards of their products and pass this information on to consumers through the **Safety Data Sheet (SDS)**. Many dental materials contain more than one chemical (Fig. 4.3).

How Chemicals Enter the Body
- Inhalation
- Direct contact with the skin or eyes
- Absorption through the skin
- Ingestion (eating or drinking)
- Invasion directly through a break in the skin

General Handling and Safety of Dental Materials in the Dental Office CHAPTER 4 37

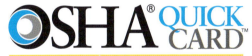

Hazard Communication Standard Labels

OSHA has updated the requirements for labeling of hazardous chemicals under its Hazard Communication Standard (HCS). As of June 1, 2015, all labels will be required to have pictograms, a signal word, hazard and precautionary statements, the product identifier, and supplier identification. A sample revised HCS label, identifying the required label elements, is shown on the right. Supplemental information can also be provided on the label as needed.

For more information:

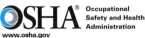 Occupational Safety and Health Administration (800) 321-OSHA (6742) www.osha.gov

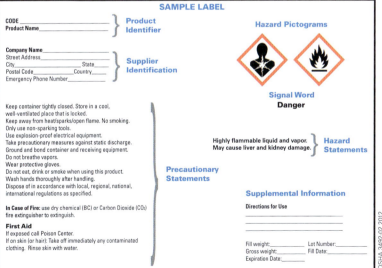

FIG. 4.3 Modern dental assisting: **(A)** Hazard Communication Standard pictograms. **(B)** Sample label. (From Occupational Safety and Health Administration. Available at http://www.osha.gov/dsg/hazcom/index.html.)

SKIN AND EYES

The skin is an effective barrier for many chemicals; however, some chemicals are absorbed through the skin. In general, the skin must be in direct contact with the chemical for this to occur. Absorption also may happen directly through a break in the skin, such as cuts, open sores, or chapped hands. After repeated contact with some chemicals, a skin disease called *dermatitis* may result. Adverse occupational reactions in the form of hand or facial dermatitis are not uncommon in dental personnel. These reactions seem to be most often associated with exposure to acrylates, formaldehyde, latex, and rubber additives that can be the result of exposure to dental materials or the components that make up PPE.

Other chemicals, such as acids, can break down the outer layer of the skin, causing burns, and are extremely harmful to the eyes. In the bonding technique for all ceramic crowns, hydrofluoric acid is used to etch the prosthesis to enhance the bond to the tooth. Hydrofluoric acid (HF) is extremely dangerous; anyone handling this acid must be well informed about the risks and safety requirements in handling the material and how to handle potential accidental exposure. Eye exposure may result in permanent damage or even blindness. Flushing the eyes at the eyewash station for at least 15 minutes and immediate medical attention are recommended. Exposure to HF is not limited to contact with the skin and eyes; inhalation of this potent acid is of equal concern. Adequate ventilation must be used when manipulating this material.

INHALATION

Inhalation of materials via gases, vapors, or dusts is a common route of chemical exposure for dental personnel. Some chemicals can cause damage directly to the lungs in the form of pneumoconiosis. Among dental personnel, prolonged exposure to dusts containing metal or silica has led to pneumoconiosis. Other chemicals may not directly affect the lungs but are absorbed by the lungs and sent via the bloodstream to other organs, such as the brain, liver, or kidneys, where they may cause damage. PPE such as masks or a proper respirator and adequate ventilation must be considered and used as appropriate for each procedure.

INGESTION

Ingestion (swallowing) is another way that chemicals can enter the body. Eating in an area where chemicals are used, and eating with hands that are contaminated with chemicals, are common ways of ingesting harmful chemicals. In the dental laboratory, many procedures are performed that produce contaminants such as metal grindings and gypsum products. It is essential to not eat in the clinical or laboratory area and food should not be stored in the same refrigerator as other dental materials. It is also important to wash your hands thoroughly after contact with any chemical. In many cases, the use of special protective gloves is indicated, and they must be removed and the hands washed before food is handled.

EXPOSURE TO BISPHENOL A

Bisphenol A (BPA) is a chemical currently used to harden plastics and to line water pipes and metal food and beverage cans. It is also found in very low levels in the resin used in some dental sealants and composite resins, especially those containing a BPA derivative, bis-DMA. Higher BPA levels in the urine of young adults and children have been associated with development of type 2 diabetes, cardiovascular disease, and reproductive abnormalities, possibly the result of BPA's weak estrogenic properties. However, the current position of the US Food and Drug Administration is that low BPA levels found in dental composites and sealants is not a health concern. Dental products are less likely to cause exposure to BPA than consumer products made with plastic and epoxy resin (see Chapter 8).

EXPOSURE TO MERCURY

There is a known health risk to dental health care personnel from exposure to elemental mercury. This risk has long been established and each office using mercury-containing amalgam procedures must take precautions to eliminate exposure to the dental personnel. Precautions must be taken in the dispensing, placement, condensing, and carving of amalgam, as well as handling and storage of amalgam scrap and removal of existing amalgam restorations (see Chapter 11).

ACUTE AND CHRONIC CHEMICAL TOXICITY

The toxicity of a chemical, and thus its harmfulness, depends directly on the dose, length of exposure, and frequency of exposure.

ACUTE CHEMICAL TOXICITY

Acute chemical toxicity results from high levels of exposure over a short period of time. This is frequently caused by a large chemical spill in which the exposure is sudden and unexpected. The effects of this type of toxicity are felt right away. The symptoms of acute overexposure to chemicals may include dizziness, fainting (syncope), headache, nausea, and vomiting.

CHRONIC CHEMICAL TOXICITY

Chronic chemical toxicity results from repeated exposures, usually to lower doses, over a much longer period of time, such as months or years. The effects of chronic toxicity can include cancer, neurologic deficits, and infertility.

For example, a single exposure to a high concentration of benzene may cause dizziness, headache, and unconsciousness; long-term daily exposure to low levels of benzene may eventually cause leukemia.

Another example is that of beryllium, a metal used in partial denture frameworks. When grinding beryllium frameworks for adjustment, one must avoid inhaling the dust because it is a toxic hazard that can lead to lung disease. A proper mask or respirator must be worn.

PERSONAL AND CHEMICAL PROTECTION

HAND PROTECTION

Appropriate hand hygiene is the most important step that health care personnel can take to prevent the transmission of infectious diseases in any healthcare setting. When routine dental treatment is being performed, hand-washing with plain soap, hand antisepsis with antimicrobial soap, or cleansing with an alcohol hand rub should be utilized. Alcohol handrubs may be effective; however, soap and water are necessary to clean the hands when they are visibly soiled with dirt, blood, or bodily fluids.

Fingernail integrity is an integral part of hand hygiene. Nails should be short, with smooth edges not extending beyond fingertips. Artificial nails, tips, and extenders are not recommended as they may harbor bacteria. If nail polish is worn, it should be maintained with a smooth appearance. Once fingernail polish has become chipped or nails grow out, showing margins of the polish at the cuticle, bacterial growth is encouraged.

Procedure gloves (patient treatment gloves) worn during patient care do not provide adequate protection when chemicals are handled. When exposed to chemical disinfectants, antiseptics, resins, and bonding agents, patient treatment gloves may degrade. When degradation of gloves occurs, contaminants and chemicals can be pulled through the glove and onto the hands. Chemical-resistant gloves such as nitrile utility gloves are recommended for wear during chemical handling (Fig. 4.4). With many materials on the market, the manufacturer's SDS instructions should be consulted to determine the compatibility of the glove material with various chemicals. Some individuals develop sensitivity to latex; however, a proper dermatologic diagnosis is required before a latex reaction can be distinguished from sensitivity to some other chemical. To ensure patient treatment gloves maintain their integrity and protective features, they should be worn no longer than 60 minutes and be changed when moisture on the internal surface is visible, become tacky on the exterior surface, or become ripped or torn.

EYE PROTECTION

Serious damage to the eyes, including blindness, may result from chemical accidents. It is necessary to protect the eyes from exposure to all dental materials including fumes and splashes while chemicals such as alcohol or methyl methacrylate monomer, acid, or other solvents are poured. The acids used for bonding procedures can be splashed into the eyes during rinsing from the etched teeth. Protective eyewear with side shields and splash shields are available from many manufacturers and must be worn when handling materials and in patient care settings.

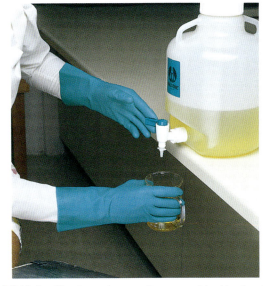

FIG. 4.4 Nitrile utility gloves, because they are resistant to chemicals, are used to handle disinfectants, acids, and hazardous chemicals. (Courtesy Lab Safety Supply, Janesville, Wisconsin.)

PROTECTIVE CLOTHING

Protective clothing such as disposable overgowns or laboratory jackets should be worn over uniforms and personal clothing to protect the clinician from blood-borne pathogens and dental materials. The most effective overgowns and laboratory jackets button up to the neck, cover the legs to the top of the knee when in both a seated or standing position, and have elastic at the wrist. Water-resistant overgowns are more effective in protecting the clinician than laboratory jackets as the lab jackets are not impervious to liquids. Overgowns and lab jackets are not to leave the dental facility once worn and potentially contaminated by blood-borne pathogens. Overgowns should be disposed of or sterilized as indicated by the manufacturer. Lab jackets should be laundered in the dental office or processed by a laundry service that specializes in handling biohazardous items.

When manipulating chemicals, the type of chemical that is being used should guide the selection of protective clothing. A rubber or neoprene apron should be worn when one is mixing or pouring chemicals that are caustic; can stain; or would saturate, penetrate, or damage regular fabric.

INHALATION PROTECTION

Patient treatment masks are necessary to protect the clinician not only from the spread of infection but particulate matter described earlier in the chapter. During routine dental treatment, the mask should be changed after every patient, every 60 minutes, or when it becomes damp or wet. The necessity to change masks frequently stems from the mesh in the mask beginning to break down after 20 minutes, which causes the protection of the clinician to decrease the longer the mask is worn.

The masks worn during patient care may or may not provide adequate protection when one is working with chemicals, depending on the quality of the mask. The facemask should be fluid repelling and provide respiratory protection. If the job requires frequent pouring or mixing of chemicals, sensitive or allergic individuals might need a National Institute of Occupational Safety and Health–approved dust and mist respirator facemask. Several masks are on the market for personnel with sensitive skin; these masks are free of dyes and chemicals and have a lint-free cellulose inner layer.

CONTROL OF CHEMICAL SPILLS

MERCURY SPILL

Mercury spill kits should be available in all dental offices that use amalgam for restorations (Fig. 4.5). Exposure to even small amounts of mercury is very hazardous to workers' health. Mercury can be absorbed through the skin or by the inhalation of mercury vapors.

The spill kit for small amounts of mercury should contain mercury-absorbing powder, mercury sponges, and a disposal bag. A mask and utility-type gloves should be worn when cleaning a mercury spill (see Chapter 11). Large mercury spills are infrequent because of the way mercury and amalgam alloy powder are currently prepackaged in enclosed capsules.

FLAMMABLE LIQUIDS

Many solvents used with dental materials have a very low **flash point** and can easily ignite when used near an open flame such as a Bunsen burner or an alcohol torch. Take extreme caution when using flammable products (e.g., the liquid monomer for acrylic or acetone). The SDS for each product describes the flammability of that product.

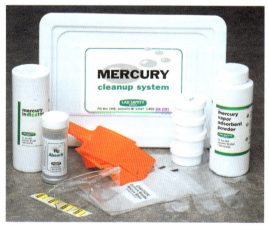

FIG. 4.5 Mercury spill kit. Note its compact size for convenient storage. (Courtesy Lab Safety Supply Inc., Janesville, Wisconsin.)

ACIDS

As mentioned previously, phosphoric, hydrofluoric, and hydrochloric acids are used during the manipulation of various dental materials. Splashing any of these acids on the skin, eyes, or clothing can cause severe burns or damage. Flushing with water immediately is essential to prevent severe injury.

EYEWASH

OSHA regulations require an eyewash unit to be installed in every place of employment where chemicals are used. A wide variety of styles are available. (Fig. 4.6) The standard eyewash unit attaches directly to existing faucets for emergencies, yet still allows normal faucet use. When turned on, the eyewash unit will irrigate the eyes with a soft, wide flow of water as necessary to flush away contaminants without causing additional damage. As an employee, you must be trained in proper use of the eyewash station. It is recommended that eyewash stations be inspected frequently to ensure water flow. Some manufacturers suggest running them for several minutes periodically to discharge any potential built-up biofilms or infectious agents. A posting of suggested times for eyewashing after an exposure (Table 4.1) and directions for the proper use of the particular type of eyewash unit should be placed near the eyewash station.

VENTILATION

Good ventilation is a necessity when dealing with any type of chemical. Dental offices should be equipped with special exhaust systems for fumes and dust in the laboratory and in radiographic processing areas if traditional processing methods are utilized. Laboratory areas may be covered with fine dust particles from grinding or chemical vapors such as from acrylic monomer or pickling acid (used to remove oxides from cast metals).

 Do You Recall?

How can improper handling of dental materials affect the safety of the dental staff and patients?

Table 4.1 OSHA Recommendations for Eyewashing

CHEMICAL EXPOSURE TO THE EYE	TIME PERIOD FOR EYEWASHING (MIN)
Nonirritants or mild irritants	5
Moderate-to-severe irritants	15–20
Nature of contaminate unknown	20
Corrosives	30
Strong alkalies (sodium, potassium, or calcium hydroxide)	60

OSHA, Occupational Safety and Health Administration.

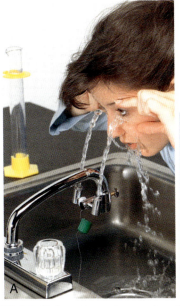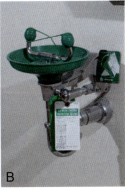

FIG. 4.6 **(A)** Faucet-mount eyewash and eye/face-wash station. **(B)** Wall-mounted eyewash station showing inspection record. (A, Courtesy Lab Safety Supply Inc., Janesville, Wisconsin; B, Courtesy Dr. Mark Dellinges.)

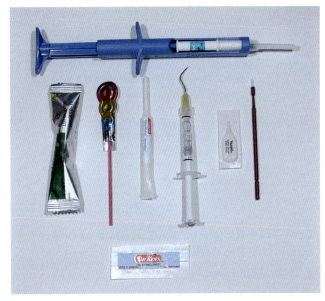

FIG. 4.7 Examples of single-use items (dental floss, fluoride varnish, temporary restorative materials, cement cartridge, and etching solution).

GENERAL PRECAUTIONS FOR STORING AND DISPOSING OF CHEMICALS

STORAGE

All dental materials contain chemical components, and some are more hazardous than others. Careful use and storage of dental materials are essential to ensure these products retain their therapeutic activity and identity. Changes in the chemical composition of materials can occur for many reasons. When changes take place, the product may no longer retain its effectiveness. Expiration dates must be monitored and out-of-date material should be disposed of properly. A basic "safe" policy for the storage of dental medications and chemicals is to keep them in original containers when possible and a dry, cool, dark place where they are not exposed to direct sunlight. Many single-dose products have been developed to eliminate cross-contamination and deterioration of the product due to evaporation or contamination (Fig. 4.7).

DISPOSAL OF CHEMICALS

EMPTY CONTAINERS

Even empty containers can be hazardous because they often hold residues that can burn or explode. Never fill an empty container with another substance because a dangerous chemical reaction could occur. Follow the label and the SDS on how to dispose of empty containers. (Safety Data Sheets are discussed later in this chapter.)

Tips to Aid in the Safe Use and Effectiveness of Dental Materials

Follow instructions: The manufacturer has already determined the best methods of protective packaging and storage. Therefore the manufacturer's instructions for storage, manipulation, and protection should be followed.

Light, heat, and air: Exposures to light, heat, and air are the prime factors in the deterioration of many bonding solutions. Changes in color, viscosity, or curing time are the most common signs of deterioration.

Expiration date: The substance's expiration date should always be noted. To maintain the proper chemical reactions, materials should be replaced when the expiration date is reached. Also, new supplies should always be stocked behind the current inventory so that the oldest product is used first.

Hazardous Waste Disposal

 KEY POINTS: Hazardous Waste Disposal

1. Waste is considered hazardous if certain properties or chemicals could pose dangers to human health and the environment after being discarded.
2. Waste is classified as hazardous if it has any of the following characteristics:
   - *Ignitable*
     - The substance is **ignitable** if it is flammable or combustible.
   - *Corrosive*
     - The substance is **corrosive** if it is highly acidic (pH less than 2.0) or basic (pH greater than 12.5). (Water has a pH of 7.0, which is neutral.)
   - *Reactive*
     - The substance is **reactive** if it is chemically unstable or explosive, reacts violently with water, or is capable of giving off toxic fumes when mixed with water.

> **KEY POINTS: Hazardous Waste Disposal—cont'd**
>
> - *Toxic*
>   - The substance is toxic if it contains arsenic, barium, chromium, mercury, lead, silver, or certain pesticides. (*Note:* Dental amalgam, asbestos, lead foil, and radiographic processing solutions are examples of hazardous waste that may be regulated differently by individual states and provinces.)
> - *Listed by the US Environmental Protection Administration (EPA) and the Canadian Environmental Protection Agency (CEPA):* Several hundred chemicals are listed by the EPA/CEPA as hazardous chemicals.

Guidelines for Minimizing Exposure to Chemical Hazards in the Dental Office

- Keep a minimum amount of hazardous chemicals in the office
- Read the labels and use only as directed
- Store according to the manufacturer's directions
- Keep containers tightly covered
- Avoid mixing chemicals unless consequences are known
- Wear appropriate personal protective equipment (PPE) when handling hazardous substances
- Wash hands immediately after removing gloves
- Avoid skin contact with chemicals; immediately wash skin that has come in contact with chemicals
- Maintain good ventilation
- Do not eat, drink, smoke, apply lip balm, or insert contact lenses in areas where chemicals are used
- Keep vaporizing chemicals away from open flames and heat sources
- Always have an operational fire extinguisher handy
- Know and use proper cleanup procedures
- Keep neutralizing agents available for strong acid and alkaline solutions
- Dispose of all hazardous chemicals according to SDS instructions

REGULATIONS FOR HAZARDOUS WASTE DISPOSAL

Regulations for hazardous waste disposal vary among states and provinces, and heavy fines may be imposed for those individuals who knowingly violate regulations. More important than the legal penalties are the environmental damage and the pollution of surface and groundwater that can result from improper handling, transportation, and disposal of hazardous wastes. The solutions from the wet processing of dental radiographs are not permitted in the public sewer systems, and if they are disposed of in private septic systems, they can cause those systems to fail. The disposal limits, either down the drain or in a landfill, of x-ray film, lead foil, disinfectants, and acid etch are also regulated by either county or state regulatory agencies and can vary widely throughout the United States.

In July 2017 the EPA mandated under the Clean Water Act that dental practices must control amalgam waste through the use of amalgam separators certified by the International Organization for Standardization (Standard 11143).

DENTAL LABORATORY INFECTION CONTROL

OSHA mandates that the dental laboratory have the same infection control protocols as the dental office. Dental laboratories may be a part of the dental office or may be off-site and owned and operated by dental laboratory technicians not employed by the office. Effective communication must be established with facilities within the office or off-site to prevent disease transmission from contaminated items entering the dental laboratory. In addition, dental laboratories are obligated to make sure that the products delivered back to the dental operatory are free of contaminants.

Dental laboratory technicians must adhere to the same standard precautions for the prevention of health-related diseases from the materials they handle. For example, impressions, casts, and dental prostheses are often moved back and forth between laboratories and dental operatories. These items may be contaminated with blood and saliva, which allows microorganisms to be transferred to the laboratory environment and back to the dental operatory. Microbes have been cultured from set gypsum dental casts for up to seven days.

Good communication and standardized protocols are essential for effective infection control. If there is ever a doubt as to the status of an incoming or outgoing case, the appropriate disinfection process must be completed before the item may be handled or placed in the patient's mouth.

> **Do You Recall?**
>
> What are the various consequences of not handling hazardous wastes properly?

Infection Control Communication between Laboratory and Dental Office

- Disinfection status of incoming and outgoing cases
- Utilization of appropriate shipping and receiving containers
- Designated receiving and shipping areas and protocols
- Designated production areas

All equipment used in the dental laboratory must be single-use items or handled with standard precautions for prevention of cross-contamination. Even though cases are appropriately disinfected before entering the production area, dental lathes, handpieces, burs, brushes, rag wheels, and other laboratory equipment should be disinfected or sterilized daily. The dental lathe should be protected with a functional shield surrounding the lathe to prevent spatter, aerosols, and the possibility of flying debris (Fig. 4.8).

Appropriate PPE must be worn in the dental laboratory to protect individuals from biological contaminants, bioaerosols, and chemical contact and inhalation. Appropriate ventilation and/or air-suction motors are important for these areas.

The dental office and dental laboratory must follow the same infection control guidelines to protect health care personnel and patients from blood-borne pathogens. Standard precautions, appropriate personal protective equipment, and good communication between the laboratory and the office are all components of successful infection control protocols.

HAZARD COMMUNICATIONS

OCCUPATIONAL SAFETY AND HEALTH ADMINISTRATION HAZARD COMMUNICATION STANDARD

OSHA has created standards to protect the safety of workers. Dental office personnel should be very familiar with the Blood-borne Pathogens Standard. This section addresses the standard that protects workers who are at risk of chemical exposure: the Hazard Communication Standard.

OSHA issued the Hazard Communication Standard because employees have "the right and the need to know" the identity and hazards of chemicals that they use in the workplace. The Hazard Communication Standard, also known as the Employee Right to Know Law, requires employers to implement a hazard communication program.

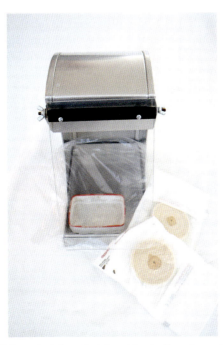

FIG. 4.8 Picture of a lathe splash hood lined with a disposable bag, a removable dish for a new mix of pumice, and sterilized rag wheels attached.

HAZARD COMMUNICATION PROGRAM

OSHA has been enforcing a Hazard Communication Standard (HCS) since 1983. A chemical hazard communication program has five parts: the written program, the chemical inventory, the SDS, labeling of containers, and employee training.

Written Hazard Communication Program

The written program must identify by name all employees who are exposed to hazardous chemicals and identify the person responsible for the program. In addition, it must describe how chemicals are handled in the workplace, must include a description of all safety measures and an explanation of how one should respond to chemical emergencies such as spills or exposures, and include staff training.

Chemical Inventory

The chemical inventory is a comprehensive list of every product used in the office that contains chemicals, including amalgam, bonding agents, disinfectants, and impression materials. Each time a new product is added to the office, it must be added to the chemical list and the SDS for that product must be placed in the SDS file.

The office will frequently appoint a staff member to be the hazard program coordinator. This person will be responsible for maintaining the chemical inventory and updating the SDS file.

Safety Data Sheets

The basic elements of the safety sheet use a combination of signal words and standardized pictograms to communicate hazards associated with a specific chemical (Fig. 4.3). SDSs contain health and safety information about each chemical in the office. SDSs provide comprehensive technical information and are a resource for employees/providers who work with chemicals. They describe the physical and chemical properties of a material; health and environmental health hazards; protective measures; precautions for safe handling, use, and storage; emergency and first-aid procedures; and spill-control measures. The manufacturers of products must provide SDSs, and an SDS must be obtained for every chemical used in the office. Manufacturer's typically enclose the SDS in the box with delivery of the product. SDSs should be organized in binders so that employees/providers have ready access to them and can easily locate a particular SDS (Box 4.1).

Necessary Parts of a Hazard Communication Program

- Written hazard communication program
- Inventory of hazardous chemicals
- Safety Data Sheet for all chemicals
- Labeling of containers
- Employee training

Box 4.1 Explanation of the Safety Data Sheet

HAZARD COMMUNICATION SAFETY DATA SHEETS

The Hazard Communication Standard (HCS) requires chemical manufacturers, distributors, or importers to provide Safety Data Sheets (SDSs) (formerly known as Material Safety Data Sheets) to communicate the hazards of hazardous chemical products. As of June 1, 2015, the HCS will require new SDSs to be in a uniform format, and include the section numbers, the headings, and associated information under the headings below:

Section 1, Identification includes product identifier; manufacturer or distributor name, address, phone number; emergency phone number; recommended use; restrictions on use.

Section 2, Hazard(s) identification includes all hazards regarding the chemical; required label elements.

Section 3, Composition/information on ingredients includes information on chemical ingredients; trade secret claims.

Section 4, First-aid measures includes important symptoms/effects, acute, delayed; required treatment.

Section 5, Fire-fighting measures lists suitable extinguishing techniques, equipment; chemical hazards from fire.

Section 6, Accidental release measures lists emergency procedures; protective equipment; proper methods of containment and cleanup.

Section 7, Handling and storage lists precautions for safe handling and storage, including incompatibilities.

Section 8, Exposure controls/personal protection lists OSHA's Permissible Exposure Limits (PELs); ACGIH Threshold Limit Values (TLVs); and any other exposure limit used or recommended by the chemical manufacturer, importer, or employer preparing the SDS where available as well as appropriate engineering controls; personal protective equipment (PPE).

Section 9, Physical and chemical properties lists the chemical's characteristics.

Section 10, Stability and reactivity lists chemical stability and possibility of hazardous reactions.

Section 11, Toxicological information includes routes of exposure; related symptoms, acute and chronic effects; numerical measures of toxicity.

Section 12, Ecological information
Section 13, Disposal considerations
Section 14, Transport information
Section 15, Regulatory information
Section 16, Other information, includes the date of preparation or last revision.

NOTE: Since other agencies regulate this information, Occupational Safety and Health Administration (OSHA) will not be enforcing Sections 12 through 15, (29 CFR 1910.1200(g)(2)). Employers must ensure that SDSs are readily accessible to employees. See Appendix D of 1910.1200 for a detailed description of SDS contents. From OSHA.gov.

LABELING OF CHEMICAL CONTAINERS AND SAFETY DATA SHEETS

The manufacturer or distributor is responsible for labeling of chemicals. Containers must be labeled to indicate manufacturer's name, address, and telephone number; product name or identifier; signal words for warning or hazards; hazard statements; and precautionary statements and pictograms (Fig. 4.9).

All chemicals in the dental office must be labeled. In many cases, the manufacturer's label is suitable. However, when the chemical is transferred to a different container, the new container must also be labeled. For example, when a concentrated chemical such as acrylic monomer is transferred to a small bottle for use in the treatment area or laboratory, the bottle must be labeled. No official labeling system is required, and a variety of styles are available on the market (Fig. 4.10) (Procedure 4.1). Even affixing to the new container, a photocopy of the label from the original container is acceptable. The most important considerations are that the labeling system should be easy to use, in legible condition, and provide all the information from the original label, including words, pictures, and symbols. All employees must be properly trained to understand and read the labels.

LABELING EXEMPTIONS

Some products, such as pharmaceuticals directly dispensed to the patient by the pharmacy and drugs intended for personal consumption by the employee for use in the workplace (such as aspirin), are exempt. Other examples of exempted products are food, alcoholic beverages, and cosmetics packaged for consumer use.

National Fire Protection Association Labels

The National Fire Protection Association has a labeling system that is frequently used to label containers of hazardous chemicals. This system consists of blue, red, yellow, and white diamonds filled with numerical ratings from 0 to 4. Categories are identified as follows: health (blue); flammability (red); reactivity (yellow); and special hazard symbols, such as "OXY" for oxidizers (white).

 Do You Recall?

Why must all chemicals in the dental office be labeled correctly?

Guidelines for Chemical Labeling

The label must contain the following information:
- Name, address, and phone number of the manufacturer or responsible party
- Product name or identifier
- Signal word for warning or hazard
- Hazard statement
- Precautionary statement
- Pictogram(s)

General Handling and Safety of Dental Materials in the Dental Office **CHAPTER 4** 45

HAZARDOUS MATERIALS CLASSIFICATION

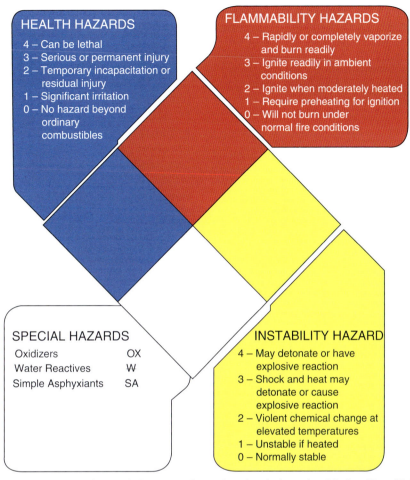

HEALTH HAZARDS
- 4 – Can be lethal
- 3 – Serious or permanent injury
- 2 – Temporary incapacitation or residual injury
- 1 – Significant irritation
- 0 – No hazard beyond ordinary combustibles

FLAMMABILITY HAZARDS
- 4 – Rapidly or completely vaporize and burn readily
- 3 – Ignite readily in ambient conditions
- 2 – Ignite when moderately heated
- 1 – Require preheating for ignition
- 0 – Will not burn under normal fire conditions

SPECIAL HAZARDS
- Oxidizers   OX
- Water Reactives   W̶
- Simple Asphyxiants SA

INSTABILITY HAZARD
- 4 – May detonate or have explosive reaction
- 3 – Shock and heat may detonate or cause explosive reaction
- 2 – Violent chemical change at elevated temperatures
- 1 – Unstable if heated
- 0 – Normally stable

FIG. 4.9 Hazard Communication Standard pictograms. Secondary chemical container labeling. (From Bird DL, Robinson DS: *Modern Dental Assisting,* ed 11. St. Louis, 2015, Elsevier.)

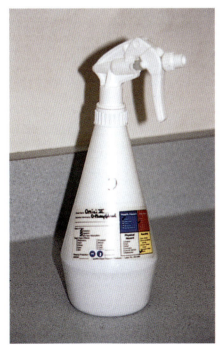

FIG. 4.10 Labeling of chemical transferred to a secondary container. (From Bird, D, Robinson D: *Modern dental assisting,* ed 12, St. Louis, 2018, Elsevier.)

Employee Training

> **KEY POINTS: Employee Training**
>
> 1. Employee training is essential for a successful hazard communication program.
>   Staff training is required:
>   - When a new employee is hired
>   - When a new chemical product is added to the office
>   - Once a year for all continuing employees
> 2. Records of each training session must be kept on file and retained for at least 5 years.
>   - Although the dentist is responsible for providing the training, the hazard program coordinator is responsible for routinely following these safety precautions.
> 3. The chemical training program for employees must include the following:
>   - Use of hazardous chemicals
>   - All safety practices, including all warnings
>   - Required personal protective devices
>   - Safe handling and disposal methods

Outline for a Hazard Communication Training Program

1. Discuss requirements of the Hazard Communication Standard
2. Prepare a written communication plan for the office (location, use, etc.)
3. Explain the hazards of the chemicals
4. Ensure that employees can interpret warning labels and the Safety Data Sheets
   a. Product identifier, chemical name, code number, or batch number
   b. Signal work—indicates the severity of the hazard
   c. Pictogram—Occupational Safety and Health Administration (OSHA) has designated eight pictograms (Box 4.2 provides examples of two of the eight pictograms)
   d. Hazard statement—nature of the hazard
   e. Precautionary statements—how to minimize or prevent adverse effects resulting from exposure, storage, or handling of a hazardous chemical
   f. Name, address, and phone number of the manufacturer, distributor, or importer.
5. Discuss how to obtain more information
6. Discuss taking measures to protect oneself and others:
   a. Office safety procedures
   b. Available personal protective equipment
   c. Instructions for reporting accidents and emergencies
   d. Information about first aid
   e. Information regarding proper storage
7. Present methods and observations that can be used to detect the presence or release of a hazardous chemical
8. Provide a question-and-answer opportunity
9. On completion, ask employees to sign a training record that will remain in their personnel file

Responsibilities of the Hazard Program Coordinator

- Read and understand the Hazard Communication Standard
- Implement the written hazard communication program
- Compile a list (chemical inventory) of products in the office that contain hazardous chemicals
- Obtain Safety Data Sheets (SDSs)
- Update the SDS file as new products are added to the office inventory
- Inform other employees of the location of the SDS file
- Label containers appropriately
- Provide training to other employees

ECO-CONSCIENCE GREEN PRACTICES

What about protecting your office and the environment? The process of preventing the transmission of disease and performing dental procedures involves equipment and products that produce waste, consume excess energy, and use toxic chemicals. To accomplish this, there are traditional and environmentally friendly products, supplies, and procedures available. The average dental practice disposes of hundreds of pounds of paper and plastic waste each year. There must be effective compromises to maintain an eco-friendly practice while not compromising the safety of the patient. Chris H. Miller (Indiana University School of Dentistry, Indianapolis, Indiana) has developed a list of green infection control "do's and don'ts" as they relate to recyclable and biodegradable materials, energy and water conservation, waste management, and infection control standards.

Eco-Friendly Do's and Don'ts

THE DO'S
- Choose reusables instead of disposables when possible
- Use alcohol hand rubs instead of hand-washing. If hands are visibly soiled, clinical staff must perform hand-washing as alcohol hand rubs will not physically remove debris
- Use trigger/pump sprays instead of aerosols
- Establish better inventory control to eliminate discarding excess product past its expiration date
- Ensure accurate mixing of chemicals and prepare amounts based on use life and shelf life
- Switch to digital instead of film x-ray
- Ensure sterilizers and cleaning units are full to reduce number of cycles per day
- Use products made from recycled materials
- Use products that are recyclable

THE DONT'S
- Do not use paper (i.e., biodegradable) instead of plastic surface barriers, because paper will allow penetration of moisture and microbes
- Do not reuse standard sterilization wraps and pouches because they were not designed to maintain sterility after more than one use
- Do not use woven cloth (e.g., denim) as sterilization wraps and then reuse it, because it is not a good microbial barrier
- Do not use a disinfectant that has a reduced concentration of an active ingredient unless there is evidence of its efficacy
- Do not shorten cleaner or sterilization cycles just to save energy
- Do not reuse items that are sold as disposable

Dental facilities can do their part to sustain the environment while continuing to prevent disease transmission. We are all encouraged to "reduce, reuse, recycle, and rethink."

BOX 4.2 OSHA Pictograms

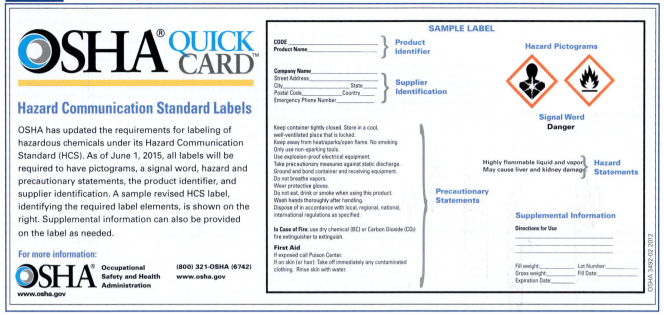

American Dental Association Council on Dental Practice "Go Green" Subcommittee Recommendations

Top 10 Initiatives
- Install an amalgam separator
- Turn off equipment when not in use
- Reuse paper scraps
- Use recycle bins and create a "Green Team" to bring items to recycle centers
- Recycle shredded confidential patient information
- Convert to digital technology
- Install solar or tinted shades
- Install locked or programmable thermostats
- Install high-efficiency lightbulbs
- Use nontoxic cleaners and do not use too much disinfectant

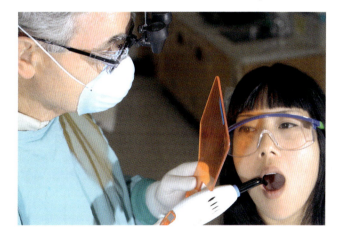

FIG. 4.11 Patient and clinician wearing protective eyewear; a protective light shield is being used.

The dental auxiliary is most frequently responsible for ordering supplies. Choosing cost-effective greener options to address environmental contamination and waste may begin with small steps and gradually build to an office that is environmentally responsible.

PATIENT SAFETY

It is extremely important for the health care provider to consider the safety of the patient while providing care and when various materials and chemicals are used. First, consideration should be given to protection of the patient's eyes. It is recommended that protective eyewear be supplied to the patient even if they wear glasses as the patient's glasses may not be shatter resistant. The same type of general protective eyewear used by the practitioner will do. Patient protective eyewear should be washed and disinfected between patients. Although some patients prefer dark glasses to shield their eyes from the dental unit light, most providers prefer to use clear lenses so they can observe the patient's eyes and facial expressions during treatment as a clue to the patient's level of comfort (Fig. 4.11).

 Caution

Be certain that protective eyewear has been dried thoroughly after treatment with disinfectant to avoid inadvertent contamination of the patient's skin or eyes.

Another vital safety consideration is the patient's airway. The use of high-velocity evacuation and a rubber dam whenever possible is excellent practice.

During rinsing of chemicals such as acid for etching, the patient may experience an unpleasant, bitter taste and may have a gagging reaction. The patient should be warned of this taste, and the rinse should be controlled to minimize discomfort.

Patients are more aware than ever before of the various chemicals and filling materials that are used in the dental practice. It is essential that the dental auxiliary be as familiar as possible with hazards and reactions that can occur when these materials and chemicals are used. The SDS is the best source of this information, along with the directions for use supplied by the product manufacturer.

 Do You Recall?

How can the dental auxiliary best prepare to answer questions patients might have related to hazards and reactions of dental materials used in the office?

SUMMARY

The management of a safe environment in the dental office is the responsibility of the employer and all employees. The safe use of any chemical or material is the responsibility of the user during the time of use. The safety of the patient is the responsibility of the dental team. Familiarity with each material or chemical used by the dental team is a must. This text provides general and technical information, but specific hazards are best determined by referring to the manufacturer's instructions and the SDS. Keep yourself informed, keep up to date with the standards, and continue to inquire "how can I protect myself, patients, coworkers, and the environment"?

INSTRUCTIONAL VIDEOS

See the Evolve Resources site for a variety of educational videos that reinforce the material covered in this chapter.

Procedure 4.1 Safety Data Sheet and Label Exercise

See Evolve site for Competency Sheet.

Consider the following with this procedure: *PPE is required for the operator, ensure appropriate safety protocols are followed, and check your state guidelines before performing this procedure.*

Use the information found on the SDS for acid etchant (conditioner) for pit and fissure sealant.

EQUIPMENT/SUPPLIES

SDS for product and labeled product
Pen
Secondary label (Refer to Fig. 4.3)

PROCEDURE STEPS

1. What is the product name and identifier? (This information is found in the product identification section of the SDS.)
2. What is the manufacturer's name, address, and emergency phone number? (This information is found in the product identification section of the SDS.)
3. What precautionary statements should be included on the label? (This information is found in the exposure controls/personal protection section of the SDS.)
4. What hazard pictograms and signal word should be included? (This information is found in the hazards identification section of the SDS.)
5. What is the hazard statement(s) associated with this product? (This information is found in the hazard identification section of the SDS.)
6. What supplemental information should be included?

Get Ready for Exams!

Review Questions

Select the one correct response for each of the following multiple-choice questions.

1. When working with dental materials, what are the most common work-related health and safety hazards?
   a. Exposure to mercury, exposure to particulate matter, exposure to perfume, and exposure to airborne contaminants
   b. Exposure to particulate matter, exposure to biological contaminants, exposure to noise, exposure to perfume, and exposure to airborne contaminants
   c. Exposure to particulate matter, exposure to biological contaminants, exposure to perfume, and exposure to airborne contaminants
   d. Exposure to mercury, exposure to particulate matter, exposure to biological contaminants, and exposure to toxic effects of chemicals
2. The proper PPE to be worn during handling of dental materials that can generate particulate matter consists of:
   a. Safety glasses, surgical or special dust mask, heavy-duty utility gloves, and overgloves
   b. Lab coat or overgown, surgical or special dust mask, heavy-duty utility gloves, and vinyl examination gloves
   c. Safety glasses, lab coat or overgown, surgical or special dust mask, and heavy-duty utility gloves
   d. Safety glasses, lab coat or overgown, and surgical or special dust mask, patient treatment gloves
3. There are multiple hazards associated with the use of the dental lathe in the laboratory. Which is NOT a hazard associated with the use of the dental lathe?
   a. Flying debris
   b. Aerosols
   c. Spatter
   d. Mercury vapor
4. Ways in which chemicals can enter the body include:
   a. Inhaling, through cuts in the skin, and by touching the product of a reaction
   b. Swallowing, inhaling, and by touching the product of a reaction
   c. Swallowing, inhaling, and through cuts in the skin
   d. Swallowing, through cuts in the skin, and by touching the product of a reaction
5. What is the most important step the dental auxiliary can take to prevent the transmission of infectious disease?
   a. Wear a dust and mist respirator face mask
   b. Utilize nitrile utility gloves
   c. Practice appropriate hand hygiene
6. Eyewash stations are:
   a. Never to be tested because they create a mess
   b. Best used at the end of the day for tired eyes
   c. Required to have a posted set of instructions
   d. Best used in an emergency only if the employee has had training in their use
7. What are the best ways to minimize exposure to chemical hazards in the dental office?
   a. Read the label and place in a secondary container to keep the original fresher
   b. Place in a secondary container to keep the original fresher, and keep a log of all chemicals ever purchased
   c. Read the label and store according to the manufacturer's directions
   d. Place in a secondary container to keep the original fresher, and store according to the manufacturer's directions

For answers to Review Questions, see the Appendix.

Case-Based Discussion Topics

1. Discuss the various items in an SDS. Take out an SDS for a sealant kit and identify all of the precautions required for handling the various components and identify the pictograms used.
What if it is light-cured versus chemical-cured?
2. Regarding secondary labeling:
Discuss the requirements and exceptions to the use of secondary labels.
3. Discuss some of the aerosols and bioaerosols used in the dental office.
Give examples of procedures that are most likely to generate these aerosols, and describe how they can be eliminated or reduced. (Hint: Don't forget about disinfecting and sterilizing procedures and the treatment performed on patients.)
4. Patient safety:
Discuss the various procedures that must be in place to ensure patient safety.
5. Cross-contamination:
Describe the procedures used to control cross-contamination and health care personnel exposure to the various materials that may be passed from a dental office to a dental laboratory. For example, what can you do to prevent cross-contamination and bacterial exposure of the dental office and laboratory personnel and patient from a dental impression?

BIBLIOGRAPHY

American Dental Association (ADA): Best management practices for amalgam waste. Available from http://www.ada.org/media/ADA/Member%20Center/Files/topics_amalgamwaste_brochure

Association (ADA) Council on Dental American Dental Association (ADA) Council on Dental Practice, American Dental Assistants Association (ADAA): Go green: it's the right thing to do. *The Dental Assistant* March/April 2012.

Bird DL, Robinson DS: *Modern Dental Assisting,* ed 13, St. Louis, 2021, Elsevier/Saunders.

Cuny E: Changes to the OSHA hazard communication standard: are you ready? *Inside Dental Assisting,* November/December 2013.

Donaldson K: Is your office environmentally responsible? *RDA Magazine,* 2011.

Jacks M: Protecting yourself, *Dimen Dent Hyg* 9(8):26–29, 2011.

MacDonald G: Chemical hazards: regulations, identification and resources, *J Calif Dent Assoc* 17(12), 1989.

Miller C, Long T, Molinari J: Protect against oral aerosols and splatter, *Dental Products Report*, 2009.

Miller CH: *Infection Control and Management of Hazardous Materials for the Dental Team,* ed 6, St. Louis, 2009, Mosby.

Mount GJ, Hume WR: *Appendix 1. Preservation and Restoration of Tooth Structure,* St. Louis, 1998, Mosby.

Powers JM, Wataha JC: *Dental Materials: Foundations and Applications,* ed 11, St. Louis, 2017, Elsevier.

Terézhalmy GT, Huber MA: Environmental infection control and in oral healthcare settings. A Continuing Education Course offered at dentalcare.com. Available from http://www.dentalcare.com/en-US/dental-education/ce-courses/ce363

Terézhalmy GT: Clinical practice guideline for an infection control/exposure control program in the oral healthcare setting. A continuing education course offered at dentalcare.com. Available from http://www.dentalcare.com/en-US/dental-education/ce-courses/ce342

U.S. Department of Labor: *Hazard communication standard: labels and pictograms,* 2013. [OSHA Brief] DSG BR 3636.

Wallace S, St. Cyr W: Sustainability challenge, *Dimen Dent Hyg,* 12(3):23–24,26, 2014.

Impression Materials

5

http://evolve.elsevier.com/Eakle/materials/

Chapter Objectives

On completion of this chapter, the student should be able to:
1. Describe the purpose of an impression.
2. Identify the three basic types of impressions.
3. Explain the importance of the key properties of impression materials.
4. Explain why alginate is an irreversible hydrocolloid.
5. List the supplies needed to make an alginate impression and explain how they are used.
6. Select trays for obtaining alginate impressions on a patient.
7. Demonstrate proper mixing of alginate, loading and seating the tray, and removing the set impression.
8. Evaluate upper and lower alginate impressions to ensure criteria for acceptability has been met.
9. Identify proper methods to disinfect alginate impressions and prepare them for transport to the office laboratory.
10. Identify and troubleshoot problems experienced with alginate impressions.
11. Compare and contrast the physical and mechanical properties of polyvinyl siloxane (PVS) and polyether impression materials.
12. Discuss the advantages and disadvantages of using polyether impression material for a crown impression.
13. Explain the difference between a hydrophobic and a hydrophilic impression material.
14. Determine acceptability of cord placement and gingival retraction.
15. Identify how the use of ferric sulfate astringent can control gingival bleeding before making an impression.
16. Demonstrate the proper steps to make registration of a patient's bite in centric occlusion.
17. Assemble the cartridge of impression material with mixing tip and load into the dispenser.
18. Explain what a digital impression is and how it is used.
19. Describe the advantages and disadvantages of digital impressions.
20. Demonstrate proper disinfect of PVS and polyether impressions and prepare them for transport to the dental laboratory.

KEY TERMS

Diagnostic Casts positive replicas of the teeth and surrounding oral tissues and structures produced from impressions that create a negative representation of the teeth; commonly called *study models* and used for diagnostic purposes and numerous chairside and laboratory procedures

Preliminary Impression an impression of the dentition or edentulous arch and surrounding tissues taken as a precursor to other treatment; often used to make casts (models) of oral structures for planning, and to construct custom trays or provisional restorations

Final Impression a detailed impression of oral structures used to make an accurate cast from which restorations or prostheses are made

Bite Registration an impression of the upper and lower teeth in the patient's normal bite relation

Dimensional Stability ability of a material to maintain its size and shape over a period of time

Accuracy ability of a material to adapt to and flow over the surfaces of the oral structures to record fine detail

Tear Resistance ability to avoid tearing when the material is in thin sections

Colloid glue-like material composed of two or more substances in which one substance does not go into solution but is suspended within another substance; it has at least two phases: a liquid phase called a *sol* and a semisolid phase called a *gel*

Hydrocolloid a water-based colloid used as an elastic impression material

Reversible Hydrocolloid an agar impression material that can be heated to change a gel into a fluid sol state that can flow around the teeth, and then cooled to gel again to make an impression of the shapes of the oral structures

Irreversible Hydrocolloid an alginate impression material that is mixed to a sol state and, as it sets, converts to a gel by a chemical reaction that irreversibly changes its nature

Agar a powder derived from seaweed that is a major component of reversible hydrocolloid

Sol liquid state in which colloidal particles are suspended; by cooling or a chemical reaction, it can change into a gel

Gel a semisolid state in which colloidal particles form a framework that traps liquid (e.g., Jell-O)

Alginate a versatile irreversible hydrocolloid that is the most used impression material in the dental office; it lacks the accuracy and fine surface detail needed for impressions for permanent restorations such as crown and bridge procedures

Elastomers highly accurate elastic impression materials that have qualities similar to rubber; they are used extensively in indirect restorative techniques, such as crown and bridge procedures

Imbibition the act of absorbing moisture

Surfactant a chemical that lowers the surface tension of a substance so that it is more readily wetted; for example, oil beads on the surface of water, but soap acts as a surfactant to allow the oil to spread over the surface

Polysulfide an elastic impression material that has sulfur-containing (mercaptan) functional groups; it has also been referred to as *rubber base impression material*

Condensation Silicone a silicone rubber impression material that sets by linking molecules in long chains but produces a liquid by-product by condensation

Addition Silicone a silicone rubber impression that also sets by linking molecules in long chains but produces no by-product; the most commonly used addition silicones are the polyvinyl siloxanes

Polyvinyl Siloxane (PVS) (also referred to as vinyl polysiloxane) is a very accurate addition silicone elastomer impression material; it is used extensively for crown and bridge procedures because of its accuracy, dimensional stability, and ease of use

Polyether a rubber impression material with ether functional groups; it has high accuracy and is popular for crown and bridge procedures

Astringent a chemical used in tissue management during gingival retraction to control bleeding and constrict tissues

Flash a common term for the cuff of impression material that extends apical to the margin of a crown preparation and represents an impression of the root or unprepared tooth

Digital Impression detailed digital images of the oral cavity or preparation, surrounding and opposing teeth, and tissues taken by a digital scanner for the purpose of making a restoration or to record baseline data for new patients

Intraoral Scanner a type of camera that takes digital images (typically in continuous video form) of oral structures

---

In dentistry, an impression material is used primarily to reproduce the form of teeth, including existing restorations and preparations made for restorative treatments, as well as the form of the arches and other hard and soft oral tissues for removable prostheses. Impression materials are also used by maxillofacial prosthodontists to make molds of facial defects resulting from cancer, trauma, or congenital defects for the purposes of constructing facial prostheses to restore facial form. Many different types of impression materials have been developed over the years, allowing the dentist to select materials according to the demands of the treatment and the oral environment.

Participation in making of impressions is one of the most frequently performed patient contact functions of the dental auxiliary. It is important for the auxiliary to have an understanding of the clinical applications, handling characteristics, physical properties, and limitations of these materials. In addition, they must know proper techniques and materials for disinfecting the impressions. In some states, dental auxiliaries can be licensed in expanded functions that include making final impressions for crowns and bridges, implants, and partial denture procedures.

OVERVIEW OF IMPRESSIONS

Making impressions of oral structures is a daily occurrence in a busy dental practice. Selection of the impression material is determined by what the impression will be used for. To replicate oral structures, the impression materials must be in a moldable or plastic state that can adapt to the teeth and oral tissues. Usually, the impression material in its plastic state is loaded into a tray for transport to the mouth and supporting it to maintain its shape. Within a specified time, the impression material must set to a semisolid, elastic, or rigid state. Elastic impression materials are used more extensively than rigid materials, because elastic materials flex from tissue undercuts when removed from the mouth, whereas rigid materials cannot. The completed impression forms a negative reproduction of the teeth and tissues. When plaster or stone is poured into the impression and hardened, the replica that is formed is a positive reproduction of the teeth and tissues (see Chapter 6). The replica is called a *cast* or *model*. In the initial diagnosis and treatment planning phase, the dentist may request that the auxiliary make impressions of the teeth and surrounding structures, so **diagnostic casts**, commonly called *study models*, can be made for further evaluation when the patient is no longer present. When an impression is made of a tooth that has been prepared for restoration, the replica of the prepared tooth is called a *die* and is used for fabrication of the restoration in the dental laboratory. Fig. 5.1 shows an impression and the mold and die made from that impression. Use of the die allows the dentist or laboratory technician to perform the procedure by the indirect technique. With the indirect technique, the restoration is not made directly on the tooth or in the mouth, as with the direct placement of amalgam, but is constructed in the laboratory (indirectly) and is cemented on the tooth later.

 Do You Recall?

What is the positive reproduction replica of the teeth and tissues called?

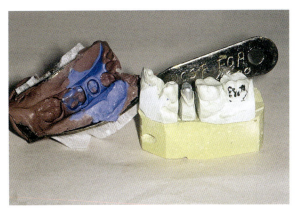

FIG. 5.1 A double-bite impression and the cast from the impression with a die of the crown preparation that can be removed by the laboratory technician to facilitate the creation of a wax pattern.

TYPES OF IMPRESSIONS

Dental impressions can be categorized into three basic types based on utilization. These types include the following:
1. Preliminary impressions
2. Final impressions
3. Bite registration (occlusal) impressions

While the dentist has a wide variety of materials to choose from to make these impressions, the choice will likely be alginate, silicone rubber (polyvinyl siloxane), polyether, or digital impressions. It is possible that traditional impression material may not be selected; instead, a digital image of the oral structures may be utilized as the technology is becoming more popular in modern dental practices. Digital impressions are discussed later in this chapter (see Digital Impressions section).

Preliminary Impressions

Preliminary impressions are made prior to another treatment. Casts made from preliminary impressions are often used for:
- Planning purposes, such as for diagnostic casts (study models)
- To make working casts from which custom trays or provisional (temporary) restorations can be made
- To create casts for pre- and post-treatment records.

Alginate is a useful, inexpensive material that is excellent for preliminary impressions but lacks the detail and accuracy to be used for a final (e.g., crown) impression.

Final Impressions

Final impressions are impressions that are more accurate in their replication of the oral structures. A very detailed and accurate impression of the preparation and surrounding structures is needed to provide a good fit and marginal integrity for a permanent restoration, such as:
- Crown
- Bridge
- Implant
- Partial denture
- Complete denture

Polyvinyl siloxane and polyether are the two most commonly used materials for final impressions.

> **? Do You Recall?**
>
> What is the difference between a final impression and preliminary impression?

Bite Registration

A replication of the patient's bite is needed to establish the proper relation between a restoration or prosthesis and the opposing teeth. A **bite registration** is an impression:
- that captures the occlusal relationship (see Procedure 5.3)
- Can be used in the office
- Sent to the dental laboratory where the restoration will be fabricated
- Used to help mount diagnostic casts in their proper relationship on an articulator

Although wax has been used for bite registration for decades (see Procedure 5.4), polyvinyl siloxane is currently more popular for this purpose. A wax bite registration can be easily distorted.

IMPRESSION MATERIAL TYPES

Impression materials can be categorized into two major groups:
1. Elastic materials
2. Inelastic materials

Elastic impression materials include:
- Hydrocolloids (agar and alginate)
- Polysulfides
- Silicone rubber materials (condensation and addition; e.g., polyvinyl siloxane)
- Polyethers
- Hybrid of polyether
- Polyvinyl siloxane

Of the elastic materials, agar hydrocolloids, polysulfides, and condensation silicone rubbers are not used much anymore. Alginate, polyvinyl siloxane (PVS), and polyether are the most commonly used elastic impression materials. Alginate is used extensively for preliminary impression, whereas PVS and polyether are used primarily for final impressions.

Inelastic materials are the older impression materials and include:
- Dental compound
- Impression plaster
- Zinc oxide eugenol
- Impression wax

Because of the superior properties of the elastic materials, inelastic materials are seldom used in dentistry today.

Key Properties

Although impression materials must have a degree of strength, their key properties are as follows:

- **Accuracy:** When the impression is made, the impression material must closely adapt to and flow over the surface of the tooth preparation and tissues to record the minute details to be accurate. The material will tend to flow if it has low viscosity and there is pressure on the material as the tray is seated.
- **Tear resistance:** After the impression material sets, it must have good tear resistance to prevent tearing during removal from the mouth. With a crown impression, the material in the gingival sulcus is very thin and will tear if the tear resistance is poor.
- **Dimensional stability:** After the impression is removed, the set material must remain dimensionally stable; otherwise, casts and dies poured from it will be inaccurate.

IMPRESSION TRAYS

Impression trays are used to:
- Transport the impression material to the mouth
- Provide support to the impression material until it sets and removed from the mouth
- Provide support and structure to the pure dental plaster or stone

Trays should be rigid to prevent distortion of the impression. The impression trays can be made for arches with teeth or edentulous ridges.

STOCK TRAYS

Impression trays can be premanufactured, called *stock trays*, which are purchased in a variety of sizes (small, medium, large, and extra large) for both adults and children (Fig. 5.2). Stock trays can be metal or plastic, and solid or perforated. Plastic trays are inexpensive and disposable, whereas metal trays are more expensive and must be cleaned and sterilized between uses. Plastic trays can be heated to manipulate the fit around exostoses and tori and they can be sized with a laboratory handpiece and bur.

Perforated trays have holes throughout to help retain impression material as it extrudes through the holes and locks into place. Solid trays often have raised borders on the internal surfaces that help lock in the impression material. These are called "rim-lock" trays. Impression materials used in solid trays require the application of an adhesive to further retain them and prevent distortion of the impression.

Stock Sectional Trays

In addition to full-arch impression trays, metal and plastic stock trays can be used for sectional impressions as well. Sectional trays can be shaped for:
- Quadrants
- Anterior segments
- Half-mouth

TRIPLE TRAYS (CLOSED-BITE TRAYS)

The triple tray (also called *closed-bite*, *double-bite*, *dual-arch*, or *check-bite tray*) is a stock sectional tray that is used to make an impression of the teeth being treated, the opposing teeth, and the patient's occlusion simultaneously. If used properly, the impression will capture the correct centric occlusion (bite) of the patient. Quadrant trays will fit a quadrant of the mouth or one-half of an arch.

BITE REGISTRATION TRAYS

Bite registration trays are typically U-shaped plastic frames with a thin fiber mesh stretched between the sides of the frame. The mesh retains the impression material (called *bite registration material*) and is thin enough so as not to interfere with closure of the upper and lower teeth in proper bite relationship. Bite registration material is placed on both sides of the mesh, the frame is positioned over the teeth to be recorded, and the patient closes into the normal bite relationship until the material sets (see Procedure 5.3). They can encompass a full arch or be limited to a quadrant or anterior section.

CUSTOM TRAYS

Because of the wide variation in size and shape of patients' arches, stock trays may not fit some patients well. Ideally, the properly fitted tray should conform to the:
- Length, size, and height of the arch
- Depth of the palatal vault
- Position of the teeth

To get the best fit, it may be necessary to custom make the tray to fit the patient's mouth (Fig. 5.3). Custom trays used with elastomeric impression materials provide a uniform thickness of the impression material, producing dimensional stability and reducing inaccuracies. The result is highly accurate working models and, ultimately, well-fitting restorations.

Custom trays are usually constructed in the laboratory with chemical-cured or light-cured resins. Custom trays can be made for full-arch or sectional impressions. A stock tray can be customized by lining it with a putty impression material that is adapted to the dental arch of the individual, and then an impression is made in this customized stock tray.

Do You Recall?

What are the different types of impression trays available for impressions and what types of impressions are they used for?

HYDROCOLLOIDS

A **colloid** is a glue-like material composed of two or more substances in which one substance does not go into solution but is suspended within another substance. **Hydrocolloids** are water-based colloids that function as elastic impression materials. The two hydrocolloids used in dentistry are:
- Agar hydrocolloid (or **reversible hydrocolloid**)
- Alginate hydrocolloid (or **irreversible hydrocolloid**)

Impression Materials CHAPTER 5   55

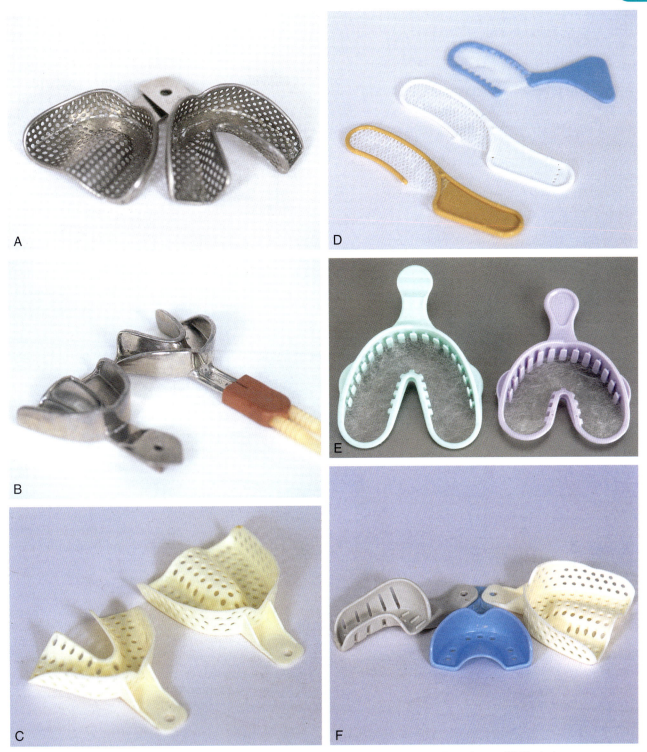

FIG. 5.2 Variety of metal and plastic stock impression trays. **(A)** Full-arch metal perforated trays. **(B)** Rim-lock metal tray with option for water cooling (tray on the right has water hose attached). **(C)** Disposable plastic perforated trays. **(D)** Bite registration trays. **(E)** Triple trays take impression of prepared teeth, opposing teeth, and bite. **(F)** Quadrant (*left*), anterior section (*middle*), and full-arch (*right*) trays. (From Bird DL, Robinson DS. *Modern Dental Assisting.* 11th ed. Elsevier; 2015.)

REVERSIBLE HYDROCOLLOID (AGAR)

Much like gelatin, when **agar** powder is mixed with water, it forms a glue-like suspension that entraps the water, making a colloidal suspension called a **sol**. Heating the material will disperse the agar in the water faster. When the agar sol is chilled, it will **gel**, becoming semisolid or jelly-like (like Jell-O). When the agar gel is heated, it will reverse into a liquid suspension (sol). Therefore it is a reversible hydrocolloid. Agar's main clinical use is for impressions of operative and crown and bridge procedures. It also has uses in the laboratory for the duplication of casts (models). Its use has declined over the years as elastic (rubber) impression materials have been introduced. Detailed information about reversible (agar) hydrocolloid can be found on the student resource section of the Evolve website.

IRREVERSIBLE HYDROCOLLOID (ALGINATE)

Alginate, also called *alginate hydrocolloid* or *irreversible hydrocolloid*, is by far the most widely used impression material. It is inexpensive, easy to manipulate, requires no special equipment, and is reasonably accurate for many dental procedures.

Alginate is used for making impressions for:
- Diagnostic casts
- Partial denture frameworks
- Repairs of broken partial or complete dentures
- Fabrication of provisional restorations
- Fluoride and bleaching trays
- Sports protectors
- Preliminary impressions for edentulous arches
- Removable orthodontic appliances

Alginate is not accurate enough for the final impressions for inlay, onlay, crown, and bridge preparations. It does not capture the fine detail of the preparation needed for a precise fit of such restorations. Additionally, it is thick and does not flow well into embrasures or occlusal surfaces.

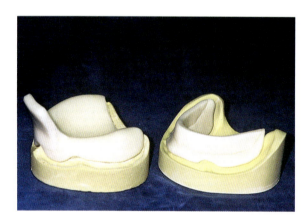

FIG. 5.3 Custom acrylic trays that were fabricated on edentulous casts.

Composition and Setting Reaction. Alginate is produced from derivatives of seaweed with the main active ingredient being potassium or sodium alginate, which makes up 15% to 20% of the powder. Proportions of ingredients vary by manufacturer and with fast-, regular-, and slow-set materials. See Table 5.1 for the components of alginate and their functions. The "dustless" alginate powders have organic glycols or glycerin added to keep powder from becoming airborne when it is dispensed. The dust contains silica particles, which can be a potential health hazard if inhaled.

When alginate powder is mixed with water, calcium sulfate dihydrate reacts with sodium alginate to form calcium alginate. Calcium alginate is insoluble and causes the sol of mixed powder and water to gel. Because this occurs by a chemical reaction, it cannot be reversed back to the sol state; therefore it is a reversible hydrocolloid. A variety of chemicals are added to alginate to provide various qualities useful in dentistry:
- Trisodium phosphate is added as a retarder to delay the reaction. The amount of retarder that is added will control the time of the set and determine if fast- or regular-set alginate.
- Diatomaceous earth is added as a filler to increase stiffness and strength and to prevent the surface from being sticky.
- Potassium sulfate is added to keep the alginate from interfering with the set of the gypsum products used to pour the impression.
- Some manufacturers have added chemicals to the alginate that change color as the chemical reaction progresses to indicate when it is time to insert the impression, and the color changes again when it is time to remove the impression.

Working Time. Alginates have varying working times which start from the combination of materials to seating in the mouth. Working times are as follows:
- Regular-set alginates—2 to 3 minutes
- Fast-set alginate—1.25 to 2 minutes (American Dental Association specification no. 18 sets the minimum at 1.25 minutes).

TABLE 5.1 Composition of Alginate Impression Material

MATERIAL	PERCENTAGE (APPROXIMATE)	PURPOSE
Sodium or potassium alginate	15%–20%	Colloidal particles as basis of the gel
Calcium sulfate dihydrate	14%–20%	Creates irreversible gel with alginate
Potassium sulfate	10%	Ensures set of gypsum materials
Trisodium phosphate	2%	Retarder to control setting time
Diatomaceous earth	55%–60%	Filler to increase thickness and strength
Other additives:	Very small quantities	
• Organic glycols		To reduce dust when powder is handled
• Flavoring agents		To improve taste of material
• Coloring agents		To provide pleasant colors
• Disinfectants		To cause antibacterial action

The longer the time used to mix the alginate, the faster it must be loaded into the tray and seated in the mouth.

Setting Time. Setting time can be lengthened by using cold water or shortened by using warm water. Adjusting the powder-to-water ratio can affect the set, but also adversely affects the physical and mechanical properties and therefore is not recommended. When the material is mixed according to manufacturer instructions, the following times will be observed:
- Regular-set alginates set in 2 to 5 minutes
- Fast-set alginates set in 1 to 2 minutes.

It is advisable to leave the impression in the mouth for an additional minute after it appears set, because the tear strength and the ability to rebound from undercuts without permanent deformation increase during this time.

Do You Recall?
How can the water temperature change the setting time of alginate?

Clinical Tip
For patients with sensitive teeth, alginate mixed with cool water can be painful. Use regular-set alginate with warm water. The working and setting times will be shortened, but the patient will be more comfortable.

Important Properties of Alginate
Permanent Deformation. Alginate will be compressed when it is removed from undercuts in the mouth. The greater the compression, the more likely the alginate will be permanently deformed to some degree. A certain thickness of alginate (2–4 mm) is needed between the impression tray and the teeth or tissue undercut; alginate that is too thin will deform more and tear more easily. When an alginate impression is removed, it should be done with a rapid "snap" to prevent the deformation of critical surfaces. If 8 to 10 minutes are allowed to elapse from the time an alginate impression is removed from the mouth until pouring the model, some recovery or rebound will occur from the deformation. That deformation that does not recover is the *permanent deformation*, and it will be recorded in the poured gypsum cast as a distortion. As long as the distortion is small, it may not be clinically significant. Usually, the time needed for disinfecting the impression is at least 10 minutes, and most of the rebound will have occurred by then.

Dimensional Stability. Alginate is very sensitive to moisture loss and will shrink as a result. Once the impression is removed from the mouth, it should be:
- Rinsed and disinfected (Procedure 5.5)
- Wrapped in a damp (not dripping wet) paper towel
- Sealed in a zippered plastic bag.
  - An alternative to wrapping in a damp paper towel would be to put a few drops of water in the plastic bag. Alginate could imbibe water from a towel that is very wet and swell.
  - Enclosing the impression this way will create an environment with 100% humidity to minimize water loss from the alginate.

Some moisture will be lost from the impression even in 100% humidity from syneresis. Syneresis occurs with many gels that are left standing, whereby they contract and some of the liquid is squeezed out of the gel, forming a wet film on the surface. This loss of water changes the properties of the material. Ideally, the impression is poured after it is disinfected. If the impression must be stored until it can be poured a few hours later, then it must be kept at 100% humidity (as with the zippered plastic bag and a few drops of water). The longer that pouring is delayed, the more likely that some distortion will occur in the alginate.

Tear Strength. The tear strength of alginate is more important than its compressive strength because most commercial alginates far exceed the minimal allowable value for compressive strength. Factors that contribute to the strength of alginate are as follows:
- Alginate mixed with too much water will be weaker and more likely to tear on removal from the mouth.
- Thin sections of alginate are also prone to tearing.
- Slow removal of the alginate from the mouth will contribute to tearing.

If the impression can be left in the mouth for an additional minute beyond the point when it is set, it will increase in tear strength. When properly handled, alginate has adequate tear strength for most purposes for which it is used. Some alginates have silicone polymers added to increase the strength.

MAKING ALGINATE IMPRESSIONS
Objective
The objective of impression making is to reproduce the oral structures with acceptable accuracy while practicing proper infection control and maintaining patient comfort. The dental auxiliary can make alginate impressions and need to do the following during the process:
- Explain the procedure to the patient to best prepare them for what to expect
- Dispense, mix, and load alginate into impression trays
- After removal of the impression, properly disinfect and handle the impression until it is poured with the appropriate gypsum material
- Clear residual alginate from the mouth and face of the patient

Tray Selection

Stock trays work well with alginate because they provide plenty of room for an adequate thickness of alginate. Alginate must be tightly adapted to the tray to be accurate. If the alginate pulls loose from the tray, a distortion will occur. Both perforated and solid trays can be used to obtain an alginate impression. If disposable plastic trays are used, they should be rigid. Flexible plastic trays have the potential to distort under the weight of the wet gypsum during pouring or when used in areas of undercuts in the mouth.

A properly selected full-arch tray should:
- Cover all of the teeth
- Extend into the facial and lingual vestibules without impinging on the tissues
- Extend posteriorly to include the retromolar area for a mandibular tray and the hamular notch area for a maxillary tray
- Be deep enough to provide at least 2 mm of space for alginate beyond the incisal and occlusal surfaces of the teeth and wide enough to allow approximately 5 mm of alginate between the sides of the tray and the tissues

On occasion, standard stock trays will not cover all of the desired areas for the impression and must be modified with utility wax to create appropriate extensions of the tray and support the alginate. A common area for this to occur is the third molar area of an individual with large jaws. Wax may also be added to the mid-palatal area of the tray to support the alginate when the patient has a very deep palatal vault (see Procedure 5.1). Usually, the patient is asked to rinse the mouth to remove loose debris and thick saliva before the impression is made. An antimicrobial rinse may be used to reduce the number of oral pathogens.

 Do You Recall?

Why are disposable impression trays not sterilized after use?

Dispensing. Manufacturers supply measures for powder and water for their alginates. Use the appropriate measures and adhere to the recommended proportions of powder and water to maintain the desired physical properties of the alginate. Powder measures (also called *scoops*) and water measures will vary among manufacturers, so do not interchange them with other manufacturers' measures.

 Clinical Tip

Water and powder measures can vary in size among manufacturers. If your office uses more than one brand of alginate, color code the measures so they are not intermixed.

During shipping or prolonged periods of sitting, the powder in the canister may pack tightly and some of the ingredients may settle out, so that they are not evenly distributed throughout the powder. Because of the compacting of powder particles, the amount of powder scooped will be greater than the manufacturer intended when developing the measuring scoop. When the compacted powder is incorporated into the recommended volume of water, the resulting mix will be too thick and will often set too rapidly. To prevent this from happening, containers of alginate such as cans or plastic containers should be turned end-over-end a few times to decompress (fluff) the powder and mix the ingredients. Some alginates are supplied in premeasured, watertight packages with a quantity suitable for a medium-sized arch (equivalent to two scoops with most manufacturers) (Fig. 5.4). Prepackages are more expensive, but some practitioners find it to be convenient, to provide a more consistent mix, and to minimize cross-contamination.

 Caution

Be sure to wear a mask while dispensing and mixing alginate. Alginate dust is potentially hazardous to inhale because it contains silicon dioxide in the diatomaceous earth fillers, as well as other chemicals. Using dustless alginate will minimize but not eliminate this risk.

Mixing. The recommended amount of alginate for various size trays is as follows:
- Upper adult arch
  - Large—three scoops
  - Medium—two to three scoops
  - Small—two scoops

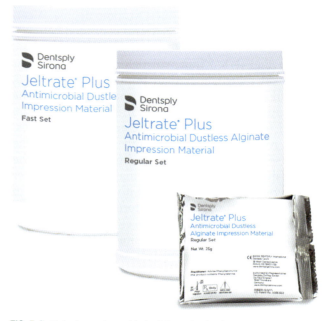

FIG. 5.4 Alginate packaged in bulk in a plastic drum or premeasured packets equivalent to two scoops with many manufacturers. (Courtesy Dentsply Sirona.)

- Lower adult arch
  - Large—two to three scoops
  - Medium—two scoops
  - Small—two scoops
- One unit of water is required per scoop of alginate

Water is placed in the flexible mixing bowl, and the powder is added to it. The powder is stirred into the water so that the powder becomes wet. Next, the wet powder is aggressively mixed against the sides of the bowl with a wide-bladed spatula. Some operators prefer to rotate the bowl in one hand while mixing with the other. Some offices use mechanical mixing machines for rapid mixing, ease of use, and a consistent mix (Fig. 5.5). With both mechanical and hand-mixing, the water-powder mixture is forced against the sides of the bowl to further incorporate the powder into the water and to force out entrapped air. Mixing should be completed within 45 seconds for regular-set alginate and within 30 seconds for fast-set alginate. The completed mix should have a creamy consistency (see Fig. 5.5C). If it appears grainy, it has not been mixed thoroughly.

Loading the Tray. Mixed alginate is picked up on the spatula and pushed into the depth of the tray. This action forces out air, thus preventing large voids in the impression. The alginate should be loaded in large increments as quickly as possible to reduce the chance of entrapped air. The tray should be loaded until the alginate is even with the top of the sides of the tray. A wet, gloved finger is used to smooth the surface of the alginate and to create a shallow trough over the ridge area of the alginate that reduces the chance for entrapped air and helps to orient the tray over the teeth when it is seated.

Seating the Tray. Once the tray is loaded, the operator should take some alginate from the bowl on the gloved index finger and spread it on the occlusal surfaces and

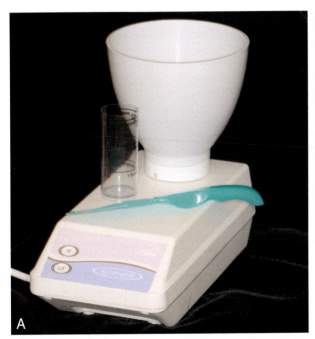
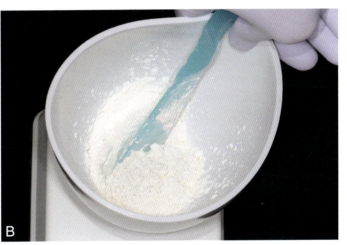
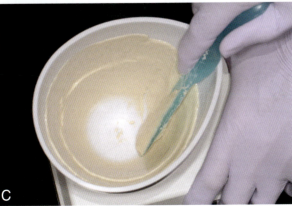

FIG. 5.5 Mechanical mixer used to mix alginate for an impression. **(A)** Mechanical mixer with water measure and spatula. **(B)** After water is added to the powder in the bowl, a spatula is used to wet all of the powder. **(C)** Spatula presses the wet powder against the rotating bowl until a smooth, creamy mixture is achieved. (From Powers JM, Wataha JC. *Dental Materials: Properties and Manipulation.* 11th ed. Elsevier; 2017.)

embrasures of the teeth to force air out from the occlusal grooves and embrasure spaces.

When seating the impression tray, the clinician should:

- Place the patient in the upright position to prevent the flow of alginate down the throat.
- Stand in front of the patient to one side at 7 o'clock for right-handers and 5 o'clock for left-handers when obtaining lower impressions.
- A right-handed operator stands just behind the patient at 11 o'clock position while the left-handed operators should reverse the positions and stand at the 1 o'clock position for maxillary impressions (Fig. 5.6).
- The right or left side of the tray is used to retract the corner of the mouth, and a finger retracts the opposite corner (see Procedure 5.1).
- The tray is rotated into the mouth, aligned over the teeth with the handle positioned at the midline.
- The tray is seated first in the posterior then seated anteriorly to allow the impression material to flow from the back to the front.
- As the tray is seated anteriorly, the lower lip is pulled out to allow the alginate to flow into the vestibular area.
- The patient is asked to lift the tongue to the roof of the mouth on mandibular impression and move side to side (Fig. 5.7). This allows alginate to flow into the lingual vestibule and defines the lingual frenum attachment.
- The clinician stabilizes the tray with the index and middle fingers on both sides of the arch.
- For both impressions, the posterior aspect of the tray should be inspected for proper seating and for excess alginate. Excess alginate should be swept away quickly with a mouth mirror or cotton swap to prevent gagging or breathing problems for the patient.

Clinical Tip

Controlling the gag reflex:
1. Place topical anesthetic on a cotton swab, and put it on the back of the tongue for 1 to 2 minutes, or spray the back of the mouth with topical anesthetic spray.
2. Place a small amount of salt on a cotton swab and put it on the back of the tongue (do not use this method with patients with a history of hypertension).
3. Place utility wax on the posterior extent of the upper tray to help contain the material.
4. Use fast-set alginate. Accelerate the set with warm water, if you can work fast enough to load and seat the tray.
5. Properly proportion the water and powder so that the mix is not too runny.
6. Do not overfill the tray.
7. Seat the tray in the posterior first, then anterior. Look at the palatal area and clear excess material with a quick sweep of the mouth mirror or cotton roll.
8. Position the patient's head forward slightly so that saliva will not pool in the back of the throat.
9. Use distraction (e.g., have the patient lift one leg during the impression and hold it up, and breathe slowly and deeply through the nose).

Removing the Tray. Alginate left in the mixing bowl can be checked for completeness of set. The impression should be left in the mouth for approximately 1 minute after the set, because it gains tear strength during this time. This may not be possible with patients who gag easily. When ready to remove the tray, use a finger at the top of the side of the tray to apply pressure to break the seal while pulling the tray quickly away from the teeth with a snap. Protect the teeth in the opposing arch with fingers placed on top of the tray.

Handling the Impression. The following steps should be utilized when handling the impression:

- The impression should be rinsed thoroughly under running water to remove adherent saliva or food debris. Rinsing is the first step to the disinfection process.
- Evaluate the impression to determine whether the impression is acceptable for its anticipated use.
- If determined to be acceptable, the impression is held inside a plastic bag (to prevent the inhalation

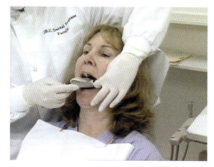

FIG. 5.6 To place the maxillary impression the right-handed operator stands in the 11 o'clock position (1 o'clock position for left-handers) and retracts the right corner of the mouth with the side of the tray while retracting the left corner of the mouth with the mirror or index finger of the other hand. (From Robinson DS, Bird DL. *Essentials of Dental Assisting*. 6th ed. Elsevier; 2017.)

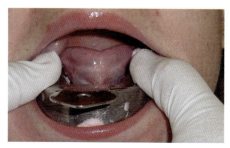

FIG. 5.7 Mandibular tray seated and patient has lifted the tongue to allow alginate to flow into the lingual vestibule and to shape the lingual frenum attachment. (Courtesy Gwen Essex.)

of disinfectant spray) and sprayed with a suitable disinfecting solution.
- An alternative to spraying the impression is to immerse it for 10 minutes in a suitable disinfectant. Immersion for up to 30 minutes in 1% sodium hypochlorite or 2% glutaraldehyde has been shown not to significantly affect the dimensions (by swelling) or surface detail of alginate.
- A laboratory knife is used to remove excess, unsupported alginate from the back of the tray.
- Any pooled fluid is drained or shaken off because the alginate can imbibe moisture and swell.
- If the impression is not poured promptly, it is placed into a zippered plastic bag labeled with the patient's name with a few drops of water or wrapped in a damp paper towel until ready to pour.
- Ideally the impression should be poured within 30 minutes but no later than an hour, because it is not dimensionally stable.

CRITERIA FOR CLINICALLY ACCEPTABLE IMPRESSIONS

Alginate impressions should be evaluated immediately after they are removed from the mouth and rinsed. The determination should be made whether or not the impression should be repeated, so it can be done while the patient is still seated and the operatory is set up. An acceptable impression will:
- Cover all areas of interest (teeth, ridge form, muscle attachments, palate, etc.)
- Have structures recorded with sufficient detail to be clearly identified
- Have a surface that will not be grainy, which is usually the result of inadequate mixing
- Have minimal voids caused by entrapped air
- Have alginate that is fully seated in the tray and should not have pulled free or distorted (Fig. 5.8)
- Have an impression that should be free of debris

Table 5.2 lists the criteria used to assess an alginate impression for clinical acceptability. When problems are found with an impression, refer to Table 5.3 for a troubleshooting guide that suggests possible causes and solutions for a variety of problems.

TWO-CONSISTENCY ALGINATE SYSTEM

An alternative to traditional alginate is a two-consistency system. Compatible alginates with two different viscosities are used together to make impressions with improved accuracy and surface detail. This combination is particularly useful for complete and partial denture impressions. The light-bodied gel flows well from the large-diameter tip of the delivery syringe and does not slump. It is placed into the peripheral vestibule of the upper or lower arch and acts as a border, molding material. The thick tray gel completes the impression of the remainder of the arch while supporting the syringe gel (Fig. 5.9). The two materials meld together without

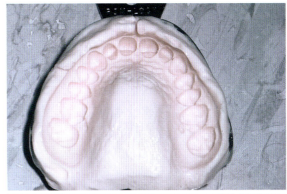
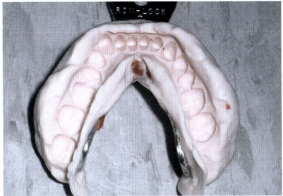

FIG. 5.8 Acceptable upper and lower alginate impressions that have met the established criteria. (Courtesy Dr. Steve Eakle.)

TABLE 5.2 Criteria for an Acceptable Alginate Impression

Both Maxillary and Mandibular Impressions
All teeth and alveolar processes recorded
Peripheral roll and frenums included
No large voids and few small bubbles present
Good reproduction of detail
Free of debris
No distortion
Alginate firmly attached to tray
Maxillary Impression
Palatal vault recorded
Hamular notch area included
Mandibular Impression
Retromolar areas included
Lingual extensions recorded

seams. The tray material resists flowing and is more likely to stay in the tray and out of the patient's throat, avoiding the gag reflex in many patients.

The two materials come in premeasured packaging and they are fast setting. However, the syringe material has a slightly longer setting time to allow it to be mixed first, loaded into the syringe, and put aside while the tray material is mixed and loaded into the tray. The tray material undergoes a color change to indicate when setting has started.

TABLE 5.3 Troubleshooting Alginate Impressions

PROBLEM	CAUSE	SOLUTION
Premature set	Too much powder in mix Prolonged mixing/loading time Water or room too warm	Fluff powder in container; use correct measures for powder and water Use timer to gauge working time Use cool water to slow the set
Slow set	Water too cold Too much water	Use warmer water Use correct water/powder measures
Grainy, lack of surface detail	Incomplete mix of powder and water	Wet all of powder, and mix to creamy consistency
Incomplete coverage of teeth or tissues	Tray too small or too short for arch Tray incompletely seated	Select larger tray or extend borders with rope wax Use a mouth mirror to check for complete seating of the tray
Voids on occlusal surfaces	Trapped air when tray is seated	Wipe alginate on occlusal surfaces before seating tray
Large voids at vestibule or midpalate	Trapped air Not enough alginate in tray Improper seating of tray Lip in the way	Place alginate in vestibule or palate before seating tray Use adequate amount of alginate Seat tray in posterior first, allow alginate to flow forward into vestibule, seat tray in anterior Pull lip out to create room for alginate
Small voids throughout	Air trapped in mix during spatulation	Press alginate against sides of bowl when mixing with wide-blade spatula to force out air
Distortion or double imprint	Impression removed too soon Tray moved while alginate was setting	Check residual alginate in bowl for set; let stand an additional 1 minute Hold the tray steady until set; do not have patient hold the tray
Torn alginate	Impression removed too slowly Thin mix	Remove impression quickly with a snap Use proper proportions of water and powder
Excess alginate at back of tray	Tray seated in anterior first, then posterior, forcing alginate out the back Tray overfilled with alginate	Seat tray in posterior first, forcing alginate anteriorly Load tray level with sides Create shallow trough for teeth Remove excess alginate from the back of the tray

KEY POINTS—Impressions

1. Various materials available for requirements of specific procedures.
2. Impression trays used depend on procedure.
   - Available as:
     - Stock
       - Disposable
       - Reusable (sterilizable)
     - Custom
3. Manufacturer's manipulation instructions should be followed.
   - Factors can alter working and setting time:
     - Temperature of the air or oral cavity
     - Temperature of the water
4. Material should have strength, flexibility, and accuracy.

ELASTOMERS

Elastomers are highly accurate elastic impression materials that have qualities similar to rubber and hence are often called *rubber materials*. They are used extensively in restorative dentistry for fabrication of:
- Metal castings
- Ceramic restorations
- Bridges
- Implant restorations
- Partial denture frameworks
- Complete dentures

The four types of elastomers are as follows:
- Polysulfides
- Condensation silicones
- Addition silicones (polyvinyl siloxane)
- Polyethers

The two most widely used elastomers are polyvinyl siloxane (PVS) and polyether. More recently, a hybrid material, vinyl polyether, has been introduced that combines the best properties of polyethers and polyvinyl siloxane.

The elastomers share a general formulation that includes a flexible matrix and because they are not water based, they are not as sensitive as the hydrocolloids to water loss or **imbibition** (water uptake). The shelf life is typically 12 to 18 months. Storage of these materials in a refrigerator will lengthen the shelf life. Stored materials should be allowed to return to room temperature before use, unless an extended working time is needed.

USE OF ADHESIVE

The rubbery nature of elastomers means that they do not adhere well to solid metal or custom acrylic impression trays. An adhesive is placed in the tray to prevent the set material from separating from the tray

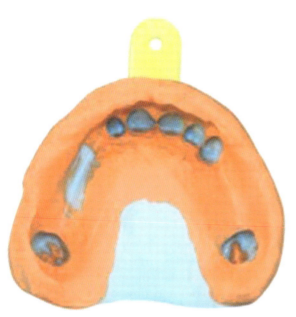

FIG. 5.9 Maxillary impression with the two-consistency alginate system for a partial denture framework. The syringe material (*orange*) has been used to establish the peripheral borders and to capture an imprint of the rest seats for the framework. (AccuDent XD, Courtesy Ivoclar Vivadent.)

and causing distortion (Fig. 5.10). Each type of elastomer has its own adhesive with which it is compatible; therefore adhesives should not be interchanged among different types of impression materials. The tray adhesive should be applied in a thin layer and allowed to dry. If the adhesive is not applied well in advance of tray use, then a stream of air can be used to accelerate the drying process.

ELASTIC RECOVERY

Elastomers have a certain amount of elastic recovery, or "rebound," from deformation due to their rubbery nature. Rebound reduces distortion in the cast that is poured from the impression. PVS impression material has the best elastic recovery of the elastomers.

WETTABILITY

Elastomers generally are not wet well by water (and are therefore called *hydrophobic*), because water forms a high contact angle with them. Of the elastomers, the polyether is the most hydrophilic, or wettable. Wettability can be seen clinically when impression materials are able to capture the detail of a tooth preparation when the surface is moist (but not submerged in water or saliva). It also means that wet gypsum materials will flow better into the fine details of the preparation when the impression is poured.

> **Clinical Tip**
>
> Each type of impression material has its own specific tray adhesive. Do not use an alginate tray adhesive for an elastomer. Likewise, do not interchange polysulfide adhesive with an adhesive for PVS or polyether material.

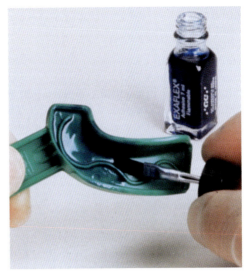

FIG. 5.10 Adhesive is applied to the interior of the tray to aid in retaining the elastomeric impression material. (From Rosenstiel SF, Land MF, Fujimoto J: *Contemporary fixed prosthodontics*, ed 4, St Louis, 2006, Elsevier.)

POLYSULFIDES

Polysulfides are the oldest of the elastomers and are commonly referred to as "rubber base." They are more dimensionally stable and have greater tear strength than hydrocolloids. They are more accurate than alginate but not as accurate as the other elastomers. Polysulfides have been used successfully for crown and bridge impressions and for partial and complete denture impressions. They cannot be used in automixing cartridges and must be hand-mixed. They are messy and have an unpleasant sulfur odor. When polyethers and PVSs came on the market, most practitioners abandoned the polysulfides for these more accurate, dimensionally stable, and pleasant materials. Detailed information for the polysulfides can be found on the student resource page of the Evolve website.

> **Clinical Tip**
>
> Alginate can be used in a moist field because it is hydrophilic. For the most part, elastomers are hydrophobic. Polyethers are the most hydrophilic of the elastomers and are more forgiving of a little moisture, but not to the degree of the hydrocolloids. A well-isolated field for elastomers is essential.

SILICONE RUBBER IMPRESSION MATERIALS

Two types of silicone impression materials have been developed and are named according to the type of polymerization reaction they undergo during setting:
- Condensation reaction
- Addition reaction

Condensation Silicone

Condensation silicone was developed in the 1960s and is useful for crown and bridge procedures. It has more desirable characteristics than polysulfide, such as:

- Ease of mixing
- Pleasant taste
- No odor
- Shorter working times
- Shorter setting times

The material sets through a condensation reaction that produces ethyl alcohol as a by-product. The ethyl alcohol is rapidly lost by evaporation, leading to a relatively high dimensional instability from shrinkage. Condensation silicones have been replaced by the more accurate and stable addition silicones.

Addition Silicone

The addition silicone impression materials were introduced in the 1970s and are an improvement over the condensation silicone materials. Their properties provide greater dimensional stability and accuracy. They are clean and easy to use, with no foul odor or taste. As a result of these improvements, addition silicones have become the most popular materials for crown and bridge procedures. They are also among the most expensive of the impression materials.

POLYVINYL SILOXANE (VINYL POLYSILOXANE)

Polyvinyl siloxane (PVS) or vinyl polysiloxane (VPS) is an additional silicone impression material that undergoes a polymerization reaction of chain lengthening (called an *addition reaction*) and cross-linking with reactive vinyl groups that produces a stable silicone rubber. The addition reaction does not produce a liquid by-product that can evaporate and cause shrinkage as with the condensation silicones. Of the elastomers, PVS has the smallest dimensional change (0.05%) on setting. PVS materials have high elastic recovery after removal from undercuts, and they resist tearing (high tear strength).

Some PVS materials produce hydrogen gas through a secondary reaction. If the impression is poured during the first two hours when the hydrogen is being released, the cast that results will have a very porous surface and will be unsuitable for most procedures. To counter the release of hydrogen, manufacturers have incorporated scavengers, such as palladium powder, to absorb the hydrogen before it gets to the surface.

PVS impressions can be poured in stone several times and are dimensionally stable for a least a week without distortion. The PVS materials exhibit little flow (deformation when subjected to a load after setting). This accounts for their accuracy even after repouring.

Hydrophobic Nature

PVS impression materials are hydrophobic by nature and must be used in a dry field. A little moisture on the prepared tooth will result in loss of surface detail in the impression because the impression material cannot displace the moisture and establish close contact with the surface (it has a high contact angle and low wetting of the surface).

Viscosities of the Material

PVS is manufactured in extra-light, light, regular, and heavy viscosities. A monophase (regular) viscosity is available from most manufacturers that is used as both a tray material and a syringe material. It is not as viscous as the tray material but is thicker than the light-body material, yet it flows well enough to be used in a syringe to be injected around a tooth preparation. Some PVS materials are also available in a two-part putty form, consisting of base and catalyst. Powdered silica is added as a filler to give thickness to the base or catalyst pastes or putties.

Surface Detail

The accuracy of an impression material is measured by how well it captures the surface detail of a structure. To capture the surface detail, the material must wet (have a low contact angle) and flow over the surface well. Low-viscosity materials (wash/syringe materials) wet and flow better than high-viscosity (tray/heavy-body) materials and, therefore, capture more detail.

Dispensing System

The most popular dispensing system for the extra-light, light, regular, and heavy materials involves a cartridge with two chambers—one with base and one with catalyst. A mixing tip fits on the end of the cartridge (Fig. 5.11). A hand-operated gun-type dispenser or a motor-driven dispenser (see Fig. 5.14) pushes both the base and the catalyst through the mixing tip at the same time. They pass through an intertwined spiral that mixes appropriate amounts of each material together thoroughly by the time they exit the end of the tip. These mixing devices ensure the proper ratio of the two materials without the creation of bubbles or voids, which are common with hand-mixing. It is important for the operator to make certain that the openings of the cartridges are cleaned of any residual set material that might block the flow of the base or catalyst before applying the mixing tip. Otherwise, proper proportions of the base and catalyst may not be mixed.

One manufacturer (Dentsply Sirona) packages the wash material in a small unit dose called a *digit* (see Fig. 5.11). The digit has enough material for a single-unit restoration and has a shorter, smaller mixing tip to minimize waste. The digit is mounted in a palm-sized syringe and the material is delivered directly to the preparation. There is also a larger digit available with enough material for about three preparations.

 Clinical Tip

Before placing the automixing tip on the impression cartridge, express a small amount of the material to make sure the openings for the two chambers are not blocked by set material.

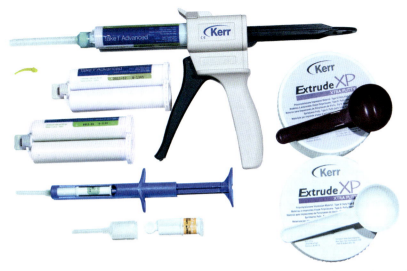

FIG. 5.11 PVS impression material in a variety of viscosities (light, regular, heavy body) in cartridges with mixing tip and mixing gun (*top left*) with unit-dose impression material (digit; Dentsply Caulk/Dentsply International) in a delivery syringe (*bottom left*) and putty (base and catalyst) in plastic jars (*right*).

Working and Setting Time

Because of the popularity of the PVS materials, manufacturers have put much effort into improving their properties to make them more appealing than other impression materials. The working time of PVS (from start of mix until it can no longer flow) is approximately 2 minutes. The setting time is the time measured from the start of mix to the time the material is hard and can be removed from the mouth. Setting times have been adjusted so that the practitioner has an assortment of materials from fast to regular set. Setting times vary among manufacturers and range from approximately 2 minutes (fast set) to 6 minutes (regular set). The working and setting times are affected by temperature. Working and setting times can be increased by refrigerating the material before use.

Some newer materials have been introduced with a setting time of 75 seconds. To achieve this fast set, a chemical reaction occurs after the working time has passed that warms the material quickly to body temperature, which accelerates the set.

Putty/Wash Techniques

Some clinicians like to use putty for the tray material and a light-body wash material to syringe around the prepared teeth. They feel that with subgingival margins on the preparations, the stiff putty causes hydraulic pressure that forces the wash material into the gingival sulcus to better capture the margins of the preparation. These materials can be used with a one- or a two-step technique.

One-Step Technique. The putty is mixed and loaded into a tray by the auxiliary while the operator injects the syringe material around the prepared teeth. An indentation should be made in the putty in the area and about the size of the preparation to allow wash material to cover the preparation without being displaced by the putty. The tray is seated while the putty and syringe material are still unset, allowing them to bond together.

 Clinical Tip

With the one-step putty/wash impression technique, be sure to make an indentation into the putty in the area of the preparation. Otherwise, the stiff putty will displace much of the wash material from the prepared tooth.

Two-Step Technique. The putty in essence is used to create a custom tray within a stock tray. In the first step, the putty is mixed and placed in a stock tray. It is seated over the teeth with a plastic sheet placed between the putty and the teeth to create room for light-body material. Some practitioners prefer to cut away some of the putty after it has set to create space for the light-body material rather than using the plastic sheet. In the second step, light-body material is syringed around the prepared teeth, and some is injected into the space in the putty created by the teeth. The tray with the putty is seated over the teeth.

 Caution

With the two-step putty/wash technique, putty should *not* show through the wash material in the impression of the preparation. Show-through areas are pressure spots where the preparation hits the putty. The putty will compress while the tray is in the mouth, and then rebound after the tray is removed. This will cause distortion in the impression.

Potential Putty/Wash Distortions. Both one-step and two-step putty techniques can result in distortions in the impression if care is not taken during the impression procedure. With the one-step technique, because putty does not flow well:
- Voids may result.
- There is a pulled appearance of the wash material when wash and putty do not flow and join together completely.

With the two-step technique, because the putty is set before the wash is added:
- Any areas where the putty shows through the wash material potentially have distortion.
- Flexible-set putty may have been compressed by contact with the tooth structure and then rebounded to its original shape when the impression was removed from the mouth. This is particularly critical if it occurs in the area of the prepared tooth.

To avoid these problems with putty, some clinicians use a one-step technique in which putty has been replaced with a heavy-body tray material that flows better.

> **Clinical Tip**
>
> PVS putty should *not* be mixed while latex gloves are worn. Sulfur products from the gloves can interfere with the set of the material. Washed hands covered with vinyl gloves should be used.

Removing the Set Impression.
- Read the manufacturer's instructions on setting time.
- Immediately after seating the impression, place a small portion of the tray and wash materials on the bracket table. When they have set, the materials in the mouth should also be set because the heat of the patient's mouth should accelerate the set.
- Determine that the impression materials are fully set prior to removing. Removing the impression prematurely can cause distortion.
- Remove the impression quickly to minimize the potential for plastic deformation (permanent deformation) of the impression.
- Quick removal of the tray applies stress quickly and allows it to release without deforming. However, it takes a few minutes for complete recovery to occur. For PVS materials, it is best to wait 20 to 30 minutes before pouring the impression.

Bite Registration. A registration of the patient's bite is typically made using elastomers (PVS or polyether) or wax.

Polyvinyl Siloxane Bite Registration. PVS is used for bite registration because of its accuracy, dimensional stability, and ease of use. It offers no resistance to biting down; therefore it does not risk shifting the direction of the patient's bite as a hard material might. It can be used for this purpose in two ways:

1. Most practitioners use automatic mixing cartridge systems and inject material from the mixing tip directly onto the occlusal surfaces of the mandibular teeth. Then the patient closes into centric occlusion (Fig. 5.12). Bite registration materials are viscous materials that stay in place when applied to the occlusal surfaces of teeth. This property makes it easier to register the bite and remove the material from the mouth.
2. Some practitioners use a bite tray (Fig. 5.2D) that is usually a disposable plastic frame with a gauze-like material stretched between the arms of the frame. Material is dispensed on both sides of the gauze, the frame is seated over the teeth, and the patient closes into centric occlusion until the material sets (see Procedure 5.3).

Wax Bite. Wax is a less expensive material used by some clinicians to register the bite (see Procedure 5.4). Baseplate wax or utility wax can be softened by heating and then folded several times into a wide rope about 4 or 5 mm thick that is bent into the shape of an arch (horseshoe shaped). Premade horseshoe-shaped bite wafers are commercially available and come with or without a thin aluminum foil between two layers of wax (Fig. 5.13). The foil prevents biting all the way through the wax.

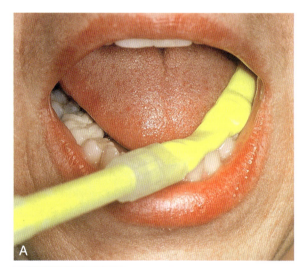
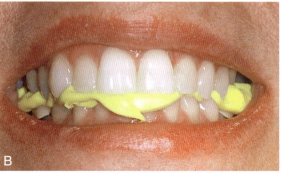

FIG. 5.12 Bite registration: **(A)** Applying bite registration material to the teeth. **(B)** Patient closed into centric occlusion.

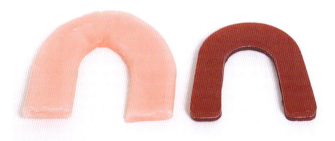

FIG. 5.13 Wax bite wafers. On the left is a wafer made by the heating and folding baseplate wax and on the right is a preformed commercially available wax wafer.

Polyvinyl Siloxane Alginate Substitutes. Relatively inexpensive PVS materials and Counter-Fit (Clinician's Choice Dental Products) have been developed as substitutes for alginates. They are much more dimensionally stable for long periods and do not need to be poured right away.

Silicone Die Technique. Some practitioners use a specially formulated addition silicone material in an automatic mixing cartridge system to make dies for indirect composite inlays. A tooth is prepared for a composite inlay, and an alginate impression is made of the preparation. The silicone die material is injected into the alginate impression and sets within 2 minutes.

Polyethers

Polyethers are elastic impression materials that came to the European market in 1965 and gradually became popular in the United States. Polyethers are very accurate materials with good flow and tear strength and are excellent for use in crown and bridge procedures. They are more hydrophilic than PVS. The hydrophilicity gives polyethers good wetting properties for making detailed impressions in the presence of a small amount of moisture, which makes them particularly useful for impressions of preparations with subgingival margins. They do not release hydrogen gas and can be poured immediately with gypsum products without the formation of bubbles on the surface of the cast. They have excellent mechanical properties with good elastic recovery, and they do not shrink.

Consistency and Setting Reaction. Polyethers are supplied as light-, medium-, and heavy-body viscosities. Equal lengths of material are dispensed from two unequal-sized tubes of base and catalyst onto a mixing pad, or the materials are provided in cartridges with automixing tips, similar to the PVS materials. The catalyst can cause skin and tissue irritation. Therefore thorough mixing of the base and catalyst is necessary to avoid any irritation of the oral tissues. When polyethers go through their final reaction, they set very quickly.

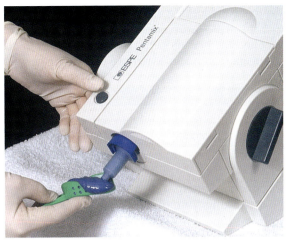

FIG. 5.14 Polyether impression material mixed and dispensed from the mixing machine (Pentamix; 3M ESPE) directly into a tray.

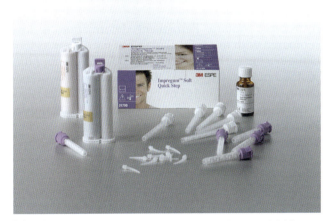

FIG. 5.15 Softer formulation of polyether impression material. Kit contains three cartridges of tray (heavy-body) material and a cartridge of syringe (light-body) material, bottle of tray adhesive, and mixing tips and delivery tips that snap on to the end of the mixing tips. (Impregum Soft Quick Step, Courtesy 3M ESPE.)

Mechanical Mixing. In addition to tubes or cartridges, both polyethers and PVS impression materials come in large pouches of the base and catalyst that are placed into a mechanical mixer and delivered directly into the impression tray (Fig. 5.14). The mixer handles a much larger volume of material than cartridges used in the automatic mixing guns and is more economical.

Properties. The original polyethers were stiff and in 2000, newer formulations of polyether were introduced and are much more flexible and have a more pleasant taste (Fig. 5.15). They are easier to remove from the mouth, and it is easier to separate the cast from the impression without breaking teeth.

Block Out Undercuts. With all of the elastomers, undercuts around bridge pontics, open embrasures around periodontally involved teeth, large and bony tori, and fixed implant fixtures should be blocked out with utility wax. This will prevent the impression material from flowing under them and locking the impression tray in the mouth (Fig. 5.16). It is an unpleasant experience for both the patient and the practitioner to have locked-in impression trays cut apart with burs to remove them from the mouth.

 Do You Recall?

What happens to the impression material when it flows and locks into an undercut?

Working and Setting Times. Regular set polyethers have a working time of 2 to 3 minutes and a setting time (total time from start of mix) of 5 to 6 minutes. Fast-setting polyethers have a working time of 1 minute and the setting time is 4 minutes. Polyethers have a "snap" set, meaning that the initial viscosity remains the same throughout the working time, but changes rapidly during the remainder of the setting process.

Hydrophilic Nature. Permanent deformation is low compared with the polysulfides, but not as low as that of the silicones. This material is somewhat hydrophilic, so it is more forgiving of a little moisture on the preparation than polysulfides or polyvinyl siloxanes. Also, because of this hydrophilic nature, they must not be stored in water or disinfecting solution because they will swell from the uptake of moisture.

Impressions from this material can be poured repeatedly for up to a week and can be shipped to a dental laboratory and remain dimensionally stable for up to 14 days if properly stored. Table 5.4 compares the features of elastic impression materials.

VINYL POLYETHER SILICONE HYBRID

In the 2000s, a new class of elastomers was introduced. The new material is a hybrid of PVS and polyether. The purpose of the hybrid is to obtain the best features of each type of material. The material is composed of polyether and siloxane groups combined in a polymer. The polyether component makes the material hydrophilic, so it can tolerate a little moisture around the preparation and can be poured easily without the need to spray the impression with a **surfactant**. The siloxane component provides dimensional stability and recovery from deformation (caused by removal of the impression from the mouth). The material flows well and has a high tear strength. It is available in regular and fast sets and in five viscosities, including light and extra light, regular, heavy, and rigid heavy body.

 KEY POINTS—Elastomers

1. Highly accurate elastic impression materials.
2. Used extensively in restorative dentistry.
3. Most commonly used elastomers:
   - Polyvinyl Siloxane (PVS)
   - Polyether
   - vinyl polyether
     - Hybrid material that combines the best properties of both polyethers and PVS
4. Must use adhesive in impression trays
5. Materials have a certain amount of elastic recovery which reduces distortion
6. Materials do not wet well; however, of the elastomers, polyether is the most hydrophilic or wettable.

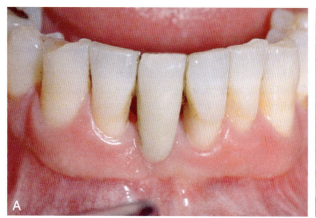
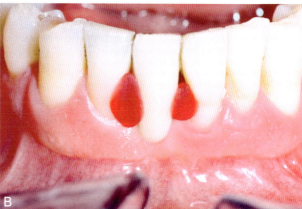

FIG. 5.16 Wax to block out undercuts: **(A)** teeth with gingival recession that has created large embrasure spaces where impression material may lock in place. **(B)** Soft, red utility wax placed in spaces to prevent impression material from entering.

TABLE 5.4 Features of Elastic Impression Materials

IMPRESSION MATERIAL	COST	SURFACE DETAIL	DIMENSIONAL STABILITY	TEAR STRENGTH	EASE OF USE	POUR WITHIN	ABILITY TO REPOUR
Alginate	Low	Lowest	Low	Low	High	1 hr	No
Addition silicone (polyvinyl siloxanes)	High	High	Highest	Medium	High	1 wk	Yes
Polyether	High	High	High	Low to medium	High	1 wk	Yes

COMPONENTS OF IMPRESSION MAKING FOR CROWN AND BRIDGE PROCEDURES

Auxiliaries are frequently involved in the impression-making process. Those that are licensed or certified in expanded functions may actually pack retraction cords, use astringents, and make the impressions for crowns and bridges according to the state dental practice act. All of those involved in assisting with taking the impression or with making it need to be knowledgeable about the materials and the process.

GINGIVAL RETRACTION

Retraction of the marginal gingiva is often needed for impressions of teeth prepared for restorations such as crowns and bridges, especially when the preparation extends subgingivally. The objective of gingival retraction is to provide a space in the gingival sulcus of adequate dimensions to receive the wash (syringe) impression material so that the entire margin can be captured in detail and at least 0.5 mm of the tooth (usually the root) beyond the margin.

Methods of Retraction

There are several ways to achieve the desired space in the sulcus for the impression material. Methods include use of cord, retraction paste, or a minor surgical procedure with a laser or electrosurgery to produce a small trough in the sulcus.

Retraction Cord

Placement of gingival retraction cords is among the most common methods of displacing the gingival tissue away from the tooth preparation to create space for the impression material. Cord placement should not cause damage to the gingival tissue or tear the epithelial attachment of the gingiva to the root. It should produce mild lateral displacement of the free gingival tissue.

Retraction cords come in a variety of forms and thicknesses. The cords can consist of:
- Twisted strands
- Braided strands
- Woven strands
- Knitted strands

The various thicknesses of the cord are numbered to aid selection. Typically, the smaller the number, the smaller the diameter of the cord. For example, 000 cord is very small and number 3 is very large (Fig. 5.17). Cords can also be plain or impregnated with an astringent.

Bleeding should be controlled before attempting to place retraction cords. Bleeding control can be accomplished in several ways:
1. A local anesthetic containing epinephrine can be injected into each gingival papilla to constrict the blood vessels.
2. An astringent can be applied to the sulcus to stop the bleeding.
3. Coagulation can be obtained with a laser or by electrocautery.

Prepacking the Sulcus

Bleeding caused by trauma to the gingiva from the bur during preparation of the tooth can be minimized by packing a cord of medium diameter before finalizing the margins. The cord displaces the gingiva away from the tooth and provides some protection for it (Fig. 5.18). It also begins the retraction process, making it easier to pack the cords for the impression.

> 💡 **Clinical Tip**
>
> Bleeding of the gingival tissue is the number-one reason for an inadequate impression. It must be controlled **before** attempting to make the impression.

Astringents/Hemostatic Agents

Astringents are topically applied chemicals that constrict tissues and are useful in gingival retraction. Because they also constrict small blood vessels and produce mild coagulation of blood, they are also hemostatic agents. They are commonly applied to the tissues on a:
- Cotton pledget
- Retraction cord
- Cotton-tipped cannula attached to a syringe (Fig. 5.19)

Astringents and hemostatic agents used to control bleeding in the gingival sulcus will adversely impact the surface detail of a PVS impression. Ferric sulfate may also interfere with the set of the material. Astringents should be washed off the tooth before applying wash material.

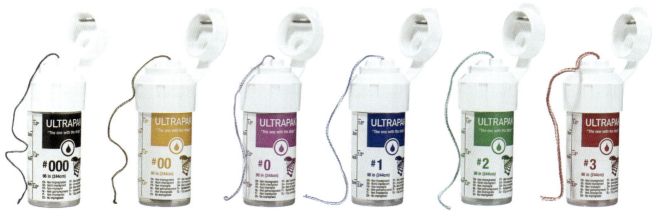

FIG. 5.17 A series of sizes of knitted gingival retraction cord. (Ultrapak, Courtesy Ultradent Products.)

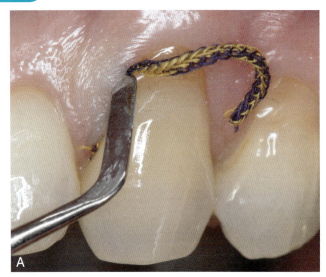

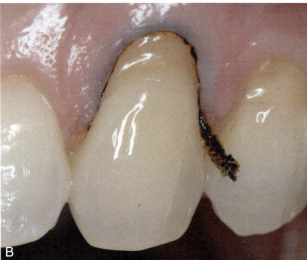

FIG. 5.18 Prepacking the gingival sulcus: **(A)** Cord is being packed into the gingival sulcus. **(B)** Cord is placed prior to an operative procedure to place a restoration in the sensitive root abrasion lesion. It keeps the gingival tissue away from the rotating bur and helps prevent bleeding. (From Heymann H, Swift E, Ritter A. *Sturdevant's Art & Science of Operative Dentistry*. 6th ed. Elsevier; 2013.)

> **⚠ Caution**
>
> Racemic epinephrine hemostatic agents should be used with caution for patients with hypertension or cardiac problems. A cord soaked in racemic epinephrine and applied to the gingival sulcus can spike the blood pressure and increase the heart rate!

Two-Cord Retraction Technique

A gingival retraction technique using two cords has become popular. A small cord is placed first in the sulcus and functions to help control bleeding and minimize the flow of gingival fluid from the sulcus. Often the first cord is dampened with an astringent before it is placed. Once it is in the sulcus, any overlapping edges are cut so it fits end to end. The second (top) cord is larger in diameter and does the bulk of the retraction.

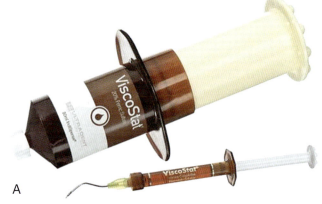

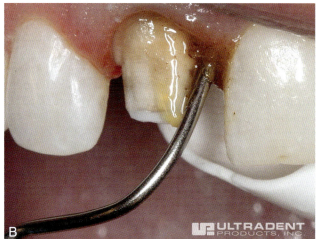

FIG. 5.19 Astringent is used to control bleeding gingival tissues prior to making the impression (ViscoStat, Ultradent Products): **(A)** Large syringe of astringent is used to fill individual smaller syringes. **(B)** Ferric sulfate astringent is scrubbed into the bleeding tissue with a cotton-tipped cannula to form blood clots over the capillaries.

The largest cord that fits into the sulcus should be used and placed so that it is at the level of the margin or slightly apical to it. The top cord should have some overlap so that a "tail" of cord sticks out of the sulcus. This provides something easily grasped when the cord is removed. If the sulcus is very shallow, it may not be possible to use two cords. In this case, an appropriately sized single cord should be used to achieve retraction.

Evaluation of Cord Placement

Once the top cord is in place, cord placement should be evaluated. First, the working field should be well isolated, and isolation should be maintained throughout the impression-making process. If the prepared tooth is wet and the cords become wet, they will be slippery and very difficult to place in the sulcus. In addition, if isolation is not maintained after the cords are placed, they tend to float out of the sulcus and retraction will be lost. Next, an inspection is made of the top cord. It should be at the level of the margin (unless the margin is supragingival) and should be visible 360 degrees around the tooth. If gingival tissue is leaning over the cord, it should be retracted by placement of an additional piece of cord or a cotton pledget in that area. The cord should remain in place for approximately 5 to 8 minutes to achieve good retraction. Time is needed for the cord to stretch the gingival fibers to relax the gingiva away from the preparation, and any astringent/hemostatic agent used needs time to produce hemostasis.

Cord Retraction Checklist: Before proceeding to making the impression, a properly placed retraction cord checklist should include:
1. Good isolation
2. No bleeding
3. Cord at the level of the margin and visible entirely around the tooth (Figs. 5.20 and 5.21)

Evaluation of Retraction

When you are ready to remove the top cord, dampen the cord slightly so it does not stick to tissues and cause bleeding when it is removed. Grasp the "tail" of the cord with cotton forceps and gently peel the cord out of the sulcus to minimize the risk of bleeding.

Now, evaluate whether or not the gingiva is adequately retracted. You should be able to see a space between the gingiva and the margin. There should be no bleeding. The bottom cord should have remained apical to the margin. If any of these criteria are not met, do not proceed! If there is inadequate space, repack the cords and determine whether a larger cord is needed. If there is bleeding, pick up a syringe of astringent (ferric sulfate is a good one for this) and scrub the tissues with the cotton-tipped applicator (where allowed by state law). Rinse and dry the tooth, and look to see whether the bleeding has stopped. If not, you may need to inject (where allowed by state law) a local anesthetic with epinephrine into the papillae. If the bottom cord has lifted, pack it back down. Once these criteria have been met, you are ready to start the impression process.

See Fig. 5.22 for an illustration of "stop signs" or evaluation points for cord placement and gingival retraction. The first "stop sign" is after placement of the cord. Evaluate its placement. The second "stop sign" is after removal of the top cord. Evaluate whether retraction is adequate. Do not proceed with the impression until each step is adequately performed!

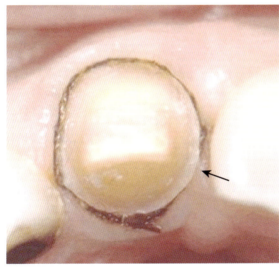

FIG. 5.20 Retraction cord improperly placed: Gingiva rests against the tooth in one portion *(lower right)*.

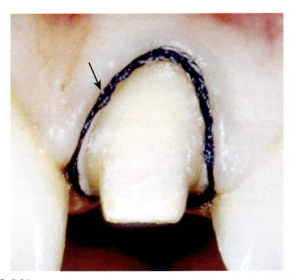

FIG. 5.21 Retraction cord has come partly out of the sulcus and rests on the margin *(upper left)*. The cord should be tucked back in the sulcus to ensure adequate retraction.

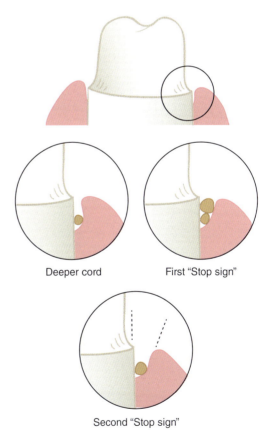

FIG. 5.22 Evaluation points (stop signs) for cord placement and gingival retraction. Top: Prepared tooth before cord placement. Left: Small cord placed to help control gingival fluids and bleeding. Right: Top cord is placed to displace gingival crest away from the margins of the prepared tooth. At this point, cord placement is evaluated (first "stop sign"). Bottom: Top cord has been removed. At this point, the retraction is evaluated (second "stop sign"). If evaluation at either "stop sign" indicates a problem, it should be corrected before proceeding to the next step. (Courtesy Dr. John Ino, University of California, San Francisco, California.)

Retraction Paste, Silicone, or Gel

Alternatives to cord for gingival retraction are retraction paste, silicone (PVS), or gel. The material displaces the gingiva laterally, and the astringent produces some tissue shrinkage and helps to control bleeding. The material remains in place a minimum of 2 minutes, and then is rinsed out thoroughly and dried before placing the wash material (Fig. 5.23).

MAKING THE IMPRESSION

(See Procedure 5.2 for detailed instructions.)

Criteria for a Successful Impression

A final impression made for a permanent restoration such as a full crown must meet certain criteria to be considered useable.

First—the impression must capture the fine detail of the prepared tooth, especially at the margins. A lack of detail at the margins may result in an ill-fitting restoration with recurrent caries or continued tooth sensitivity.

Second—the impression should be free of voids, folds, pulls, and tears. The impression should capture an accurate representation of the other teeth and tissues in the impression site.

Third—if the impression is a double-bite impression (using a triple tray), it should capture the opposing teeth and a representation of the patient's acquired bite (where their teeth ordinarily fit together).

Criteria for a Good Impression for a Restoration

- Rigid tray selected and tried in mouth for fit and coverage
- Appropriate adhesive applied to tray
- Material mixed accurately
- Tray adequately filled with material
- Impression free of voids, tears, pulls—no critical errors
- Fine detail of preparation, margins with "flash" (impression beyond the margin)
- Accurate representation of other teeth and tissues in the impression site
- Teeth do not contact tray

Evaluating the Impression

Before attempting to evaluate an impression:
- Continue wearing gloves when handling impression
- Wear magnifying loops
- Rinse impression thoroughly to remove blood, saliva, and debris
- Dry impression throughly
- Bring the operatory light over the impression at about a 70-degree angle to the plane of the teeth to cast a slight shadow on portions of the impression to help you read the impression
- Rotate the impression to read all aspects of it
- Ask yourself the following:
  - Did the impression capture all of the teeth and tissues needed for the restoration?
  - Can I see the preparation clearly?
  - Is the margin visible clearly all the way around the tooth?
  - Has the impression captured at least 0.5 mm of the unprepared tooth just apical to the margins (producing a cuff of syringe material that is often referred to as the "flash").

Some flaws may be present in the impression. Most impressions are not perfect. It is important to know which of the flaws represent critical errors (must remake the impression) and which ones are considered minor errors that will still allow the impression to be used for the fabrication of the restoration.

Critical errors in impression making include the following:
- A portion of the margins is missing or torn.
- The margins look shiny and rounded rather than clearly demarcated. This is usually caused by moisture (blood, saliva, or fluid from the sulcus) on the margin.

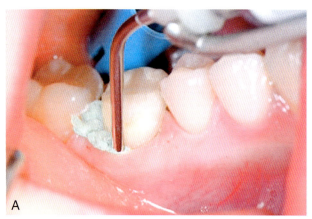
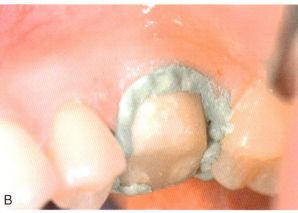
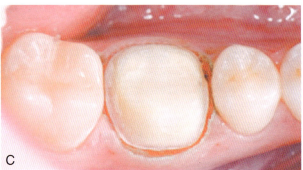

FIG. 5.23 Clay retraction material Expasyl; Courtesy Kerr Corporation, Orange, California) contains aluminum chloride astringent: **(A)** isolate, dry thoroughly, and inject material slowly into sulcus. **(B)** Leave material in sulcus for 2 minutes. **(C)** Wash material away and dry. Retraction has been obtained.

- A fold or crease is present in the margin or wall of the preparation. A fold occurs at the junction of two portions of materials that do not flow together.
- A pull (or drag) is present in the area of the preparation. A pull occurs when the wash material starts to set before the tray is placed.
- A large void is present in the preparation or the teeth needed to articulate with the opposing cast to establish the proper bite relationship. Voids on the margins are often caused when the syringe tip loses contact with the tooth surface. As the syringe tip bounces away and comes back to the tooth, some air is trapped in the wash material.
- Set impression material separates from the tray. This will cause a distortion.
- Lack of a good union between the heavy-body or putty material used in the tray and the light-body/syringe material placed around the teeth (often caused by one material starting to set before the other material is placed).

See Fig. 5.24 for clinical images of critical errors in impression making.

Minor errors in impression making include the following:
- Small voids (<1 mm) not on the margin
- Small folds not on the walls or margins of the preparation
- A pull on buccal or lingual surfaces of teeth that are away from the preparation
- A slight separation of the material from the tray at a site not involving the preparation or teeth critical to establishing the occlusal relationship with the opposing teeth

Fig. 5.25 shows examples of acceptable impressions.

> **Clinical Tip**
>
> When using the two-cord technique, the bottom cord often will come out and be embedded in the impression (Fig. 5.25B). *Do not* try to remove it! That may tear the impression into the margins. Simply cut off any loose ends. The remaining cord will end up in the cast and can be easily removed when a removable die is made.

Factors That Limit Obtaining an Accurate Impression

- Selecting a poorly fitting tray
- Not using enough tray adhesive or not letting it dry adequately before loading the tray
- Inadequate control of bleeding
- Incomplete retraction of the gingiva
- Selecting impression material for syringing that is too thick to flow around the preparation or into the gingival sulcus
- Using mixed impression material that is starting to set
- Tearing of impression material on removal because the material is too weak or the sulcus was not opened adequately and the material flowing into it was too thin

> **Key Points: Impressions for Indirect Restorations**
>
> 1. Gingival retraction is often needed when preparations extend subgingivally.
> 2. Astringents or local anesthesia can be used to control bleeding of tissues around the preparation
> 3. A dry field is needed during the impression taking to ensure the retraction cord remains in place and saliva does not distort the impression
> 4. The impression must capture fine detail of the preparation to ensure the final restoration fits properly

DIGITAL IMPRESSIONS

As outlined in this chapter, traditional impression materials for crown and bridge procedures are required to be dimensionally stable, accurate in reproducing fine detail, strong in tear resistance, sufficiently flowable, easy to remove, able to rebound rapidly from distortion, pleasing in taste and smell, and easy to disinfect and store. The impression process is technique sensitive and often unpleasant for the patient. Computer-assisted design/computer-assisted machining (CAD/CAM) dentistry (see Chapter 10) introduces the capture of digital images of the preparation, adjacent structures, and opposing dentition and structures, and this process is known as the **digital impression**. The digital impression removes many of the requirements and pitfalls of traditional impressions.

LEARNING CURVE

As with any new technology introduced into the dental practice, the use of digital impressions requires some thought as to how it will be incorporated into the practice, who will use the **intraoral scanner** (the image capture device), who will maintain it, and how training and practice will occur. Some accommodations must be made to allow team members to practice the new techniques before they can become proficient, as there is a learning curve. Some manufacturers of the intraoral scanners provide training in the dental office and others provide it at their headquarters. With proper education, the dental auxiliary can perform image capture and transmission of the images to the laboratory. Most state dental boards have not yet regulated the use of intraoral scanners by dental auxiliaries. Check to see if any regulations have been implemented in your state.

Intraoral Scanning: Originally, intraoral scanning cameras were part of a complete in-office CAD/CAM system. The digital images captured by the scanner were used with computer software to design the restoration and the design file was sent to an in-office milling unit to cut out the ceramic restoration. Later, stand-alone scanners were developed that could capture the desired images and send the file to a laboratory for processing. Stand-alone scanners do not have the capability to design the restoration, but some scanning systems let the clinician mark the

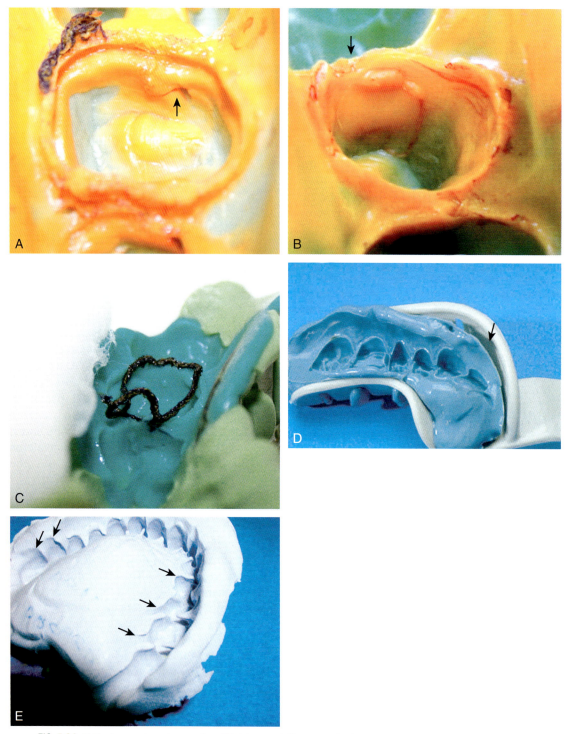

FIG. 5.24 Critical errors in an impression: **(A)** A large void is present in the wall of the molar. The adjacent premolar impression has shiny rounded margins lacking detail from contamination with blood. **(B)** A portion of the margin is missing. **(C)** The bottom cord from a two-cord technique was not packed apical to the margin and is caught in the impression of the margins. **(D)** The set impression material has separated from the tray, likely from inadequate tray adhesive. **(E)** Facial (left molars) and lingual (right molar and premolar) pulls of material. Syringe material was starting to set before the tray was seated. (Courtesy Dr. Steve Eakle.)

location of the margins. Captured images can be transmitted through a secure Internet portal to a commercial laboratory and copies of the file stored on the computer as part of the dental record. Not all dental laboratories are equipped for CAD/CAM processing, so there may be designated laboratories to which the images are transmitted. Another variation is to send the images to a central processing center that makes the models from those images and sends the models to a standard laboratory where the restoration is made.

SCANNING DEVICES

Complete in-office CAD/CAM systems with digital scanners, computer with design software, milling

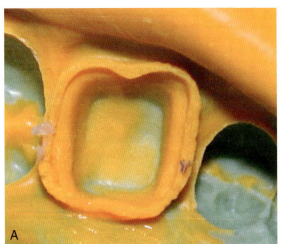 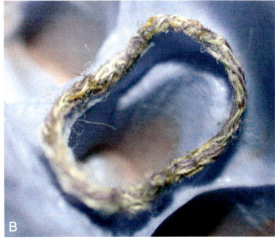

FIG. 5.25 Examples of good impressions: **(A)** Clear margins with "flash," no voids, and fine detail. Adjacent structures are captured well. **(B)** Bottom cord has been retained in the impression but is not sitting on the margins. Good detail, no voids, and "flash" is present at the margins. (Courtesy Steve Eakle, University of California School of Dentistry, San Francisco, California.)

device, and firing/glazing oven are available as well as stand-alone intraoral scanners. Most of the scanners are connected to the computing unit by a cord, but some new scanners are cordless.

Image Capture: Intraoral scanners are handheld, but their methods of capturing images differ. Older scanners capture images by taking multiple still images and stitching them together by software. Newer scanners use streaming video to capture images of the teeth and surrounding structures.

For most single restorations, images are needed of the prepared tooth, adjacent teeth, and opposing teeth. A buccal bite registration image is used by many scanners to establish the proper occlusal relationship, but the type of bite registration may vary from scanner to scanner. All scanning systems are capable of scanning full arches, not just quadrants.

Use of Powder: Some systems require that the teeth be coated lightly with an opaque powder (usually titanium oxide) to provide contrast for the best image reproduction; however the use of powered has decreased over time. The powder provides uniform reflective surfaces so the camera can accurately record the many contours present in the preparations or teeth. Other systems do not need to use the powder due to a variance in their imaging mechanisms.

Scanner Positioning: Some systems require that the intraoral portion of the scanner with the camera portal be held just off the teeth when capturing the images, whereas others allow the scanner to rest on the teeth to increase steadiness for a clear image (Fig. 5.26). Scanning times vary from system to system and range from about 3 to 8 minutes, depending on operator skills, the number of teeth being scanned, whether powder is needed, and the demands of the scanning unit.

Correcting the Scan: Some units have an erase software tool that allows the operator to erase a portion of a scan and rescan only that portion. Some clinicians have their assistant scan the arch before the preparation and

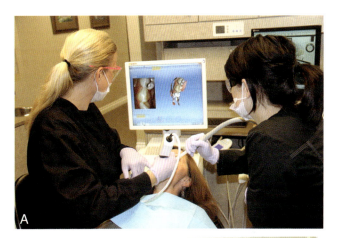

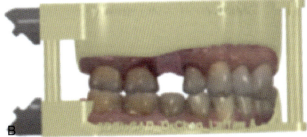

FIG. 5.26 Intraoral digital scanner used by the auxiliaries: **(A)** obtained a digital impression and opposing arch. **(B)** Virtual bite registration. (A, From Rosenstiel SF, Land MF. *Contemporary Fixed Prosthodontics*. 5th ed. Elsevier; 2016. B, From Powers JM, Wataha JC. *Dental Materials: Properties and Manipulation*. 11th ed. Elsevier; 2017.)

scan the opposing arch. The assistant erases the portion of the scan that has the unprepared tooth and then just scans the prepared tooth. The software fills in the prepared tooth in the correct location. There is no need to redo the entire scan.

Open or Closed Software Platform: Some manufacturers have a closed software platform meaning that the scanned images can only be used with that manufacturer's CAD/CAM products (design software and milling). The trend is for manufacturers to use open software platforms that allow images to be transferred and milled on platforms produced by different manufacturers.

From Table 5.5 with scanners from major manufacturers, the trend with the newest versions of intraoral scanners is that they use continuous video to capture images in full color without the use of powder and the captured images can be used with other manufacturers' CAD/CAM chairside or laboratory equipment.

Shade Taking: Some scanning systems incorporate shade taking with their ability to take digital intraoral photographs. The scanner takes the shades of the adjacent teeth during the scan, eliminating the potential human error in interpreting shades. The shades are mapped out on the images at several locations and can be seen on the computer monitor. This is a time-saving feature since it eliminates separate steps for shade taking and writing a shade description for the laboratory.

ADVANTAGES AND DISADVANTAGES OF DIGITAL IMPRESSIONS

A significant advantage is the ability of the clinician to view the preparation magnified on a computer monitor and see it from multiple angles by rotating the image. Undercuts, uneven or rough margins, and areas of under-reduction can be detected and corrected before the image is transferred to the laboratory. The evaluation of the preparation before sending the images to the laboratory eliminates many potential errors that would result in remakes of the restorations. The images themselves can be reviewed and retaken if judged inadequate. In many states this important function can be delegated to a properly educated auxiliary, allowing the dentist to perform other functions. When digital impressions are used in conjunction with an in-office milling device, the restoration can be completed in one visit instead of two.

For the patient, the digital impression process is easier, particularly for those patients with a strong gag reflex or severe tissue undercuts or tori. A few studies have been done comparing the accuracy of digital impressions to traditional impressions. The studies concluded that digital impressions were as accurate as or better than traditional impressions. See all advantages and disadvantages to digital impressions in the bulleted list below.

Digital Impressions: Advantages and Disadvantages

Advantages
- Creates permanent 3D color pre- and postoperative models that can be stored and reused indefinitely and do not take up space in the office.
- Digital images can be used to point out problems to the patient and better communicate treatment needs.
- At least as accurate as traditional impressions, possibly better.
- Does not need impression materials, adhesive, trays, pouring impressions, and packaging them for the lab.
- The prepared tooth/teeth can be viewed on the computer monitor and corrections can be made before sending images to the lab or in-office milling.
- Images can be sent to the lab instantly.
- Scanning can be stopped and restarted at will (e.g., to control moisture).
- Images can easily be remade if necessary.
- Images can be made by properly trained dental auxiliaries in most states.
- Eliminates messy cleanup.
- More comfortable for the patient.
- Fewer adjustments needed on the restoration and fewer remakes.

Disadvantages
- Cost of the scanner is significant.
- Specialized education and practice are needed.
- There may be a fee for processing digital images.
- Some scanners may be too large to fit in posterior regions of small mouths or patients with a limited opening.
- Very few manufacturers have closed-system software so that the scanner only works with their CAD/CAM systems.

SOFT TISSUE MANAGEMENT

Although many of the components of traditional impressions are not needed when taking digital impressions, there is still a need for management of the gingival tissues. If the margins of the preparation

TABLE 5.5 Digital Impression Systems

SYSTEM	IMAGING CAPTURE	COLOR IMAGE	DIRECT IMAGE TRANSMISSION TO LABORATORY	POWDER NEEDED	USE WITH ANY MANUFACTURERS' PRODUCTS (OPEN PLATFORM)
CS 3600 (CareStream Dental)	Continuous video	Yes	Yes	No	Yes
CEREC Omnicam (Sirona Dental Systems)	Continuous video	Yes	Yes	No	Yes
Planmeca Emerald (E4D Technologies)	Continuous video	Yes	Yes	No	Yes
Lava Chairside Oral Scanner (3M ESPE)	Continuous video	Yes	Yes	No	Yes
iTero Element (Align Technology)	Continuous video	Yes	Yes	No	Yes
TRIOS 3 (3Shape)	Continuous video	Yes	Yes	No	Yes

are all supragingival, there may be no need for gingival retraction and likely there will be no bleeding. However, most crown preparations involve the replacement of old restorations where at least some of the margins are at or below the gingival crest. The digital image of the preparation needs to capture the margins and approximately 0.5 mm of the tooth apical to the margin. So, some form of gingival retraction and use of astringents/hemostatic agents (as previously discussed) may be needed. As with any restorative impression, good isolation is also required. The preparation must be kept free of blood, saliva, and debris, as the scanner cannot distinguish between extraneous material and the prepared tooth. Any debris could result in a restoration with faulty margins.

EXPANDED USE OF DIGITAL IMPRESSIONS

As the technology has improved and more clinicians and manufacturers have discovered the capabilities of digital impressions, their applications have expanded beyond the uses for traditional crown and bridge procedures. Many clinicians are applying the technology to:
- Implant impressions for surgical guides
- Custom abutments and crowns
- Complete denture impressions to produce digital models of the ridges and design software to fabricate dentures
- Orthodontic impressions, such as for orthodontic aligners and appliances

The models needed for these applications can be milled from large blocks of acrylic or generated from digital impression using software-directed 3D printers that spray fine acrylic particles in layers to build up the models to the desired form (Fig. 5.27).

Offices Without Scanners

For clinicians who do not have scanners in their offices, there are still options to have CAD/CAM restorations fabricated. A traditional impression can be taken and the laboratory can scan it to create a digital impression or they can pour up the traditional impression to produce a gypsum model that the laboratory can scan and use to design and mill a restoration.

> **KEY POINTS: Digital Scanners**
> 1. Digital scanners remove the need for traditional impression taking
> 2. The process of digital scanning is more comfortable for the patient especially those with a gag reflex
> 3. There is a learning curve for the use of the scanner by the dental personnel
> 4. The equipment can be expensive and require regular software updates
> 5. The technology allows for shade taking and editing of images to improve the quality of the final restoration
> 6. Scanned images can be sent to other dental offices or dental laboratories via email or a connection through the software

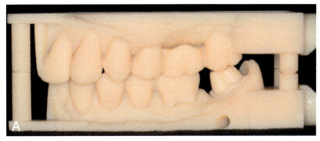
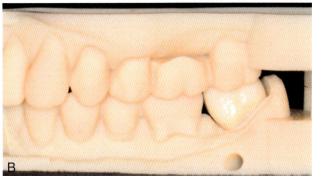

FIG. 5.27 Model and die created from a digital scan that was sent to a 3D printer: **(A)** Digital scan of the quadrant with the crown preparation and opposing quadrant articulated by a digital bite registration. **(B)** CAD/CAM ceramic crown is seated on the die. (From Powers JM, Wataha JC. *Dental Materials: Properties and Manipulation.* 11th ed. Elsevier; 2017.)

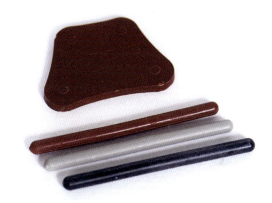

FIG. 5.28 Types of impression compounds: cake and sticks.

INELASTIC IMPRESSION MATERIALS

Inelastic impression materials in the form of dental impression compound, impression plaster, zinc oxide eugenol, and impression wax are among the oldest impression materials used in dentistry. For the most part, the elastic impression materials have replaced inelastic materials in modern dentistry.

DENTAL IMPRESSION COMPOUND

Uses

An impression compound is a rigid thermoplastic material that softens when heated and becomes firm again at mouth temperatures. An impression compound is most commonly used as thick sheets (sometimes called *cakes*) or sticks (Fig. 5.28).

Some dentists use, and some dental schools still teach the use of, compound sticks to mold the

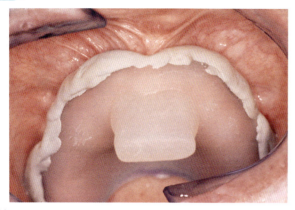

FIG. 5.29 Stick compound used for border molding of a custom impression tray. (Courtesy Mark Dellinges, University of California School of Dentistry, San Francisco, California.)

peripheral borders of a custom tray and to form the palatal seal in impressions for complete dentures (Fig. 5.29). After the peripheral borders are established, an impression is taken in the tray with one of the elastomers.

IMPRESSION PLASTER

Impression plaster is seldom used today but was used mainly for complete denture impressions. When used as the primary impression material, a wet mix (high water-to-powder ratio) was used to make it more fluid. After it set in the mouth, it was scored with a knife or bur, fractured along the score lines, and removed. The pieces were reassembled in the laboratory and poured into dental stone to form the cast. Because of the complexity of its technique, impression plaster has been replaced by elastic materials that are easier to use and more accurate.

ZINC OXIDE EUGENOL IMPRESSION MATERIAL

Zinc oxide eugenol (ZOE) impression material, like impression plaster, is seldom used today. In its day, ZOE was favored as an impression material for mucostatic (does not displace the tissues) impressions. When a patient had loose tissue over an edentulous ridge and the operator did not want to displace these tissues with a stiff or heavy viscosity impression material, ZOE was often chosen.

IMPRESSION WAX

Waxes are often stiff at room temperature and become moldable when heated. They lack accuracy for final impressions for restorative treatments and distort easily on removal from tissue undercuts or when affected by temperature fluctuations after removal from the mouth.

Some waxes with low melting temperatures remain moldable at mouth temperatures. These waxes are used to correct minor voids in impressions for complete dentures or to build a posterior seal (post dam) for the maxillary denture by adding wax to the impression in the area of the juncture of hard and soft palates, and then reseat the impression in the mouth.

INFECTION CONTROL PROCEDURES

DISINFECTING IMPRESSIONS

Dental impressions should always be considered contaminated. They are usually contaminated with oral fluids. Although most infectious agents, such as human immunodeficiency virus, do not survive for long periods of time outside of the body, many pathogens, such as the hepatitis viruses, can survive for several days. When impressions are not disinfected before they are poured, microorganisms can get into the gypsum and survive for a week or longer. Spores can survive even longer.

> **! Caution**
>
> Impressions are potentially infectious. They must be disinfected before being handled in the office laboratory or sent to a commercial laboratory.

Disinfection of impressions should begin chairside once the impression is removed from the mouth. Dental personnel should wear PPE while handling and disinfecting the impressions. The dental office has the primary responsibility for disinfection. Although the Occupational Safety and Health Administration allows transportation of contaminated items, regulations require proper packaging and labeling of these contaminated items. Dental offices should discuss with the dental laboratory the protocol they will use to disinfect items sent to the laboratory and how restorations returning from the laboratory should be handled.

The material that is to be disinfected must be compatible with the disinfectant used and the procedure employed. Incompatible disinfection materials and procedures can cause significant distortion of the impression and failure of the restoration to fit correctly.

After removal from the mouth, impressions should be:
- Rinsed thoroughly with water to remove debris and oral fluids
- Excess water should be shaken off before the disinfectant is used
- Disinfection should occur through the application of the disinfectant via immersion of the impression or by spraying its surfaces
  - Spraying may be preferred for impression materials that tend to distort with immersion
  - Spraying has two main disadvantages:
    – First, it creates airborne particles of the disinfecting chemicals that could be inhaled by the staff or patients
    – Second, it may not adequately reach all surfaces if severe tissue undercuts are present
- Immersion can cause distortion of some impression materials because they are prone to imbibe water and they swell
  – Alginate can be immersed in appropriate disinfectants for up to 30 minutes, typical disinfection time is 10 minutes
- The length of time these sensitive materials are immersed must be monitored carefully

- Rinsed after the recommended contact time with the disinfectant to remove residual chemicals
- Placed in a closed container or a sealed plastic bag if they are being transported to the dental laboratory

Do You Recall?

Why is rinsing the impression the most critical step in the disinfection process?

Clinical Tip

Spraying an impression should be done inside a plastic bag or headrest cover to contain the spray and protect the handler from inhaling droplets. Spraying the impression inside a plastic bag does not eliminate the need to wear a mask for protection from aerosols.

Selecting Disinfecting Solution

Impression materials differ from each other in their composition. Thus each type of impression material may require its own disinfecting solution and procedure. Manufacturer recommendations for disinfection should be followed. See Table 5.6 for disinfecting times and materials for impressions. Procedure 5.5 describes processing methods for impression materials.

DISINFECTING CASTS

On rare occasions, it may be necessary to disinfect the cast produced from an impression that could not be properly disinfected because of the nature of the contaminants or an impression material that could not be immersed in the proper disinfectant. Casts should be completely set and stored for at least 24 hours before disinfection to prevent attack by the chemicals on the surface of the cast. Casts seem to be minimally affected by the use of 1:10 sodium hypochlorite, iodophors, or chlorine dioxide. Casts should be sprayed rather than immersed in disinfecting solutions because some studies have shown damage to the surface in only a few minutes in water-based solutions. Manufacturers have added antimicrobial agents to some gypsum materials, but studies are not conclusive as to their effectiveness.

TABLE 5.6 Disinfection of Impressions

IMPRESSION MATERIAL	COMPATIBLE DISINFECTANTS	IMMERSION TIME
Alginate	Iodophors or chlorine compounds (1:10 dilution of household bleach)	10 (up to 30) minutes or spray
Polyvinyl siloxane	Iodophors, glutaraldehydes, complex phenolics, chlorine compounds	10–30 minutes or spray
Polyether	Iodophors, glutaraldehydes, chlorine compounds	<10 minutes or spray

STERILIZING IMPRESSION TRAYS

Reusable impression trays (aluminum, chrome-plated, and stainless steel) must be sterilized properly after their use and after a tray is tried in the patient's mouth for fit. Disposable plastic trays are recommended when they can meet the demands of the impression material being used. Plastic trays should be discarded when the procedure has been completed. Custom acrylic trays should be discarded when the procedure has been completed or should be immersed in an acceptable disinfectant if they will be reused at the patient's next appointment.

SUMMARY

In almost all phases of dentistry, impressions are an integral part of the procedures needed for delivering comprehensive care to patients. In most offices, impressions are made daily, and the various selection, manipulation, and disinfection of impression materials must be understood. With the improvements made in the impression materials over the past several decades, many of the older materials, such as agar hydrocolloid, polysulfide, condensation silicone, and the inelastic materials, have been replaced by more accurate, dimensionally stable elastic materials. PVSs and polyethers are the most popular impression materials for final impressions for restorations and removable prostheses. Alginate is still the material of choice for preliminary impressions.

Each category of the impression materials has its own handling characteristics. Changes in temperature and humidity will influence the materials in different ways, so operators must take these factors into consideration when making impressions. Dimensional changes over time, water loss and gain, deformation, and rebound are among the many physical and mechanical properties that must also be considered when impression materials are handled and disinfected.

Dental auxiliaries who have been properly educated and licensed in their states can pack retraction cord and make final impressions using elastic materials or digital images for crowns, bridges, implants, and removable prosthetics when the state dental practice act allows. It is imperative that clinicians have a reliable approach to making impressions, including soft tissue management.

CAD/CAM technology and digital impressions are being used more and more as an alternative to impression materials. Digital impressions are much easier for patients, and they eliminate many of the requirements needed in the impression materials. Digital impressions can be transmitted to the dental laboratory within minutes of capturing the images or may be used to design and mill restorations in the dental office.

INSTRUCTIONAL VIDEOS

See the Evolve Resources site for a variety of educational videos that reinforce the material covered in this chapter.

Procedure 5.1 Making an Alginate Impression

See Evolve site for Competency Sheet.

Consider the following with this procedure: *safety glasses are recommended for the patient, PPE is required for the operator, ensure appropriate safety protocols are followed, and check local state guidelines before performing this procedure.*

EQUIPMENT/SUPPLIES (FIG. 5.30)
- Basic examination setup
- Alginate, powder scoop, and water-measuring cylinder (supplied by manufacturer)
- Flexible rubber mixing bowl, wide-bladed spatula
- Impression trays (perforated) or solid trays including rim-locks (require alginate adhesive)
- Utility wax ropes
- Saliva ejector, disinfecting solution, zippered plastic bag, paper towels

PROCEDURE STEPS

1. *Patient preparation:* Seat the patient. Cover the patient's clothes with a plastic-backed patient napkin. Explain the procedure to the patient to obtain consent. Inquire about the gag response and ability to breathe through the nose. Remove dental prostheses unless needed in the impression. Have the patient rinse his or her mouth with antiseptic mouthrinse.
   NOTE: If the patient has bridges or fixed implant prostheses, block out around pontic spaces with utility wax as those areas are likely to lock alginate in place and make removal of the impression difficult. Orthodontic bands, brackets, and arch wires may also need to be blocked out. If the patient has very loose teeth, block out embrasures around these teeth to prevent removal of the teeth with the impression. Take precautions for gagging (as highlighted in the clinical tip on controlling the gag reflex). Patients who cannot breathe through the nose may feel threatened if alginate runs out the back of the tray and blocks the airway; therefore seat the tray in the posterior first and rock the tray forward to force material to the front of the mouth and tray. On occasion, the dentist may want the prosthesis left in during the impression to examine the occlusion later on. Check with the dentist. Rinsing before making the impression removes debris and ropy saliva. An antibacterial rinse will reduce the number of pathogens.

2. *Tray selection:* Quickly examine the patient's mouth, arch size and shape, and palatal depth. Select a tray of the appropriate size. Try it in the mouth for fit. Add utility wax as needed for comfort and extension of the tray.
   NOTE: If the tray border is short or the palate deep, add wax to extend the tray and support the alginate (Fig. 5.31).

3. *Mixing alginate:* Tumble the container of alginate to fluff the powder. Measure three level scoops of powder for a large upper arch or two scoops for a medium or small arch. Two scoops are adequate for the average lower arch. Place in a flexible rubber mixing bowl one measure of room-temperature water for each scoop of powder. Add powder to water and stir to wet the powder. Vigorously mix and press the wet powder against the sides of the bowl with a spatula while rotating the bowl with the other hand. The final mix should appear smooth and not grainy (Fig. 5.32).
   NOTE: Prepackaged alginate does not require fluffing because it is already present in the correct proportions. Mix by wiping vigorously against the sides of the bowl is intended to remove entrapped air, and thoroughly mix the powder and water. Water that is cooler than room temperature lengthens working and setting times, whereas warm water shortens these times. Complete the mix within 45 seconds for regular-set or within 30 seconds for fast-set alginate to allow enough time to load the tray, paint occlusal surfaces, and seat the impression before initial set.

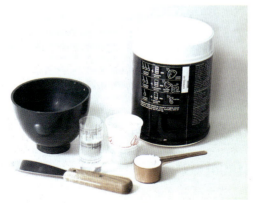

FIG. 5.30 Alginate, powder scoop, eater measurer, flexible rubber mixing bowl, wide-bladed spatula, and paper cup.

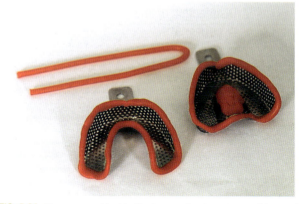

FIG. 5.31 Rope wax added to the impression trays to provide comfort and accommodate the depth of the palate.

Procedure 5.1 Making an Alginate Impression—cont'd

4. *Loading the tray:* Load the tray in large increments, pressing each increment into the tray until level with the sides. Use a wet, gloved finger to smooth the surface of the alginate and create a shallow indentation where the teeth will go (Fig. 5.33). Remove excess alginate.

   NOTE: Fewer increments will trap less air. Force out entrapped air by pressing alginate into the depth of the tray. Indentation for the teeth helps to orient the tray when seating. Extra material added to the anterior part of the tray helps to fill the vestibule and get a good peripheral roll.

5. *Seating the tray:* Take alginate from the bowl on a finger, and wipe it over the occlusal surfaces and into the embrasures. For upper impression: From behind and to the side of the patient (right-handed—11 o'clock position; left-handed—1 o'clock), retract the right cheek with the posterior corner of the tray and the left cheek with the index finger (reverse for left-handed). For lower impression: From the front and to the side of the patient (right-handed—8 o'clock position; left-handed—4 o'clock), retract the left cheek with the side of the tray and the right cheek with the left index finger (reverse for left-handed) (Fig. 5.34). Both impressions can be made with the operator seated and the patient reclined, or with the operator standing with the patient upright. Many offices request the patient to be upright for impressions to decrease the possible need for suction as impression materials clog suction lines. If the patient is reclined, seat the patient upright immediately after the tray is placed. For both upper and lower impressions: Rotate the tray into the mouth, and align the tray over the teeth with the handle at the midline. Seat the back of the tray first and complete seating to the anterior as the lip is gently pulled out of the way. Inspect the back of the tray for excess alginate and remove with a quick sweep of the mouth mirror. For lower impression: Have the patient lift the tongue and move it side to side once the tray is seated, and relax it again once alginate has flowed into the lingual areas.

   NOTE: Seating the posterior of the tray first allows alginate to flow forward rather than back into the patient's throat. Lifting the lip allows alginate to flow into the vestibule. Quickly removing excess alginate minimizes the gag response. Employ distraction techniques for gaggers. Once the tray is in place, have the patient position the head forward, breathe through the nose deeply and slowly, and use the saliva ejector to prevent pooling of saliva.

6. Stabilize the tray until the alginate is fully set. Allow an additional minute before removing the tray.

   NOTE: Check alginate remaining in the bowl to confirm set. Tray movement during setting will cause distortion in the impression. Allowing 1 minute after set helps to increase tear strength.

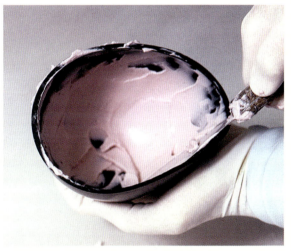

FIG. 5.32 Alginate being pressed against the sides of the flexible rubber mixing bowl.

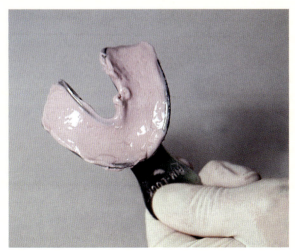

FIG. 5.33 Smooth surface of the alginate created by a wet, gloved finger.

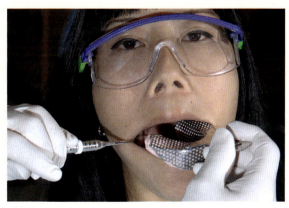

FIG. 5.34 Seating of a lower impression tray.

Continued

Procedure 5.1 Making an Alginate Impression—cont'd

7. *Removing the tray:* Break the seal by running a finger around the tray in the vestibule and then press down (or up for a lower impression) on the side of the tray with a finger, or have the patient close his or her lips around the tray handle and blow to puff out the cheeks. Hold the handle in the hand, grasping with the index finger and thumb, and remove the tray with a snap.
   NOTE: Protect the patient's teeth in the opposing arch with fingers of the other hand. Rapid removal minimizes distortion and tearing of alginate.
8. *Handling the impression:* Rinse the impression under running water to remove saliva and debris. This is the first step in the disinfection process. Shake off pooled water. Inspect the impression, using criteria for acceptability (see Table 5.3) (Figs. 5.35 and 5.36).
9. *Disinfecting the impression:* Spray thoroughly with disinfectant. Allow to sit for 10 minutes in the zippered plastic bag to allow disinfection to occur.
   NOTE: When the impression is sprayed inside a bag or headrest cover, the aerosol is better contained (Fig. 5.37). Alginate will imbibe liquid and swell, so pooled liquid should be removed.
10. Once disinfection has occurred, cut off unsupported alginate at the back of the tray. Drain off the pooled liquid. If the impression will not be poured immediately, wrap the impression in a damp paper towel or place a few drops of water in a zippered plastic bag marked with the patient's name (Fig. 5.38) and seal it.
    NOTE: If the tray is laid on the bench top, unsupported alginate at the back of the tray may lift a portion of the impression and dislodge it from the tray. This will cause a distortion in the impression. If alginate is left in the air, water will evaporate, causing distortion. Ideally, the impression should be poured within 30 minutes because it is not dimensionally stable for long periods. It will lose water (by synersis) even in 100% humidity.
11. Help the patient remove alginate from the face with a damp towel. Have the patient rinse their mouth. Inspect the patient's mouth and remove trapped alginate from the embrasures with an explorer and floss when necessary.

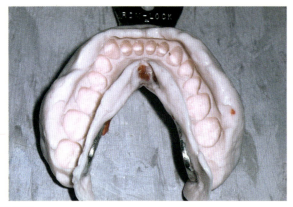

FIG. 5.35 Acceptable mandibular alginate impression

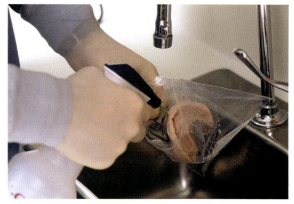

FIG. 5.37 Alginate impression being sprayed with disinfectant in a zippered plastic bag

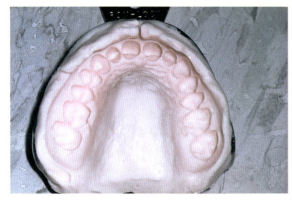

FIG. 5.36 Acceptable maxillary alginate impression

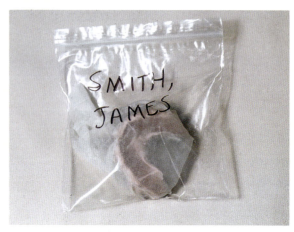

FIG. 5.38 Disinfected alginate impression wrapped in a damp paper towel and sealed in a zippered plastic bag marked with the patient's name.

Procedure 5.2 Making a Double-Bite Impression for a Crown

See Evolve site for Competency Sheet.

Consider the following with this procedure: *safety glasses are recommended for the patient, PPE is required for the operator, ensure appropriate safety protocols are followed, and check local state guidelines before performing this procedure.*

NOTE: In some states, the dental auxiliary may be permitted to place a retraction cord and make the impression. In states where these functions are not permitted, it is assumed that the auxiliary will assist the dentist.

EQUIPMENT/SUPPLIES (FIG. 5.39)
- Basic crown and bridge setup
- Double-bite tray (paper insert for metal trays), tray adhesive
- Elastomeric impression material in cartridges: Heavy-body tray material and light-body syringe material
- Dispenser gun and mixing tips
- Impression syringe

PROCEDURE STEPS

1. Assemble the cartridge in the appropriate dispenser gun and extrude a small amount of impression material onto a paper towel to ensure that the openings are not clogged. Place the mixing tip.
   NOTE: Clogged or partially clogged openings will result in an improper mix of the material, with alteration of setting time and physical properties.
2. Inform the patient of the procedure and have the patient practice closing into centric occlusion (patient's "normal" bite) with the tray in place (Fig. 5.40).
   NOTE: Choose opposing teeth that are easily seen, such as the canines on the opposite sides of the mouth, and note their position when they occlude. This relationship will be checked when the impression is made to ensure proper closure.
3. Maintain isolation in the quadrant in which the impression will be made.
   NOTE: Saliva can saturate the retraction cord and may cause it to displace from the gingival sulcus.
4. Confirm that cord retraction around the crown preparation is adequate (Fig. 5.41).
   NOTE: This is the first "stop sign." The clinician should be able to see the preparation, the cord, and the gingiva displaced from the preparation. In other words, the cord should not be placed so deeply into the gingival sulcus that the gingival crest has collapsed over it and is resting on or near the preparation or the cord should not be placed so shallowly that it is resting on top of the margin.

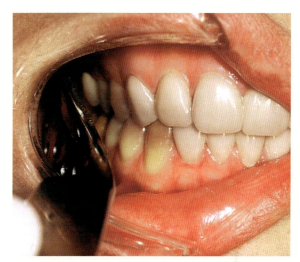

FIG. 5.40 Patient closing in centric occlusion.

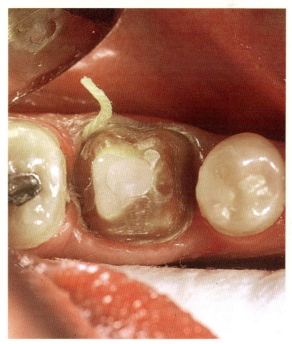

FIG. 5.41 Adequate tissue retraction around the crown prep with retraction cord.

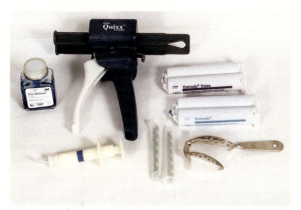

FIG. 5.39 Elastomeric impression material in cartridges, dispenser gun, mixing tips, tray adhesive, double bite tray, and impression syringe.

Continued

Procedure 5.2   Making a Double-Bite Impression for a Crown—cont'd

5. Carefully remove the retraction cord after it has been in place for about 5 minutes (8 minutes if the tissue had been bleeding prior to cord placement). Rinse and dry the tooth.

   NOTE: If the retraction cord is dry, lightly wet it before removal. A dry cord may stick to tissues and cause bleeding when removed. To prevent bleeding, the cord should be gently lifted from the sulcus rather than ripped out quickly.

6. Inspect the gingiva, sulcus, and preparation before proceeding with the impression. Check to see that the tissue is adequately retracted in *all* areas around the preparation, that it is not bleeding, and that the margins of the preparation are free of debris, blood, and astringent. (This is the second "stop sign.")

   NOTE: The tissues will stay retracted long enough to control the field. The impression syringe should not be loaded until the field is dry, bleeding is controlled, and retraction is adequate. If a two-cord retraction technique is used in which a smaller cord is left in the sulcus during the impression, check to see that the smaller cord has stayed in place and has not lifted over the margins. If it has lifted, pack it back into place. If blood is oozing from the sulcus, control bleeding by scrubbing the sulcus with ferric sulfate astringent on a small cotton pellet or applicator. Then, rinse residual astringent away, because compounds that contain sulfur can interfere with the set of polyvinyl siloxane impression materials.

7. With the preassembled dispenser gun and mixing tip, load the impression syringe with the light-body material. Change cartridges and mixing tips. Load both the preparation and opposing arch sides of the double-bite tray with the heavy-body material.

   NOTE: The gun-type mixing system ensures a thorough mix with minimal waste of material. For efficiency of time and motion, two guns could be used and preassembled rather than having to unload the light body and load the heavy body with a single gun. Impression putty could be used in place of the heavy starting with the tip just apical to the margin. With the material continually flowing, keep the tip in contact with the tooth while slowly tracing the margin and filling the gingival sulcus. Circle the entire tooth to completely cover the margins, and then continue circling while covering the axial walls and finally the occlusal surface (Fig. 5.42).

   NOTE: Establishing a good finger rest will help stabilize the impression syringe. Some manufacturers provide a delivery tip that can be attached to the mixing tip to deliver the light-body material directly to the preparation from the cartridge. This method can be awkward in the posterior part of the mouth because the end of the long mixing tip is far away from the operator's

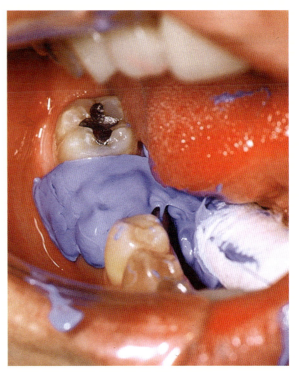

FIG. 5.42 Light bodied impression material covering the crown prep.

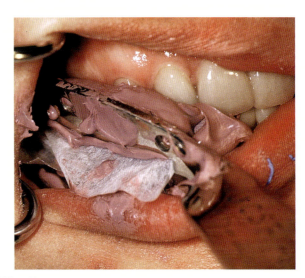

FIG. 5.43 Patient biting together into impression while in centric occlusion

hand, making fine control of the tip difficult. Without good hand control, the tip frequently bounces out of contact with the preparation during injection of light-body material around the tooth, creating air voids in critical parts of the impression. For retention grooves, the syringe tip should be placed at the bottom of the groove and the groove filled from the bottom to the top.

8. Place the impression tray over the teeth and instruct the patient to close into the rehearsed bite. Check the reference teeth to ensure that the patient has closed into the proper position (Fig. 5.43).

Procedure 5.2 Making a Double-Bite Impression for a Crown—cont'd

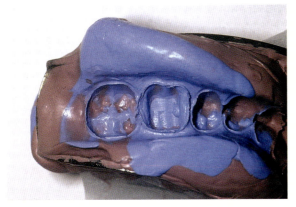

FIG. 5.44 Double bite impression of crown preparation.

Instruct the patient not to shift the bite or open until instructed to do so.

NOTE: A missed bite relation will result in a crown that is grossly high.

9. When the two viscosities of impression material have set, remove the impression. Rinse and dry the impression to remove saliva, blood, and debris. Inspect it for completeness of the preparation detail. There should be a slight excess of impression material extending beyond the margins and no folds or voids (Fig. 5.44). Minor air bubbles in noncritical areas such as the occlusal surface might be acceptable. Check with the dentist.

NOTE: Folds on axial walls are often the result of material that did not join together at the start and end of the circling process around the tooth because the material had started to set or because the circle was not completed with new material flowing into first-placed material. Air entrapment resulting in small or large voids is often the result of loss of contact of the syringe tip with the tooth during syringing of the material. If a two-cord retraction technique was used and the cord left in place during the impression comes out attached to the impression, do not attempt to remove it. The impression could tear. Cut off with scissors any loose ends of cord hanging from the impression and leave the cord that is embedded in the impression material.

10. Hold the impression up to the operatory light and inspect for proper occlusal contacts. The impression material will be very thin where there is contact between opposing teeth, and light can be seen through the material. If contacts are not in the proper locations, a separate bite registration may need to be made.
11. Spray the impression with a suitable disinfectant while it is contained within a plastic bag, seal it in a zippered plastic bag that has been labeled with the patient's name, and transport it to the laboratory (see Figs. 5.37 and 5.38 in Procedure 5.1).

Procedure 5.3 Bite Registration With Elastomeric Material

See Evolve site for Competency Sheet.

Consider the following with this procedure: *safety glasses are recommended for the patient, PPE is required for the operator, ensure appropriate safety protocols are followed, and check local state guidelines before performing this procedure.*

EQUIPMENT/SUPPLIES
- Basic examination-setup
- Plastic bite tray
- Elastomeric bite registration material in dual cartridge
- Automatic mixing extruder (gun type) and mixing tips (Fig. 5.45)

PROCEDURE STEPS
1. Assemble the cartridge in the gun and extrude a small amount of bite registration material onto a paper towel to ensure that the openings are not clogged.

NOTE: Clogged or partially clogged openings will result in an improper mix of the materials, with alteration of setting time and physical properties.

2. Place the mixing tip on the cartridge.

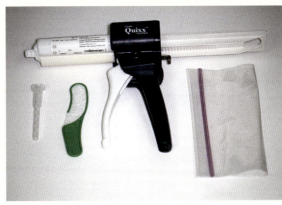

FIG. 5.45 Plastic bite registration tray, dual cartridge of elastomeric bite registration material in automix extruder with mixing tip, and zippered plastic bag.

Continued

Procedure 5.3 Bite Registration With Elastomeric Material—cont'd

3. Inform the patient of the procedure and have the patient practice closing into centric occlusion (the patient's "normal" bite) with the tray in place.

   NOTE: Choose opposing teeth that are easily seen, such as the canines, and note their position when they occlude. This relationship will be checked when the bite registration is taken.

4. Dry the teeth to be included in the bite registration.
5. Extrude mixed material onto each side of the bite registration tray until the gauze in the center of the tray is evenly covered with material, about 2 mm thick (Fig. 5.46).
6. Center the tray over the mandibular teeth to be included in the bite registration and have the patient close into the practiced bite (Figs. 5.47 and 5.48).

   NOTE: Now is the time to check the relationship of the opposing teeth (i.e., canines) to see if they are properly occluded.

7. Instruct the patient to hold the teeth together until the material is set (in 3 minutes or less).

   NOTE: If the patient moves the teeth during the setting stage, a distortion will likely occur and will often be seen as imprints wider than the teeth.

8. Remove the bite tray when the material is set. Inspect impression to see that all of the teeth needed for the registration are included and that there are no major voids (Fig. 5.49).

   NOTE: When set, the material should not indent and should feel firm.

9. Check for correct occlusion. Hold the bite registration material to the operatory light and see that light shines through in areas of contacting teeth. Gauze with a thin layer of material should be present in these areas.

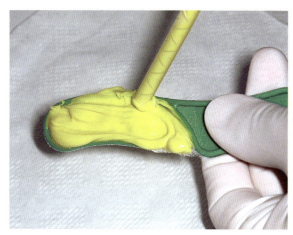

FIG. 5.46 Extruded mix material covering both sides of the bite registration tray.

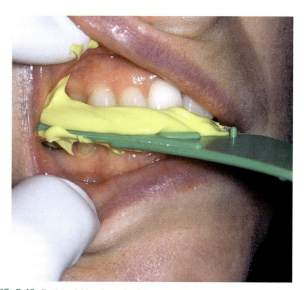

FIG. 5.48 Patient biting into the bite registration impression in centric occlusion

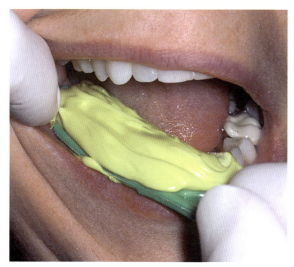

FIG. 5.47 Bite registration tray centered over the mandibular teeth to be included in the bite registration impression.

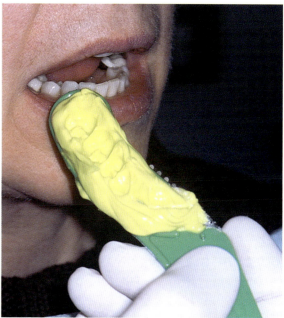

FIG. 5.49 Inspection of set bite registration to ensure all teeth needed for the registration are included.

Procedure 5.3 Bite Registration With Elastomeric Material—cont'd

NOTE: If the material is thick in areas where there should be contact of opposing teeth, the patient may not have closed properly. Inspect the patient's occlusion and compare it with the bite registration. If there is an error, rehearse bite closure and repeat the procedure. If the tray is not inserted far enough posteriorly, the patient may bite on the back edge of tray rather than biting together completely.

10. Rinse the material under running water to remove saliva and debris.
11. Spray the bite registration material with a suitable disinfectant while it is contained within a plastic bag. Seal it in a zippered plastic bag labeled with the patient's name, and transport it to the laboratory.

Procedure 5.4 Wax Bite Registration

See Evolve site for Competency Sheet.

Consider the following with this procedure: safety glasses are recommended for the patient, PPE is required for the operator, ensure appropriate safety protocols are followed, and check local state guidelines before performing this procedure.

EQUIPMENT/SUPPLIES (FIG. 5.50)
- Bite registration wax or utility wax
- Heat source
- Laboratory knife

PROCEDURE STEPS

1. Heat utility wax sheets until pliable and fold several times to get three to four layers of wax.
   NOTE: You will need a thickness of 3 to 4 mm to avoid distortion when removing.
2. Form the wax into a horseshoe shape.
   NOTE: You may need to reheat the wax to keep it pliable (Fig. 5.51).
3. Try the wax into the mouth, cutting the ends to fit only to the middle of the last tooth in the arch.

NOTE: If you are using preformed wax bite registration blocks, then you will need to trim them only for length (Fig. 5.52).

4. Seat the patient in the upright position and give them instructions on closing in centric occlusion.
   NOTE: Concerning patients in the supine position: if the patient's mouth has been open for a long time or is numb, the patient may close in an abnormal position.

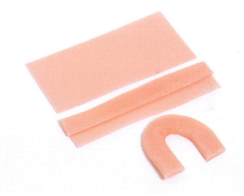

FIG. 5.51 Example of wax sheets folded several times to form a sheet 3–4 mm thick and formed into a horseshoe shape similar to that of the dental arch.

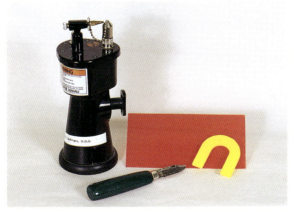

FIG. 5.50 Heating element, laboratory knife, and utility and bite registration wax.

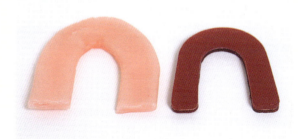

FIG. 5.52 Wax arch on left was fabricated in the dental office utilizing a sheet of wax. Wax arch on right is an example of a preformed wax bite registration block.

Continued

Procedure 5.4 Wax Bite Registration—cont'd

5. Heat the wax again until softened.
   NOTE: If using a flame source, assure the patient that the wax will not burn their tissues (Fig. 5.53).
6. Place the wax horseshoe onto the occlusal surfaces of the maxillary teeth (Fig. 5.54).
7. Instruct the patient to bite gently, yet firmly, into the wax.
   NOTE: If the patient bites too firmly, the wax may be distorted and torn. If not firmly enough, the teeth may not make adequate indentations in the wax (Fig. 5.55).
8. Allow the wax to cool in the patient's mouth for 1 to 2 minutes.

NOTE: Use an air syringe to hasten cooling by gently spraying the area around the wax.

9. Have the patient open with a straight snap to avoid distortion of the wax.
10. Remove the wax bite registration carefully, being sure not to break or distort the wax (Fig. 5.56).
11. Disinfect the wax bite and store it in a bag labeled with the patient's name (Fig. 5.57).
    NOTE: Follow the manufacturer's recommendations for use of this material. Some disinfecting agents may break down the wax.
12. Store the wax in a cool area (ideally at slightly less than room temperature).

NOTE: You should try to use the wax as soon as possible to articulate models and to avoid distortion due to relaxation of residual stress.

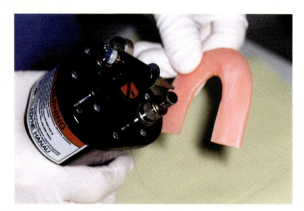

FIG. 5.53 Wax being softened by a heating element.

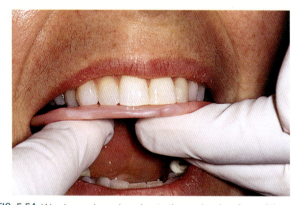

FIG. 5.54 Wax horseshoe placed onto the occlusal surface of the maxillary teeth.

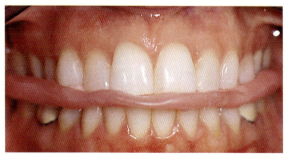

FIG. 5.55 Patient biting into the surface of the wax bite registration.

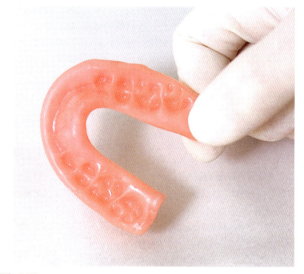

FIG. 5.56 Completed wax bite registration.

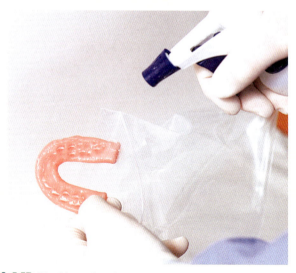

FIG. 5.57 Wax bite registration being sprayed with disinfectant.

Procedure 5.5 Disinfection of Impression Material or Bite Registration

See Evolve site for Competency Sheet.

Consider the following with this procedure: *safety glasses are recommended for the patient, PPE is required for the operator, ensure appropriate safety protocols are followed, and check local state guidelines before performing this procedure.*

EQUIPMENT/SUPPLIES

- Impressions/bite registration
- Various disinfecting solutions in appropriate containers
- Zippered plastic bags

PROCEDURE STEPS

1. Rinse the impression under running tap water and shake off the excess.
   NOTE: Rinsing is considered the first step in the disinfection process as it removes much of the saliva, blood, and other biological debris that can interfere with disinfection.
2. Immerse or spray the impression with an acceptable disinfectant prepared according to the manufacturer's instructions. If spraying, hold the impression within a plastic bag to contain the spray (see Fig. 5.37 in Procedure 5.1).
   NOTE: Polyethers can be sensitive to immersion. ZOE should not be disinfected with chlorine-containing solutions because it breaks down the material.
3. Leave the solution on the sprayed impression or leave the immersed impression in solution for the recommended time period.
   NOTE: Polyethers should not be immersed for longer than 10 minutes because they imbibe water and swell. Spraying is preferred.
4. Rinse with water and gently shake off the excess to remove any residual chemicals.
   NOTE: Residual chemicals can adversely affect the surface of the cast when the impression is poured.
5. Package properly for transport (see Fig. 5.38 in Procedure 5.1). A zippered plastic bag is usually satisfactory. Label with the patient's name.
   NOTE: Alginate and agar hydrocolloid should be wrapped in a damp paper towel (or place a few drops of water in the plastic zipper bag) to keep them from losing moisture and distorting. It is not necessary to wrap elastomers. They should be dried after the disinfectant is rinsed off.

Get Ready for Exams!

Review Questions

Select the one correct response for each of the following multiple-choice questions.

1. What best describes a dental impression material?
   a. Forms a positive imprint of the oral structures involved
   b. Allows the creation of a replica of the structures involved
   c. Is always flexible for easy removal from the mouth
   d. Is used only for crown and bridge procedures and for diagnostic casts (study models)
2. Which one of the following impression materials is transformed from a sol to a gel state when set?
   a. Alginate
   b. Polysulfide
   c. Polyether
   d. Polyvinyl siloxane
3. All of the following are elastic impression materials *except* one. Which one?
   a. Alginate
   b. Polyether impression material
   c. Dental compound
   d. PVS impression material
4. The types of impression materials that are considered hydrophilic have what type of quality?
   a. Have a lot of water in them
   b. Can be immersed in water without absorbing it
   c. Cause water to bead on their surface
   d. Have good surface-wetting characteristics
5. Hydrophobic impression materials:
   a. Absorb moisture only after their final set
   b. Are the best type of material to use in the mouth because they repel saliva and blood
   c. Need a dry field to get the best results
   d. Provide the best surfaces on gypsum casts because they resist the uptake of water during curing of the gypsum
6. Which statement best describes alginate impression material?
   a. Is accurate enough to be used for crown and bridge procedures
   b. Has very few uses in the modern dental practice
   c. Is dimensionally stable during the first 24 hours
   d. Can be immersed in an appropriate disinfectant for up to 10 minutes without distorting

Continued

Get Ready for Exams!—cont'd

7. An irreversible hydrocolloid:
   a. Goes from a gel to a sol when it is heated
   b. Is no longer in common use
   c. Is hydrophobic
   d. Cannot reverse from a gel to a sol because a chemical reaction prevents it
8. The elastic recovery (or rebound) of alginate impression material can be increased by which one of the following?
   a. Leaving the impression in the mouth for 1 minute beyond its set
   b. Using a thicker mix of material
   c. Using cold water in the mix
   d. Removing the impression slowly from the mouth
9. Which one of the following would a preliminary impression not be useful for?
   a. Diagnostic casts (study models)
   b. All-ceramic inlays
   c. Custom trays
   d. Provisional restorations
10. Which one of the following impression materials is not commonly used?
    a. Polysulfide
    b. Polyether
    c. Polyvinyl siloxane
    d. Alginate
11. The three key properties that materials used for final impressions must possess include all of the following except one. Which one?
    a. Accuracy
    b. Dimensional stability
    c. Wettability
    d. Tear resistance
12. Which one of the following impression materials has the lowest tear strength?
    a. Polyvinyl siloxane
    b. Polyether
    c. Vinyl polyether hybrid
    d. Alginate
13. What quality does a clinician not want to see in a tray to aid in obtaining an accurate impression?
    a. Too smooth
    b. Too flexible
    c. Too rigid
    d. Perforated
14. Which one of the elastomers has the highest natural (no chemicals added) wettability?
    a. Polyvinyl siloxane
    b. Polysulfide
    c. Polyether
15. As the viscosity of the impression material increases, which one of the following properties decreases?
    a. Accuracy
    b. Tear strength
    c. Dimensional stability
    d. Setting time
16. Which of the following elastomers will absorb water when stored in it and change dimensions?
    a. Polysulfides
    b. Polyethers
    c. Addition silicones

17. Which one of the following statements is true about the addition silicones?
    a. They are good materials for complete denture impressions but are not accurate for crown and bridge procedures.
    b. They are very dimensionally stable.
    c. They cost about the same as alginate.
    d. They require the use of custom acrylic trays.
18. The least accurate of the elastic impression materials is:
    a. Polyvinyl siloxane
    b. Polyether
    c. Vinyl polyether silicone hybrid
    d. Alginate
19. After removing a PVS impression from the mouth, it is found that the surface has unset material on it. What can cause this to happen?
    a. Incomplete mixing of the material
    b. Residual ferric sulfate astringent on the teeth
    c. Contamination from latex gloves
    d. All of the above
20. Which of the following is not an advantage of PVS substitutes for alginate?
    a. Dimensionally stable for long periods
    b. Less expensive than alginate
    c. Can be repoured several times
    d. Do not have to be poured right away
21. At present, the most common conservative method of creating space in the gingival sulcus of a prepared tooth for wash (syringe) material is which one of the following?
    a. Retraction paste
    b. Retraction cord
    c. Laser troughing
    d. Electrosurgical troughing
22. Which one of the following astringents has the potential to be dangerous to patients with cardiovascular disease?
    a. Racemic epinephrine
    b. Ferric sulfate
    c. Aluminum chloride
    d. ViscoStat
23. Which one of the following is not a reason the wash material may tear when removing the set impression from the mouth?
    a. Narrow sulcus width (<0.2 mm)
    b. Very deep sulcus
    c. Sharp edges on the preparation
    d. Removing the impression with a snap
24. A successful double-bite impression for a crown on tooth 30 includes all of the following except one. Which one?
    a. The margins of the preparation are shiny and rounded.
    b. The margins and a little of the tooth beyond are captured in the impression.
    c. No large voids are present in the walls of the preparation.
    d. Opposing teeth are captured in the proper bite relation.

Get Ready for Exams!—cont'd

25. Which *one* of the following is *not* an advantage of digital impressions over traditional impressions?
    a. Impression material and associated supplies are not needed.
    b. Digital impressions can be electronically transferred to the laboratory.
    c. Images of the preparation can be viewed from multiple angles before being sent to the laboratory.
    d. Gingival retraction is not needed for preparations with subgingival margins.
26. Which *one* of the following impression materials is *least* affected by soaking it in a disinfectant solution for two hours?
    a. Alginate
    b. Polyether
    c. Polyvinyl siloxane
27. Disinfecting of impressions:
    a. Is done to protect the patient from surface bacteria
    b. Must be done for all impressions
    c. Is done only with impressions for patients with known infectious diseases
    d. Does not need to be done for the new alginates that have bactericidal chemicals incorporated into them

For answers to Review Questions, see the Appendix.

Case-Based Discussion Topics

1. A 30-year-old retail store manager comes to the dental office to have impressions made for home whitening trays. The patient indicates that they have a moderate gag reflex.
What impression material is well suited for making whitening trays? What steps can be taken to minimize gagging and to shorten the length of time the impression material remains in the mouth? How should the impression material be handled from the time it is removed from the mouth until it is poured with dental plaster or stone?
2. A dentist practicing in California decides to use the services of a dental laboratory located in New York City. The office plans to mail all impressions to the laboratory rather than pour them in the office.
What types of impression materials can be used under these circumstances and still produce accurate casts and dies? Which materials definitely cannot be used? What properties of the materials are most important? How should the impressions be handled before they are shipped to the laboratory?
3. A 53-year-old mail carrier comes to the dental office with a broken buccal cusp on tooth 31. Adjacent to 31, the patient has a fixed bridge from 28 to 30 that has a hygienic pontic replacing tooth 29. The dentist will prepare 31 for a porcelain-bonded-to-metal crown, and the dental auxiliary will make an impression. Isolation is difficult because the patient salivates profusely, and the gingiva is bleeding because the patient is taking blood thinners. The clinician will be able to control most of the saliva. The bleeding will be greatly reduced when a local anesthetic with a vasoconstrictor is injected into the gingival papillae around the tooth. However, the preparation will not be completely dry.
Which elastomer, by its nature, is somewhat hydrophilic and could be used? Which materials are not naturally hydrophilic but may have surfactants added to make them more hydrophilic? What precautions should be taken before the impression is made to ensure that it can be easily removed from the mouth?
4. The dentist in your office will replace an existing crown on tooth 5 for a young college student because of recurrent caries under the distal margin. The dentist likes to use a two-step PVS putty/wash technique. You will be asked to prepare an acrylic custom provisional crown for the patient.
How should you prepare for this before the dentist removes the crown, using the materials at hand? What types of impression trays can the dentist use with this technique? Can a polysulfide tray adhesive be used with the PVS putty? How soon does the PVS impression have to be poured? What disinfectants are safe to use with PVS materials?
5. The dentist uses polyether in the office for crown and bridge impressions. This afternoon, a call came in from the dental laboratory indicating that the laboratory's delivery person had been in an automobile accident yesterday; the dies picked up from the dentist's office were broken.
Can the dentist repour the impression and send new dies? Why or why not? Which of the impression materials are good for this purpose? Which elastomer has the greatest accuracy for the longest time?
6. A variety of impression materials may be used in the dental office on a daily basis. It is important to protect all dental personnel who might handle the impressions by proper disinfection. In addition, the accuracy of the impressions might be adversely affected by improper disinfection techniques.
Describe the procedures for disinfecting alginate, PVS, and polyether impression materials.
7. A licensed dental hygienist with an expanded functions credential is preparing to make a PVS impression of tooth 19 for a gold crown. The hygienist has packed retraction cord according to the two-cord technique. The hygienist needed to scrub the gingival sulcus with ferric sulfate astringent to control bleeding.
Before making the impression, what criteria should the hygienist use to determine whether the top cord is properly placed? Once the top cord is removed, what criteria should be used to determine whether the next steps for making the impression can be taken? What should be done to the prepared tooth surfaces once the bleeding has been controlled with ferric sulfate? When the impression has been completed, what criteria will the hygienist use to determine whether the impression can be used for the crown?

BIBLIOGRAPHY

Alghazzawi TF: Advancements in CAD/CAM technology: options for practical implementation, *J Prosthodont Res* 60: 72–84, 2016.

Boksman L, Cowie RR: Making polyvinyl impressions: success lies in the details, *Contemporary Dental Assisting*:28–32, 2007.

Bilir H, Ayguzen C: Comparison of digital and conventional impression methods by preclinical students: efficiency and future expectations, *J Int Soc Prevent Commun Dent*:402–409, 2020.

Burgess JO: Impression material basics, *Inside Dent* 1(1), 2005.

Burgess JO, Lawson NC, Robles A: Comparing digital and conventional impressions, *Inside Dent*:68–74, 2013.

Burgess JO, Lawson NC, Robles A: Digital impression system considerations, *Inside Dent*:72–76, 2015.

Kelsch NB: Dental laboratories and infection control, *RDH Mag*, 2012.

Powers JM, Wataha JC: *Dental Materials: Foundations and Applications*, St. Louis, 2017, Elsevier.

Robinson DS: *Modern Dental Assisting*, Philadelphia, 2022, Elsevier.

Sakaguchi RL, Ferracane J, Powers JM: *Craig's Festorative Dental Materials*, St. Louis, 2018, Mosby.

Shen C, Rawls HR, Equivel-Upshaw JF: *Phillips' Science of Dental Materials*, St. Louis, 2022, Elsevier.

Wilkins EM, Wyche CJ, Boyd LD: *Clinical Practice of the Dental Hygienist*, ed 13, Philadelphia, 2021, Wolters Kluwer.

Yuzbasioglu E, Kurt H, Turunc R: Halenur B: Comparison of digital and conventional impression techniques: evaluation of patients' perception, treatment comfort, effectiveness and clinical outcomes, *BMC Oral Health* 14:10, 2014.

Gypsum and Wax Products

6

http://evolve.elsevier.com/Eakle/materials/

Chapter Objectives

On completion of this chapter, the student should be able to:

1. Differentiate between negative and positive reproduction of oral structures.
2. Differentiate among diagnostic cast, working cast, and dies.
3. Describe the chemical and physical nature of gypsum products.
4. Explain the manufacturing process for gypsum products and how this affects their physical characteristics.
5. Compare the following properties and behaviors of gypsum products: strength, dimensional accuracy, solubility, and reproduction of detail.
6. List the American Dental Association–recognized gypsum products and their most appropriate uses.
7. Explain initial and final set of gypsum and the factors that affect the setting time, setting expansion, and strength.
8. Explain the procedure for mixing and handling gypsum products to create diagnostic casts.
9. Identify the common components of dental waxes.
10. Compare the properties of waxes.
11. Describe the clinical/laboratory significance of each of the properties of waxes.
12. Discuss the three classifications of waxes.
13. Differentiate between direct and indirect waxings and identify which property of dental waxes is most important in their difference.
14. Describe the usual color, form, and use of inlay, casting, baseplate, boxing, utility, and sticky waxes.
15. Prepare model plaster or stone for pouring.
16. Pour the anatomic and base portions of maxillary and mandibular diagnostic casts.
17. Trim maxillary and mandibular diagnostic casts.
18. Obtain a bite registration, using bite registration materials or utility wax.

KEY TERMS

Casts replicas of hard and soft tissue of the patient's oral cavity, made from gypsum products; also referred to as *models*

Diagnostic Casts casts generally made from dental plaster or stone and used for patient education, treatment planning, and tracking the progress of treatment, as with orthodontic models; these casts are also known as *study models*

Working Casts casts generally made from one of the dental stones that are strong enough to resist the stresses of fabricating an indirect restoration or prosthesis; these casts are also known as *master casts* or *working models*

Dies replicas of the prepared teeth that are generally removable from the working cast

Model Plaster the weakest, most porous form of gypsum product used in dentistry

Dental Stone a stronger, less porous form of gypsum product used in dentistry

Die Stone the densest form of gypsum product used in dentistry

Pouring *pouring the cast* refers to the process of vibrating the flowable gypsum product into an impression; this process must produce a cast that is an exact replica of the structures captured in the impression

Trimming the process of removing excess hardened gypsum from the cast for ease in working with the cast and appearance in presentation

Melting Range a range of melting points of the individual components of wax that starts when the first part begins to liquefy and finishes when the wax is completed melted.

Flow the movement of wax as it approaches the melting range

Excess Residue a wax film that remains on an object after the wax is removed

Wax Pattern a duplicate of a restoration carved in wax

Lost Wax Technique a technique for fabricating a metal restoration by encasing the wax pattern in stone and then vaporizing the wax under high temperatures to leave an empty impression space once occupied by the wax; molten metal is then cast into the space and takes the shape of the pattern

Gypsum is a mineral widely found in nature that has been used for making dental casts since 1756. Dental casts and dies are used as replicas of the hard and soft tissues of the patient's oral cavity. First, an impression, the negative reproduction of the patient's mouth, is taken using a soft, elastic material. This impression is filled with a gypsum material made from a fine powder that is mixed with water to form a flowable mass. Once hardened, this material will be a hard, stable positive reproduction, or cast, of the hard and soft tissues (Fig. 6.1). These hard replicas are used to plan and track the progress of treatment. They are also used in laboratory procedures, where they serve as the replicas on which dental procedures, either unsafe or too difficult to do directly in the mouth, are performed.

The dental auxiliary is frequently called on to produce these replicas. In some states, the assistant or the hygienist may fabricate intraoral prostheses on these replicas. Both auxiliaries may also find the resultant model useful in presenting information for patient education. The production of gypsum casts requires meticulous attention to detail, a well-thought-out process in their production, and knowledge of the advantages and limitations of each gypsum material in order to select the appropriate material. Inaccurate, incomplete, or weak casts are of little use and are likely to produce costly mistakes in patient treatment procedures.

Dental waxes are used in a wide variety of clinical and laboratory dental procedures. Clinically, they may be used to fabricate direct wax patterns for cast restorations, alterations and adaptations for impression trays, and wax bite registrations. In the laboratory, they may be used to box an impression before pouring a gypsum product, as baseplates for full and partial dentures, to hold components together before articulation, and to provide indirect patterns for casting.

The dental assistant and hygienist typically will not fabricate the actual direct or indirect wax pattern for a dental casting, but they do need an appreciation for the many steps in the procedure known as the lost wax technique (described later in this chapter). The assistant and the hygienist will frequently manipulate waxes in making alginate impressions, pouring impressions, and making a wax bite registration for articulation of models.

GYPSUM MATERIALS

USES OF GYPSUM MATERIALS

Gypsum products are most frequently used to make replicas of the patient's mouth. These replicas are called *diagnostic casts, working casts,* and *dies*. Each of these has a specific purpose in the treatment planning or fabrication of intraoral appliances, prostheses, or restorations.

Diagnostic casts: Also called *study models*, these are used to plan treatment and observe the oral structures of the mouth. Orthodontists use study models extensively as they plan and treat for the alignment of the teeth (Fig. 6.2).

Working casts: Also called *working models*, these are used to fabricate appliances such as an orthodontic retainer or bleaching tray or a removable prosthesis such as a partial or full denture (Fig. 6.3).

Dies: Dies are replicas of individual teeth or groups of teeth and are used to fabricate crowns and bridges (Fig. 6.4).

Diagnostic casts, working casts, and dies are not subjected to the same stresses; therefore they do not have the same physical property requirements. The accuracy of each of these replicas is dependent on the accuracy of the impression from which they are poured. The accuracy and use of the replica also depend on the gypsum material used and the properties of this material.

DESIRABLE QUALITIES

There are several desirable qualities for gypsum products used in the making of diagnostic and working

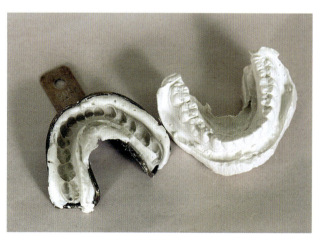

FIG. 6.1 Impressions (negative reproductions) are poured into gypsum to form casts (positive reproductions).

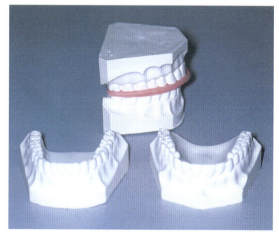

FIG. 6.2 Diagnostic casts made from plaster. (From Bird DL, Robinson DS. *Modern Dental Assisting.* 12th ed. Elsevier; 2018.)

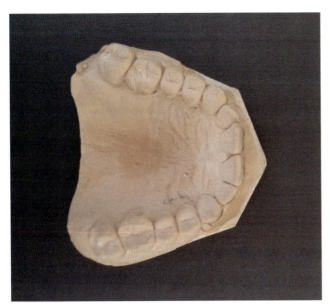

FIG. 6.3 Working cast made of dental stone used to fabricate appliances. (Courtesy Steve Eakle.)

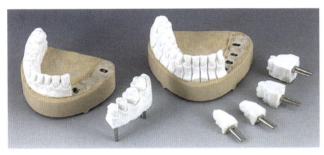

FIG. 6.4 Dies, which are replicas of individual teeth, are used to fabricate crowns and bridges. (Courtesy Pocket Dentistry.)

casts or dies. These qualities have differing significance depending on the stresses applied to the product. The importance of the qualities listed below depend on the application of the product:
- Accuracy
- Reproduction of fine detail
- Dimensional stability
- Hardness, strength, and resistance to abrasion
- Solubility
- Ease of use
- Cost
- Color
- Safety

All casts and dies must be accurate, hard, and dimensionally stable under normal conditions of use and storage. Because working casts and dies are used to fabricate intraoral prostheses and restorations, they must also have excellent reproduction of fine detail, strength and resistance to abrasion, and minimal solubility. Color is important in the identification of the material and to provide contrast between the die material and the waxed inlay pattern. The amount of expansion of the gypsum material during its set is important to the overall accuracy of the cast. The cost, ease of use, and safety are practical considerations in the manipulation of the product and how often it is used.

BEHAVIORS OF GYPSUM PRODUCTS

Chemically, the mineral gypsum is a dihydrate of calcium sulfate ($CaSO_4 \cdot 2H_2O$), which is mined as solid mass.

FORMATION OF GYPSUM

To transform the mined gypsum into a useable form, the manufacturer completes the following steps:
- Heats the dihydrate, which causes it to lose water.
- Grinds it ground to produce a powdered hemihydrate, $CaSO_4 \cdot \frac{1}{2}H_2O$.
  - This process is referred to as *calcination*.

The powder can now be used for dental purposes:
- Mix the powder with water to produce a viscous product capable of flowing.
- A chemical reaction occurs that converts the hemihydrate back to a dihydrate and it becomes a solid mass again useful for making casts and dies.

The by-product of the chemical reaction is heat, so it is called an *exothermic reaction*. The amount of water required to mix with the calcium sulfate hemihydrate is greater than the amount required for the chemical reaction. This excess water produces a mix that can flow into the details of dental impressions. The excess water evaporates on setting, and a mass of interlocking gypsum crystals is produced. Between the gypsum crystals are small voids of air that were once occupied by the water that has evaporated. The amount and size of the air voids remaining affects the hardness, strength, and resistance to abrasion of the final product.

The components of all gypsum products are chemically the same; the physical differences in the materials are due to the differences in calcination and the resulting amount of water that is drawn off the dihydrate.

> 💡 **Clinical Tip**
>
> Plaster contains the most excess water of the various gypsum mixes and therefore produces bigger and more numerous air voids resulting in a weaker product that abrades easily; die stone contains the least excess water and therefore produces fewer, smaller air voids resulting in a stronger product that is more abrasion resistant.

PRODUCTION OF GYPSUM PRODUCTS

Production of the various forms of gypsum is basically the same. With some modifications, they are used for several different purposes.

Ground gypsum (i.e., calcium sulfate dihydrate) is heated during the manufacturing process until it loses water and becomes calcium sulfate hemihydrate.
- If the heating process occurs in open vats at a temperature of approximately 115°C (239°F), the resulting hemihydrate is porous and irregular in shape. This process will form **model plaster,** commonly used for diagnostic casts (study models).

- If the heating process is done under pressure, in the presence of steam, and at a higher temperature (125°C [257°F]), a more uniformly shaped and less porous form of hemihydrate, referred to as **dental stone**, is produced. Dental stone is used for working casts (master casts).
- If the gypsum rock is boiled in a 30% calcium chloride solution, a high-density raw material called *densite* is produced. The densite is then washed and heated with a greater increase in pressure. Then even more refining of the powder by grinding results in the densest stone known as high-strength or **die stone**. This additional refining makes even more regular particles with better packing ability, thus reducing the amount of water required for mixing and increasing the final density of the product.
- If high-strength stone is mixed with silica, it forms *dental investment*, a material able to withstand the high heat and stress produced when molten metal is forced into molds to form indirect restorations by the lost wax technique (described later in this chapter).

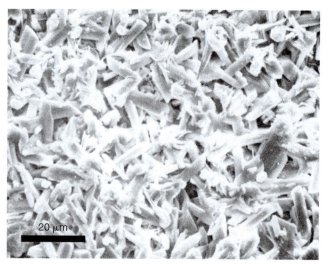

FIG. 6.5 Scanning electron micrograph of the surface of set high-strength dental stone (die stone). The surface is porous with many interlocking crystals of calcium sulfate dihydrate. To the naked eye, this surface would appear smooth. (From Powers JM, Wataha JC. *Dental Materials: Properties and Manipulation.* 10th ed. Elsevier; 2013:115.)

> **Clinical Tip**
>
> The increase in water necessary to mix a gypsum product also increases the setting time and reduces the strength and hardness of the set gypsum.

PHYSICAL PROPERTIES

Physically, gypsum products are manufactured as:
- Plaster
- Stone
- High-strength stone
- Gypsum-bonded investment

The main differences in the physical forms are dependent on the variations in size, shape, and porosity of the powders produced by the different manufacturing processes. The larger, more irregular, and porous the particles of powder, the weaker and less resistant to abrasion the final product becomes (Fig. 6.5).

Its properties and behavior determine the specific use of the gypsum product. Depending on the application, the following properties vary in importance:
- Strength
- Abrasion resistance
- Solubility
- Behaviors of setting time
- Expansion

Diagnostic casts, for example, are placed under little stress and are usually produced from less expensive materials such as plaster or stone, both of which have lower properties of strength and abrasion resistance. Working casts and dies require materials resistant to greater stresses and thus require higher properties of strength and abrasion resistance and precise accuracy; therefore setting expansion must be carefully controlled.

Strength, Hardness, and Resistance to Abrasion

Factors that affect the strength of gypsum products also affect their hardness. Two factors contribute to the strength and abrasion resistance of the final product:
- The shape of the particles and their porosity
  - Increased porosity of the particles makes it necessary to use more water to convert the hemihydrate particles back to dihydrate particles.
  - A product with less water has a higher density of crystals and is therefore a denser and stronger product.
  - The larger, more irregularly shaped particles are prevented from fitting together densely.
    - As an example: plaster particles are both porous and irregular, requiring more water to mix. The resulting product has more air space because of the less densely packed particles, making plaster considerably weaker than the less porous and more densely packed stone products.
- The amount of water needed to mix the product
  - The strength of gypsum products is related to the amount of water, and more critically, excess water, used in producing the study or working cast.

Factors that affect the strength of gypsum products also affect their hardness. Because gypsum products require varying amounts of water to wet and incorporate the powder into a workable mixture, it follows that the more water that is used, the weaker the cast will be.

The strength of the gypsum product is an indicator of its ability to resist fracture. Compressive strength of plaster is four times less than that of densite and three times less than that of stone. The tensile strength of plaster is half that of stone. American Dental Association (ADA) specifications require that the material reach minimal compression strength (i.e., wet strength) 1 hour after setting.

> **Clinical Tip**
>
> To reach maximal strength (i.e., dry strength), the cast may need to set in a dry environment for several hours or overnight.

Dimensional Accuracy

Setting expansion occurs with all gypsum products:
- Plaster expands the most, at 0.30%
- High-strength stone products the least, at 0.10%

Setting expansion is a result of the growth of crystals as the particles join. Controlling setting expansion is critical for the production of accurate models and dies. It is important that expansion be held to a minimum, particularly when the material is being used to fabricate restorations and dental prostheses. If expansion were excessive, any die fabricated from the gypsum material would eventually result in an oversized restoration. Although some expansion is acceptable for models fabricated from plaster, expansion of die materials would be a source of costly errors. Strict proportioning of water and powder, and of the chemical additives provided by the manufacturer, is required to produce dies with the required level of accuracy. High-strength stone produced by mechanically mixing under a vacuum will expand less than if the stone is hand-mixed with no vacuum. Setting expansion occurs only during the hardening of the gypsum product. No changes occur under normal conditions of use and storage once the product has reached its final set.

Reproduction of Detail

The greater the porosity of the final gypsum product, the less surface detail is produced. Even products that have the least amount of porosity have surface irregularities visible at the microscopic level.

Surface detail will be affected by contamination of an impression with:
- Blood
- Food debris
- Saliva

The impression should be rinsed with water and closely inspected for extraneous materials, and all water used in this rinsing should be thoroughly removed before pouring the impression. Compressed air via the air/water syringe is the best method for removing all the water from the impression prior to pouring. However, overdrying may produce distortion in alginate impressions.

Compatibility of impression material and gypsum material can influence the quality of surface reproduction. Gypsum materials flow best when there is compatible wetting with the surface of the impression. *Wetting* describes the ability of a material to flow and not bead up, like water on a waxed surface. A decrease in wetting may prevent the gypsum material from flowing into all the details of the impression, leaving air voids from bubbles. Impression materials that are water based work better with water based gypsum materials: for example, agar and alginate impression materials are water based and generally form the best surface detail with gypsum products. It is always important to follow the manufacturer's directions in selecting gypsum products that are compatible with impression materials.

Silicone, Polyvinyl Siloxane (PVS), and polyether impression materials, which are not water based, may benefit from the addition of a surfactant sprayed into the impression before pouring to aid the gypsum in wetting the impression material. The surfactant helps in the wetting of the impression, thus allowing the gypsum material to flow more easily on the impression surface. Spray surfactants should be used sparingly, as pooling of the surfactant in the impression will result in chalky areas on the model.

A material (Wonderadmix; Dental Creations) (Fig. 6.6) is marketed to distribute surfactant throughout the gypsum product to ensure an equal distribution of surfactant to the entire impression. It helps to eliminate pouring bubbles by breaking the surface tension and allowing the gypsum to glide over the surface of the impression. Wonderadmix is added to the water before the gypsum powder is introduced.

Solubility

Set gypsum products are not highly soluble in water. Solubility is directly related to the porosity of the material; therefore plaster is much more soluble than

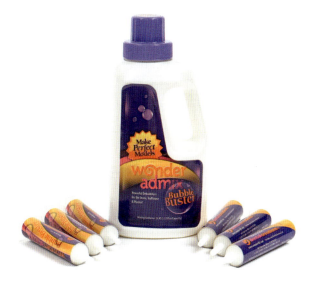

FIG. 6.6 Surfactant that can be added to gypsum to prevent bubbles from occurring. (Courtesy WonderAdmix.)

stone. Exposing models to water for prolonged periods should be avoided (Table 6.1), as they will lose much surface detail as they begin to dissolve.

Clinical Tip
If gypsum needs to be soaked in water, the soaking should be done in *slurry water*, which is water saturated with plaster particles to prevent the loss of surface detail.

Do You Recall?
Which gypsum product is the least soluble in water?

Clinical Tip
Computer-aided design and computer-aided machining (CAD/CAM) technology (see Chapter 10) uses a digital image of the preparation and can avoid the use of stone dies when the restoration is made in one visit without the use of models. Therefore many of the problems mentioned regarding strength, abrasion, dimensional accuracy, and solubility can be avoided.

CLASSIFICATION OF GYPSUM PRODUCTS

The desired physical properties and behavior necessary for a particular use determine the criteria for selection of a gypsum product. If strength is desired, the choice of a stone or high-strength stone material is important. If a diagnostic cast is being fabricated, plaster or stone is adequate. ADA specification number 25 identifies the following five gypsum products.

IMPRESSION PLASTER (TYPE I)

Impression plaster is rarely used by today's dentists, having been replaced with the less rigid, elastic impression materials. If selected, it would be used as a final impression wash for edentulous arches. Impression plaster may also be used to mount casts on an articulator, which is a mechanical device used to place maxillary and mandibular casts in occlusion and in a fixed position (Fig. 6.7). This device is used in the fabrication of removable and fixed prosthodontic appliances.

MODEL PLASTER (TYPE II)

Model plaster is frequently used for diagnostic casts and articulation of stone casts. It has a water-to-powder (W/P) ratio of approximately 0.45 (i.e., 0.45 mL of water per 100 g of powder), which produces a durable but relatively weak cast when compared with the stone categories. The irregular shapes of the particles prevent them from fitting together tightly. These study casts do not require a significant amount of strength or abrasion resistance. Model plaster is available in fast and regular sets and is easy to manipulate. This product is traditionally produced in a white color to distinguish it from dental stones. Because of its simple manufacturing processes, plaster is the least costly of all the gypsum products.

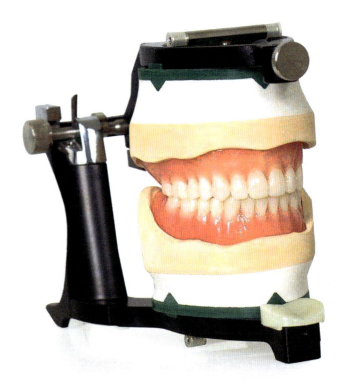

FIG. 6.7 Articulated working casts with full upper and lower removable prosthodontics. (Courtesy Keystone Industries.)

Table 6.1 Properties of Gypsum Products

TYPE[a]	POROSITY	COMPRESSIVE STRENGTH (MPA)	ABRASION RESISTANCE	SETTING EXPANSION
Type II: model plaster	High	8.8	Low	High
Type III: dental stone	Moderate	20.6	Moderate	Moderate
Type IV: high-strength/low-expansion stone	Low	34.3	High	Low
Type V: high-strength/high-expansion stone	Low	48.0	High	High

MPa, Megapascal (1 MPa equals approximately 145 lb/in^2); *W/P ratio*, water-to-powder ratio (milliliters of water per gram of powder).
[a]Type I (impression plaster) is rarely used by today's dentists.

Clinical Tip

Model plaster is different from orthodontic plaster, which is a mixture of plaster and stone.

Uses of Diagnostic Casts

- Provide a 3D record of the patient's hard and soft tissues
- Facilitate study of the occlusal relationship of the dental arches
- Facilitate study of tooth size, position, and shape and arch relations
- Facilitate study of hard and soft tissues from the lingual view while teeth are in occlusion
- Provide a record of present conditions for comparison as treatment progresses
- Provide a visual aid for patient education
- Provide a legal record of the patient's arches for insurance, legal suits, and forensics

DENTAL STONE (TYPE III)

Dental stone (e.g., *Hydrocal*, USG Corporation), is ideal for making:
- Full or partial denture models
- Orthodontic models
- Casts requiring higher strength and abrasive resistance

Dental stone has uniformly shaped, relatively nonporous crystals. Because of the particle characteristics, dental stone requires less water 0.30 (i.e., 0.30 mL of water per 100 g of powder); its particles therefore pack together more tightly (i.e., the material is denser) and approximately 2.5 times stronger than plaster. Stone is easy to use, slightly more expensive than model plaster, and traditionally colored yellow or white.

DENTAL STONE, HIGH STRENGTH/LOW EXPANSION (TYPE IV)

Type IV materials are often referred to as *die stones* or *densite* because they are especially suited for fabricating wax patterns for cast restorations. A hard, abrasive-resistant surface is necessary to resist the abrasion of sharp instruments used to carve wax on these stone dies. Their crystals are slightly larger and more dense than stone. These products require very strict and detailed handling, are often colored pink or green, have a W/P ratio of 0.23 (i.e., 0.23 mL of water per 100 g of powder), and are almost two times stronger than type III stones.

DENTAL STONE HIGH STRENGTH/HIGH EXPANSION (TYPE V)

Type V has been developed in response to the need for even higher strength, high-expansion dental stones and materials that can withstand the high temperatures (1500°C [2732°F]) required by the casting process. The addition of silica, a refractory material, improves the material's resistance to heat and is the reason the material has increased thermal expansion. Higher expansion may seem to be an undesirable property, but it is needed to compensate for the greater casting shrinkage of the newer base metals used for dental castings. These materials are also referred to as *gypsum-based investment*. The increased strength is obtained from a W/P ratio of 0.20 (i.e., 0.20 mL of water per 100 g of powder). This material, colored blue or green, is the most costly of all the gypsum products.

METAL-PLATED AND EPOXY DIES AND RESIN-REINFORCED DIE STONE

Type IV and V gypsum products are commonly used die materials. These materials are very hard, but they are susceptible to abrasion during carving of wax patterns.

Electroplating

Dies are occasionally electroplated with metal to produce better surface detail and make them less susceptible to abrasion. Silver or copper plating can create metal-plated dies that are highly resistant to abrasion. Electroplating transfers metal ions from a solution by using a electric current to form a thin shell of metal on the outside of the die.

Epoxy

Epoxy dies use a resin and hardener to produce a die that is harder and has greater abrasion resistance than high-strength stone. These epoxy materials set slowly and may require 6 to 24 hours for setting. Newer fast-set epoxy materials are supplied in an automix system similar to automix impression materials. The epoxy resin and catalyst are forced through the mixing tip directly into the final impression. These fast-set products harden within 30 minutes.

Resin-Reinforced

Some gypsum product die stones have resin particles added to reinforce the high-strength stone and make them more abrasion resistant.

INVESTMENT MATERIALS

Investment materials are used to form metal castings through the lost wax technique. These materials, which combine gypsum and silica, can be used to produce molds sufficiently strong to allow molten metal to be poured into them. Investment materials have increased expansion on setting; this expansion is necessary to compensate for the shrinkage of metal castings. Expansion liquid is available to replace the use of water for mixing of investment materials. This liquid formulation is used to achieve greater expansion, allowing the dental laboratory technician to achieve optimal fit for a variety of materials.

Do You Recall?

Which gypsum product is most frequently used for diagnostic casts?

KEY POINTS – Classification of Gypsum and Uses

1. Used to make replicas of the patient's mouth
   - Diagnostic casts
   - Working casts
   - Dies
2. Must be accurate, hard, and dimensionally stable
3. Strength of material dependent on method of production
   - Type II—Model Plaster
     - Weakest material—used for diagnostic casts
     - Heating process occurs in open vats at temperature of 115°C
     - Least dimensionally accurate
   - Type III—Dental Stone
     - Stronger material compared to plaster—used for working casts
     - Heating process done under pressure in presence of steam at a temperature of 125°C
   - Type IV—High-Strength Stone
     - Stronger material compared to dental stone—used for dies
     - Boiled in a 30% calcium chloride solution to produce densite, then desite washed and heated under pressure
   - Type V—Gypsum-Bonded Investment—used for lost wax technique
     - Strongest of the gypsum materials
     - High-strength stone mixed with silica

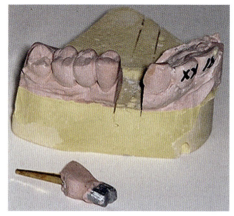

FIG. 6.8 A working cast with a stone base and high-strength stone anatomic portion, and a die made from high-strength stone with metal plating.

MANIPULATION OF GYPSUM PRODUCTS

MATERIAL SELECTION

The selection of a gypsum product should be based on the desired properties of the material.
- If a diagnostic cast is being fabricated, dental plaster is the appropriate choice because of the low physical property requirements and because of its low cost and ease of manipulation.
- If a working cast is being fabricated, dental stone would likely be used because of the requirement for higher strength, accuracy, hardness, and abrasion resistance.
- If a die is being fabricated, high-strength stone is the best choice because of its dimensional accuracy, strength, and abrasion resistance.
- In some instances, a combination of one or more gypsum products is appropriate to curtail cost and increase ease of manipulation.
  - When working models for cast restorations are being made, the die (the replica of the tooth on which, e.g., a crown is being fabricated) and surrounding teeth are poured in high-strength stone and the base is poured with type III stone (Fig. 6.8).
  - The entire working model is attached to a dental articulator with plaster.

PROPORTIONING (WATER-TO-POWDER RATIO)

The properties of gypsum products are directly related to their W/P ratio. It is important that the mixed material have sufficient flow to reproduce accurate and small surface detail; it should be remembered that an increase in the recommended water will result in:
- A thinner mix that takes longer to set
- A weaker final product
- A less accurate final product

If water is decreased:
- The mixture will be thicker
- May become difficult to manipulate, because it does not produce a flowable mix

Strict adherence to the manufacturer's suggested W/P ratio is recommended (Table 6.2).

> **Caution**
> The W/P ratio has a direct effect on the properties of the resultant product and must be carefully controlled.

Correctly Measured Proportions

Water should be measured with a graduated cylinder and powder weighed on a scale. The use of scoops to measure powder is not recommended because the powder tends to pack down over time as it sits in a container. The use of inappropriate measuring devices and measuring technique will likely lead to one of two results:
- Stone cast with a too-low W/P ratio: The stone will be too thick and detail will be lost.
- Stone cast with a too-high W/P ratio: The stone will be too thin, and its strength may be no greater than that of model plaster.

To avoid either of these scenarios, manufacturers produce preweighed envelopes of powder for critical measurements. This method enhances accuracy and saves time, but also increases the cost of the material.

MIXING: SPATULATION

Most commonly, plaster and stone are mixed in a flexible rubber mixing bowl with a broad metal or plastic plaster spatula (Fig. 6.9); this mixing process is called *spatulation*.

Table 6.2 Recommended Water/Powder (W/P) Ratios

MANUFACTURER RECOMMENDED W/P RATIOS

GYPSUM PRODUCT	WATER (IN ML)	POWDER (IN G)
Plaster (type II)	45–50 mL (0.45–0.50)	100
Stone (type III)	30–32 mL (0.30–0.32)	100
High-strength stone (type IV)	19–24 mL (0.19–0.24)	100

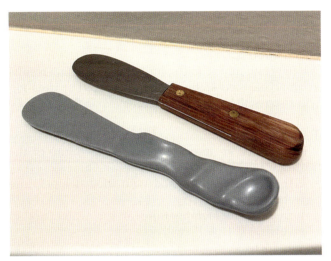

FIG. 6.9 Broad metal and plastic plaster spatula. (Courtesy Kim Bastin.)

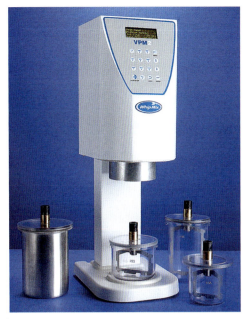

FIG. 6.10 Programmable, power-driven, vacuum-mixing unit, programmed for various types of gypsum products. The powerful vacuum quickly removes air and reduces the risk of bubbles. (Courtesy Whip Mix Corporation, Louisville, Kentucky.)

- The measured amount of water is placed into the mixing bowl and the measured powder slowly sifted into the water within 30 seconds.
  - By sifting powder into water, an even wetting of the powder particles takes place and clumps are avoided.
  - This is the reason for placing the powder in water rather than water into powder.
  - This technique will also minimize the amount of air incorporated into the mix during hand spatulation.
- The materials are spatulated by first incorporating the powder and water slightly and then vigorously wiping the mix against the sides of the bowl to force out air and ensure wetting of all the powder particles.
- Spatulation should continue for 1 minute at two revolutions per second until a smooth, homogeneous mix with a glossy surface is produced.
- An increase in the time and rate of spatulation has a definite effect on setting time and expansion: it will shorten the setting time and increase the rate of setting expansion.

Mechanical vacuum mix devices are used when the control of spatulation is critical. Many dental laboratories use mechanical spatulation with a vacuum device to reduce air bubbles and enhance the consistency and accuracy of mixing (Fig. 6.10). Hand spatulation is the most common means of mixing gypsum materials in private dental offices (Procedure 6.1).

SETTING TIMES

Initial Setting Time and Working Time

After mixing for 1 minute, the working time begins. During this time, the semifluid mixture is **poured** into the impression with the help of a mechanical dental vibrator (Fig. 6.11). As the viscosity of the mixture increases, the flow characteristics are decreased and the product loses its glossy appearance. This loss of gloss indicates that the gypsum has reached its initial set. At the time of initial set, the material has no measurable compressive or tensile strength and should not be removed from the mold. For regular-set products, the initial set occurs within 6 to 8 minutes from the beginning of the mix. With a mixing time of 1 minute, this leaves ample working time to pour the impression.

Final Setting Time

The final set is reached when the material can be handled safely, but it has minimal hardness and resistance to abrasion. At this time, the chemical reaction is complete and the model is cool to the touch, having completed the exothermic reaction. Most manufacturers recommend 45 minutes to 1 hour before the material may be safely separated from the impression. Gypsum products continue to harden and are two to three times harder after 24 hours.

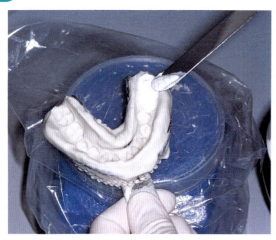

FIG. 6.11 Small increments of plaster flowing slowly from the posterior of an alginate impression on the dental vibrator to ensure air does not get trapped. (From Robinson DS, Bird DL. *Essentials of Dental Assisting*. 6th ed. Elsevier; 2017.)

Do You Recall?

What is the name of the setting reaction that generates heat as part of the process?

Clinical Tip

Before separating the impression from the cast, ensure that no part of the impression tray is connected to the gypsum. Do not pry or rock in one direction too far, or the cast will likely break because of its lack of tensile strength.

Allowing the impression and cast to remain together for more than 1 hour before separation may have a detrimental effect on the surface characteristics of the cast. Alginate will absorb water from the surface of the cast producing a weaker, more porous surface. The directions provided by the manufacturer of the impression material will indicate how long a gypsum product may remain in contact with the impression material.

Clinical Tip

If an alginate impression has dried out before the cast has been separated, soak the impression and cast in water for 15 minutes. The alginate will soften, allowing removal of the cast without breaking of the teeth or other anatomic structures. Do not leave gypsum products soaking in water longer than absolutely necessary as they will begin to dissolve.

CONTROL OF SETTING TIMES

It is important to keep in mind that it is impossible to accelerate the final set of a mixture without also accelerating the initial set, thereby reducing the working time. If it is necessary to alter the setting time, this can be accomplished by altering the water to powder ratio, spatulation, temperature or amount of accelerators or retarders.

Altering the W/P Ratio

As previously mentioned, an increase in the proportion of water will slow the setting times. However, because an increase by even one part water can reduce the strength by as much as 50%, this is not a recommended control. Decreasing the proportion of water will speed the setting time, but it also makes the mixture more difficult to manipulate, causing air bubbles and leading to an inaccurate model. Decreasing the amount of water mixed with the powder (i.e., decreasing the W/P ratio) is recommended only when the mixture is not being poured into an impression, such as when it is being used as a base to secure models on an articulator.

Spatulation

A longer and more rapid spatulation of gypsum results in an accelerated setting time. This rapid spatulation will also result in increased setting expansion.

Temperature

Within limits, an increase in the temperature of the mixing water will accelerate the setting time.
- Gypsum is ideally mixed with room temperature water.
- Increasing the temperature of the water, not to exceed 38°C (100°F), will accelerate the set.
- Any increase in temperature to above 38°C (100°F) will have a retarding effect.
- A temperature at 100°C (212°F) means no reaction takes place and the gypsum will not set.

Accelerators and Retarders

The most practical way to control setting time is through the manufacturer's addition of chemical accelerators (increased speed) or retarders (slowing).

Manufacturers add accelerators and retarders to change the solubility of the hemihydrate in water. By increasing the solubility of the hemihydrates:
- The added accelerator decreases the setting time
- By decreasing the solubility, the added retarder increases the setting time
- When accelerators are placed into the gypsum, the manufacturer can cut the time between the initial and final set by 50%
  - These materials are labeled "fast set."
  - If no accelerators or retarders are placed in the product, the product is labeled "regular set."

The clinician may also add accelerators:
- Potassium sulfate (K_2SO_4) and set gypsum ($CaSO_4$) particles are examples.
- The water and crystals from ground set gypsum, commonly retrieved from the runoff water of model trimmers, create *slurry water*.
- The dihydrate crystals in the slurry water accelerate the chemical reaction by acting as established sites for crystallization.

Using Clean Equipment and Impressions

When set materials are left in mixing bowls, on spatulas, or on other mixing equipment, these materials may inadvertently become part of the fresh mix. The result may be the same as the addition of an accelerator; however, this uncontrolled error will likely also result in an uneven setting of the material. All equipment should be thoroughly cleaned after pouring an impression to avoid this mistake.

Blood, saliva, and alginate are organic substances that can retard the set of gypsum. If these organic components are left in an impression, the surface detail of the resulting model may be easily abraded. All impressions must be rinsed free of any organic matter before the impression is poured. Alginate remains in contact with the gypsum product, so it must be noted that even though the outside surface of a cast poured from an alginate impression may seem set, the area adjacent to the teeth needs more time to fully harden.

Remember that when a change is made in the final setting time, a sacrifice is usually made in:
- The working time
- Strength
- Setting expansion of the final product (Table 6.3)

Do You Recall?

How can the setting of gypsum materials be altered if clean equipment is not utilized during the mixing process?

FABRICATING DIAGNOSTIC/WORKING CASTS

Parts of the Cast

Diagnostic and working casts have two parts: (see Fig. 6.12)
- *Anatomic portion:*
  - The anatomic portion replicates the hard and soft structures.
  - The anatomic portion is poured by vibrating small increments of flowable gypsum into the impression.
  - The mixture should be poured slowly in small increments under vibration and allowed to flow from the one tooth imprint to the next, pushing out air ahead of itself as it fills the entire impression, thus eliminating air voids.
  - To conserve costs and make the cast easier to trim, the anatomic portion may be poured with a higher-strength gypsum product and the base poured with a lower-strength product.
- *Art portion or base:*
  - The art portion aids in handling and articulating the casts.
  - The art or base portion can be poured by any of three methods (Fig. 6.13) (see Procedures 6.2 and 6.3).

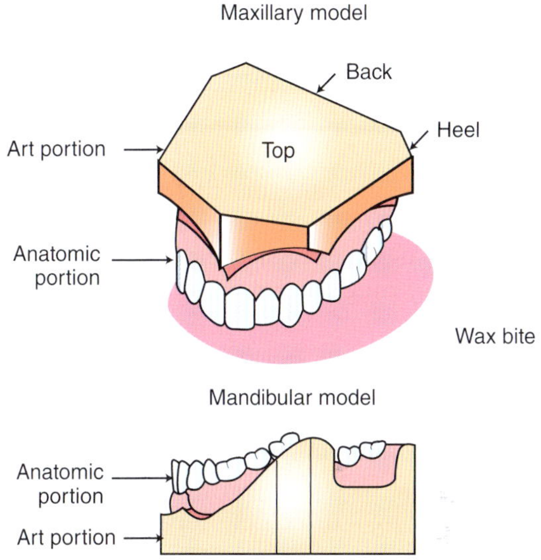

FIG. 6.12 Line drawing of parts and proportions of diagnostic casts. (From Bird DL, Robinson DS. *Modern dental assisting*, 11th ed. Elsevier; 2014.)

Table 6.3	Manipulation Factors		
FACTOR	**WORKING TIME**	**VISCOSITY**	**STRENGTH**
Increase W/P ratio	Increase	Decrease	Decrease
Decrease W/P ratio	Decrease	Increase	Increase
Increase rate of spatulation	Decrease	Increase	No effect
Increase temperature of H$_2$O	Decrease	Increase	No effect
Decrease temperature of H$_2$O	Increase	Decrease	No effect

W/P ratio, Water-to-powder ratio (milliliters of water per gram of powder).

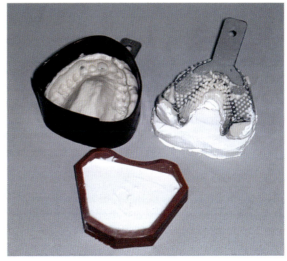

FIG. 6.13 Pouring the art portion of a cast by boxing; model former and inversion on putty base.

Methods for Pouring the Casts

Double-Pour Method. The double-pour technique involves the following.
- Two separate mixes and two separate setting times:
  - The anatomic portion of one or both arches is poured and left in the upright position.
  - Make sure you have slightly overfilled the entire impression, including the palate and borders of the impression.
  - Add a couple of additional small mounds of gypsum to the surface to make a better lock with the base.
  - Approximately 10 minutes after the loss of gloss, a second mix is produced for the art portion(s).
  - This mixture is approximately 1 inch thick and placed on a glass tile in the shape of the impression tray or into a base former.
  - The filled impression is inverted onto the base, with the handle of the tray parallel to the base, and the peripheries of the two portions are joined.
  - Care must be taken to ensure that the base material is thick enough to support the weight of the filled impression so that it does not sink into the base.
  - Avoid manipulating the filled impression once you place it on the base; overmanipulation will sink the filled impression into the base.
  - After inverting the impression, excess material may be carefully removed from the base to form a model requiring less time to trim on the model trimmer.
  - Be careful not to allow the base material to contact the impression tray as this will produce a mechanical lock between the tray and set gypsum, making it difficult to separate the tray from the model.

If the cast is being used as a working cast, the anatomic portion is frequently poured with dental stone and the base portion is poured with plaster. This gives the anatomic portion sufficient density while allowing for easier trimming of the base portion.

Single-Step Method (Inverted Pour Method). In the single-step method:
- One mix of gypsum is produced to pour both the anatomic and art portions of the cast.
- After the impression is poured, the remaining material is used for the base.
- This material is placed on a glass tile or into a base former (Fig. 6.13, lower image), the impression is inverted onto it, and the peripheries of the two portions are joined.
- This method requires better skill and timing.
- If the mixture is too wet when you finish pouring the impression, the base may flow excessively when the impression is inverted, causing the tray to become locked into the set gypsum.
- Also, the material in the inverted impression may slump away from the impression, causing distortion of the cast or trapping of air voids.
- If the mixture in the anatomic portion has reached its initial set when it is inverted onto the art portion, the union between art and anatomic portions will be incomplete.

Criteria for Evaluation of Poured Diagnostic Casts

- The anatomic portion is free of all air voids.
- The art portion is free of all air voids greater than 2 mm.
- The union between art and anatomic portions forms a continuous surface.
- The occlusal plane, at the premolar area, is parallel to the bottom of the base.
- The base is of adequate thickness but not so thick as to require excessive trimming.
- There is sufficient material extending past the mucobuccal fold and posterior to the casts to replicate all anatomic structures.
- Excess material in the tongue area has been smoothed.

Boxing the Impression. In the boxing method, a strip of boxing wax is used to surround the impression, forming a wall into which the gypsum is poured (Fig. 6.13, upper-left image). The wax should not distort the impression. It should extend at least 0.5 inch higher than the highest point of the impression and create a base that is parallel to the occlusal plane.

STORAGE

Gypsum products can absorb water from the environment. Humidity and close proximity to water sources will adversely affect the powder. Initially this exposure will accelerate the setting reaction by producing established sites of crystallization. After prolonged exposure, the setting reaction is retarded because of decreased solubility of the crystals by the formation of a dihydrate layer on the hemihydrate particles.

Gypsum should be stored in airtight, moisture-proof containers. To avoid prolonged exposure to moisture, open plaster bins are recommended only if there is rapid turnover of the products.

 Clinical Tip

Avoid reaching into the plaster bin with wet hands or spatulas. It will affect the set of the material that has been contaminated. Products offered in preweighed envelopes are commonly used in offices where the turnover of gypsum is low.

CLEANUP

Gypsum mixing and handling equipment must be kept meticulously clean. As previously mentioned, set gypsum particles inadvertently included with freshly mixed gypsum will increase the setting time. Bowls, spatulas, mechanical dental vibrators, and mixing devices should be cleaned of all traces of gypsum as soon as possible after manipulation.

> **! Caution**
> Remember that all excess material should be placed in the trash and not rinsed down sink drains, where it will likely clog pipes. Equipment should then be thoroughly rinsed under running water. Sinks in gypsum-handling areas should be fitted with plaster traps to catch any excess paster that inadvertently gets rinsed down the drain.

INFECTION CONTROL AND SAFETY ISSUES

Disinfecting the Impression and Casts

The need for infection control measures to extend into the dental laboratory has been clearly documented.

- Routine disinfection of impressions should be done in the dental office. (A discussion of disinfecting agents and procedures for disinfecting impressions are presented in Chapter 5.)
- Disinfection of impressions is the best way to prevent the introduction of contaminants into the laboratory area.
- If this has not been done, the impression and all equipment, such as plaster spatulas and dental vibrators, must be handled with proper personal protective equipment or barriers.
- Casts should be completely set and stored for at least 24 hours before disinfecting to prevent attack by the chemicals on the surface of the cast.
- Casts should be sprayed rather than immersed in disinfecting solutions, because some studies have shown damage to the surface in only a few minutes in water-based solutions.
  - Solutions such as 1:10 sodium hypochlorite, iodophors, or chlorine dioxide have been shown to have minimal effect on cast surfaces when used in this manner.

Safety Measures

Whenever working with powdered gypsum products a mask should be worn to prevent inhaling the fine powders. A mask should also be worn during trimming of casts as aerosols are produced by the model trimmer that can be inhaled. Protective glasses must always be worn for both the pouring and trimming of casts. Make sure fingers are kept away from the abrasive wheel.

SEPARATING THE IMPRESSION FROM THE CAST

Once the gypsum has set, the impression, tray, and cast must be separated (Procedure 6.4). When the impression is poured, care should be taken to make sure the gypsum does not flow onto the tray, which locks it into the set gypsum.

To separate the cast:
- Begin by cutting the excess gypsum away from the periphery of the tray
- Gently ease a laboratory knife under the tray and lift the tray slightly in several areas
- Use the impression material as a cushion to avoid gouging the anatomic portion of the cast
  - Remember, gypsum products have very low tensile strength
  - Do not rock the tray back and forth too much; this may result in breaking the teeth of the cast

TRIMMING THE CASTS

Trimming of models with a model trimmer is done to produce an attractive, symmetric model with easy access to all anatomic portions of the model and a base of sufficient bulk for stability.

- Bases made from dental stone should be soaked in water for 5 to 10 minutes before trimming to saturate the stone, making it easier to trim.
- Anatomic portions should never be soaked.
  - Saturation of the teeth may lead to a change in surface texture and, in the case of plaster, may make the teeth more susceptible to chipping.

Trimming Method

The cast should be trimmed so:
- All cuts are proportional.
- The base makes up one-third of the total depth.
- The anatomic portion is two-thirds of the total depth.
- The occlusal plane is parallel with the base.
- The periphery of the largest arch is trimmed first.
- The smaller arch is articulated with a wax bite and trimmed to match (see Procedure 5.5 for a description of wax bite registration).
- The outer borders are cut to the depth of the vestibule and include all muscle attachments, retromolar pads, and tuberosities.
  - If there are facially inclined or rotated teeth, the outside borders should be extended symmetrically to include these anatomic structures.
- The anterior portion of the maxillary arch is cut to a point at the midline, and the anterior portion of the mandibular arch is rounded from canine to canine (Fig. 6.14) (see Procedure 6.5 for detailed instruction on trimming models).

 Do You Recall?

What portion of the dental cast should be soaked prior to trimming?

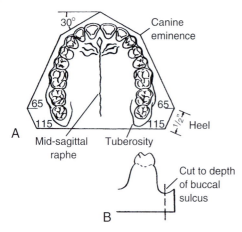
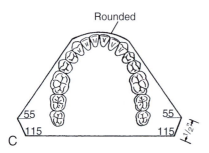

FIG. 6.14 Line drawing of landmarks, angles, and cuts of art portion of diagnostic casts: **(A)** Maxillary cast. **(B)** Cut to depth of the vestibule. **(C)** Mandibular cast. (From Bird DL, Robinson DS. *Torres and Ehrlich Modern Dental Assisting*. 9th ed. Elsevier; 2009.)

Criteria for Evaluation of Trimmed Diagnostic Casts

- Anatomic portion accounts for two-thirds of the total depth, and the base portion for one-third of the total depth.
- Bases of the maxillary and mandibular casts should be parallel with the occlusal planes and with each other.
- Posterior borders of both casts are at right angles to the base and will stand together when articulated on end.
- Posterior portions include retromolar pads and tuberosities.
- Side borders are perpendicular to the base, symmetric, and trimmed to the depth of the vestibule.
- Anterior borders are perpendicular to the base and are trimmed to the depth of the vestibule.
- Anterior borders of the maxillary cast form a point at the midline and are rounded from cuspid to cuspid for the mandibular cast.
- Mandibular casts have a smoothed tongue space.
- Maxillary and mandibular casts are labeled with the patient's name and date.

> **Caution**
> Exercise care when using the model trimmer. Always wear protective eyewear and mask, establish a flat surface 90 degrees from the abrasive wheel from which to trim, and pay attention to your hand positions. The abrasive wheel can rapidly abrade skin and fingernails! Use even, steady pressure with both hands while trimming. To maintain the abrasive surface of the trimming wheel, establish and maintain an adequate flow of water on the trimming wheel when in use so that it does not clog with gypsum. Clean the wheel and work surface of all gypsum products immediately after finishing.

COMPOSITION AND PROPERTIES OF DENTAL WAXES

COMPOSITION OF WAXES

Dental waxes are composed of a mixture of components from natural and synthetic sources.
- Natural waxes are produced from:
  - Plants—used in carnauba wax
  - Insects—used in beeswax
  - Minerals—used in paraffin and ceresin wax

These natural waxes contribute properties to the wax but are rarely used in their pure form.
- Natural waxes are combined or mixed with synthetic waxes consisting of:
  - Gums
  - Fats
  - Oils
  - Resins
  - Coloring agents

Each component is added to attain the physical properties desirable for the wax application. The components of waxes allow them to be sticky, solid, or liquid depending on the temperature of the wax. Use of the wax will determine properties that are desirable for its application.

PROPERTIES OF WAXES

Important properties of waxes in general, and of dental waxes in particular, include the following:
- Melting range
- Flow
- Excess residue
- Thermal expansion

The operator must consider these properties when selecting a wax, as well as during manipulation of the wax.

MELTING RANGE

Dental waxes have a **melting range**, a range of temperatures at which each component of the wax will start to soften and then flow. The components with lower melting points will soften first; then, as the temperature is increased, more components will soften and the wax will eventually flow and become a liquid or vaporize. Because wax is unstable, the operator must use care to prevent its distortion. Controlling the temperature of the wax allows operator control of the viscosity and flow of the wax. In many cases, the operator does not want the wax to flow but only to soften. A flame source is needed if a flowable state is desired. To prevent distortion, the melting range must be higher than the temperature of the environment. This is especially important in hot climates.

FLOW

Flow is the movement of wax as molecules slip over each other. As the temperature of the wax increases, the viscosity of the wax decreases until the wax becomes a liquid. Control of the flow and the melting range is important in manipulating wax. If a wax were capable of flowing at room temperature, it would be very difficult to control. However, even at mouth temperature, there is a point at which flow is undesirable. If you were using a wax for a wax bite registration, you would not want it to flow at mouth temperature, causing distortion of the wax. It is important that the wax not require temperatures much greater than mouth temperature to soften, or it would be uncomfortable when placed in the mouth of the patient. A melting range that is only slightly higher than mouth temperature is desirable for this wax application. For laboratory purposes, waxes may have a much higher melting range. However, even for laboratory purposes, high melting ranges may be undesirable. If you want to use a wax in the boxing of an impression, for example, it is much more desirable to mold the wax, using the heat of your hands or warm water, rather than using a flame.

EXCESS RESIDUE

It is important that all wax be removed from the object onto which it is melted. If **excess residue** remains after the wax is removed, this may result in inaccuracies in the object being produced. This is especially important in the lost wax technique, which requires that the wax pattern be completely melted out of the investment mold.

THERMAL EXPANSION

Waxes expand when heated and contract when cooled; the thermal expansion and contraction of waxes is greater than that of any other dental material. This property is especially important for pattern waxes. If a wax is heated too far above the melting range or is heated unevenly, expansion above acceptable standards will result. Manufacturers provide temperature and handling guidelines for pattern waxes to prevent inaccuracies in the final casting. In addition, if waxes are allowed to stand, dimensional changes occur from the release of residual stress. Wax patterns should be invested within minutes of carving.

CLASSIFICATION OF WAXES

WAXES ARE GROUPED AS FOLLOWS:

- *Pattern waxes:* Pattern waxes include inlay wax, casting wax, and baseplate wax.
- *Processing waxes:* Processing waxes include boxing wax, utility wax, and sticky wax.
- *Impression waxes:* Impression waxes include corrective impression wax and bite registration wax.

Manufacturers produce these waxes in several forms, such as sticks, sheets, blocks, and tins. Waxes have unique coloring to distinguish them in use (Fig. 6.15).

PATTERN WAXES

Pattern waxes are used in the construction of metal castings and bases for dentures. The three types of pattern waxes are inlay wax, casting wax, and baseplate wax.

Inlay Wax

Inlay waxes are used to produce patterns for metal casting through the lost wax technique. There are three ADA specifications for inlay wax:
- Type A can be used directly in the mouth
  - Has a much lower melting range to prevent damage to the pulp of the tooth, for the comfort of the patient and the accuracy of the wax on removal
  - Because direct waxing is performed in the patient's mouth, all the limitations of working in the mouth and patient safety measures must be considered
  - Because of these limitations, most dentists prefer to use the indirect waxing technique and call on the expertise of a dental laboratory technician to produce the wax pattern and casting
- Type B (type I)
  - Melted onto a die outside the mouth in the indirect technique (Table 6.4) (see Fig. 6.6)
- Type C (type II)
  - Melted onto a die outside the mouth in the indirect technique (see Table 6.4 and Fig. 6.6).
  - Types B and C inlay waxes are supplied in sticks, pellets, and tins, generally in dark colors of red, blue, or green.
  - They are labeled hard, medium, and soft, which refers to their melting ranges.
  - ADA specification number 4 sets standards for pattern waxes: low thermal expansion, complete removal of excess residue, and appropriate melting ranges are important properties.

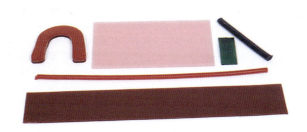

FIG. 6.15 Various forms of wax: sheets, ropes, and sticks. Impression wax *(top row, left)*, baseplate wax *(top row, middle left)*, casting wax *(top row, middle center)*, inlay wax *(top row, middle right)*, utility wax *(middle)*, and boxing wax *(bottom)*.

Table 6.4 Classification of Pattern Waxes, ADA Specification, and General Application

CLASSIFICATION OF DENTAL PATTERN WAXES

NAME OF WAX	ADA SPECIFICATION	USES
Inlay wax	Type A	Direct patterns in mouth
	Type B (type I)	Indirect patterns on dies
	Type C (type II)	
Casting wax		Construct metal framework of partial and complete denture
Baseplate wax	Type I	Impression in cool climates
	Type II	Impression in warm climates
	Type III	

This table identifies the different types of pattern waxes, the American Dental Association (ADA) specification, and uses of waxes in dentistry.

Casting Wax

Casting waxes are used to construct the metal framework of partial and complete dentures. These waxes come in sheets and preformed pieces for components of partial dentures. The physical properties of casting waxes are similar to those of inlay waxes, with the exception of melting range. Because these waxes are not softened in the mouth, the melting range is important only for laboratory procedures.

Baseplate Wax

Baseplate waxes are sheets (7.5 cm wide by 15 cm long) of wax that generally are pink in color, layered to produce the contours of the denture, and hold the position on which denture teeth are set (Fig. 6.16).

There are three ADA specifications for baseplate wax:
- Type I is softer and utilized in cool climates.
- Type II has a medium hardness and utilized in warm climates.
- Type III is harder and is also utilized in warm climates (see Table 6.4).

When the sheets of baseplate wax have been layered on resin denture bases to produce the contours of the denture and the denture teeth are set, the form is then tried into the mouth to establish denture dimensions. The wax must not distort at mouth temperatures. Baseplate wax may also be used for occlusal rims (see Chapter 14) and bite registration (see Chapter 5).

PROCESSING WAXES

Processing waxes are used primarily to aid in both clinical and laboratory dental procedures. The three types of processing waxes are boxing wax, utility wax, and sticky wax.

Boxing Wax

Boxing wax is used to form the base portion of a gypsum model. A 1.5-inch-wide red, green, or black strip of boxing wax is wrapped around an impression to produce a form into which gypsum is poured. This wax is easily manipulated and is also slightly tacky at room temperature, allowing it to adhere to itself to secure the boxed form.

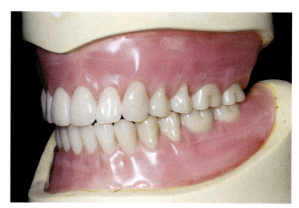

FIG. 6.16 A denture setup on baseplates.

Utility Wax

Also called *periphery wax*, comes in sticks, long square ropes, and round strips that are easily manipulated at room temperature. They may be used with boxing wax to aid in the pouring of an impression. Utility rope wax is used to adapt the periphery of the impression tray to customize the tray and aid in patient comfort (Fig. 6.17). The wax provides a better fit into the vestibule and control of movement of the impression material.

The pliable wax can also be used to block out undercuts around teeth or tissues prior to impression making to prevent the impression from locking in place (see Fig. 5.20). However, a block-out wax is available on the market for this specific purpose and is soft and pliable, allowing for easy placement into undercuts prior to an impression.

Utility wax ropes clear or ivory in color may be given to orthodontic patients to cover sharp brackets and wires that irritate lips, cheeks, and tongue. Utility wax sheets may also be layered to form a horseshoe shape and used for wax bite registrations; however, because they are pliable, they can distort easily. These waxes come in various colors of pink, white, and red.

Sticky Wax

Sticky wax comes in orange and red sticks that at room temperature are hard and brittle, but when heated under a flame become soft and sticky. Sticky wax is

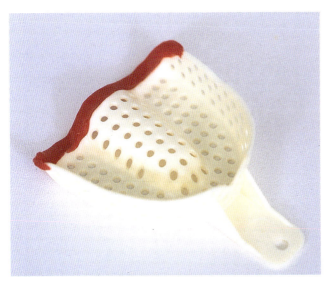

FIG. 6.17 Utility wax used on the posterior of the impression tray to extend the tray and make the fit more comfortable for the patient. (From Bird DL, Robinson DS. *Modern Dental Assisting*. 12th ed. Elsevier; 2018.)

used to adhere components of metal, gypsum, or resin together temporarily during fabrication and repair. Because of its brittle nature at room temperature, even the slightest torque will fracture the wax. This is an important characteristic because it alerts the operator that distortion has occurred during manipulation.

IMPRESSION WAXES

Impression wax and impression wax compounds are thermoplastic materials used to obtain impressions of the oral structures. When heated, they become soft and able to take on a new form in the mouth; and when cooled, they harden and can be removed. These waxes and techniques for using them to take impressions are described further in Chapter 5. The two types of impression waxes are corrective impression wax and bite registration wax.

Corrective Impression Wax

Corrective impression wax is used in conjunction with other impression materials in the process of taking edentulous impressions. This wax flows at mouth temperature and is used within another impression material to correct undercut areas, to fill in small voids or to help develop a functional posterior palatal seal for maxillary complete denture impressions.

Bite Registration Wax

Bite registration wax is used to produce wax bite registrations for articulation of models. The preformed U-shaped wax is often reinforced with metal particles to provide stability. However, similar to corrective impression wax, this wax is susceptible to distortion at temperatures only slightly higher than mouth temperature and must be carefully monitored. Because of this limitation, silicone and other more stable impression materials have largely replaced wax for bite registrations. For fabrication of a wax bite registration, see Procedure 5.5.

OTHER WAXES UTILIZED IN THE DENTAL OFFICE

There are other waxes available on the market for special uses in the dental practice or laboratory setting. They are not included in the categories listed previously due to their specialized uses.

Orthodontic Wax

This wax is utilized for patients experiencing pain and irritation of the soft oral tissues from teeth movement while wearing braces. The orthodontic wax is applied to the brackets, bands, or wires to prevent poking and scratching of the tissues. The product is clear to not be readily visible in the mouth. The wax may be provided in a portable container so the patient has access to the material regularly. A small chunk is taken out of the container and flattened out, and then the piece of wax is stuck to the area, causing the patient discomfort. The product is safe to ingest as there is a chance a small piece can become dislodged and swallowed.

Bite & Impression Wax

This wax is a composite material containing powdered aluminum to increase the heat retention, integrity of the compound, and provide the properties necessary for efficient modeling. This material is utilized when a dentist is making a new removable denture for a patient. During the jaw-registration stage, the wax is softened over an open flame and placed between the record bases (also called bite blocks). It will keep the two record bases together.

> **Do You Recall?**
>
> What type of wax is used to enclose an impression to make the base portion of the gypsum model?

MANIPULATION OF WAXES

Wax should be softened evenly:
- In dry heat
- With warm hands
- A warm water bath
- By flame
  - If a wax is softened by flame, it should be rotated above the flame so that it evenly softens or flows

Melted wax should be added in layers onto an object. As previously mentioned, because of changes caused by relaxation of residual stress, wax patterns should be invested within 30 minutes of carving. Waxes such as boxing and utility wax are slightly tacky at room temperature to help them adhere to themselves. They must remain dry if one is to take advantage of this characteristic.

To avoid distortion of waxes, they should be stored at or slightly below room temperature.

LOST WAX TECHNIQUE

Today's **lost wax technique** is much the same as those used by artisans several hundred years ago (Fig. 6.18).

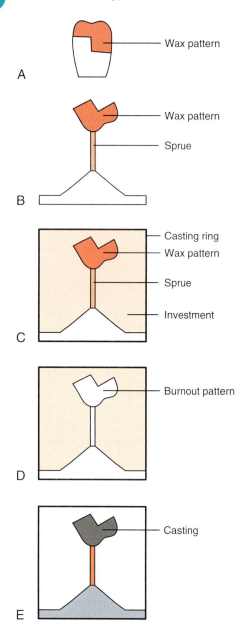

FIG. 6.18 Line drawing series on the lost wax technique: **(A)** Wax pattern on a die. **(B)** Wax pattern with sprue on a die. **(C)** Wax and sprue on sprue base and in investment ring. **(D)** Wax pattern vaporized from investment. **(E)** Metal casting of wax pattern.

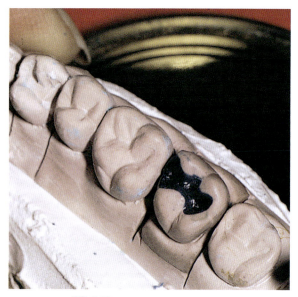

FIG. 6.19 An inlay waxing on a die.

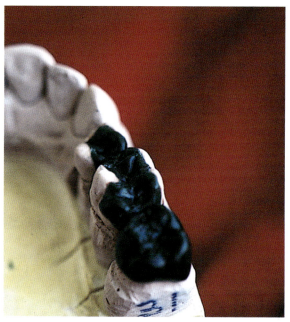

FIG. 6.20 Waxing of inlays and crown.

The process of creating a detailed wax pattern and converting it into a final restoration is known as *casting*.

The primary steps in the lost wax and casting procedure are as follows:

1. *Pouring the die:* An exact impression of the preparation is first obtained and poured into a high-strength die stone, forming the die.
2. *Waxing the die:* A detailed wax pattern of the restoration is carved on the die, including all anatomy, contours, occlusion, and proximal contacts (Figs. 6.19 and 6.20).
3. *Spruing the die:* A wax or plastic sprue is attached to the pattern to form the channel into which the molten metal will be forced. Multiple sprues may be used for a more complex wax pattern.
4. *Attaching the sprue base:* The sprue is attached to a sprue base; this forms the funnel to help guide the flow of molten metal into the wax pattern.
5. *Investing the wax pattern:* The pattern and attached sprue are encased in an investment ring into which gypsum-based investment is poured.
6. *Burning out the wax:* Once hardened, the sprue base is removed and the investment-enclosed pattern and sprue are heated in a burnout oven at high temperatures (500°C–700°C), causing the wax and the sprue to vaporize (lost wax), leaving an impression of the wax pattern in the now-empty space.
7. *Casting the restoration:* The molten metal is moved by centrifugal force through the empty channel formed by the sprue and into the empty wax pattern space.

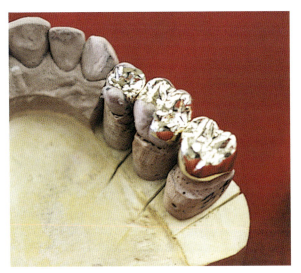

FIG. 6.21 Cleaned and polished metal castings of inlays and crowns.

8. *Final steps:* The metal cools, the sprue is removed, and the casting is cleaned and polished using a series of polishing steps to form a smooth and glossy surface. The polishing procedure must be accomplished without altering the margins, contacts, or occlusion of the restoration. It is now ready to be cemented onto the tooth (Fig. 6.21).

The accuracy of the entire casting process must be carefully executed to produce a clinically acceptable final restoration. The lost wax procedure takes several steps, each of which can cause inaccuracies in the final product. Properties of expansion and contraction in the impression material, die stone, wax, investment material, and casting must be controlled to achieve a final restoration that will have intimate contact with the tooth preparation. This accuracy will produce a cement interface of as little as 20 μm, ensuring a precise fit, with space for a very fine film of luting cement.

SUMMARY

Gypsum products are used to produce diagnostic and working models of the patient's hard and soft tissues. The properties of strength and hardness, setting expansion, and solubility are directly related to the amounts of water used in their construction. The density of the final product is related to these water amounts and to the size and shape of the particles that are manufactured. Manipulation factors such as the W/P ratio, rate of spatulation, and water temperature used in the mix have a great effect as well. The clinician must have a clear understanding of how these variables can be manipulated appropriately. The pouring of models requires meticulous attention to detail to produce a replica that accurately reflects the hard and soft tissues of the patient's oral cavity.

The dental auxiliary may have occasion to use dental waxes in a variety of clinical and laboratory procedures. Although waxes have inherent disadvantages in dimensional stability and control of flow, they are used successfully. The operator must keep in mind the limitations of each wax to use it to its best advantage.

INSTRUCTIONAL VIDEOS

See the Evolve Resources site for a variety of educational videos that reinforce the material covered in this chapter.

Procedure 6.1 Mixing Gypsum Products

See Evolve site for Competency Sheet.

Consider the following with this procedure: personal protective equipment is required for the clinician, and ensure appropriate safety protocols are followed.

EQUIPMENT/SUPPLIES (FIG. 6.22)
- Gypsum product
- Scale
- Water (room temperature)
- Water-measuring device
- Flexible rubber mixing bowl
- Broad-blade metal or plastic spatula
- Mechanical dental vibrator

PROCEDURE STEPS

1. Measure and pour the recommended amount of room temperature water into a clean, flexible, rubber mixing bowl.

   NOTE: Increasing or decreasing the water temperature is the preferred way to alter the working time.

2. Using another bowl or paper towel, weigh the recommended amount of gypsum powder onto the scale. Make sure to account for the weight of the bowl if you are using a bowl to transfer powder.

3. Sift the powder gradually into the water, allowing the particles to become wet—about 30 seconds.

   NOTE: Sifting minimizes the amount of air trapped in the mix.

4. Vigorously mix the material for about 60 seconds by wiping the spatula against the sides of the bowl to incorporate all the powder, removing excess air, until a smooth homogeneous mixture is obtained (Fig. 6.23).

   NOTE: The viscosity of the mix should be sufficient to allow the material to flow only under mechanical vibration.

5. Turn the dental vibrator on low/medium and place the bowl onto the work surface.

Continued

Procedure 6.1 Mixing Gypsum Products—cont'd

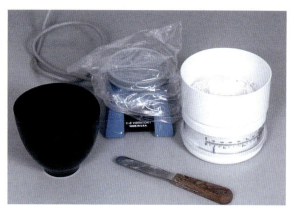

FIG. 6.22

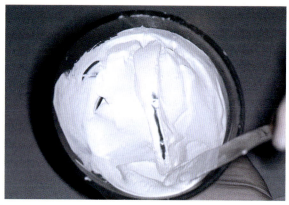

FIG. 6.23

6. Press the sides of the bowl inward with the palms of your hands, at the same time pressing the bowl downward on the work surface of the dental vibrator to remove all air incorporated during the mixing procedure. The air bubbles will rise to the surface of the mix.

NOTE: Vibrating the mix helps to remove air trapped during mixing.

7. Complete the preparation of the gypsum material within 2 minutes.

NOTE: This includes mixing and initial vibrating and allows for sufficient working time in pouring.

Procedure 6.2 Pouring the Cast: Anatomic Portion

See Evolve site for Competency Sheet.

Consider the following with this procedure: personal protective equipment is required for the clinician, and ensure appropriate safety protocols are followed.

EQUIPMENT/SUPPLIES (FIG. 6.24)
- Mask and safety glasses
- Mechanical dental vibrator
- Gypsum mixture
- Broad-blade metal or plastic spatula
- Small wax spatula
- Disinfected impression

PROCEDURE STEPS

1. Rinse the impression of all traces of disinfecting solution and tap the impression lightly over the sink until no more water can be shaken out or remove water with compressed air.
2. Holding the handle of the impression tray, place the impression tray onto the working surface of the mechanical vibrator. Rest the tray handle at an angle to the surface of the vibrator.
   Hold the tray at a slight angle to the working table of the vibrator to aid in the flow of the material. The speed of the vibrator should be adjusted only high enough to make the stone flow easily. Too much speed can incorporate bubbles into the mix. **NOTE:** To facilitate cleanup, cover the working surface of the mechanical vibrator with a disposable cover, such as a plastic bag.
3. Pick up a small increment of gypsum mixture from the flexible missing bowl, no bigger than a large pea, on the end of the small wax spatula.
   NOTE: Addition of small increments of material allows for control of the amount of material flowing into the tooth indentations.

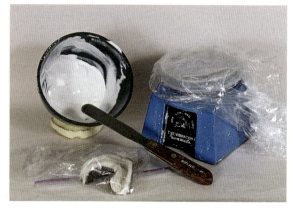

FIG. 6.24

Procedure 6.2 Pouring the Cast: Anatomic Portion—cont'd

4. Place the increment of mixture at one of the most posterior corners of the impression (Fig. 6.25).
5. Allow the mixture to flow into the tooth indentations from one side to the next of each indentation while controlling the flow of the mixture under vibration to force air out of each indentation. Use small enough increments to control the flow and tilt the impression as needed to aid the speed of the flow.

   NOTE: Air bubbles are formed when the mixture moves too fast over the tooth indentations, trapping air in the impression, or when the mixture will not flow sufficiently to fill the indentations.
6. Continue adding small increments of mixture in the same area while watching the material flow toward the anterior portion of the impression (Fig. 6.26).
7. Tilt the impression forward and continue adding increments across the anterior portion of the impression, making sure to control the flow so that air is not trapped.
8. Tilt the impression toward the opposite posterior portion and continue the addition of increments until the flow reaches the other end of the impression (Fig. 6.27).
9. When all of the tooth indentations are filled with the gypsum mixture, begin adding larger increments with the broad-blade spatula until the impression is slightly overfilled (Fig. 6.28).

   NOTE: Lift the impression from the vibrator to prevent the material from flowing over the impression tray.
10. Vibrate the entire tray for two to three seconds to settle all increments. Do not smooth the surface of the material.

    You may add an additional two or three small mounds of material to the top of the gypsum to help facilitate attachment to the base. NOTE: A roughened surface will allow for better attachment with the base.
11. Cleanup: Wipe all excess gypsum from the bowl and place the gypsum in the trash. Rinse and thoroughly clean the bowl and spatula under running water in a sink fitted with a plaster trap. Remove the plastic bag from the mechanical vibrator and clean the vibrator with a wet paper towel as needed.

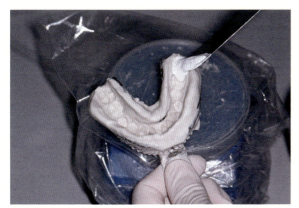

FIG. 6.25

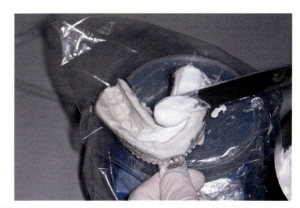

FIG. 6.27

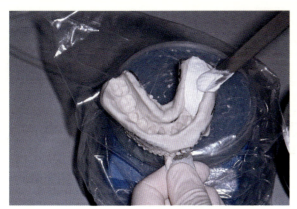

FIG. 6.26

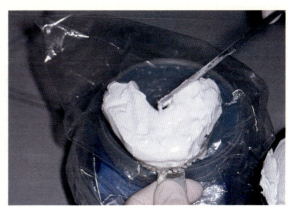

FIG. 6.28

Procedure 6.3 Pouring the Cast: Art (or Base) Portion

See Evolve site for Competency Sheet.

Consider the following with this procedure: *personal protective equipment is required for the clinician, and ensure appropriate safety protocols are followed.*

EQUIPMENT/SUPPLIES
- Mask and safety glasses
- Glass tile or base former
- Broad-blade metal or plastic spatula
- Gypsum mixture
- Poured impression

PROCEDURE STEPS: DOUBLE-POUR METHOD

1. Allow the poured impression to set for at least 10 minutes.
   NOTE: This prevents the gypsum material from "slumping" away from the impression when it is inverted, causing distortion in the cast.
2. Prepare a mixture of gypsum, using less water than typically recommended for the W/P ratio.
   You may use plaster to pour the art portion of a model even if the anatomic portion is poured with a different product. By using plaster, you will save on the cost of the more expensive stone products and if model trimming is necessary, you will save time as plaster trims much more easily than stone. NOTE: Using less water will produce a thicker mix, which is necessary to accommodate the weight of the poured impression when it is inverted.
3. Place the mixture onto the glass tile or into a base former. You should have a mass at least 0.5 inch thick and slightly larger than the dimension of the filled impression and tray (Fig. 6.29).
   NOTE: If using a base former, make sure you choose one large enough for the impression and select the correct arch shape for your impression: pointed for maxillary and rounded for mandibular.
4. Invert the poured impression onto the base, making sure the occlusal plane remains parallel with the base. Use the tray handle and the top of the impression tray as your guide.
   NOTE: If using a base former, you will also need to make sure you keep the midline centered.
5. Very gently move the impression back and forth to bring the anatomic and art portions together. Be careful to prevent the filled tray from sinking into the base.
6. Bring the base material up with a broad-based spatula to fill the heels and sides of the impression and along the tray periphery, taking care not to lock the tray in with excess material (Figs. 6.30 and 6.31).
   NOTE: Make sure there are no large air pockets trapped between the art and base portions.
7. Smooth the tongue area of the mandibular impression level with the tray periphery.
   NOTE: Some clinicians may choose to use a damp paper towel to fill the tongue area and prevent gypsum from flowing into the space.
8. You may choose to carefully remove some of the base material to begin to replicate the angle of the trimmed model. This will cut down the amount of time spent trimming the model on the model trimmer. Make sure the model has reached its initial set (loss of gloss) before attempting this.
9. Allow the gypsum to set completely before separating the model for the impression—45 to 60 minutes.
10. When the final set has been reached, the gypsum, impression, and cast are separated.

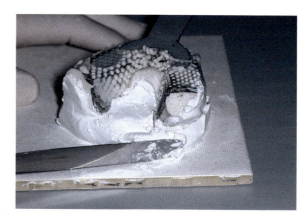

FIG. 6.30

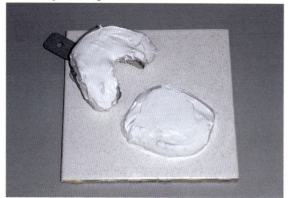

FIG. 6.29

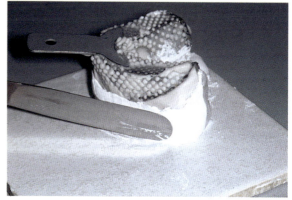

FIG. 6.31

Procedure 6.4 Separating the Impression From the Cast

See Evolve site for Competency Sheet.

Consider the following with this procedure: *personal protective equipment is required for the clinician, and ensure appropriate safety protocols are followed.*

EQUIPMENT/SUPPLIES
- Safety glasses
- Laboratory knife
- Plaster nippers

PROCEDURE STEPS
1. Remove the model from the glass tile or base former.
   NOTE: Do not allow agar-type impressions to remain longer than 1 hour without separating, as surface detail will be diminished.
2. Trim all excess gypsum from the tray at the tray edge with a laboratory knife (Fig. 6.32).
   NOTE: Ensure that no part of the tray is connected to the gypsum.
3. Loosen the tray from the impression material by placing the laboratory knife between the tray and the impression material in several areas and gently prying the two apart.
4. Attempt to lift the tray in an upward motion; if the tray does not lift, determine the location of the locked area and remove it with the laboratory knife or plaster nippers (Fig. 6.33).
   NOTE: Remember that gypsum products have very poor tensile strength; too much rocking of the tray will likely result in broken teeth.

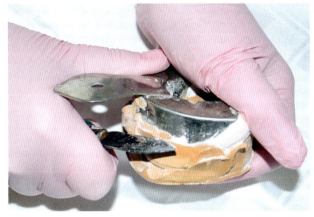

FIG. 6.32

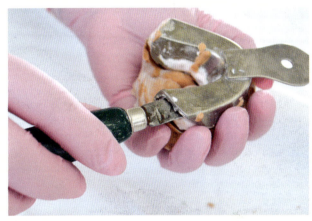

FIG. 6.33

Procedure 6.5 Trimming Diagnostic Casts

See Evolve site for Competency Sheet.

Consider the following with this procedure: *personal protective equipment is required for the clinician, and ensure appropriate safety protocols are followed.*

EQUIPMENT/SUPPLIES (FIG. 6.34)
- Safety glasses and mask
- Maxillary and mandibular diagnostic casts
- Wax bite registration
- Measuring devices; millimeter ruler and compass
- Pencil
- Laboratory knife
- Plaster nippers
- Model trimmer

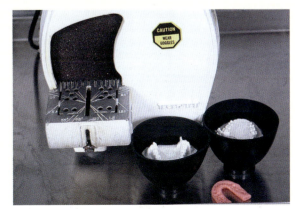

FIG. 6.34

Continued

Procedure 6.5 Trimming Diagnostic Casts—cont'd

PROCEDURE STEPS

1. Soak the art portion of casts for 5 to 10 minutes in water. The art portion of the cast should soak for a minimum of 5 minutes.
   NOTE: Do not allow teeth to soak in water, as this may cause chipping of plaster or surface roughness of plaster or stone.
2. Cut excess gypsum distal to the retromolar pads and tuberosities with plaster nippers (Fig. 6.35).
   NOTE: Excess gypsum in this area may prevent models from being articulated.
3. Remove small bubbles (blebs) of gypsum on the occlusal surfaces with a laboratory knife or pointed dental instrument.
   NOTE: Removal of excess material allows for complete articulation with the wax bite.
4. Check the working table of the model trimmer to make sure it is secure and at a 90-degree angle to the abrasive trimming wheel.
5. Adjust water flow over the trimming wheel to allow for sufficient water to clean the wheel.

Base Cut

6. Place the maxillary cast teeth side down on a cushion of evenly distributed layers of paper towels on the laboratory bench and rock forward so that the anterior teeth touch the laboratory bench. The cast should be parallel to the bench top. Measure from the teeth to the base of the cast; the anatomic portion of the cast should be two-thirds of the total height, with the art portion accounting for one-half of the total height. Mark the models with a compass to this line (Fig. 6.36).
   NOTE: The occlusal surfaces of the cast are parallel to the laboratory bench, with the anterior teeth touching the surface.
7. Trim the base to the marked line, periodically stopping to evaluate your progress. Remember: You can always continue to cut; if you cut away too much, you may need to retake and repour the impression. Removing material slowly allows the clinician the opportunity to reevaluate progress to ensure excess material is not removed.
   NOTE: You may first need to make a flat back cut to secure casts on the working table of the trimmer. Ensure you do not remove too much material if this cut is required (see step 9 below).
8. Repeat steps 6 and 7 with the mandibular cast. When occluded, the casts should be between 2 and 2.5 inches.

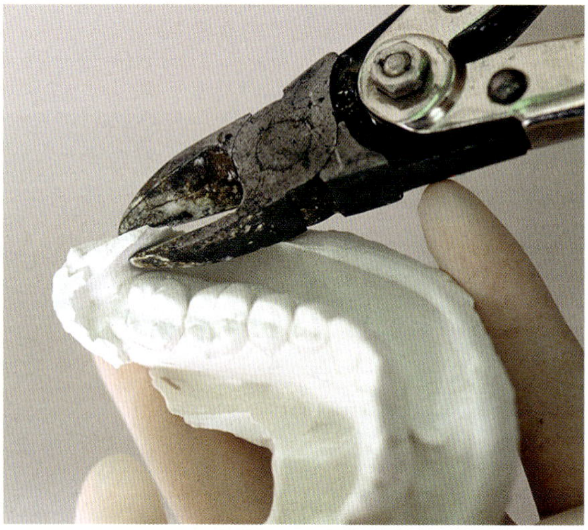

Side and Back Cuts

9. Measure the back by making a straight line 3 mm behind the retromolar pads of the mandibular cast or tuberosities of the maxillary cast.
10. Trim back to this line (Fig. 6.37). The maxillary and mandibular casts' back cuts should be parallel with one another.

NOTE: Trim the longest cast first, and then articulate casts with the wax bite, and match the opposite cast's

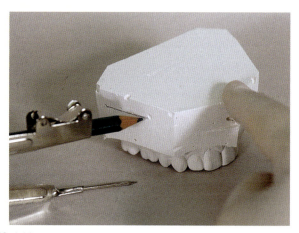

FIG. 6.36

FIG. 6.35

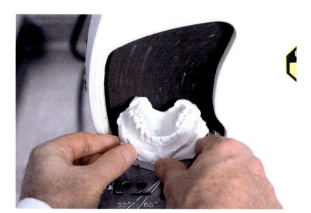

FIG. 6.37

Procedure 6.5 Trimming Diagnostic Casts—cont'd

back cut with the models articulated (Fig. 6.38). Do not trim away any anatomy on either cast.

11. Measure the sides 3 mm from the buccal bone at the widest portion of the arch (usually the molar area) and 3 mm at the canine eminence. Mark the cast with a straight edge to connect these points.
12. With the models articulated, trim the side cuts symmetrical to these lines (Fig. 6.39). Again, the maxillary and mandibular casts' side cuts should be parallel with one another.

    NOTE: Do not trim past the depth of the vestibule. It is important to maintain the anatomy inclusive of soft tissue.

Anterior Cut: Maxillary Cast

13. Measure 3 mm labial to the midline between central incisors. Measure from the depth of the vestibule or the most facially inclined tooth. Mark the casts with a straight edge to connect this point and the point 3 mm from the canine eminence.
14. Trim the anterior cuts symmetrically to form a midline point.

    NOTE: The maxillary cast forms a point between the central incisors. This is different than the mandibular arch.

Anterior Cut: Mandibular Cast

15. Measure as previously described, 3 mm from several places in the anterior region of the mandibular arch; connect these points with the point of the canine eminence to form a curved line. Trim the anterior cut of the mandible to this curved line.

Heel Cuts

16. Trim the heel cuts at a 90-degree angle to a line formed by connecting the canine eminence point to the side/back cut of the opposite side. The maxillary and mandibular casts' heel cuts should be parallel to one another.

    NOTE: This line is approximately 0.5 inch and symmetric on each side.

Optional Steps
Finishing/Polishing

17. Inspect the models for small air voids; small voids may be filled by dipping a small paint brush in water and fresh mix of gypsum. Place the brush in the water and then grab a small amount of gypsum on the brush and add to the area of the air void.

    NOTE: Unless requested by the dentist, do not fill in air voids in areas critical to the case.
18. Using a laboratory knife, trim the contours of the peripheral borders of the model above the mucobuccal fold to form soft scalloped shapes.
19. Using model polish and a soft buffing cloth, polish the cast to a shine (Fig. 6.40).

Labeling/Storage

20. Using a permanent ink marker, label the base or the back cut of the cast with the patient's name and date.
21. Place the cast in a model box labeled with the patient's name, the date of the impression, and the case number.

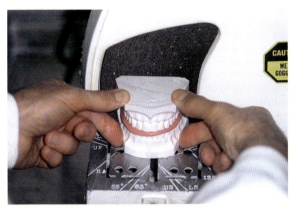

FIG. 6.38

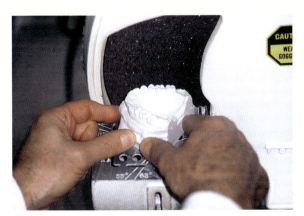

FIG. 6.39

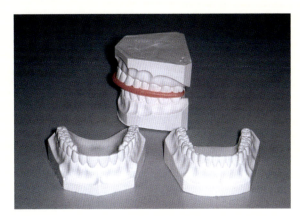

FIG. 6.40

CHAPTER 6 Gypsum and Wax Products

Get Ready for Exams!

Review Questions

Select the one correct response for each of the following multiple-choice questions.

1. What does carefully controlled calcination under steam pressure in a closed container produce?
   a. Plaster
   b. Dental stone
   c. High-strength stone
   d. High-strength, high-expansion stone
2. To decrease the working time of a gypsum product, without changing any physical properties, it is best to:
   a. Decrease the W/P ratio
   b. Increase the rate of spatulation
   c. Increase the water temperature
   d. Decrease the water temperature
3. What is the main difference between model plaster and dental stone?
   a. Chemical formula
   b. Solubility in water
   c. Particle size and shape
   d. Accelerators and retarders
4. The most appropriate type of gypsum product to use for orthodontic casts is:
   a. Type I
   b. Type II
   c. Type III
   d. Type IV
5. Initial setting can be detected clinically by:
   a. Loss of gloss
   b. The end of the exothermic reaction
   c. A change in color
   d. Testing to see whether the material is hard enough to separate from the impression
6. What is the area of the diagnostic cast that records the hard and soft tissues?
   a. Art portion
   b. Base
   c. Anatomic portion
   d. Impression
7. A study model is a positive reproduction. An impression is a negative reproduction.
   a. Both statements are true.
   b. Both statements are false.
   c. The first statement is true and the second statement is false.
   d. The first statement is false and the second statement is true.
8. Material that will act as retarders for the set of gypsum products include:
   a. Saliva
   b. Set gypsum products
   c. Slurry water from the model trimmer
   d. None of the above are considered retarders
9. It is important to consider the following statements when pouring an impression:
   a. Alginate impressions should remain unseparated from the model for only 1 hour.
   b. When the single-step method is used, the material poured into the impression must reach the initial set before the base is poured.
   c. Gypsum should be mixed as wet as possible to allow for sufficient working time.
   d. A and B.
   e. A and C.
10. What are diagnostic casts used for?
    a. Patient education
    b. Fabricating dentures
    c. Fabricating crowns
    d. Fabricating orthodontic appliances
11. The melting range for wax can best be described as:
    a. The point at which the wax flows
    b. The point at which the wax softens
    c. The required temperature of the heat source
    d. A combination of melting points of the individual components of wax
12. A direct wax pattern is fabricated in the mouth. Which property of the inlay wax is the most important?
    a. Flow
    b. Residual stress
    c. Melting range
    d. Excess residue
13. A wax pattern is invested and burned out by the lost wax procedure. Which property of the inlay wax is the most important?
    a. Melting range
    b. Flow
    c. Residual stress
    d. Removal of excess residue
14. Which wax is used to form a base into which to pour a gypsum model is?
    a. Boxing wax
    b. Sticky wax
    c. Pattern wax
    d. Baseplate wax
15. Utility wax ropes are used to:
    a. Hold components together for repair
    b. Make forms for wax bite registrations
    c. Make corrections in undercut areas of impressions
    d. Adapt the periphery of impression trays

For answers to Review Questions, see the Appendix.

Case-Based Discussion Topics

1. For each of the following situations, which gypsum material would be the best choice?
   - The assistant has taken an impression for an orthodontic case study.
   - The dentist has taken an impression for a space maintainer.
   - The hygienist has taken an impression for a custom bleaching tray.
   - The expanded-function assistant has taken an impression for a full gold crown.
2. How would each of the following situations be best handled?
   - *You need to make a custom tray for an appointment in progress and have just taken the alginate impression. How would you accelerate the setting time of the gypsum product you select?*

Get Ready for Exams!—cont'd

- You have fast-set plaster in your office and wish to mix enough material to pour two arches. How would you increase the working time?
- Several air voids are present on the surfaces of the teeth on a diagnostic cast. What factors may have caused this?
- When you are working on a cast, the teeth chip and crumble easily. What factors may have caused this?

3. A gypsum model is articulated with a wax bite registration and is left in the dental laboratory over a hot weekend. The assistant, when coming in on Monday, discovers that the model is no longer in the correct occlusion.
   - What property of the dental wax most likely caused the problem?
   - What could have been done to avoid this problem?

4. A gypsum model is being poured, using boxing wax. The wax is formed around the impression but will not hold in place.

What can the assistant do to the wax to help it adhere to itself and the tray?

5. After the problem in case 4 is corrected, the impression is poured. The hygienist, on separating the boxed model, finds that there is a thin layer of wax on the base portion.

What property of the wax most likely caused this and what property of the gypsum product contributed to this problem?

6. A final impression for an edentulous case is corrected with corrective impression wax. The impression is then sent to the dental laboratory.

What precautions must be considered when sending the impression?

BIBLIOGRAPHY

Bird DL, Robinson DS: *Modern dental assisting,* ed 13., St. Louis, 2021, Elsevier.

Brukl CE, McConnell RM, Norling BK, et al: Influence of gauging water composition on dental stone expansion and setting time, *J Prosthetic Dent,* 1984.

Darby ML, Walsh MM: *Dental hygiene: theory and practice,* ed 4., St. Louis, 2015, Saunders.

King BB, Norling BK, Seals R: Gypsum compatibility of antimicrobial alginates after spray disinfection, *J Prosthodontics,* 1994.

Kotsiomite E, McCabe JF: Experimental wax mixtures for dental use, *J Oral Rehabil.* 24:517–521, 1997.

Kotsiomite E, McCabe JF: Waxes for functional impressions, *J Oral Rehabil.* 23:114, 1996.

Powers JM, Wataha JC: *Dental materials: foundations and applications,* ed 11., St. Louis, 2017, Elsevier.

Robinson DS: *Essentials of dental assisting,* ed 7., St Louis, 2023, Elsevier.

Sakaguchi RL, Ferracane J, Powers JM: *Craig's restorative dental materials,* ed 14., St. Louis, 2019, Elsevier.

von Fraunhofer JA, Spiers RR: Accelerated setting of dental stone, *J Prosthet Dent.* 49:859–869, 1983.

Van Noort R: *Introduction to dental materials,* ed 4., London, 2013, Mosby.

7 Principles of Bonding

http://evolve.elsevier.com/Eakle/materials/

Chapter Objectives

On completion of this chapter, the student should be able to:

1. Discuss the effects of acid etching on enamel and dentin.
2. List the basic steps of bonding.
3. Explain the differences between bonding to enamel and bonding to dentin.
4. Discuss the significance of the smear layer.
5. Describe "wet" dentin bonding.
6. Compare etch-and-rinse and self-etch bonding techniques.
7. Identify how the hybrid layer is formed and its importance in bonding to dentin.
8. Explain how universal adhesives differ from etch-and-rinse and self-etch adhesives.
9. Discuss the factors that interfere with good bonding.
10. Discuss the adverse effects of microleakage at restoration margins.
11. Demonstrate proper etching of enamel and dentin with phosphoric acid as permitted by state law.
12. Apply a bonding system to etched enamel and dentin as permitted by state law.

KEY TERMS

Bond or Bonding to connect or fasten; to bind. Items are bonded together at their surfaces in three main ways: (1) mechanical adhesion (physical interlocking), (2) chemical adhesion, or (3) a combination of the two

Adhesion the act of sticking two things together. In dentistry, the term is used frequently to describe the bonding or cementation process. Chemical adhesion occurs when atoms or molecules of dissimilar substances bond together. Adhesion differs from cohesion, in which attraction among atoms and molecules of like (similar) materials holds them together

Bonding resin a low-viscosity resin that penetrates porosities and irregularities in the surface of the tooth or restoration created by acid etching for the purpose of facilitating bonding. Also called *bonding agent*

Etching the process of preparing the surface of a tooth or restoration with an acid for bonding. The most commonly used acid is phosphoric acid

Primer a low-viscosity resin applied as the first layer to penetrate etched surfaces to enhance bonding

Cure or Polymerize a reaction that links low molecular weight resin molecules (monomers) together into high molecular weight chains (polymers) that harden or set. The reaction can be initiated by strictly a chemical reaction (self-cure), by light in the blue wave spectrum (light cure), by a combination of the two (dual cure), or by heat

Wetting ability of a liquid to wet or intimately contact a solid surface. Water beading on a waxed car is an example of poor wetting

Wet Dentin Bonding bonding to dentin that is kept moist after acid etching to facilitate penetration of bonding resins into the etched dentin

Smear Layer a tenacious surface layer of debris resulting from cutting the tooth during cavity preparation. It is composed mostly of fine particles of cut tooth structure

Hydrophilic an attribute that allows a material to tolerate the presence of moisture

Hydrophobic an attribute that does not allow a material to tolerate or perform well in the presence of moisture

Hybrid Layer a resin-dentin layer formed by intermixing of the dentin bonding agent with etched dentin and the collagen fibrils exposed by acid etching. It serves as an excellent resin-rich layer onto which the restorative material, such as composite resin, can be bonded

Oxygen-Inhibited Layer (also called *air-inhibited layer*) a layer of unset resin on the surface of a polymerized resin that is prevented from curing by contact with oxygen in the air

Etch-and-Rinse Technique a clinical technique that includes etching of both enamel and dentin, then rinsing the etchant off as a separate step from the application of bonding agents. Products that use this technique are called etch-and-rinse bonding systems

Self-Etch Bonding System a bonding system that does not use a separate etching procedure with phosphoric acid. The acid is contained in the resin primer and no rinsing is needed

Selective Etching technique where enamel is etched first with phosphoric acid prior to the application of self-etch acidic primers that lack sufficient acidity to produce a good etch of the enamel

Universal Bonding System a bonding system capable of bonding to tooth structure as well as most restorative dental materials

Contamination contact with a substance that interferes with bonding or lessens the chemical or mechanical properties (e.g., contamination of the etched surface of the tooth with saliva before bonding)

Adhesive materials are used on a daily basis in the modern dental practice. They are beneficial for many restorative and preventive procedures. They provide a seal between the tooth and the restoration and seal the dentinal tubules to reduce postoperative sensitivity. They enhance retention of the restoration so that more conservative preparations can be made, and they may increase the strength of the prepared tooth to resist fracture. Materials bonded to tooth structure may themselves be more resistant to fracture than materials that are not bonded. For example, porcelain veneers are thin, brittle, and fragile until they are bonded to the tooth, and then they are very fracture resistant.

Adhesives are used for a wide variety of dental procedures. The dental auxiliary must be familiar with the terms and processes used in bonding various restorative and preventive materials to be a knowledgeable, effective member of the dental team. The auxiliary will be involved in helping the dentist perform bonding procedures many times each day. In some states, trained hygienists and assistants may etch the tooth structure and apply bonding agents and place sealants and composite resins. Additionally, the dental hygienist may perform periodontal treatments that might affect bonded restorations. Therefore it is important that the dental auxiliary understands the physical properties and handling characteristics of the bonding materials and the processes involved in their use.

BASIC PRINCIPLES OF BONDING

In dentistry the term **bond or bonding** is used in several ways. It is used to describe the process of attaching restorative materials, such as a composite resin, to a tooth by **adhesion** (the attraction of atoms or molecules of two different contacting surfaces). When describing cosmetic restorations such as porcelain or composite veneers, patients often use the term *bonding*, for example, "The dentist is bonding my front teeth." Bonding also is the basis for several other dental procedures, such as the placement of orthodontic brackets and fixed retainers. It is used to describe some of the materials used in the process of placing restorations. For example, bonding resin is placed on the etched tooth surface before light curing.

Two basic mechanisms occur to bond a restorative material to tooth structure:
- Mineral (hydroxyapatite) is removed by acid from the surface of enamel and/or dentin to create microscopic porosities.
- **Bonding resin** is infused into the porosities to create resin tags that lock into the tooth structure when hardened.

The first step in the bonding process involves removing plaque and debris from the surface. This can be done with a slurry of pumice and water applied with a bristle brush or rubber cup (Fig. 7.1). Then, an acid is used for **etching** the enamel and/or dentin to remove mineral from the surface to create roughness and microscopic porosity.

Next, a thin resin bonding agent or **primer** is flowed over the etched surface, which penetrates into the microscopic pores. When the primer hardens (**cures** or **polymerizes**), it creates projections called *resin tags* that lock into the tooth, creating a mechanical bond called *micromechanical retention*. The resin primer prepares the surface for a slightly thicker bonding resin that will chemically bond to the primer. Composite resin will chemically bond to this enamel/dentin-resin surface.

SURFACE WETTING

Acid etching also increases the ability of liquids to wet the surface of the tooth by creating high surface energy. High surface energy helps to attract the resin to the etched surface. High surface energy can also attract contaminants (such as saliva), so good isolation is important. Good **wetting** increases the intimate contact of the bonding resin with the etched tooth structure, improving the penetration of resin to form tags and thereby improving the bond. Surfaces that are poorly wetted will cause beading of the liquid, similar to water on a newly waxed car. On an unwaxed car, the water easily spreads out and has a low angle of contact (Fig. 7.2). Bonding agents are usually not very thick, so they will flow readily and wet the etched surface.

ETCHING ENAMEL AND DENTIN

ENAMEL ETCHING

Michael Buonocore introduced acid etching of enamel into dentistry in the 1950s after observing industrial applications of 85% phosphoric acid on metal to enhance adhesion of paints and resins. Enamel is composed of thousands of rods (prisms) that extend from the dentin to the tooth surface. Each rod has many millions of crystals composed of hydroxyapatite with about 20% carbonate inclusions. These carbonate imperfections add to the solubility of the crystals in acid. Proteins, lipids, and water in small quantities are found in microscopic spaces between the crystals.

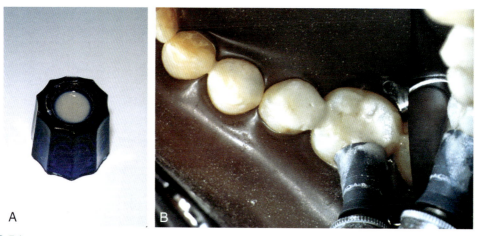

FIG. 7.1 Cleaning the tooth before bonding: **(A)** Slurry of pumice and water used to remove plaque, pellicle, and debris prior to acid etching. **(B)** Rubber cup with slurry of pumice used at low speed to clean the enamel surface before bonding procedures.

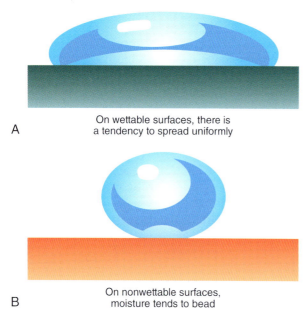

FIG. 7.2 Acid etching of enamel increases its ability to be wetted by a resin bonding agent, resulting in a stronger bond. **(A)** A low contact angle indicates good wetting as the liquid spreads over the surface. **(B)** A high contact angle indicates poor wetting as the liquid beads on the surface like water on a waxed car.

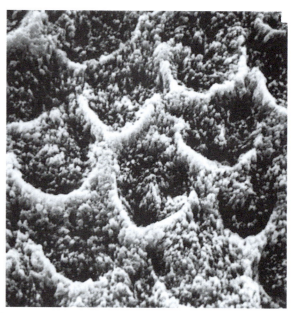

FIG. 7.3 An etched enamel surface, as seen in this scanning electron micrograph, has numerous peaks and valleys and surface roughness that provide retention and greatly increase the surface area for bonding. (From Phillips RW, Moore BK. Synthetic resins. In: *Elements of Dental Materials for Dental Hygienists and Dental Assistants.* Saunders; 1994.)

Etching of enamel removes a small portion of the surface, reduces the ends of the enamel rods, and opens microscopic porosities between adjacent rods (Fig. 7.3) creating a highly roughened surface with many tiny spaces and micropores into which the bonding resin can lock. The durability and strength of the bond to the enamel depend on how well the etch pattern is developed.

Among the many different acids tested, phosphoric acid provides the best etch pattern. It is used in concentrations ranging from 10% to 40%, but 37% is most commonly used.

> ### ⚠ Caution
> Do not rub or scrub the enamel surface with a hard instrument after etching. The portions of the enamel rods exposed by etching are very fragile and will break with light pressure. If this occurs, the available sites for resin tag formation will be greatly reduced and thus will affect the strength of the bond.

Etching Times
The enamel of permanent teeth is usually etched for 20 to 30 seconds with 37% phosphoric acid. Although etching times as short as 10 seconds appear to give

good clinical results in some teeth, research results suggest that 20 to 30 seconds is optimal. Highly mineralized teeth may be more resistant to etching and may require up to 60 seconds of etching. Primary teeth should be etched for longer periods (60 seconds or more) because the surface of the enamel has a prism pattern that is not as well structured and is irregular and thus is more resistant to deep resin tag formation.

The etched surface should have a frosty appearance when dried (Fig. 7.4). However, when a cavity preparation involves the etching of both enamel and dentin, and the preparation is left slightly moist for **wet dentin bonding**, it cannot be determined whether the enamel has a frosty appearance.

Etchant Liquid or Gel

The acid etchant comes as a liquid or a gel. Often, coloring agents are added to aid the practitioner in seeing where the etchant is on the tooth. Liquid etchants are usually applied with a brush, a small cotton pellet, or a small sponge. Gels are more popular because they stay in place, whereas liquids tend to run without control. Gels contain silica as a thickener and are usually applied by brush or dispensed from a syringe through a fine needle or brush tip (Fig. 7.5). The recommended rinsing time for acid gels is approximately 10 seconds or longer. Rinsing times shorter than 5 seconds may not remove residual silica. Rinsing times for liquid etchants can be shorter—5 to 10 seconds.

DENTIN ETCHING

The dentin has higher water and organic content (about 50% by volume) than enamel (only about 12% by volume) and lower mineral content (about 50% by volume) compared to enamel (88% by volume). Dentin contains a collagen matrix woven throughout the mineral component and a system of dentinal tubules through which fluids from the pulp flow.

Smear Layer

When a cavity preparation is cut with rotary or hand instruments, a layer of cutting debris forms on the surface of the prepared dentin and enamel. This layer, called the **smear layer**, is composed mostly of cut tooth structure and may also contain plaque, bacteria, and saliva (Fig. 7.6). The smear layer sticks tenaciously to the dentin surface, plugs the openings of dentinal tubules, and cannot be washed off with use of an air-water spray. The smear layer interferes with the formation of a bond to dentin.

Phosphoric Acid Etching of Dentin

Etching dentin with phosphoric acid dissolves the smear layer and smear plugs in the tubules first, and then dissolves portions of the hydroxyapatite crystals from the surface of the dentin, creating a porous surface and exposing the meshwork of collagen fibrils that are part of the dentin matrix (Fig. 7.7B and C). Because dentin is not as highly mineralized as enamel, it should be etched for shorter periods, typically for 10 seconds.

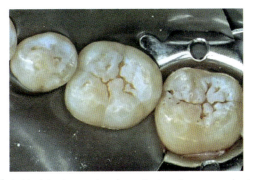

FIG. 7.4 Acid-etched enamel surfaces for bonding appear frosty white.

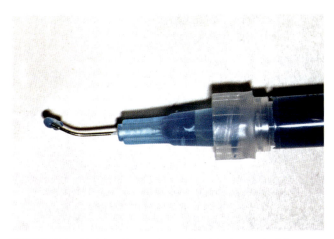

FIG. 7.5 Gel acid etchant in a syringe with a blunt cannula delivery tip. The gel has been dyed blue as a visual aid for its placement and removal.

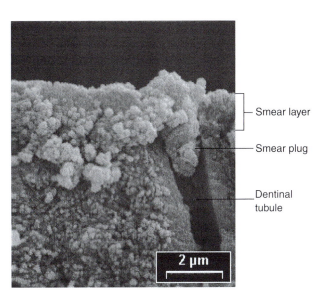

FIG. 7.6 Cutting of tooth structure with a rotary instrument forms a layer of cutting debris called the *smear layer*, as seen in this scanning electron micrograph. It is removed by acid etching so that it does not interfere with the formation of a bond. (Courtesy Grayson Marshall, University of California School of Dentistry, San Francisco, California.)

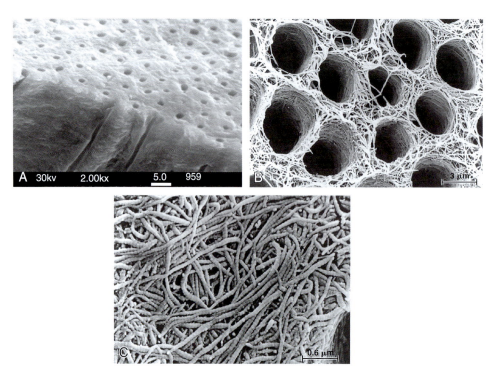

FIG. 7.7 **(A)** Normal dentin with dentinal tubules. **(B)** Acid etching of the dentin removes some of the mineral exposing the collagen fibers of the matrix, as seen in this scanning electron micrograph. **(C)** Higher magnification of collagen fibrils. (A, From Sakaguchi R, Powers J. *Craig's Restorative Dental Materials*. 13th ed. Elsevier; 2012; B and C, From Heymann H, Swift E, Ritter A. *Sturdevant's Art & Science of Operative Dentistry*. 6th ed., Elsevier; 2013.)

With a 10-second etch, mineral is removed up to 5 μm in depth. Acid that goes into the dentinal tubules is neutralized by the fluids that flow from the pulp.

When etching both enamel and dentin as in a coronal cavity preparation, it is best to apply the acid to the enamel first for 10 seconds, and then to the dentin for 10 seconds. That way, enamel will be etched for a total of 20 seconds and dentin only 10 seconds. Etching dentin for 20 seconds or longer opens the tubules too wide and removes hydroxyapatite mineral to too great a depth. Overetching will expose too much collagen matrix, causing it to act as a thick barrier and making it more difficult for the resin bonding agent to coat the dentin and seal the tubules. Overetching dentin can result in a weaker bond and posttreatment sensitivity.

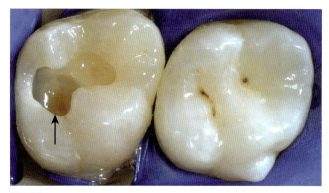

FIG. 7.8 Moist dentin for bonding after rinsing off acid. It should glisten with moisture but not have any puddles of water. (From Heymann H, Swift E, Ritter A: *Sturdevant's Art & Science of Operative Dentistry*. 6th ed. Elsevier; 2013.)

Etching Sclerotic Dentin. Sclerotic dentin is dentin in which the dentinal tubules have become highly calcified by way of mineral deposits. This can occur as a result of dental caries or from injury to odontoblasts during cavity preparation for deeper restorations.

Studies have also shown that dentin of people over 55 is more mineralized than that of younger people, making it more difficult to etch. Sclerotic dentin should be etched for an additional 10 seconds.

Moist Dentin for Bonding

Bonding to moist dentin ("wet" dentin bonding) was the first technique to achieve good bond strength to dentin. As mineral is removed from the surface of the dentin by acid etching, the fibrils of the collagen matrix are exposed. After etching, acid is removed by rinsing for at least 10 seconds. A gentle stream of air is used to remove excess water. However, the dentin is left slightly moist so that it glistens but without any puddles of water (Fig. 7.8). By keeping the dentin moist, the collagen fibrils stay spread out. However, if the dentin is dried, the fibrils collapse into a thick mass that prevents the bonding resin from penetrating the etched dentin. On the other hand, too much water remaining on the etched dentin dilutes the resin primer and makes it difficult for the resin to displace the water trapped in the collagen fibrils. Both overdrying and underdrying can produce an incomplete sealing of the dentinal tubules and a much weaker bond. A good dentinal seal helps eliminate bacterial leakage and postoperative sensitivity.

> **? Do You Recall?**
>
> Why does dentin need to be kept moist after etching for adequate bonding?

Etching Enamel and Dentin (Etch-and-Rinse Technique With 37% Phosphoric Acid)

	Enamel	Dentin
Etching Time	20 seconds	10 seconds
Rinsing Time	Total of 10 seconds	Since both are rinsed at the same time
Moisture Content for Bonding	Dry	Slightly moist (but no puddles)
Clinical Appearance	Frosty white (see Fig. 7.4)	Glistening (see Fig. 7.8)

> **💡 Clinical Tip**
>
> To restore moisture to overdried dentin, soak a cotton pellet in water and place it on the dentin for 10 to 20 seconds. Rewetting the dry dentin will allow the collapsed collagen fibrils to reexpand. If you wet it by squirting water on the dentin, then you will have to blow the excess water off and may overdry it again.

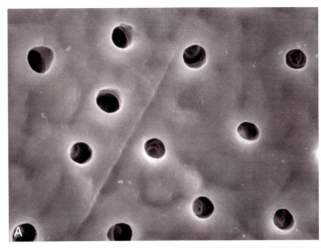
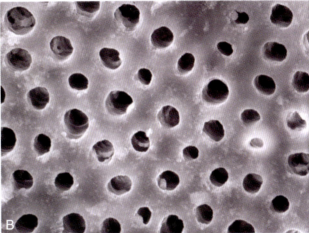

FIG. 7.9 Scanning electron micrograph of dentin. **(A)** Dentin located close to the dentinoenamel junction shows fewer tubules and they are farther apart. **(B)** Deeper dentin located closer to the pulp shows more tubules with larger openings. (Courtesy Ed Swift.)

BOND STRENGTH

The strength of the bond obtained is usually measured by determining the force needed to separate the two joined materials. Most bond tests pull the bonded materials apart (tensile bond strength) or apply forces at approximately 90 degrees to the bonded interface of the materials until the bond fails (shear bond strength). Choosing materials with good bond strength to tooth structure can enhance the longevity of the restoration.

Bonding to enamel usually achieves consistently high bond strength. The bond strength to dentin is typically much less than to enamel and varies according to how mineralized the dentin is and how deep into the dentin the cavity preparation extends. The dentin near the dentinoenamel junction has fewer dentinal tubules, and the tubules are smaller in diameter than in the dentin closer to the pulp. Deeper dentin contains more tubules that are larger in diameter (Fig. 7.9). Deeper dentin will be wetter from the flow of pulpal fluid through the larger tubules. The wetter dentin with more and larger holes (tubules) is more difficult to bond to consistently than is shallower dentin.

> **? Do You Recall?**
>
> Why is the bond to enamel stronger than the bond to dentin?

Durability of the Bond

How long the bond lasts is more important than how high the initial bond strength is. Over time, exposure of the bonding agents to moisture may cause them to degrade (hydrolyze). In addition, fatigue failure of the bond can be caused by repeated stresses on the bond caused by chewing pressures and temperature changes that cause different amounts of expansion and contraction between the restoration and the tooth structure. (Fatigue failure is similar to taking a piece of metal and repeatedly bending it back and forth until it breaks.) When composite resin is placed and polymerized, it shrinks which can put stress on the bond of the resins to the tooth. If the bond fails, the restoration could leak, causing sensitivity in the tooth or leading to recurrent caries.

> ### KEY POINTS
>
> **ETCHING ENAMEL AND DENTIN**
> Etching Enamel:
> - Enamel is mostly mineral (about 88%) and composed of thousands of enamel rods.
> - Etching with 37% phosphoric acid for 20 seconds is recommended.
> - Etching produces a microscopically porous and roughened surface with peaks and valleys.
> - Resin penetrates porosities and when cured locks into spaces around the enamel rods.
> - The bond to enamel is stronger and more reliable than the bond to dentin.
>   Etching dentin:
> - Dentin has less mineral than enamel and an organic collagen matrix woven throughout the mineral.
> - Dentin is etched for only 10 seconds to prevent exposing too much collagen.
> - Etching removes smear layer first, then some mineral, exposing collagen.
> - Bonding resin penetrates etched mineral and intermixes with exposed collagen.
> - Etched dentin must remain moist to prevent the collagen from collapsing and blocking resin penetration.

BONDING SYSTEMS

COMPONENTS OF BONDING SYSTEMS

Enamel-Bonding Resins

Bonding agents are low-viscosity resins that flow well into the microscopic porosities and irregularities of the etched surfaces. When bonding to enamel alone, the process is much simpler than bonding to dentin, and after etching and rinsing the enamel can be dried completely. Bonding to enamel alone requires only a low-viscosity liquid resin monomer that will penetrate into the spaces on and between enamel rods created by acid etching (Fig. 7.10; See Fig. 5.9).

Resin Tags. When the resin is cured by a chemical process or by light activation, it locks into the microscopic spaces and irregularities, producing resin tags (Fig. 7.11). The resin tags secure the resin to the enamel and create a very strong bond.

Dentin Bonding Resins

Resin Components. Dentin bonding resins can be viewed as two components.
- First is a resin primer that penetrates etched dentin and enamel and lays down a resin layer. The primer is composed of hydrophilic (water-tolerating) monomers and molecules that allow it to penetrate water.
- The second component is an adhesive resin that is applied over the primer.

The two resins chemically bond to each other, that is, the initial resin bonding material prepares (or primes) the tooth surface, much in the way that a primer is applied to wood before painting so that the paint will adhere better. The second resin then chemically bonds to the primer.

Solvents. For the resin to penetrate through the water on moist dentin, it must be dissolved in a solvent that can penetrate water and carry the resin with it. The solvents allow the resins to penetrate water on the dentin and in the dentinal tubules, and to penetrate around collagen fibrils and into porosities in the tooth surfaces created by etching. In general, the solvent is the largest

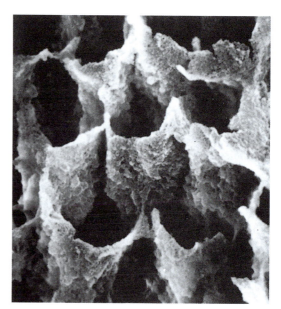

FIG. 7.11 A bonding resin placed on etched enamel penetrates the porous surface and forms resin extensions or tags that lock into the enamel and form a mechanical bond. This scanning electron micrograph shows the resin tags left after the enamel was dissolved away. (From Phillips RW, Moore BK. Synthetic resins. In: *Elements of Dental Materials for Dental Hygienists and Dental Assistants.* Saunders; 1994.)

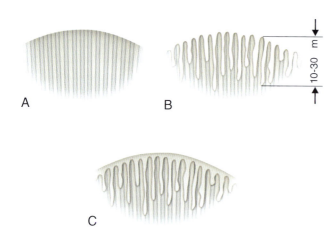

FIG. 7.10 Bonding to enamel: **(A)** Unetched enamel rods. **(B)** Etched enamel rods. **(C)** Bonding resin mechanically bonding to etched enamel rods. (© Elsevier Collection.)

portion of the bonding agent, making up 60% or more of the material.

The three basic solvents are:
- Acetone
- Ethanol (ethyl alcohol)
- Water (used more with self-etching systems)

Acetone is a highly volatile solvent. Its rapid evaporation may require that two or more coats of the bonding resin be applied to ensure adequate sealing of the dentin. Ethanol evaporates more slowly, so it may need a longer drying time.

All bottles of bonding agents should be recapped immediately after the material is dispensed to prevent evaporation of the solvent, which leads to gradual thickening of the resin left in the bottle with less ability to penetrate etched dentin. Unit-dose (single-use) packaging of bonding resins avoids some of these problems associated with bonding resins in bottles, as well as infection control issues.

After the primer is placed, it is dried before it is cured to remove the solvent and the remaining water. Next, a resin adhesive is applied over the primer. It bonds to the resin primer and provides a resin-rich layer that will chemically bond to **hydrophobic** (water-repelling) resin restorative materials such as composite resin that are placed over it. See Procedure 7.1 for bonding to enamel and dentin.

> **Clinical Tip**
>
> Bonding resins should not be dispensed before the operator is ready to place them. Otherwise, the solvent (such as acetone or ethanol) will evaporate prematurely, leaving a bonding resin with reduced ability to penetrate moist dentin.

Fillers. Some bonding resins will have added fillers. They are usually nanometer-sized silica particles that are added to increase the strength of the resin.

Hybrid Layer

The primer gets the dentin ready for the bonding resin by infusing the etched dentin and the collagen fibrils with a thin layer of resin and removing the water (wet dentin). The layer that is formed by the intermixing of dentin bonding resin with collagen fibrils and the etched dentin surface is called the **hybrid layer**, because it is a combination (or hybrid) of dentin components and resin. This resin-rich hybrid layer facilitates bonding of the composite resin to the tooth through a chemical resin-to-resin bond (Fig. 7.12).

All of the current bonding systems work by micromechanically locking into etched enamel and by forming a hybrid layer with dentin.

Benefits of Bonding Restorations

- Enhances retention of the restoration
- Allows more conservative cavity preparations
- Regains some of the strength of the tooth lost by cavity preparation
- Strengthens brittle restorative materials such as porcelain veneers
- Seals the dentinal tubules
- Reduces microleakage and the associated sensitivity or recurrent caries

HISTORY OF THE DEVELOPMENT OF BONDING SYSTEMS

Bonding systems for enamel and dentin have undergone rapid changes over the past five decades (Box 7.1). The composites that became commercially available in the early 1960s were placed without etching or bonding agents. By the beginning of the 1970s, dentists were beginning to etch the enamel with acid and place a self-cured, unfilled bonding resin on the enamel only. A number of different acids were tested, but phosphoric acid gave the best results. Great concern was expressed about putting a strong acid (like phosphoric acid) on dentin for fear of

> **Box 7.1 Time Line of Development of Bonding Systems**
>
> **Enamel Etch:** 1960s and 1970s—dentin was not etched. Bonding agents attached to etched enamel, and the smear layer blocked adhesion to dentin. First and second generations of bonding systems.
>
> ↓
>
> **Etch-and-Rinse (Enamel and Dentin Etch-and-Rinse):** 1980s—smear layer was removed by etching dentin but bonding agents could not penetrate dried, collapsed collagen layer. Third and fourth generations of bonding systems.
>
> Early 1990s—"wet" dentin bonding introduced. Two-bottle (fourth generation) bonding systems. Highest bond strengths (but technique sensitive).
>
> Mid-1990s—one-bottle systems (fifth generation). High bond strength. Unit-dose packaging available.
>
> ↓
>
> **Self-Etch (No Rinse):**
> **Sixth generation**
> Late 1990s—type I: 2 bottles. Primer applied, and then adhesive resin
>
> Early 2000s—type II: 2 bottles. Primer and adhesive mixed and applied
>
> ↓
>
> 2002—One-bottle (all-in-one, seventh generation) systems: etching, priming, and bonding combined.
>
> 2011 (approximately)—universal adhesives were introduced: capable of bonding to both tooth structure and many dental materials. Two-bottle systems were introduced first. Later, one-bottle systems were introduced.

Data from Nazarian A. The progression of dental adhesives [online continuing education]. *Dental CE Digest*. PennWell Publications; 2007.

damaging the pulp. The dentin was covered with a liner such as calcium hydroxide for protection.

By the late 1970s and early 1980s, both enamel and dentin bonding resins were being used, and they were light cured. The dentin still was not etched, so the bonding resin placed on dentin was merely bonding to the smear layer. The resulting bonds to dentin were very weak bonds.

Later in the 1980s, it was discovered that the smear layer was interfering with the ability of the bonding resins to bond to dentin. Acidic components of the bonding systems were used to remove the smear layer, but the dentin was not adequately etched and it was dried. So, bonding resins did not penetrate the dentin surface in a meaningful way. Therefore bond strengths were still relatively low.

By the start of the 1990s, etching both enamel and dentin with phosphoric acid was an accepted technique, first called the total-etch technique but now commonly called the **etch-and-rinse** technique. Not only was the smear layer removed, but the surface of the dentin was etched and kept moist ("wet" dentin bonding technique), allowing for the penetration of **hydrophilic** (compatible with water) resin primers into the etched dentin surface. The bond strength to dentin increased significantly. Primer and bonding resins were in separate bottles and applied one after the other or combined into one bottle to eliminate the extra step.

By the latter part of the 1990s, primers with acidic components that could etch enamel and dentin (called **self-etching systems**) were introduced and were light cured or dual cured (both light and chemical cures). Separate steps for etching with phosphoric acid and rinsing and drying were eliminated with the self-etching primers. These systems had primer and bonding resin in separate bottles.

In the early 2000s, improvements were made in self-etching materials so that components were contained in one bottle and did not require mixing. Around 2010, another class of bonding resins was developed that could not only bond to tooth structure but also to restorative materials such as ceramics and metal and these have been called universal bonding agents.

MODES OF CURE OF ADHESIVES

Adhesive systems are cured (polymerized) by methods similar to those used for composite resins. There are three modes of curing for the resin bonding agents:

1. Light cure—the most commonly used mode uses a light in the blue wave range to activate a chemical (a photosensitizer, camphorquinone) that reacts with an initiator (a tertiary amine) to set off the polymerization reaction (see Chapter 8 for an in-depth discussion of resin polymerization).
2. Self-cure—a chemical reaction occurs when two resins are mixed together, one of which contains benzoyl peroxide as an initiator.
3. Dual cure—uses a combination of self-cure and light-cure ingredients. Dual-cured resins can be activated by light or can cure chemically without application of the curing light.

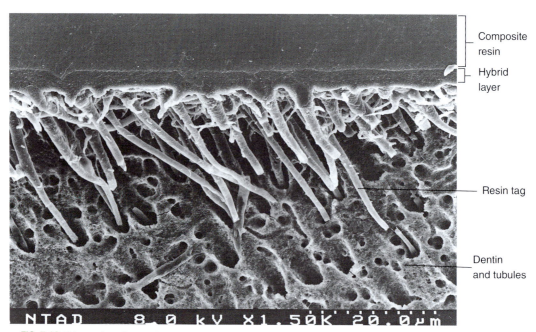

FIG. 7.12 When a bonding resin is applied to etched dentin, it penetrates the exposed collagen matrix and dentinal tubules. An intermingling of resin with etched dentin forms a hybrid layer. This layer provides a resin-rich layer for bonding with other resins such as composite resin. (Courtesy Jorge Perdigão, University of Minnesota School of Dentistry, Twin Cities, Minnesota.)

OXYGEN-INHIBITED RESIN LAYER

On the surface of the polymerized bonding resin is a very thin coating of uncured resin. The resins used for composites and sealants will also form this layer of uncured resin on their surfaces. Polymerization is inhibited where the surface is exposed to oxygen in the air (this layer is called the oxygen-inhibited layer or *air-inhibited layer*). Once the composite resin is placed over the bonding resin, its presence will exclude air, and that uncured layer on the bonding resin will cure when the composite is cured. The uncured layer will actually help facilitate a chemical bond between the bonding resin and the composite resin. When the oxygen-inhibited layer is exposed to the mouth as with sealants, many clinicians prefer to wipe it off because it can impart an unpleasant taste.

CLASSIFICATION OF BONDING SYSTEMS

Adhesive systems that bond to tooth structure can be categorized into two main categories:
- Etch-and-rinse bonding systems
- Self-etch bonding systems (Table 7.1).

These two bonding systems have three components in common:
- An acidic etchant
- A primer for the dentin
- A resin adhesive (forms a hybrid layer with dentin)

ETCH-AND-RINSE BONDING SYSTEMS

Etch-and-rinse refers to phosphoric acid etching of both enamel and dentin with a separate step that includes rinsing off the acid. After the acid is rinsed off, the dentin is left slightly moist (glistening but no water puddles), so that the collagen fibrils stay fluffed up. The etch-and-rinse technique became successful when hydrophilic resin monomers were added to the primer and adhesive. The hydrophilic monomers facilitated the penetration through the water left after rinsing and slight drying into the moist etched dentin and dentinal tubules. Drying with air is done at this stage to remove the volatile solvents from the resin and any remaining water. The resin is then light cured (or chemical cured).

Two-Bottle Adhesive Systems

Two-bottle systems have three basic steps in their procedure:
1. Acid etch (and rinse)
2. Application of primer
3. Application of bonding resin

After the etch procedure, the primer is applied, dried, and light cured. Then, the bonding resin is applied over the primer, and it is light cured. Two-bottle etch-and-rinse systems (Fig. 7.13) provide the strongest bonds to dentin of all the bonding systems, assuming the technique is followed carefully.

One-Bottle Adhesive Systems

With one-bottle systems the primer and bonding resin have been joined together in one bottle. After etching and rinsing, they are applied in one step, dried, and light cured (Fig. 7.14).

> **Clinical Tip**
>
> Good isolation is critical for good bonding. Contamination of the etched tooth surface is a major cause of bond failure leading to microleakage, recurrent caries, and loss of retention of the restoration. If the etched tooth surface is contaminated by saliva or blood, rinse thoroughly, reisolate, and reetch for 10 to 15 seconds.

TABLE 7.1 Etch-and-Rinse and Self-Etch Bonding Systems: Application and Commercial Products

ETCH-AND-RINSE		SELF-ETCH (NO RINSE)	
2 Bottles (3 steps)	1 Bottle (2 steps)	2 Bottles or chambers (2 steps)	1 Bottle (1 step)
Step 1. Etch, rinse, and gently air-dry. Leave dentin moist	Step 1. Etch, rinse, and gently air-dry. Leave dentin moist	Step 1. Etch and prime with acidic monomer, lightly air-dry	Step 1. Etch, prime, and bond (all in one bottle), gently air-dry, light cure
Step 2. Apply primer, gently air-dry	Step 2. Apply primer/bonding resin, gently air-dry, light cure	Step 2. Apply bonding resin, gently air-dry, light cure	
Step 3. Apply bonding resin, gently air-dry, light cure			
Strongest, most reliable bonds to enamel and dentin	Strong bonds to enamel and dentin	Strong bonds to dentin	Strong bonds to dentin
Reliably etches enamel	Reliably etches enamel	Bonds to enamel are not strong, especially uncut enamel. "Selective etch" advisable	Only a few products reliably etch enamel. "Selective etch" advisable

Adapted from Anusavice KJ, Shen C, Rawls HR. Table 12.1. In: *Phillips' Science of Dental Materials*, 12th ed. Elsevier; 2013.

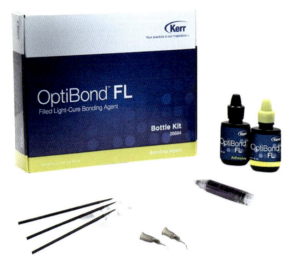

FIG. 7.13 Two-bottle etch-and-rinse bonding system. Components: primer, adhesive resin, etchant in syringe with delivery tips, microtip brushes, and disposable mixing well. (OptiBond FL, Courtesy Kerr Corp.)

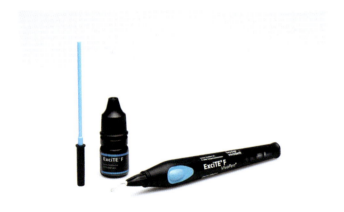

FIG. 7.14 One-bottle etch-and-rinse bonding system available in unit dose, bottle, or pen dispenser. (ExciTE F, Courtesy Ivoclar Vivadent).

SELF-ETCH BONDING SYSTEMS

Acidic Primers

Bonding systems have been developed that do not require the use of phosphoric acid etching and rinsing. One- and two-bottle bonding systems incorporate acidic groups in a resin primer that will etch enamel and dentin, then prime them with resin without the need for rinsing and drying. These are called **self-etching bonding systems**.

Water as a Solvent

The primers use water as a solvent to ionize the acidic monomer. Etching of the dentin with acidic primers dissolves the smear layer without deeply demineralizing the dentin. The acid component gradually shifts in pH to neutral and is incorporated into the polymerized resin, as are the dissolved tooth mineral and the smear layer.

Longer Drying Time

When the solvent has evaporated, the adhesive layer is thin and not very strong. Applying two coats of adhesive resin can increase the bond strength. Self-etching adhesives need a longer drying time of at least 10 seconds after application to evaporate all of the water solvent. Any water left behind will degrade the bond over time.

Postoperative Sensitivity Reduced

Self-etch systems have less postoperative sensitivity because they directly seal the dentin without rinsing and drying steps. Because self-etch systems use acidic primers to demineralize dentin and there is no rinsing, it is easier for the primer and adhesive resin to penetrate the full depth of demineralization. Self-etching bonding systems eliminate the risk of over- or under-rinsing or drying, factors that can adversely affect the bond and cause posttreatment sensitivity.

However, with etch-and-rinse systems, the phosphoric acid may be left on too long and the primer cannot penetrate the more deeply etched surface, or if the etched surface is dried too much, the collagen will collapse and prevent primer and adhesive penetration. The unsealed dentin can contribute to postoperative sensitivity.

pH of the Acidic Primers

The acidic primers are categorized as:
- Mild (pH 2 or above)
- Moderate (pH 1 to 2)
- Strong (pH 1 or less)

Systems with primers that are mildly acidic have weak bonds to enamel, especially uncut enamel, but strong bonds to dentin. Studies using the scanning electron microscope have shown that the etching pattern on enamel is shallow, resulting in poor micromechanical retention of the resin. Systems with primers that are strongly acidic demonstrate bond strengths similar to those with etch-and-rinse bonding systems.

Selective Etching

To ensure a good bond to uncut enamel, many manufacturers recommend **selective etching**, meaning that enamel only should be etched with phosphoric acid before the application of the self-etching bonding materials (Fig. 7.15). If dentin is also etched with phosphoric acid, and then a self-etching bonding system is used, a good seal with the dentin may not occur. The phosphoric acid will etch the dentin deeper than the primer and bonding resin from the self-etch system can penetrate.

Two-Bottle Self-Etch Bonding Systems

Two-bottle self-etching adhesive systems may be applied by two different methods, depending on how they were manufactured:
- Type I self-etch adhesives—an acidic water-soluble primer is applied first, and then covered with a light-cured adhesive resin (Fig. 7.16).
- Type II self-etch adhesives—a drop of acidic primer from one bottle is mixed with one drop of adhesive

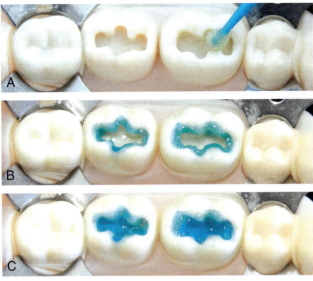

FIG. 7.15 Methods of etching (top to bottom): **(A)** Self-etch with acidic primers, **(B** and **C)** selective etch of enamel and etch-and-rinse (total etch) with phosphoric acid (seen as blue gel). (Courtesy VOCO.)

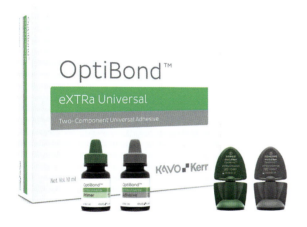

FIG. 7.16 Type 1 self-etching two-bottle adhesive system—bottle 1 is acidic primer, and bottle 2 is bonding resin. Also available in unit-dose packaging. (OptiBond eXTRa, Courtesy Kerr Corporation.)

resin from the other bottle and applied to the prepared tooth.

One-Bottle Self-Etch Bonding Systems
With one-bottle self-etch adhesive systems ("all-in-one"), the adhesive resin is already combined with the acidic primer and does not require mixing. Many of the self-etching primers require that two or more coats should be applied to the preparation, because they may not adequately cover the etched dentin with one coat.

Refrigeration
Many one-bottle self-etching bonding systems require refrigeration to prevent the bonding agent from degrading. The bottle should be removed about 30 minutes before use to allow it to return to room temperature. Cooling of the material will affect the dynamics of polymerization and also make the material so viscous that it will not flow readily.

Packaging
Most of these systems are available in a bottle or unit-dose container (Fig. 7.17).

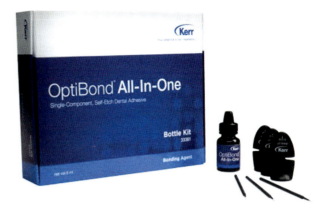

FIG. 7.17 Self-etching primer/adhesive seen in one bottle or unit-dose dispensing. (OptiBond All-In-One, Courtesy Kerr Corporation.)

> **? Do You Recall?**
> Why is selective etching needed with some self-etching bonding systems?

Fig. 7.18 illustrates self-etch adhesive systems.

Which System to Use
Some clinicians will stick with only one type of bonding system because that is what they are comfortable using and feel they get good results. Other clinicians may choose to use both systems, depending on the clinical scenario. In general, etch-and-rinse systems are preferred for indirect restorations (such as porcelain veneers) when mostly enamel is available for bonding because phosphoric acid provides the most retentive etch in enamel. Self-etch systems are preferred for direct composites when mostly dentin is available because they produce greater bond strength to dentin and reduce postoperative sensitivity. Either system will perform adequately with preparations in both enamel and dentin.

> **💡 Clinical Tip**
> One-bottle systems (that combine primer and adhesive resin), whether they are etch-and-rinse or self-etch, tend to produce a resin adhesive layer overlying the hybrid layer that is too thin. Applying at least two coats is recommended.

Universal Bonding Systems
Universal adhesives bond not only to the tooth structure but also to a variety of restorative materials such

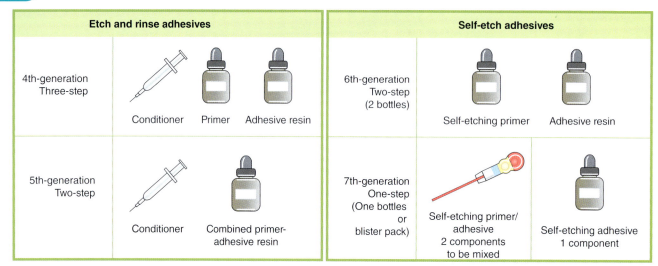

FIG. 7.18 Summary of self-etch adhesive systems. (Adapted from Cardoso MV, de Almeida Neves A, Mine A, et al. Current aspects on bonding effectiveness and stability in adhesive dentistry. *Aust Dent J.* 2011;56(Suppl 1):31–44.)

as ceramics, noble and base metals, composites, and glass ionomers. While universal adhesives can bond to these restorative materials, not all products develop a strong, lasting bond.

Universal adhesives are very versatile and most can be used with etch-and-rinse, self-etch, and selective-enamel etch techniques. The key ingredient in all **universal bonding systems** is a phosphate ester that allows them to bond to the tooth structure, ceramics, and metals. Phosphate esters are also acidic and capable of etching the tooth structure. Universal adhesives have a pH that ranges from 2.2 to 3.2, depending on the product. Products with a pH in this range are capable of etching and bonding to dentin. The ability to etch enamel adequately for bonding varies from product to product. To be safe, selective-enamel etching may be used.

Added Ingredients

Activator: Some universal bonding systems require that an activator be added to the adhesive in order for it to be compatible with other manufactures' self- and dual-cured resin restorative materials and resin cements. The acidity of the adhesive can deactivate the chemicals needed for self-curing and will not permit the resins in the self-cure/dual-cure restorative materials to cure properly without adding an activator.

Filler particles: Small quantities of microscopic particles composed of colloidal silica are added to increase the strength of the adhesive resin. The filler size ranges from 0.8 to 0.0007 μm.

Fluoride: Some universal adhesives also have fluoride compounds added to aid in the prevention of recurrent caries at the margins of restorations. However, the quantities of fluoride released are generally too small to have a therapeutic effect.

Silane: Other universal adhesive systems have silane, an agent that helps to bind the adhesive to glass-based ceramics.

Do You Recall?

What are universal bonding systems?

Clinical Tip

Some clinicians use *phosphoric acid* gel to clean the interior of ceramic restoration after trying it in the mouth. However, the etchant needed to create a surface roughness for bonding is 8% to 10% *hydrofluoric acid*.

Packaging

Universal adhesives are manufactured as one-bottle or two-bottle systems or may be packaged in unit-dose blister packs (Fig. 7.19).

Clinical Tip

For many self-etching and universal adhesive products, scrubbing the primer into the dentin for 20 seconds is recommended. Be sure to review the manufacturer's recommendations to obtain the best results with each product you use.

CLINICAL APPLICATION OF UNIVERSAL BONDING ADHESIVE

A universal bonding adhesive, when applied to a cavity preparation and to the interior of an indirect restoration, can provide resin-coated surfaces for cementation of the restoration with resin cement. The resin bonding adhesive on the tooth and restoration will bond chemically with the resin cement, forming a durable bond.

The following sequence of clinical images in Fig. 7.20 depicts how the maxillary first molar was treated for a fractured distolingual cusp. After the tooth was prepared, a digital image was made and the resin-based ceramic restoration was designed and milled using computer-aided design/computer-aided manufacturing equipment (CAD/CAM, is discussed in Chapter 10). Universal adhesive and resin cement were used to bond the restoration in place.

> **Clinical Tip**
>
> Many of the self-etch systems recommend "selective etching" of the enamel with phosphoric acid to ensure a good etch and bond to enamel.

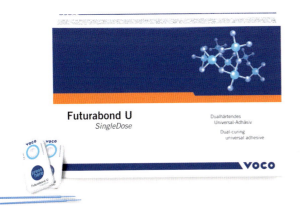

FIG. 7.19 Universal bonding system. Unit-dose package. (Futurabond U, Courtesy VOCO.)

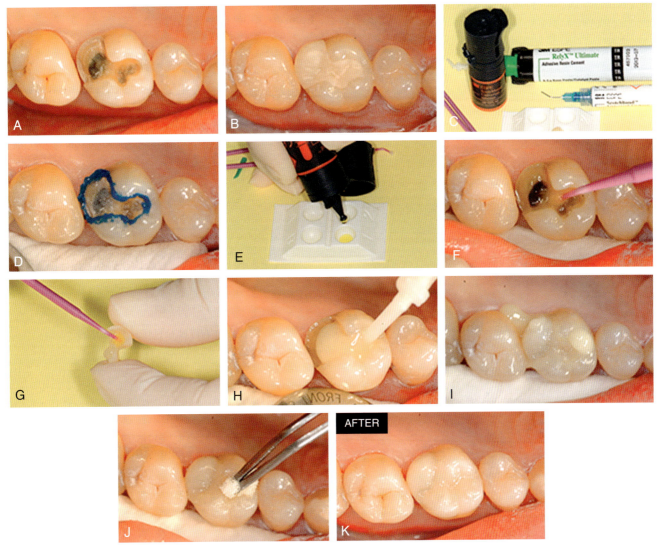

FIG. 7.20 **(A)** The tooth was prepared and a digital impression was made with the CEREC AC CAD/CAM system. **(B)** The CAD/CAM restoration was milled in the office and then tried for fit. **(C)** The universal bonding agent, adhesive resin cement, etchant, dispensing well, and microbrush applicators as setup prior to the procedure. **(D)** Selective-enamel etching with phosphoric acid was done for 10 seconds. **(E)** Universal bonding agent was dispensed into the well. **(F)** Universal bonding agent was scrubbed into the cavity preparation with a microtip applicator. **(G)** Universal bonding agent was scrubbed into the inner surface of the restoration. **(H)** Adhesive resin cement was injected into the preparation. **(I)** Cement flowed evenly from the margins on seating. **(J)** Excess cement was cleaned with a mini-sponge and removed from the interproximal with knotted floss. **(K)** The final restoration after polishing. (Courtesy *Dentistry Today* and Dr. Daniel Poticny.)

To get the best results from the bonding system you are using:

- Review the manufacturer's instructions.
- Be meticulous in your technique.
- Maintain good isolation.
- Use enough drying time with an air stream to evaporate the solvent and remove water from "wet" dentin—at least 10 seconds.
- Use fresh material. Refrigeration may extend the shelf life. Remove from the refrigerator half an hour before use.
- Use unit-dose packaging when possible. If using bottles, recap immediately after dispensing materials.

KEY POINTS

Bonding Systems

Common features of all bonding systems:
- Acid etchant
- Hydrophilic primer
- Adhesive resin

Etch-and-rinse systems
- Steps include acid etching, rinsing, and drying but leaving dentin moist
- Hydrophilic primer penetrates moisture and mixes with exposed collagen
- Air stream removes the moisture and primer's solvent
- Adhesive resin applied over primer, forming a hybrid layer (collagen and resin)
- Hybrid layer can bond to composite resin or resin cements
- 2-Bottle systems with separate primer and adhesive resin have strongest bonds to dentin
- 1-Bottle systems have primer and adhesive resin together
- Potential problems—over/underetching, over/underdrying, resin coating too thin

Self-etching systems
- Acidic primer etches enamel and dentin
- Smear layer and dissolved mineral remain within the priming resin
- No rinsing is needed
- Longer drying time to remove moisture and water solvent
- 2-Bottle systems—primer and adhesive resin applied separately
- 1-Bottle systems—primer and adhesive together
- Potential problem—some systems with weak acidic primers do not etch enamel adequately so separate enamel etching (selective etching) is needed.

Universal bonding systems
- Work with both etch-and-rinse and self-etch techniques
- Bond to both tooth and restoration (composite, ceramic, metal).

BIOCOMPATIBILITY

Acid etching dentin is unlikely to cause pulpal irritation because it is limited in its depth of penetration. The hydroxyapatite is etched less than 7 µm in depth and acid entering the dentinal tubules is buffered to neutral by components of dentinal fluids and hydroxyapatite. However, acid and acidic primers should not be placed directly on a pulpal exposure.

Bonding and restorative materials are well tolerated by the teeth. However, components of the bonding systems can irritate the skin, mucosa, and eyes. Acidic components can cause burns. Some dental personnel develop allergies to the components. PPE should be used when handling these materials. Use of the rubber dam will minimize contact with the patient's oral mucosa. Any area of contact with the skin should be washed with soap and water. An eyewash station should be available to treat accidental exposure to the eyes. Most of the undesirable effects are the result of contact with the unpolymerized components. Once the materials are polymerized, the risks of untoward reactions are much less.

Caution

Resins, solvents, and acids in the bonding systems can irritate the skin, mucosa, or eyes, and therefore caution should be taken when these materials are applied. Materials on the skin or mucosa should be washed thoroughly. Eye protection should be worn by the patient and PPE worn by the operator and assistant.

Caution

A small portion of the population may have an allergic response to acrylate resins. Precautions are to be followed because these resins may penetrate commonly used gloves.

COMPATIBILITY WITH OTHER RESINS

Etch-and-Rinse Systems

Two-bottle bonding systems are compatible with light cure, self-cure, and dual cure composites. One-bottle bonding systems are compatible with light-cure composites. They are not compatible with self-cure composite core materials or resin cements because the bonding agents are acidic and that interferes with the set of the composite or resin cement. One-bottle bonding systems require an activator to be mixed with the bonding resin in order for it to be compatible with self-cure and dual-cure composites and resin cements.

Self-Etch Systems

Type I self-etching bonding systems (primer applied first followed by bonding resin) are generally compatible with light-cure, self-cure, or dual-cure composites, but type II bonding systems (primer and bonding resin mixed together, then applied) are not.

> **Clinical Tip**
>
> Before placing a composite core for a crown preparation, check the manufacturer's fact sheet for compatibility of the bonding system with self-cured and dual-cured composite core materials.

Three Main Steps of Bonding Systems

All bonding systems have three main steps in common:
- Etching with either phosphoric acid or an acidic primer
- Priming with hydrophilic monomers in a solvent that penetrates etched surfaces
- Bonding with hydrophobic bonding resins to seal etched surfaces and to chemically bond to composite resin or resin luting cements

CONTAMINATION OF BONDING SITE

For successful bonding, good isolation and soft tissue management are essential. **Contamination** from saliva, blood, smear layer, or oils from the dental handpiece or prophy paste can interfere with the enamel or dentin bonding. Contaminants can contribute to microleakage when they are not properly removed before and during the bonding process. Microleakage (leakage at a microscopic level) occurs at gaps in restoration margins and permits fluids, bacteria, and debris to enter the cavity preparation (Fig. 7.21). Microleakage can contribute to decay under the restoration and increase sensitivity of the tooth. Pulpal irritation comes more from bacteria entering from microleakage than from chemical components of the bonding or restorative materials.

If the newly etched surface becomes contaminated, rinse it thoroughly and reetch for 10 to 15 seconds.

Factors That Prevent Good Bonding

- A surface that is overly wet does not allow good penetration of the bonding resins into the etched enamel and dentin.
- An overly dry etched dentin surface causes the collagen fibrils to collapse and cover the dentin surface so that the bonding resins cannot penetrate to reach the etched dentin and the tubules.
- Blood or saliva on the etched enamel or dentin will interfere with the ability of the bonding resin to penetrate the surface.
- Failure to saturate dentin with a bonding resin will result in voids and incompletely sealed dentin. This can result in reduced bond strength and sensitivity because tubules are open.
- Failure to adequately cure the bonding resin will cause the resin to separate from the enamel or dentin.
- Moisture from the air-water lines can wet the enamel and dentin at the wrong step in the bonding process, resulting in loss of a proper bond and seal.
- Oil lubricants expelled from the handpiece onto the tooth during preparation will prevent the bonding resins from adhering to the etched enamel and dentin.
- Recently applied whitening or topical fluoride agents can affect the enamel so that it is more difficult to etch or to bond to. Studies have shown that the bond to recently whitened enamel is not as strong. Fluoride makes the surface of the enamel more resistant to being etched by acid.
- Eugenol in cements for provisional restorations will interfere with the set of resin bonding agents and composite resins.
- Aluminum chloride– and ferric sulfate–containing astringents used to control gingival bleeding will interfere with the set of the bonding agents.

> **Clinical Tip**
>
> When bonding to preparations with large areas of enamel remaining, etch-and-rinse systems are preferred. When bonding mostly to dentin, self-etch systems are preferred. Selective etching (with phosphoric acid) of enamel when using self-etching systems is recommended to ensure satisfactory enamel etch pattern for bonding.

BONDING OF RESTORATIONS

After the initial bonding resin is cured on the tooth, other adhesive bonding resins or resin cements can be used to attach restorations to the tooth by way of resin-to-resin chemical bonds (Procedure 7.1). Restorations that are not made of resin, such as metal or ceramic products, require treatment of their surfaces to allow them to bond to the resin on the tooth. A description of bonding with composite restorations and glass ionomers can be found in Chapters 8 and 9.

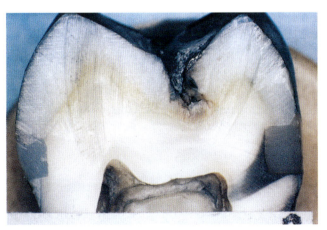

FIG. 7.21 A longitudinal section through a molar that has cervical composite restorations on the right- and left-hand sides. When a good bond is not formed between the tooth and the composite, fluids and bacteria can seep between them, a process called *microleakage*. The tooth was soaked in a dark dye to show areas of microleakage. The restoration on the right shows leakage, as indicated by dye penetration; the one on the left does not. (Courtesy Larry Watanabe, University of California School of Dentistry, San Francisco, California.)

SUMMARY

Bonding has a wide variety of uses in the modern dental practice. Present-day bonding systems bond to enamel by micromechanical retention into the etched enamel surface, and they bond to etched dentin by formation of a resin-rich hybrid layer. This resin-rich layer allows other resins to bond to it by chemical resin-to-resin bonding. Thus composite resins can be retained by bonding to the hybrid layer and to the etched enamel that has been primed with resin. Non-resin materials such as ceramic and metal restorations can be bonded to the hybrid layer and to resin-primed enamel by resin adhesives (cements) after their surfaces have been appropriately prepared.

Etch-and-rinse and self-etching bonding systems bond to the tooth structure. Universal bonding systems bond to both the tooth structure and restorations. Etch-and-rinse systems generally provide stronger bonds to enamel and dentin but are prone to postoperative sensitivity. Some self-etch systems have weaker bonds to uncut enamel and require selective etching, but other systems have solved that issue by using primers that are more acidic. Since they require no rinsing, the self-etching systems have less postoperative sensitivity. Universal systems can be used with etch-and-rinse, self-etch, and selective etch techniques, and they can bond to most restorative materials. To get good results with any bonding system, careful attention to the manufacturer's recommendations is required.

INSTRUCTIONAL VIDEOS

See the Evolve Resources site for a variety of educational videos that reinforce the material covered in this chapter.

Procedure 7.1   Enamel and Dentin Bonding Using the Etch-and-Rinse Technique

See Evolve site for Competency Sheet.

Consider the following with this procedure: Safety glasses are recommended for the patient, personal protective equipment (PPE) is required for the clinician, ensure appropriate safety protocols are followed, and check your local state guidelines before performing this procedure.

EQUIPMENT/SUPPLIES (FIG. 7.22)

- Rubber dam setup or cotton rolls and absorbent pads
- Dappen dishes or wells for bonding agents
- Disposable micro-brushes for applying bonding agents and 37% phosphoric acid (if not in a dispenser)
- Bonding agent, curing light
- Restorative material—composite

PROCEDURE STEPS

1. Isolate the field.
   Moisture interferes with the formation of a good bond.
   Etch cavity preparation with phosphoric acid: 10 seconds for dentin and 20 seconds for enamel (Fig. 7.23). **NOTE:** Rubber dam is preferred because it can provide the best isolation for the longest time. Cotton rolls and absorbent pads can also be used.
   NOTE: Start applying the etchant to the enamel first for 10 seconds and then to the dentin for 10 seconds. Total etching time for enamel is 20 seconds. Overetching dentin will open the tubules too much and remove too much mineral (hydroxyapatite) from the dentin surface.
2. Rinse with water for 10 seconds.

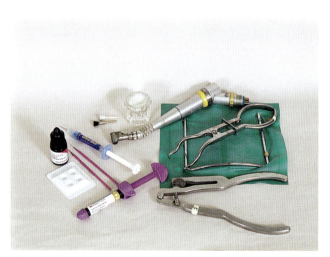

FIG. 7.22

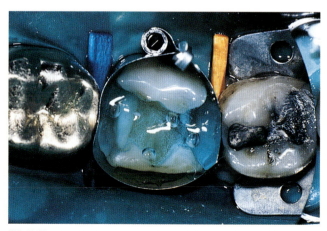

FIG. 7.23 The cavity preparation is etched with phosphoric acid. (Courtesy Alton Lacy, University of California School of Dentistry, San Francisco, California.)

Procedure 7.1 Enamel and Dentin Bonding Using the Etch-and-Rinse Technique—cont'd

3. Blot or gently air-dry enamel and dentin for 2 to 3 seconds (removing any puddles).

   Dentin should be glistening (moist) with no puddles. If only enamel is etched, it should be dried thoroughly and should appear frosty.

   Saturate the etched surface with the bonding resin (Fig. 7.24). **NOTE:** Do not overdry the dentin because the collagen matrix will collapse and prevent adequate penetration of the bonding resin into the tubules and etched dentin.

   NOTE: Some bonding resins are administered as a one-bottle/one-step application and others require two bottles/two steps—with each component applied separately. If the bonding resin contains acetone as its solvent, it is particularly volatile. Do not dispense bonding until you are ready to apply it to the etched tooth or most of the solvent may have evaporated. Also, be sure to recap the bottle immediately to keep from changing the consistency of the bonding resin and its ability to penetrate moist etched dentin. Use of unit-dose ampules eliminates this problem.

4. Apply a gentle air stream to thin the resin and to remove volatile solvents and water.

   The solvent that the bonding resin was dissolved in must be removed by applying a stream of air, otherwise the resin may not set completely. Likewise, air is used to evaporate any remaining water from the moist dentin. **NOTE:** The bonding resin is not as strong as the composite, so it should not be allowed to puddle in the preparation and cause weakness in the restoration.

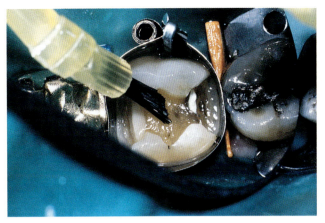

FIG. 7.24 The etched enamel and dentin are coated with bonding resin. (Courtesy Alton Lacy, University of California School of Dentistry, San Francisco, California.)

5. Light cure all surfaces with bonding agent for 10 to 20 seconds. The cavity preparation is now ready for placement of a restoration. The enamel and dentin surfaces have been physically bonded with resin bonding agent and will bond to resin restorative materials, such as composite, placed on top of them by resin-to-resin chemical bonding.

   NOTE: The tip of the light wand is usually held about 1 mm from the surface. The curing time may vary with newer, high-intensity curing lights. If the light tip cannot be placed close to the restoration surface, then a longer curing time may be needed. Follow the manufacturer's recommendations.

Get Ready for Exams!

Review Questions

Select the one correct response for each of the following multiple-choice questions.

1. Which acid is most commonly used to etch the tooth structure for a bonding procedure?
   a. Citric acid
   b. Hydrochloric acid
   c. Hydrofluoric acid
   d. Phosphoric acid

2. Which one of the following statements about bonding to **enamel** is true?
   a. Bonding is achieved by micromechanical retention.
   b. Bonding is achieved by chemical bonds.
   c. Bonding is achieved by resin tags penetrating the collagen matrix.
   d. Bonding to enamel is less reliable than bonding to dentin.

3. Bonding to **dentin** by the etch-and-rinse technique:
   a. Is best on dentin that has been etched with 37% phosphoric acid for 30 seconds
   b. Is stronger when the dentin is well dried after etching
   c. Is inhibited by formation of the hybrid layer
   d. Is best accomplished when the dentin is kept moist after etching

4. One of the following statements about etch-and-rinse bonding resins is true. Which one?
   a. Water is the most common solvent used with these bonding resins.
   b. They form the best hybrid layer with dry dentin.
   c. They chemically bond to the composite resin.
   d. They chemically bond to the dentin.

5. Self-etching bonding systems:
   a. Use 37% phosphoric acid as the etchant
   b. Use acidic primers to etch the tooth structure
   c. Require rinsing after etching
   d. Generally etch enamel equally as well as dentin

Get Ready for Exams!—cont'd

6. Etch-and-rinse bonding systems:
   a. May result in tooth sensitivity caused by overdrying or overetching
   b. Do not require a separate etching and rinsing step
   c. Do not require drying of the primer
   d. Do not provide a good etch of uncut enamel
7. With the etch-and-rinse system, when bonding to dentin, one of the following statements is true. Which one?
   a. The dentin surface should be thoroughly dried after etching and rinsing.
   b. The surface of the etched, rinsed, and lightly dried dentin should be "glistening."
   c. The surface of prepared dentin should have visible water droplets.
   d. Once you have dried the etched surface, it cannot be rewetted.
8. The smear layer:
   a. Is a tenacious layer of cut tooth debris on the surface of prepared enamel and dentin
   b. Is easily removed by rinsing with water
   c. Is necessary for good bonding
   d. Is not removed when bonding by the etch-and-rinse technique
9. Which one of the following does *not* interfere with the formation of a good bond?
   a. Saliva on the etched enamel or dentin
   b. Oil lubricant from the handpiece
   c. Moist dentin after rinsing etchant off and lightly drying
   d. Flavoring agents in prophy paste
10. Which type of bonding system has been shown to consistently provide the greatest bond strengths to enamel and dentin?
    a. Three-step, two-bottle etch-and-rinse
    b. Two-step, one-bottle etch-and-rinse
    c. Two-step, two-bottle self-etch
    d. One-step, one-bottle self-etch

For answers to Review Questions, see the Appendix.

Case-Based Discussion Topics

1. A 24-year-old graduate student needs two occlusal sealants on the lower first molars and a composite resin restoration to repair toothbrush abrasion on the facial root surface of the maxillary left canine.

   Discuss the similarities and differences in bonding to enamel for the sealants and to dentin for the composite resin.

2. A 42-year-old factory worker comes to the dental office with a chief complaint of discolored maxillary incisors. The patient has tried tooth whitening but that did not work. The dentist has planned for porcelain veneers to cover the discoloration. The preparations will be entirely in enamel.

   Which type of bonding system works best for etching and bonding to enamel? Why is it more effective than other systems?

3. A 65-year-old retired schoolteacher needs restoration of both mandibular first molars, which have root caries on the facial root surfaces. The caries extend beneath the crest of the gingiva so that isolation with a rubber dam is not possible. The patient wants tooth-colored restorations.

   Discuss the requirements for ensuring a good bond.

4. A 23-year-old college student comes to the dental office complaining of sensitivity to cold foods and air in the area of the lower-right first molar. The pain is limited to the cervical part of the tooth at the gingival crest, which has receded 3 mm. The problem appears to be caused by toothbrush abrasion of the root. The patient is a needle phobic and does not want an injection of local anesthetic. The dentist wants to apply a bonding resin to the area.

   Discuss which bonding materials to select. Which technique (etch-and-rinse or self-etch) will likely cause the patient the least amount of pain? Why?

BIBLIOGRAPHY

Alex G: Universal adhesives: the next evolution in adhesive dentistry? *Compend Contin Educ Dent*, Jan 2015.

Bird DL, Robinson DS: *Dental liners, bases and bonding systems.* In *Modern dental assisting,* ed 13, St. Louis, 2021, Elsevier.

Farah JW, Powers JM: Bonding agents—2008, *Dent Advis* 25(1–9), 2008.

Ferracane JL: *Direct esthetic anterior restoratives.* In *Materials in dentistry,* Philadelphia, 2001, Lippincott Williams & Wilkins.

Lane JA, Hughey SJ, Gregory PN, et al: Is your dental adhesive forgiving? How to address challenges, *Compend Contin Educ Den.* 37(10), 2016.

Nakabayashi N, Nakajima K, Masuhara E: The promotion of adhesion by resin infiltration of monomers into tooth structure, *J Biomed Mater Res.* 16:265, 1982.

Nazarian A: *The progression of dental adhesives [online continuing education].* In *Dental CE Digest,* 2007, PennWell Publications.

Ozer F, Blatz MB: Clinical applications of self-etching and etch-and-rinse adhesive systems, *Inside Dentistry,* Jan 2013.

Phillips RW, Moore BK: *Adhesion and elasticity.* In *Elements of dental materials for dental hygienists and dental assistants,* Philadelphia, 1994, Saunders.

Poticny D.J.; Adhesive systems continue to evolve: a case report. *Dentistry Today.* Available at http://www.dentistrytoday.com/dental-materials/9217-adhesive-systems-continue-to-evolve-a-case-report, 2013.

Powers JM, Wataha JC: *Bonding agents.* In *Dental materials: foundations and applications,* ed 11, St. Louis, 2017, Elsevier.

Retief DH: Effect of conditioning the enamel surface with phosphoric acid, *J Dent Res.* 52:333, 1973.

Ritter AV, Boushell LW, Walter R: *Adhesive Dentistry.* In *Sturdevants's art and science of operative dentistry,* ed 7, St. Louis, 2019, Elsevier.

Sakaguchi RL, Ferracane J, Powers JM: *Materials for adhesion and luting.* In *Craig's restorative dental materials,* ed 14, St. Louis, 2019, Mosby.

Shen C, Rawls HR, Esquivel-Upshaw JF: *Bonding and bonding agents.* In *Phillips' science of dental materials,* ed 13, St. Louis, 2022, Elsevier.

Silverstone LM: *The acid-etch technique: In vitro studies with special reference to the enamel surface and the enamel-resin interface.* In *Proceedings from the International Symposium on Acid Etch Technique,* St. Paul, 1975, North Central Publishing.

Strassler HE: Contemporary resin adhesives, *Inside Dent,* October 2014.

Composites

8

http://evolve.elsevier.com/Eakle/materials/

Chapter Objectives

On completion of this chapter, the student should be able to:

1. Describe the various types of composite resin restorative materials.
2. Identify the advantages and disadvantages of each type of composite resin.
3. Discuss the similarities and differences among chemical-cured, light-cured, and dual-cured composite resins.
4. Describe how fillers affect the properties of composites.
5. Describe the important physical properties of composites.
6. Explain why incremental placement of composite resin is recommended.
7. Describe the factors that determine how long an increment of composite resin should be light-cured.
8. Demonstrate proper placement of a sectional matrix for a class II composite.
9. Identify the appropriate type of composite for a class II cavity preparation.
10. Describe the process of selecting an appropriate shade of composite for a patient's restoration.
11. Demonstrate proper placement and light curing of a composite in a class II cavity preparation as permitted by the state dental practice act.
12. Light cure a composite resin restoration following recommended exposure times
13. Demonstrate proper use of eye/retina protection.
14. Finish and polish a class III composite restoration as permitted by the state dental practice act.

Key Terms

Direct-Placement Esthetic Materials tooth-colored materials that can be placed directly into the cavity preparation without being constructed outside of the mouth first

Composite Resins direct-placement, tooth-colored materials composed of an organic resin matrix, inorganic filler particles, a coupling agent, and coloring pigments

Organic Resin Matrix thick liquids made up of two or more types of organic molecules (polymers) that form a matrix around filler particles

Inorganic Filler Particles fine particles of quartz, silica, or glass that give strength and wear resistance to a material

Silane Coupling Agent a chemical that helps to bind the filler particles to the organic matrix

Pigments coloring agents that give composites their color

Monomers organic molecules that act as building blocks to link together to form larger, complex molecules known as polymers

Polymerization a chemical reaction in which organic monomers link to form chains or networks of polymers often causing the material to harden

Self-Cured Composites composites that polymerize by a chemical reaction when two filled resin pastes are mixed together; one paste with an initiator and the other with a catalyst

Light-Cured Composites single-paste composites that polymerize when a photosensitive chemical is activated by light in the blue wave range

Depth of Cure the depth to which light from a curing unit can penetrate and cure composite resin

Dual-Cured Composites composites that contain components of light-activated and chemically activated materials. When the two parts are mixed together, it polymerizes by a chemical reaction that can be accelerated by blue light activation

Incremental Placement a technique for composites that places and cures small increments individually to reduce the overall polymerization shrinkage in the restoration

Elastic Modulus a measure of the stiffness of a material; the higher the elastic modulus, the stiffer the material

Macrofilled Composites an early generation of composites that contained large filler particles ranging from 10 to 100 microns (μm)

Microfilled Composites composites that contain very small filler particles averaging 0.04 μm in diameter but do not contain a large volume of filler

Hybrid Composites composites that contain both fine fill (2–4 μm) and microfill (0.04–0.2 μm) particles to obtain the strength of a macrofill and the polishability of a microfill

Microhybrids hybrid composites that contain fillers that are smaller fine-particle (0.04–1 μm) and microsized fillers

Nanohybrids microhybrids to which nanosized fillers (less than 100 nm) have been added

Universal Composites composites that have physical and mechanical properties such as strength and polishability that allows them to be used in both the anterior and posterior parts of the mouth

Nanocomposites composites that contain all nanosized fillers to enhance physical properties

Flowable Composites light-cured, low-viscosity composite resins

Bulk-Fill Composites composites with greater depth of cure that permit placement in large increments up to 4 mm thick instead of the standard 2 mm; their use speeds up the filling process

Hue the color of a material such as a tooth (e.g., yellow-brown)

Chroma the intensity of color (i.e., bold yellow is more intense than pastel yellow)

Value the amount of lightness or darkness of a material such as a tooth (i.e., a high value is brighter and a low value is darker)

Indirect-Placement Esthetic Materials tooth-colored materials that are used to construct restorations outside of the mouth in the dental laboratory or at chairside on replicas of the prepared teeth. They are later cemented into the prepared teeth

---

Composites have overtaken amalgams as the most frequently placed direct restorations. In 1999 approximately 86 million composites were placed in the USA. By 2006 approximately 146 million composites were placed in the USA (ADA Survey of Dental Services). Manufacturers have continually improved composites by making them easier to handle, more durable, esthetic, and color stable. Advances in esthetic materials and techniques have improved the ability of the dental team to deliver the esthetic results that patients demand. Good listening skills are needed to determine the types of esthetic services the patient is requesting so that the dental team and the patient are working together toward a common goal. Esthetic materials must be carefully selected so that their properties are compatible with the patient's oral condition and occlusion. As important members of the dental team, dental auxiliary must understand the properties of these materials, so they can help the dentist to assess the soundness of the restorations and alert the dentist when they perceive that a restoration may be failing. The auxiliary need to be familiar with the physical properties of the materials so they do not damage the restorations during routine oral hygiene, coronal polishing, and preventive procedures. Knowledge of the handling characteristics of the esthetic materials is important so the auxiliary can assist the dentist in placement of the material or can perform steps in their placement, finish, and polish as permitted by state dental practice acts.

This chapter describes the composition, physical and mechanical properties, clinical applications, advantages, and shortcomings of directly placed composite resin materials. Guidelines for selection of the shade of these materials to obtain satisfactory cosmetic results also are discussed.

HISTORY OF THE DEVELOPMENT OF COMPOSITE RESIN FOR DENTISTRY

For the first half of the 20th century, amalgam and gold were the primary restorative materials for posterior teeth. Some anterior teeth also had metal restorations that were visible when the patient smiled. In the latter half of the 20th century, various direct-placement tooth-colored restorative materials were introduced. Initially, chemical-cured, unfilled acrylic resins were used, but they leaked, wore down quickly, and became discolored.

In 1962 Rafael L. Bowen developed bis-GMA resin monomer that is still used in many composites today. Silica particles were added to bis-GMA to reinforce it and make it more wear resistant. In 1963 chemical-cured composite resin was introduced. The early composite resins were available in a very limited number of shades, were rough and worn out quickly, discolored, and shrank excessively when they cured. Resin bonding agents had not been developed yet, so the restorations leaked and postoperative sensitivity and recurrent caries were common occurrences. In an effort to have more control over the working time, composites cured by ultraviolet light were developed. Later, composites cured by visible blue light were introduced. Most of the improvements that have occurred in composites to the present have been related to reducing shrinkage, using smaller fillers to enhance polishing and wear resistance, improving the selection of colors, increasing durability, improving handling properties, and delivery methods.

DIRECT-PLACEMENT ESTHETIC RESTORATIVE MATERIALS

Esthetic materials are those that are tooth colored. Direct-placement esthetic materials are those that can be placed directly into the cavity preparation or onto the tooth surface by the clinician without first being constructed outside of the mouth and match the appearance of the tooth. The direct-placement esthetic materials used most commonly are as follows:

- Composite resin
- Glass ionomer cement
- Resin-modified glass ionomer cement (also called *hybrid ionomer*)
- Compomer

This chapter will limit the discussion to composite resin. Chapter 9 will cover the other direct-placement esthetic materials.

COMPOSITE RESIN

A composite is a mixture of two or more materials with properties superior to any single component. Composite resins are tooth-colored restorative materials that are used in both the anterior and posterior parts of the mouth. They are composed mainly of
- An organic resin matrix
- Inorganic filler particles
- A silane coupling agent that sticks the particles to the matrix

Additional components are initiators and accelerators that cause the material to set and pigments that give color to the material and match tooth colors. Composite resins are commonly called *composites* and also can be referred to in the dental literature as *resin composites*.

COMPONENTS

Resin Matrix
The most commonly used resins for the matrix of composites are dimethacrylate monomers such as bis-GMA (bisphenol-A-glycidyl dimethacrylate) or UDMA (urethane dimethacrylate). These monomers are organic molecules that, when activated, link together to form a long chain called a polymer.

Filler Particles
Fillers are small particles composed of:
- Glass
- Quartz
- Silica
- Ceramic

Filler particles have several functions:
1. Fillers make the composite stronger and more wear resistant.
2. When fillers are added to the resin, it reduces the amount of resin present in the final product. The amount of shrinkage that occurs when the resin matrix sets is less because there is less resin to shrink.
3. Fillers help to control the translucency of the composite by their effect on the scattering of light.
4. The amount of filler and its size and shape affect the viscosity of the composite and how it handles.
5. Adding filler reduces the amount of resin, thereby reducing thermal expansion and contraction and decreasing water sorption (uptake) that softens the resin and makes it more likely to wear.

Coupling Agents
A coupling agent is used to provide a stronger bond between the fillers and the resin matrix. This coupling agent is silane, which reacts with the surface of the filler and with the organic matrix to allow the two to adhere to each other. Good adhesion of the two is necessary to minimize loss of filler particles from the resin matrix and thereby reduce wear.

Pigments
Inorganic pigments (usually metal oxides) are added to the resin matrix in varying amounts to develop a variety of colors that approximate the basic colors of teeth or specialized colors. Pigmented resins (also called *coloring resins*) can be used to cover discolorations or dark dentin, or to hide the graying effect of a metal post in a root canal–treated tooth. Pigments are also used to characterize a restoration. For example, a white pigment can be added to parts of the restoration to mimic white spots that occur on the tooth. Coloring resins are usually lightly filled and come in a variety of colors, including blue, white, orange/yellow, pink, light and dark brown, ochre, and clear.

 Do You Recall?

What role does each of the components of the composite play?

POLYMERIZATION

Polymerization is the chemical reaction that occurs when low-molecular-weight resin molecules called *monomers* join together end to end to form long-chain, high-molecular-weight molecules called *polymers*.

Activation of the polymerization process can be done by three processes:
- Chemically (chemical cured)
- By light (light cured)
- By a combination of the two (dual cured)

During polymerization, regardless of method, an activator (chemical or light) causes an initiator molecule to set off the chain reaction that joins the monomers.

Cross-Linking of Polymer Chains
Polymer chains have small *branches* of atoms hanging off their sides. When branches of adjacent polymer chains bond together (called *cross-linking*) (Fig. 8.1), the cross-linked chains produce a stronger, stiffer material.

Modes of Cure
Chemical Cure. Chemically cured composite resins, also called self-cured composites, are two-paste systems supplied in screw-type syringes or cartridges. One paste, called the *base*, contains composite and an initiator (benzoyl peroxide). The other paste, called the *catalyst*, contains composite and an activator (tertiary amine). Equal parts of these two pastes are mixed together, and the polymerization reaction begins. The reaction could go to completion very quickly, but chemicals called *inhibitors* are added to each paste to slow down the reaction. The operator has a limited amount of time (working time—usually about 2 minutes in the mouth) to place the restoration before it becomes too stiff to manipulate. Once the initial set occurs, the material should not be manipulated or the properties of the restoration will be degraded. Chemical-cured composites packaged in two-chamber cartridges are

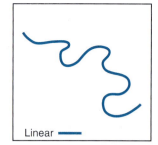 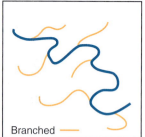 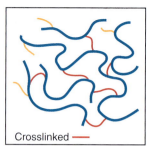

FIG. 8.1 Diagrams of linear, branched, and cross-linked polymers. Adjacent linear polymer chains are linked by covalently bonded atoms from short side chains (branches). (From Shen C, Rawls HR, Esquivel-Upshaw JF. *Phillips' Science of Dental Materials.* 12th ed. Elsevier; 2013.)

extruded from the cartridge by a gun-type apparatus that forces the two pastes through a mixing tip that automatically mixes the materials (see Fig. 8.12). This automixing greatly reduces the introduction of air into the mixed composite and provides the correct proportions of each material. The composites most commonly found in cartridges are those used as core materials for crowns.

Light Cure. **Light-cured composites** are the most common type of composite resin used in private practice. Many clinicians prefer light-cured composite resin, because it requires no mixing and the operator can control the working time by deciding when to apply the curing light. An intense visible light in the blue wave range activates these materials. Blue light with a wavelength of about 470 nm activates an initiator (camphorquinone) that, in the presence of an accelerator (an organic amine), causes the resin to polymerize. These components are both present in the composite but do not react until the light triggers the reaction. Inhibitors are also present to reduce the effects of the operatory light on premature setting. However, some manufacturers' materials are sensitive to direct exposure of the operatory light. The operator may choose to turn the operatory light away from the mouth when placing the composite.

Depth of Cure. The ability of the light to penetrate the composite and cure it is limited in depth (called the **depth of cure**). Just how far the light can penetrate and cure is affected by several factors:
1. The length and intensity of the light application
2. The distance the composite is located from the light
3. The thickness of the composite
4. The color of the composite
5. The amount and type of filler used
6. The type of material the light must pass through to reach the composite (such as enamel, dentin, ceramic).

A composite restoration that is not completely cured can lead to microleakage, recurrent caries, or loss of the restoration from the cavity preparation.

Dual Cure. **Dual-cured composites** are two-paste systems that contain the initiators and activators of both light-activated and, to a lesser extent, chemically activated materials. The advantage is that when the two pastes are mixed together and placed in the tooth, the curing light initiates the setting reaction, and the chemical setting reaction continues in areas not reached by the light to ensure a complete set.

 Do You Recall?

Why do clinicians prefer light-cured composites?

 KEY POINTS

COMPOSITE COMPONENTS AND CURING
Composites have three main components:
- Resin matrix
- Filler particles
- Coupling agent

Resin matrix contains pigments to provide tooth-like colors or to characterize the restoration. It also contains activators and initiators to set off the curing process. Additionally, accelerators and inhibitors control the speed of the reaction.
Curing occurs in three modes:
- Chemical cure—has limited working time.
- Light cure—has operator-controlled working time.
- Dual Cure—assures a complete cure when the curing light cannot reach all of the composite.

 Do You Recall?

What can happen if a composite restoration is not cured completely?

PHYSICAL AND MECHANICAL PROPERTIES OF COMPOSITE RESINS

Important properties of composites include the following:
- Biocompatibility
- Strength
- Wear
- Polymerization shrinkage
- Thermal conductivity
- Coefficient of thermal expansion
- Water sorption
- Elasticity
- Radiopacity

Biocompatibility

Newly placed composite resins can release chemicals that, in deep cavity preparations, could pass through the dentinal tubules into the pulp, causing an inflammatory reaction. When the tubules are sealed by dentin bonding agents or protected with a base or liner, the opportunity for this pass-through is eliminated. Composites can release components into the oral cavity as well. Water or other solvents in the diet can dissolve out unbound monomers and other additives, and some components can leach out as the composite degrades over time.

Bisphenol A is a polymer that can be found in some composites and fissure sealants. The concern with bisphenol A is that it can mimic the effects of estrogen and cause the development of secondary female characteristics or stimulate certain cancer cells. Research reports suggest that the level of bisphenol A released by composites and sealants is very low and does not represent a health threat to individuals.

Polished composites are well tolerated by surrounding soft tissues. Very few individuals may be allergic to one or more of the components of the material, and for these individuals another restorative material must be chosen.

Steps to reduce the incidence of bisphenol A (BPA) exposure during sealant and composite placement:

- Properly cure the resin. Undercured resin can release BPA.
- Wipe off the uncured resin film on the surface of sealants or composites.
- Use good isolation techniques such as rubber dam or four-handed delivery with high-volume suction.
- When adjusting sealants or composites, use high-volume suction.

Strength

Most of the composites commonly used today are similar in compressive strength. They are not as strong in compression as amalgam but are stronger than glass ionomers.

Wear

Composites wear faster than amalgams. Recent improvements have made the latest generation of composites more wear resistant than early composites.

Wear of the composite is related to the filler particle size, the amount of filler in the resin, and the amount of resin between particles. Large filler particles tend to get pulled from the resin matrix at the surface (called *plucking*) when the restoration is under function or abraded by food and tooth brushing, resulting in wear of the remaining resin matrix and a rough surface. Smaller particles are not as easily plucked from the resin and therefore cause fewer voids that contribute to wear. The smaller the particles, the smoother the surface of the composite will be after finishing and polishing and the longer it will be able to retain its luster (Figs. 8.1 and 8.2).

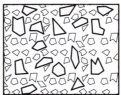 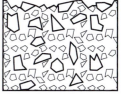

Smooth surface at time of placement and surface polish

Irregular surface due to erosion and loss of filler particles

FIG. 8.2 Wear of composite surface. At left, smooth surface at the time of placement and surface polish. At right, rough surface caused by wear and loss of filler particles at the surface.

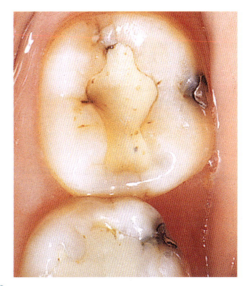

FIG. 8.3 Worn composite with staining at the margins indicative of microleakage. Opposing occlusion has worn the composite down, and numerous pits have developed as bits of the composite have fractured out.

Composites with a lower volume of filler (microfills and flowables) wear faster than more heavily filled materials. Wear from the opposing teeth can abrade composites quickly especially in people who grind their teeth (Fig. 8.3).

Polymerization Shrinkage

Polymerization shrinkage refers to the shrinkage that occurs when the composite is cured (polymerized). As the monomers link together into chains (polymers), the volume of resin decreases, so the net result is shrinkage.

Clinical Consequences of Polymerization Shrinkage.

As light-cured composite polymerizes and shrinks it tends to pull toward the walls of the cavity preparation that are bonded. This can create problems such as:

- Stress created on bonds when two opposing walls (e.g., buccal and lingual walls of class I occlusal preparation) are connected with composite and cured
- Enamel cracking or a gap at the margins of the restoration
- Microleakage (leakage at a microscopic level) at the shrinkage gap that allows fluids and bacteria to travel through dentinal tubules into the pulp causing sensitivity

- Microleakage that leads to recurrent caries or staining at the margins

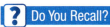

Do You Recall?

What are the undesirable effects of composite shrinkage when composites shrink when they are cured?

Methods of reducing polymerization shrinkage:

- When possible use composites with a high filler content such as hybrids
- Place composite in small (2-mm) increments (**incremental placement;** Fig. 8.4)
- Use composite with low-shrinking monomers
- Make the composite in the laboratory from an impression; then cement in place

Thermal Conductivity

Composite resin will transmit hot and cold temperatures much like the natural tooth structure. So, its thermal conductivity is compatible with the teeth and much lower than that of metal, such as amalgam or gold. Therefore it is a biologically protective material for the dental pulp.

Coefficient of Thermal Expansion

The coefficient of thermal expansion (CTE) is the rate at which a material expands when heated. With composite resin, the CTE is greater than that of the tooth structure, and therefore it will undergo a greater change in dimension than the adjacent tooth structure. This change can result in debonding and leakage of the restoration. The greater the filler content, the lower the CTE.

Elastic Modulus

The **elastic modulus** (also referred to as the *E-modulus* or *Young's modulus*) is a measure of the stiffness of a composite and is determined by the amount of filler. The greater the volume of filler, the stiffer (higher elastic modulus) the composite will be and the more wear resistant the restoration will be.

Water Sorption

The resin matrix absorbs water from the oral cavity over time. The greater the resin content, the more water is absorbed. The water can soften the resin matrix, leading to gradual degradation of the material (called *hydrolysis*). Water also causes some expansion (hydroscopic expansion) of the composite over the first week after placement.

Radiopacity

Metals such as lithium, barium, or strontium are added to the filler to make a restoration more opaque when viewed on a radiograph. However, some older composite materials do not have any of these additives and might appear radiolucent on radiographs (Fig. 8.5). Clinicians may have a difficult time determining whether there is recurrent caries around such radiolucent composites because the caries also appears somewhat radiolucent on radiographs.

KEY POINTS

PHYSICAL PROPERTIES

Knowing about the physical properties of the various composites is useful in determining which composite to select for restorations in the anterior and posterior parts of the mouth. Composite heavily filled with small particles will have these benefits:

- Increased strength
- Increased wear resistance
- Reduced polymerization shrinkage
- Increased stiffness
- Thermal expansion close to that of the tooth
- Reduced water sorption

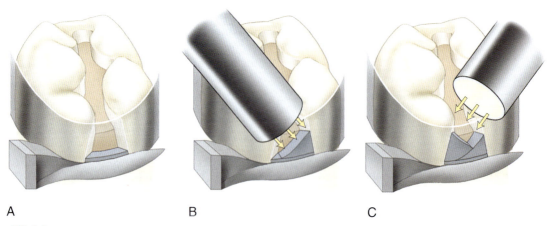

FIG. 8.4 Incremental placement of composite to minimize polymerization shrinkage and ensure complete cure of composite. **(A)** First increment has been placed horizontally *(gray area)* in a thin layer on the gingival floor and light-cured. **(B)** Second increment has been placed diagonally and light-cured. **(C)** Third increment has been placed diagonally on the opposite wall and light-cured. (From Shen C, Rawls HR, Esquivel-Upshaw JF: *Phillips' Science of Dental Materials*, ed 13, St. Louis, 2022, Elsevier.)

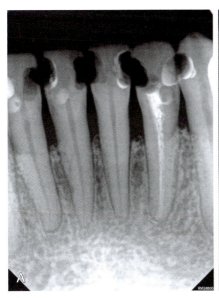
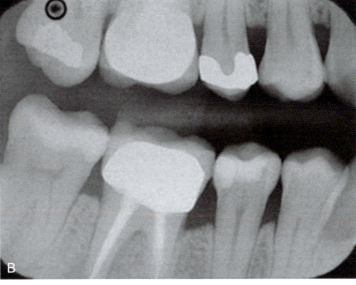

FIG. 8.5 X-rays of two types of composites. **(A)** Older anterior composites that lacked heavy metals in the filler particles so they are radiolucent and appear to be missing. **(B)** A class II composite on tooth 29 DO that is radiopaque. (Courtesy Dr. Steve Eakle, University of California, San Francisco.)

CLASSIFICATION OF COMPOSITES BY FILLER SIZE

Composite resins have undergone a steady progression in their development to improve their properties. Over time, the filler particle size has become smaller and smaller, the number of filler particles placed in the resin has increased, and polymerization shrinkage has decreased. As a result, composite restorations have become more durable, leak less, polish better, and match the teeth better. One way to classify composites is by the size of the filler particles they contain (Fig. 8.6).

MACROFILLED COMPOSITES

The first generation of composite resins used relatively large particles as fillers, ranging in size from 10 to 100 μm. By comparison, a human hair is about 70 μm in diameter. These composites are called **macrofilled composites**. The large particles make these composites difficult to polish. They become rough as filler particles are lost at the surface under function or as the resin wears, exposing the large particles. Because of their roughness and rapid wear, macrofilled composites are no longer used.

MICROFILLED COMPOSITES

Microfilled composites were developed to overcome the problems that arose with larger particle size. Microfill particles average about 0.04 μm in diameter and range in size from 0.03 to 0.5 μm. It is difficult to load a large volume of microfillers in the resin matrix. Therefore the volume of filler in microfilled composites is only 35% to 50%, as opposed to 70% to 85% with many other composites. A lower filler volume results in a composite with poorer physical properties (i.e.,

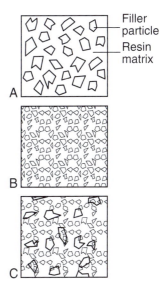

FIG. 8.6 Variety of filler sizes that are combined in the composite resins and contribute to their classification names: **(A)** macrofilled, **(B)** microfilled, and **(C)** hybrid—a combination of microfillers (about 0.4 μm) and small fillers (about 1–4 μm).

weaker, with greater polymerization shrinkage, and more wear). When polished, the microfilled composites produce a very smooth, shiny surface, unlike the rougher macrofilled composites. However, because of their poorer physical properties, they are not suitable for stress-bearing sites, such as for class I, II, and IV (incisal edge repair) restorations (Table 8.1).

HYBRID COMPOSITES

Hybrid composites get their name because they contain both large fillers (2–4 μm) and 5% to 15% microfine fillers (0.04–0.2 μm). The combination of the two filler sizes produces a strong composite that polishes well. The microfine particles fill in between the larger

Table 8.1 Classification of Dental Caries (or Cavity Preparations)

CLASSES OF CARIES	LOCATION OF CARIES	ILLUSTRATION OF CARIES LOCATION
Class I	Pits and fissures—posterior teeth; lingual of maxillary incisors	
Class II	Proximal surfaces of posterior teeth	
Class III	Proximal surfaces of anterior teeth	
Class IV	Proximal plus incisal angle of anterior teeth	
Class V	Cervical third of anterior and posterior teeth	
Class VI	Cusp tips of posterior and incisal edge of anterior teeth	

particles to allow higher filler content (70%–80% by weight). These composites have universal application in that they can be used well in both the anterior and posterior parts of the mouth. Improved products have reduced the demand for hybrids.

MICROHYBRIDS

Hybrids were improved by the use of even smaller particles (75% are smaller than 1 μm). These hybrids are called **microhybrids**, because they contain a mixture of small particles (0.04–1.0 μm) and microfine particles (0.01–0.1 μm). Microhybrids contain high filler content (70% by volume).

NANOHYBRIDS

Nanohybrids were introduced shortly after microhybrids. **Nanohybrids** are microhybrids with nanosized particles added. Their particle sizes range from 0.005 to 0.020 μm. The ability to add increased numbers of filler particles reduces the amount of resin. With less resin, these composites shrink less when polymerized. Shrinkage has been reduced from roughly 2% to 3% with earlier composites to about 1% with nanohybrids. They are strong composites that can be polished to a high shine, and they retain that shine better than earlier composites. The nanohybrid composites are called **universal composites** because they are esthetic, wear resistant, and strong which allow them to be used in both the anterior and posterior parts of the mouth.

NANOCOMPOSITES

Nanofilled composites, or **nanocomposites**, have filler particles that range in size from 5 to 75 nm. The nanocomposite filler particles are about a thousand times smaller than conventional fillers, which are approximately 1 μm. It is difficult to imagine how small these particles are. One nanometer is one-billionth of a meter. Nanocomposites have a combination of individual spheroidal particles and clusters of these particles produced by fusing the particles together at their edges (Fig. 8.7). The spaces between the particles in the cluster are filled with silane, which helps bind the clusters to the resin matrix. Nanoclusters range in size from 0.6 to 1.4 μm. The extremely small size of the filler particles allows for many more of them to be packed into the resin and more closely together than in the other types of composites. This high filler content (about 78% by weight) reduces polymerization shrinkage and provides strength so that they can be used in both anterior and posterior applications. They have excellent polishability and with improved wear resistance will maintain their luster long term. They have handling characteristics and physical properties similar to micro- and nanohybrids.

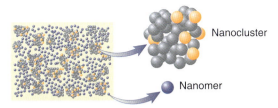

FIG. 8.7 Illustration of nanofilled composite with nanomers and nanoclusters. (From Sakaguchi R, Ferracane J, Powers J. *Craig's Restorative Dental Materials.* 14th ed. Elsevier; 2019.)

Optically, the nanocomposites are very esthetic because light passes through rather than being absorbed and is also scattered by the multitude of particles, so the composite tends to blend in better with the surrounding tooth structure.

 Do You Recall?

Which types of composites should not be used on chewing surfaces of posterior teeth?

Composite Kits

Composite kits may contain anywhere from 10 to 30 or more shades (colors). Most kits have shades that are slightly translucent to mimic enamel and shades that are more opaque to mimic dentin. Shades that are more translucent are available to mimic incisal translucency, and opaque shades are available to block out or hide discolorations or darker dentin. Very light shades have been made to match teeth that have been whitened.

 KEY POINTS

COMPOSITES' PROPERTIES
- Composites have evolved from rough materials with very large particles and rapid wear to materials with nano-sized particles that better match the color of the teeth, polish to a smooth surface with a high shine, and have reduced wear.
- Polymerization shrinkage has been reduced from around 3% to approximately 1–1.5% with improved resins and increased volume of nanosized particles.
- Nanohybrids and nanocomposites are considered universal composites in that they can be used in both the anterior and posterior parts of the mouth.

OTHER COMPOSITE TYPES

Flowable Composites

Flowable composites are low-viscosity, light-cured resins that may be lightly filled (about 40%) or more heavily filled (up to 70%). Initially, the particle size was in the range of those for hybrid composites. However, nanosized fillers are also being used in flowable composites.

Delivery. These composites flow readily and can be delivered directly into cavity preparations by small needle cannulas attached to the syringes in which they are packaged. Because of their low viscosity, they adapt well to cavity walls and flow into microscopic irregularities created by diamond and carbide burs.

Uses. Flowable composites are well suited for use in conservative dentistry (i.e., minimal preparations), where they readily flow into the narrow preparations created with small-diameter burs, diamonds, or lasers. Many dentists use them in place of conventional pit and fissure sealants because they are more wear resistant than lightly filled sealants. They are also useful as liners in large cavity preparations, because they adapt to the preparation better than more viscous composites.

Flexibility. Their low elastic modulus allows them to cushion stresses created by polymerization shrinkage or heavy occlusal loads when they are used as an intermediate layer under hybrid and packable composites. They are used for restoration of cervical noncarious lesions caused by acid erosion. (Fig. 8.8). In cervical restorations flowable composites tend to flex if the tooth flexes slightly. Stiffer composites often fall out when the tooth flexes.

Properties. Lightly filled flowable composites wear more readily, are weaker, and shrink more (about 4%–6%) when polymerized than hybrid composites (<3%), However, flowable composites too are being improved to make them stronger and more durable with less shrinkage. Some manufacturers have developed self-adhesive flowable composites that bond directly to dentin because the bonding agent is incorporated into the composite. See Table 8.2 for classification of composites by four different criteria.

Pit and Fissure Sealants

Pit and fissure sealants are low-viscosity resins that vary in their filler content from no filler to more heavily filled resins that are essentially the same as flowable composites. They are used to prevent dental caries in pits and fissures of teeth (see Chapter 18).

Bulk-Fill Composites

Bulk-fill composites were developed to speed up the placement process of the composite restoration. Instead of having to place and cure multiple small increments, the clinician can place one large increment and cure it. This provides a significant time savings.

Depth of Cure. The challenges of the bulk-fill composite are to have a depth of cure that permits increments of 4 mm or more, to not shrink excessively, to

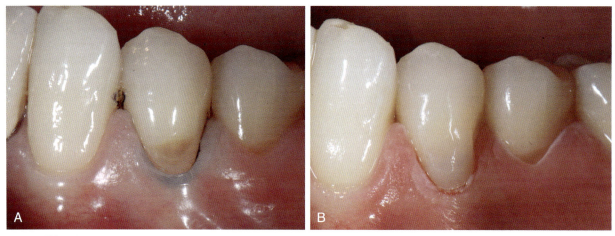

FIG. 8.8 Restoration of class V erosion lesion: **(A)** erosion lesion pretreatment and **(B)** lesion restored with flowable composite. (From Powers JM, Wataha JC. *Dental Materials: Properties and Manipulation.* 11th ed. Elsevier; 2017.)

TABLE 8.2 Four Classification Methods for Composites

CLASSIFICATION METHOD	MICROFILL	MICROHYBRID	NANOCOMPOSITE	FLOWABLE HYBRID
1. Filler amount (volume %)	30–50	60–70	78	30–55
2. Particle size (μm)	Macro (10–100)	Fine (0.1–10)	Micro (0.01–0.1)	Nano (0.001–0.01)
3. Matrix composition	Bis-GMA	Bis-GMA or UDMA	Silorane (low shrinkage)	Bis-GMA or UDMA
4. Polymerization method	Self-cured or light cured	Self- or light-cured	Light cured	Light cured

Bis-GMA, Bisphenol-A-glycidyl dimethacrylate; *UDMA*, urethane dimethacrylate.

flow well into all aspects of the preparation without voids, to have acceptable physical properties, and to be esthetic with good polishability. To achieve a greater depth of cure manufacturers, have done one or more of the following:
1. Increased the translucency
2. Reduced the amount of filler
3. Changed the chemical makeup to enhance polymerization when curing is initiated

Because the bulk-fill composites are more translucent, they do not match the tooth shade very well. Additionally, with reduced filler, they wear more readily. For these two reasons, bulk-fill composites may need to be covered with a layer of a more wear-resistant and color-matching composite.

Polymerization Shrinkage. Polymerization shrinkage of bulk-fill composites has been reduced by adding special modifiers that relieve stress in the restoration during curing or by adjusting the size, number, and composition of the filler. The shrinkage for bulk-fill composites is in the range found with other high-viscosity composites (about 1.3%–2.4%).

Formulations. Bulk-fill composites are found in two consistencies: flowable and viscous nanohybrids. Flowable bulk-fills adapt well to the internal portions of the preparations, whereas viscous nanohybrids must be carefully manipulated into the line angles and undercut areas. In general, shade selection is very limited, with most manufacturers offering only one to four shades.

Light-Curing Bulk-Fill Composite. To achieve the desired depth of cure, the curing light must be used for the recommended time. Check the light wand tip to make sure it is free of residual composite debris that could limit the transmission of light.

Packable Composites

Packable composites are highly viscous materials that contain a high volume of filler particles (as much as 90% by volume). The filler particles are long, rough, irregular fibers (about 100 μm in length) that bind on each other as the composite is packed into the preparation giving them a stiff consistency and make them less likely to stick to the composite placement instrument. They are used in posterior teeth for class I and II restorations, because they are slightly stronger and more wear resistant than most hybrids that contain less filler. Their physical properties show no significant improvement over traditional universal composites. They are not widely used.

Core Buildup Composites

Core buildup composites are heavily filled composites used in badly broken-down teeth needing crowns. They replace missing tooth structure lost from dental caries or tooth fracture, so that there is adequate structure to retain a crown. These composites can be light cured, self-cured, or dual cured. They often contain pigments that colorize them so that they can be easily differentiated from the natural tooth structure (Fig. 8.9). Dentin-colored core materials are used when all-ceramic crowns are to be placed to avoid an esthetically unacceptable dark discoloration under the all-ceramic crown, as light passes through the ceramic and reflects off the core buildup.

Core buildup composites are strong and can be bonded to the tooth structure to minimize bacterial leakage and increase retention. However, mechanical retention in the remaining tooth structure is necessary, because bonding alone is not strong enough to resist the forces placed on the crown. The tooth can be prepared immediately after the composite core is placed and polymerized.

The materials are packaged in compules, syringes, and cartridges with automixing tips similar to impression materials (see Fig. 8.16 in the section on Dispensing). Some dual-cured core materials are supplied in syringes that have two chambers (one for the base and one for the catalyst). An automixing tip is attached to the syringe to mix the material. A small delivery tip can be added to the mixing tip to deliver the mixed composite directly into the preparation.

> **Clinical Tip**
>
> Not all light-cured bonding agents are compatible with chemical-cured composites, so follow the manufacturer's recommendations when selecting a bonding agent for the core material.

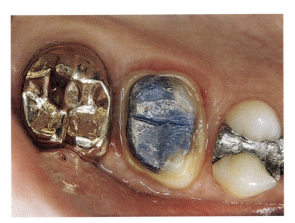

FIG. 8.9 Composite core material with color contrasting to the tooth structure for easy identification during crown preparation. (Courtesy Dr. Dennis J. Weir, Novato, California.)

Provisional (Temporary) Restorative Composites

Provisional (temporary) crowns and bridges hold the prepared teeth in position so they do not drift and change their proximal contact position or occlusal relation with the opposing teeth (see Chapter 15). Provisional composite restorations also have the following functions:

1. They provide esthetics in the smile zone
2. Maintain proper speech
3. Allow proper function for chewing
4. Maintain proper form for oral hygiene
5. Protect exposed dentin
6. Provide a good marginal seal

Provisional materials made with bis-acrylic and rubberized urethane are more popular than acrylic resins because of their ease of handling, reduced shrinking on setting, and do not generate the heat found with acrylic resin. Flowable composites can be used to add contacts or repair margins. These materials are covered in more detail in Chapter 15.

See Table 8.3 for a description of composite resin types on the basis of their properties.

> **KEY POINTS**
>
> **COMPOSITES VISCOSITIES**
>
> A variety of viscosities for special applications:
> - Flowables are easily dispensed from a syringe through a needle cannula and they flow readily into tight spaces and undercuts. However, generally they are weaker, wear faster, and shrink more when cured than hybrids.
> - Bulk-fills speed up placement time compared to multiple small increments. However, it is difficult to cure large increments to their full depth. Longer curing times are needed.
> - Packables are thick and stiff and were marketed as esthetic replacements for amalgam using similar packing techniques. They are not widely used.
> - Core buildups are heavily filled composites used for making solid substructures for crowns. They have mostly replaced amalgams for this purpose.
> - Provisional restorative composites are used to make temporary crowns and bridges. They shrink less and generate less heat when cured than acrylic resins. Flowables can be used to add contacts and margins when needed.

TABLE 8.3 Comparison of Properties of Composite Resins

COMPOSITE	POLYMERIZATION SHRINKAGE	FLEXURAL STRENGTH	COMPRESSIVE STRENGTH	POLISHABILITY	WEAR RESISTANCE
Macrofills	Low	High	High	Low	Low
Microfills	Moderate	Moderate	Moderate	High	Low
Hybrids (nano)	Low	High	High	High	High
Bulk-fill	Low	High	High	Moderate	Moderate
Flowables	High	Low	Low	High	Low

CLINICAL HANDLING OF COMPOSITES

USES OF COMPOSITE RESINS

Although initially used mostly on the anterior teeth, composite resins now are very popular for posterior teeth as well. Composites are used in all classes of restorations, from class I through class VI. Advantages and disadvantages of posterior composites can be found in Table 8.4.

In addition to use for restorations, composites can be used for esthetic applications. They can be applied to the facial surfaces of teeth as veneers to cover discolorations, reshape chipped or worn teeth, or provide a more even and brighter smile. They can also be used to close spaces (diastemas) between anterior teeth (Fig. 8.10). Special composite materials are also used for fiber-reinforced posts and laboratory-fabricated onlays and bridges.

SELECTION OF MATERIALS

Several criteria can be used for the selection of composite resins for restorations. When used in the anterior part of the mouth in non–stress-bearing areas, selection is usually based on the ability of the material to match the color of the teeth and to achieve a high polish. Microfills, microhybrids, and nanohybrids are well suited for this purpose. When incisal edges or other stress-bearing areas are being restored, one of the micro- or nanohybrids should be considered (Fig. 8.11) because they are stronger than microfills. In stress-bearing areas of the posterior part of the mouth, use a microhybrid, nanohybrid, or nanocomposite for strength and wear resistance. Flowable composites should not be used in areas subjected to stress or abrasion because they are relatively weak and wear more rapidly. See Table 8.5 for a summary of uses for composites.

HOW TO MATCH THE SHADE

Selecting the Shade

The dental auxiliary may be asked to assist the dentist in obtaining the appropriate shade for a restoration. A poorly chosen shade will likely result in replacing the restoration to satisfy the patient's esthetic expectations. This is disappointing for all involved and usually results in additional chair-time and possibly an additional appointment. Therefore it is important for all members of the dental team performing clinical procedures to have an understanding of what goes into the perception of color and how to match the variation of shades within a single tooth.

COLOR CHARACTERISTICS: HUE, CHROMA, AND VALUE

When teeth are viewed for shade taking, three characteristics should be taken into consideration: hue, chroma, and value (see Chapter 2):

- **Hue** is the color of the tooth and may include mixtures of colors, such as yellow-brown. It is determined by the wavelength of light that is reflected from or transmitted through the tooth.
- **Chroma** is the amount or intensity of color present; for example, a bold yellow has more chroma than a pastel yellow. The more chroma, the more intense the color (hue) will be.

TABLE 8.4 Posterior Composite Resins: Advantages and Disadvantages

ADVANTAGES	DISADVANTAGES
Durable (but not for as long as amalgam)	More costly than amalgam
Placed in one appointment	Wear is slightly greater than with amalgam
Good compressive strength	Shrinks when cured
Tooth colored	May leak, especially on root surfaces
Preparation more conservative than amalgam	Technique sensitive—patient may have sensitivity to cold or biting if restoration is not properly placed
Bonding helps to support the surrounding tooth	Not a good choice for very large restorations

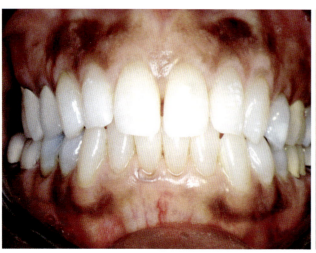 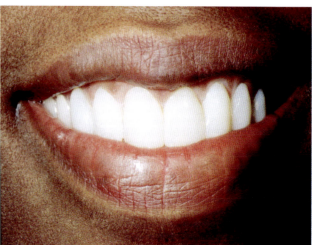

FIG. 8.10 Microhybrid composite was used to close the space (diastema) between teeth 8 and 9 and also to veneer the six anterior teeth. (Courtesy Dr. Stephan Eakle.)

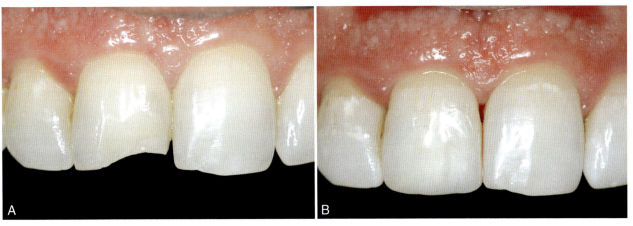

FIG. 8.11 **(A)** Fractured incisal edge tooth 9. **(B)** Fracture was repaired with microhybrid composite. (From Ritter AV, Boushell LW, Walter R. *Sturdevant's Art and Science of Operative Dentistry.* 7th ed. Elsevier; 2019.)

TABLE 8.5 Uses for Composites

COMPOSITE TYPE	USES
Macrofills	High-stress areas No longer used (high wear, poor polish)
Microfills	Class III, V cavity preps (low stress–bearing areas)
Micro- and Nanohybrids	Class I–VI (Universal)
Nanocomposites	Class III, V, low-stress areas
Flowables	Class I minimal preparations, V, as a sealant, cavity liner and where improved flow is needed
Bulk-fills	Class I, II, large cavity preparations, often veneered with micro- or nanohybrid for better color match
Packables	Class I, II
Provisionals	Temporary crowns, short-span bridges

- **Value** is the amount of lightness or darkness of the tooth (some describe it as the grayness of the tooth). A tooth with low value is darker and one with high value is brighter. Also, as the chroma increases, the value will decrease.

Patients tend to notice differences in value (or brightness) more than differences in hue or chroma when they assess how well a restoration matches their own teeth. So, if a restoration is the same value as the natural dentition but is slightly off in its color or chroma, it will be better accepted by the patient.

Involving the Dental Auxiliary and the Patient

The dentist often relies on the dental auxiliary (chairside assistant or hygienist) to help obtain a good color match for restorations with composite or ceramics. Three pairs of eyes (doctor, auxiliary, and patient) are usually better than one. Each person may interpret color differently. In addition, color-blindness (or the inability to correctly perceive certain colors) is more common in males (about 8% of males) than females. Involving the patients in shade taking helps the clinician in determining whether their expectations can be met. Matching shades can be very difficult because many teeth do not match the standard shade guides.

Lighting for Shade Taking

The lighting in which the shade is viewed is very important. Shade matching should be done in two different types of light because the perception of shade may vary in different lights, a phenomenon called *metamerism*.

Most dental offices have fluorescent or incandescent lights (or both). Fluorescent lights emit more blue light, and incandescent lights emit more yellow light. Some dentists install color-corrected light bulbs to help in shade taking. Ideally, the laboratory should also have color-corrected lighting.

A natural north light is considered a good light for shade taking. However, early-morning and late-afternoon natural light contains more yellow and orange light and less green and blue. If possible, the shade should also be taken while in the type of lighting that the patient is in most often. The bright light from the dental unit will tend to increase the perceived brightness of the shade and decrease the color intensity, so it should be turned off or moved away from the mouth.

Matching the Shade

A neutral background is important so that the colors do not distract the eye and alter the perceived shade. A pastel-blue patient bib is a good color for shade taking. Female patients should be requested to remove lipstick and colorful makeup because these colors may influence the shade. Colorful clothes should be covered. The room in which the shade is selected should not have brightly colored walls or decorations. The ideal color for the area in which the shade will be matched is a neutral gray.

In general, the shade should be taken before the tooth is prepared and before a rubber dam or other isolation is placed. The color of the rubber dam can interfere with accurate matching, and teeth dry out and become lighter when under the dam or when isolated with cotton rolls. For best shade matching, the teeth should be clean, free of stain, and moist.

> **Clinical Tip**
>
> Prior to Taking the Shade:
> - Have the patient remove lipstick and colorful makeup
> - Cover bright, colorful clothing with a neutral-colored bib, such as pastel blue
> - Place the patient in a neutral-colored room
> - Remove debris and surface stain from the teeth
> - Do not isolate the teeth; keep them moist
> - Move the dental unit light away from the mouth

Shade Guides

Select the appropriate shade guide for the material that will be used. Many manufacturers of composites include a shade guide with color tabs that can be used to help in shade selection. Sometimes these color tabs are not an exact match to the composites they represent. Therefore it is a good practice to apply and cure a small quantity of the composite selected onto the clean, moist tooth to verify the color match before the tooth is isolated and dried. The shade tab should be moist and held in the same plane as the surface of the teeth being matched, not in front of the teeth or behind them; otherwise the light reflected off the tooth and the tab will be slightly different (Fig. 8.12). The tab should be viewed under different lighting conditions. Do not stare at the color for longer than a few seconds at a time, because the retina adjusts for red and yellow colors, and the brain's perception of the color will be off. Looking at a pastel-blue object (such as a pastel-blue patient bib) after each shade tab was once recommended, but it causes blue color retinal fatigue. Instead, look at a neutral gray color for a few seconds.

The patient, dentist, and auxiliary should view the tabs and rank them as to the closest match for lightness or darkness (value) and color intensity (chroma). If the color intensity of the tooth is low, it may be more difficult to determine the color. In this case, the cervical area of a tooth with a more intense color, such as a maxillary canine, should be used to help pick

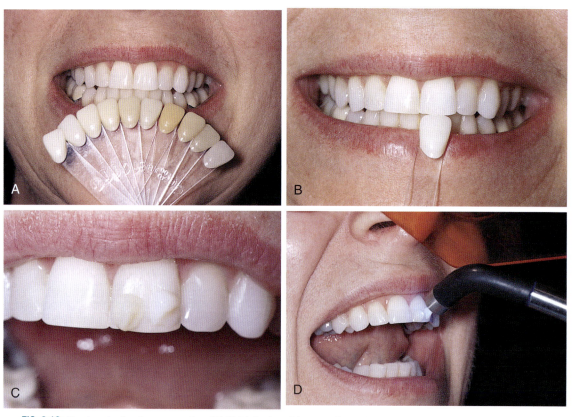

FIG. 8.12 Shade selection for composites: **(A)** Hold shade guide up to the teeth and look for the shade that is the closest match. **(B)** Hold that shade tab next to the tooth to be restored to confirm the match. **(C)** If unsure of an exact match, place a small amount of composite in the two closest shades on the tooth. **(D)** Light cure the composite so that its final shade can be compared with the tooth. Select the closest match. On occasion, a couple of shades will need to be mixed together to get a good match. (Note: The patient has naturally reddish lips and no lipstick.)

the initial color. It is often necessary to take separate shades for the cervical portion of the tooth, for the occlusal surfaces of posterior teeth, and for the incisal edges of anterior teeth.

Some clinicians find it helpful to arrange the shade guide tabs by value from lightest to darkest, and then they select the three shades closest to the tooth in value. From there, they narrow the selection to the one that most closely matches the tooth color.

Clinical Tip

A good use of time is to take the shade after the injection of local anesthetic, while you are waiting for the patient to get numb.

Do You Recall?

What are factors to consider when selecting a shade for a composite restoration?

KEY POINTS

SHADE MATCHING

Three characteristics should be considered when shade matching:
- Hue—the color of the tooth
- Chroma—the intensity of the color present
- Value—the lightness or darkness of the tooth
Factors for shade matching in the office environment:
- Artificial light is often more yellow.
- Natural light is good but early-morning and late-afternoon light has more yellow or orange.
- Do not use the bright dental unit light.
- Eliminate color distractions such as lipstick, colorful clothing, bright-colored walls. Use pastel blue or gray patient bibs.
- Take shade before isolating or preparing teeth for restoration.
- Use an appropriate shade guide, moisten shade tabs, and hold them next to the teeth.
- Do not stare at the shade tab and teeth for more than a few seconds to avoid color fatigue of the retina.

PLACING THE COMPOSITE

Thickness of Composite Increments

Most composites should be placed in small increments about 2 mm thick (Fig. 8.13). Bulk-fill composites can be placed in increments about 4 mm thick.

Light-Curing the Increments

If the composite resin is placed in too thick an increment, the light might not penetrate completely, and the composite might not cure all the way to the bottom. Longer curing times may be required for increments greater than 2 mm thick. Even with a long curing time, some light-curing units may not have the output needed to cure to the bottom of large increments (>4 mm). More powerful curing lights might be able to cure greater thicknesses of material.

Interproximal areas may need additional time to cure completely because of the more difficult access of the area to the direct path of the light. It is good practice to cure the interproximal composite restoration again from both facial and lingual surfaces after the metal matrix band is removed to ensure complete curing in the bottom of the box form of the preparation.

Darker shades also require a longer curing time because the light is more readily absorbed by the dark color and does not transmit through the material as readily as through lighter-colored materials. Composites that are heavily filled also will take longer curing times because the filler tends to disperse the light rather than allowing it to transmit through the composite to its full thickness.

RESIN-TO-RESIN BONDING

Etched enamel and dentin are infiltrated with resin bonding agents to form a resin-rich layer. The resin-infiltrated dentin is called the *hybrid zone* or *hybrid layer* (see Chapter 7). The initial increment of composite resin will chemically bond to the resin bonding agent on the enamel and dentin. Each additional increment will bond to the previously placed increment of composite as long as good isolation is maintained and no contaminants are introduced.

When resins polymerize, the thin layer of unpolymerized resin on the surface (caused by with oxygen in the air) looks shiny and feels slippery. This thin, unset layer facilitates chemical bonding with the next layer of composite. It will set when the layer placed over it excludes air and then is cured.

The completed restoration comprises a series of layers of resin-based materials that are all chemically bonded to each other and micromechanically bonded to the tooth structure. The layers of resin seen when starting from the dentin side of the restoration and progressing toward the composite are the following:
- Resin tags in the dentinal tubules
- Resin-rich hybrid layer (dentin and resin)
- Adhesive resin layer
- Composite resin restoration (Fig. 8.14)

Do You Recall?

When placing composite material in increments, how does one increment stick to the following increment?

CONTAMINANTS

Newly etched dentin is kept moist for "wet" dentin bonding. However, before and after bonding, any form of extraneous moisture (water, saliva, fluid from the gingival sulcus [i.e., space between the gum and tooth], or blood) should be kept away from the tooth until the restoration has been completed. Contamination requires removal of the contaminant and re-etching for 10 to 15 seconds.

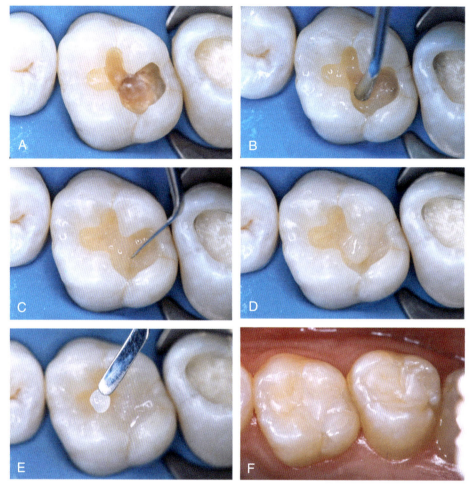

FIG. 8.13 Incremental insertion of composite in maxillary first molar: **(A)** class I occlusal preparation for composite. **(B)** A glass ionomer base was placed before the first increment of composite. **(C–E)** Additional increments are applied and light cured. **(F)** Final restoration finished and polished. (From Ritter AV, Boushell LW, Walter R. *Sturdevant's Art and Science of Operative Dentistry.* 7th ed. Elsevier; 2019.)

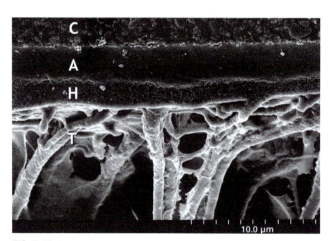

FIG. 8.14 Scanning electron micrograph of a traverse section of bonded composite restoration after the tooth has been dissolved away. Layers from the top are *(C)* composite, *(A)* adhesive layer, *(H)* hybrid layer, and *(T)* resin tags that had gone into the dentinal tubules. (From Sakaguchi R, Ferracane J, Powers J: *Craig's Restorative Dental Materials,* ed 14, St. Louis, 2019, Elsevier.)

Alcohol should not be used to wet the composite placement instrument to keep the composite from sticking because it weakens the composite. Use of a little of the bonding agent or other unfilled resin on the instrument to prevent sticking can dilute and thin the composite, making it weaker and more likely to wear. Special composite instruments are made with a coating of nonstick materials to help with the stickiness problem. They should be reserved for composite placement because once they get scratched, they lose their nonstick quality.

LAYERING (STRATIFICATION) OF COMPOSITE

Many dentists prefer to apply layers of composite of different shades or degrees of opacity or translucency to obtain a good match to the natural teeth. This process is called *layering* or *stratification*.

Teeth are usually not one color throughout, but a variety of colors and can be described as three general areas:

1. The cervical part of the tooth is closest to the dentin color. The translucent enamel is thinnest in the cervical part of the tooth, and light passing through it reflects back the color of the dentin. The dentin color is the bulk of the color of the tooth and can range from yellow to orange to red or mixtures of those colors. The dentin color of composite is usually the most opaque and is useful for blocking out stains from amalgam or tooth discolorations.
2. The middle of the tooth is called the *body area*. Its color is a result of light interacting with both enamel and dentin. The enamel in this area is thicker than in the cervical area.
3. The incisal part of the tooth is mostly enamel and will be more translucent. Often the interplay of the light with the translucent enamel will produce a bluish tint to the enamel (Fig. 8.15). Cusp tips of posterior teeth are not translucent like anterior teeth but will appear lighter in color than the cervical or body areas.

Dentists can select dentin, body, and enamel shades and apply them in layers to simulate the natural tooth colors with their opacities and translucencies. When faced with a challenging color match, dentists may choose to do a trial run or mock-up on the unetched tooth. The colors selected are applied in the desired layers and light cured. The results can be seen and modified before the tooth is restored. Because the tooth has not been etched, the mock-up material will come off easily.

The restoration can be characterized to replicate white spots, stains in occlusal fissures, or bluish incisal translucency. Special tints or stains made for composite can be used.

SHELF LIFE

The shelf life of composites varies with the type of resin used and the manufacturer. In general, avoiding heat and light can extend shelf life. Manufacturers usually recommend refrigerating the material. The average shelf life is two to three years, if stored properly. Check the label on the container that the composite came in to see the expiration date.

DISPENSING AND CROSS-CONTAMINATION

Light-cured composites are supplied in compules or syringes. All of these containers are opaque so that the material is not affected by light. Some offices prefer single-use (unit-dose) items such as composite compules (small containers of composite resin that fit into a delivery gun) that can be disposed of after the procedure to minimize the risk of cross-contamination. Reusable syringes require careful handling to ensure that they are not contaminated during the procedure. The delivery tip on syringes of flowable composites should be disposed of in a sharps container after use, and the syringes should be recapped and sprayed or wiped with disinfectant. Composite in screw-type syringes should be dispensed after the shade is selected and covered in a light-protected container until use (Fig. 8.16).

Chemical-cured composites come in screw-type tubes or two-container cartridges. They require similar dispensing measures to prevent cross-contamination.

If the composite is stored in the refrigerator, it should be removed an hour or more before its planned use to allow it to return to room temperature. Cold composite will be stiff and less likely to stick to the placement instruments, but more difficult to adapt to the wall of the cavity preparation. Composite syringes or compules can be placed in warm water to increase the flow of the material.

> **Clinical Tip**
>
> Placing a composite syringe or compule in warm water will increase its flow. Putting it in the refrigerator before use will make it stiffer; consequently, it will not stick to the placement instrument as much.

> **KEY POINTS**
>
> **COMPOSITE PLACEMENT**
> - Use 2-mm increments (4 mm for bulk-fill).
> - Check curing light manufacturer's recommendations for curing time.
> - Increase curing time for thick increments, dark shades, and composite farther away from the curing light.
> - A thin film of uncured resin on the surface (air-inhibited layer) of one increment allows the next increment to chemically bond to it.
> - Contamination of the tooth preparation requires cleaning, re-etching, and reisolation.
> - Composite shades for dentin and enamel can be added in layers to mimic the natural tooth.
> - To prolong shelf life, store composite in the refrigerator.
> - Good infection control practices should be followed to prevent cross-contamination. Disposable items help facilitate this process.

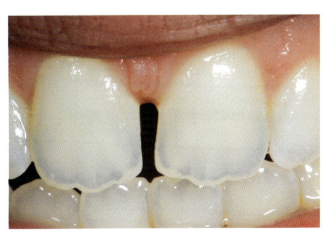

FIG. 8.15 Several different colors are seen in the central incisors. The color is slightly darker in the cervical part of the teeth and gets progressively lighter toward the incisal. The incisal edges show translucency, which gives the enamel a bluish tint. From Ritter AV, Boushell LW, Walter R. *Sturdevant's Art and Science of Operative Dentistry.* 7th ed. Elsevier; 2019.

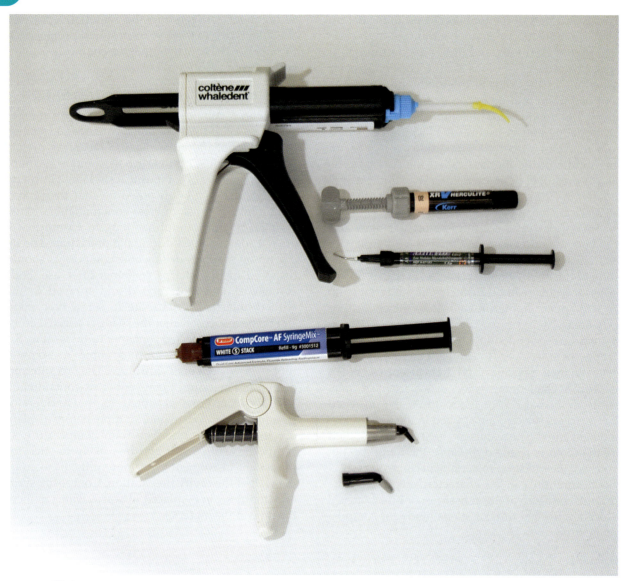

FIG. 8.16 Dispensing systems for composites. *Clockwise from top to bottom:* Dual cartridges with automixing tip, screw-type syringe, injection-type syringe, dual syringe with automixing tip, and compules delivered by a dispensing gun.

MATRIX SYSTEMS

Matrix systems for operative dentistry are comprised of components such as metal or plastic bands, wedges, and pressure rings (also called *separator rings*) that help to adapt and shape the restorative material. The matrix is used most often when restoring the proximal surface of a tooth. It is also used for extensive direct restorations such as complex composites or amalgams and crown buildups. On occasion, a matrix is used when restoring cervical lesions with composite or glass ionomer cement.

Matrix Bands

The purpose of the matrix band is to help contain the restorative material within the preparation during placement and to develop natural contours and proximal contact areas. Matrix bands for anterior teeth are usually clear plastic (polyether or celluloid), and they may be precontoured to help shape the proximal surface of the restoration or straight strips (Fig. 8.17). Precontoured forms are also available for repairing a proximal surface involving an incisal angle.

Matrix bands for posterior teeth are made of soft metal (typically stainless steel in thicknesses ranging from 0.02 to 0.045 mm) that is flat or precontoured or of clear precontoured polyester. The bands may go entirely around the tooth (circumferential) or just on a proximal surface (sectional). Sectional bands fit only on one proximal surface at a time, as with mesioocclusal or distoocclusal cavities.

Whole crown forms can be used when the entire crown must be built up. The stock crown form is trimmed to fit the remaining tooth structure, and then filled with composite. After etching and application of bonding agent, it is pressed onto the remaining tooth structure and cured from multiple directions. Then the crown form is slit and peeled away.

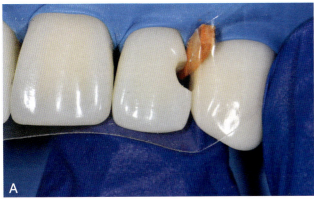
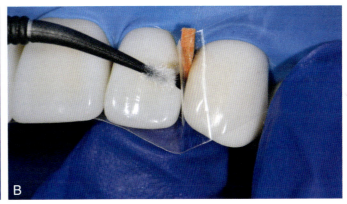
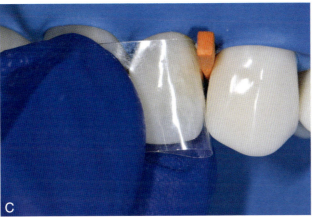

FIG. 8.17 Matrix system for class III composite on 7D: **(A)** a transparent plastic strip is placed interproximally and a wedge is applied to hold the band against the gingival margin of the preparation and slightly separate the teeth. The strip is folded back to provide access to the preparation. **(B)** After etching, a bonding agent is applied and light cured. **(C)** Composite is inserted into the preparation and the matrix strip is folded across the facial surface to form the proximal surface in the composite. The band is held on the lingual by the index finger. (From Ritter AV, Boushell LW, Walter R. *Sturdevant's Art and Science of Operative Dentistry.* 7th ed. Elsevier; 2019.)

Circumferential Matrix Systems

The Tofflemire circumferential matrix system is well established and very popular for amalgam restorations (see Chapter 11). It is very difficult to use this system with class II composites and achieve a good proximal contact area. Composite shrinks when it cures, and it cannot be condensed against the matrix band as amalgam can, so more separation of the teeth is needed to create a firm contact area. If a circumferential band, like the Tofflemire band, is used, wedges must be inserted heavily into the interproximal space to create enough separation of the teeth to make up for the thickness of the band in both mesial and distal interproximal spaces. In addition, the band is flat and needs to be contoured to the adjacent tooth to help form an anatomic proximal contact area. Some of the bands have cervical extensions used for proximal boxes that extend subgingivally.

Circumferential metal bands can also be pre-welded into loops or spot-welded in the office to the desired diameter. With the T-band, flanges of metal that form the T shape can be folded and crimped around the band at the desired diameter. T-bands are thin, soft brass or stainless steel and have been used in pediatric dentistry for decades (Fig. 8.18).

Criteria for a well-placed matrix band for proximal box:

- Band extends beyond the gingival margin of the box at least 1 mm
- Side of the band contacts the gingival margin of the box
- Band contacts the adjacent tooth
- Band establishes contours for the restoration (facial—lingual, gingival—occlusal and proximal)
- Band extends no more than 1 mm above the marginal ridge to be restored

Do You Recall?

What is the purpose of the matrix band?

Clinical Tip

Circumferential bands may be difficult to fit around a tooth that has only one proximal surface prepared. A tight proximal contact with the adjacent tooth on the unprepared proximal side makes it difficult to slip the band down between the teeth. Insert a wedge under heavy pressure in the interproximal space to separate the teeth. This can help in slipping the band between the prepared and unprepared teeth.

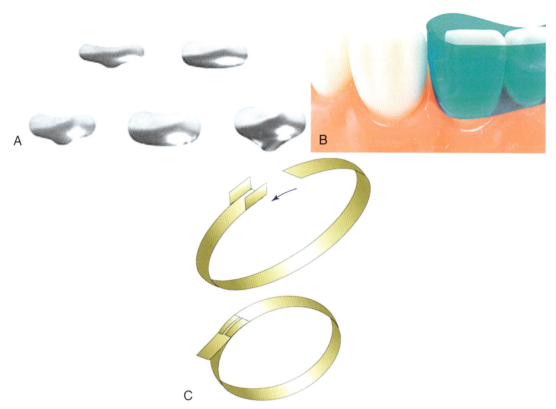

FIG. 8.18 Matrix bands: **(A)** sectional metal matrix bands with some having cervical extensions. **(B)** Clear plastic band. **(C)** T-bands. (A and B, Courtesy Garrison Dental Solutions, Spring Lake, Michigan and C, From Bird DL, Robinson DS. *Modern Dental Assisting.* 13th ed. Elsevier; 2021.)

Sectional Matrix Systems

Sectional matrix systems used for class II composite resins usually are equipped with a selection of precontoured sectional bands of various widths appropriate for premolars or molars, a pressure ring, and ring placement forceps (Fig. 8.19). Some systems also supply forceps for handling the matrix band. Some of the bands have cervical extensions for deep proximal box forms (see Fig. 8.18A). The matrix systems have a metal ring that is opened with forceps (similar to those for a rubber dam clamp) and placed on the tooth to engage the interproximal embrasures of a class II cavity preparation. The ring has metal tines or soft rubber that holds the sectional matrix band firmly against the buccal and lingual surfaces of the tooth, and it applies pressure to the teeth to cause some separation (see Fig. 8.19B and D). Some pressure rings have a notch in the cervical extent of the ring so they fit right over the wedge (see Fig. 8.19C). The matrix bands are anatomically contoured to shape the contact areas and embrasures. Once the band, wedge, and ring are in place, the band should be burnished against the adjacent tooth surface to ensure firm contact.

If more than one proximal surface on a tooth is to be restored (i.e., a mesio-occluso-distal restoration), a sectional band could be placed on each proximal surface and pressure rings could be stacked one over the other. Otherwise, one proximal surface could be restored, and then the other.

Cervical Matrices

Plastic matrices are available for cervical composite or glass ionomer restorations (Fig. 8.20). These matrices are placed over the composite or glass ionomer (including resin-modified glass ionomer cement) to give it form, and then the restorative material is cured. These matrices are not always needed. The clinician may be able to contour the composite with an instrument.

Wedges

Tapered, triangular-shaped wedges of wood or plastic are placed interproximally and hold the matrix band against the tooth to seal the gingival margin of the proximal box, so that the restorative material does not extend out of the cavity preparation and cause an overhang. Wedges are usually placed from the lingual side, because the lingual embrasure is usually the widest. On occasion, wedges will need to be placed from both buccal and lingual approaches to secure the band against the tooth without gaps at the gingival margin. Wedges are usually inserted with pressure to create some separation of the teeth to make up for the thickness of the matrix band. Otherwise, when the band is

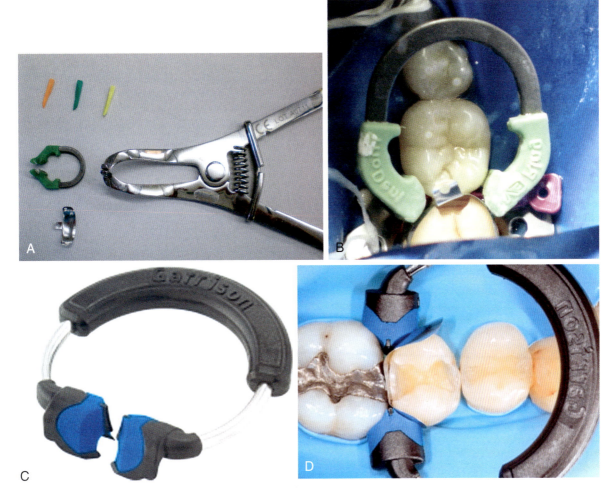

FIG. 8.19 Sectional matrix systems: **(A)** sectional matrix setup with wedges, pressure ring (Triodent V3, Dentsply Caulk), sectional matrix band, and ring forceps. **(B)** Sectional matrix system applied clinically. **(C)** Pressure ring (Composi-Tight 3D XR, Garrison Dental Solutions), for sectional matrix to create slight separation of the teeth to ensure a firm contact. **(D)** Pressure ring and sectional matrix band in place. (Courtesy Garrison Dental Solutions, Spring Lake, Michigan.)

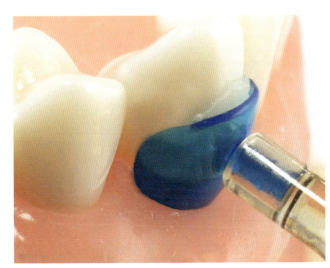

FIG. 8.20 Cervical matrices. (BlueView Cervical Matrix, Courtesy Garrison Dental Solutions, Spring Lake, Michigan.)

removed from the interproximal area after placement of the restoration, a space will exist between the restoration and the adjacent tooth (an open contact) leading to food impaction and periodontal disease. Placing a wedge before cavity preparation will help protect the gingival papilla and prevent bleeding during the preparation. It also initiates separation of the teeth.

Wooden and plastic wedges may be color coded for their size (Fig. 8.21). Plastic wedges may be opaque or transparent. Some plastic wedges have an advantage over wooden wedges, because they are shaped to conform better to the embrasure space and to the tooth. Transparent wedges are used on proximal surfaces when a clear matrix band is used for restoration of light-cured composites. The clear wedge allows light transmission to cure the material at the gingival margin; an opaque wedge would block the light.

Criteria for a well-placed wedge:

- Placed at or slightly below the gingival margin of the proximal box
- Placed firmly to produce separation of the teeth
- Seals the matrix band against the gingival margin of the box
- Does not distort the matrix band

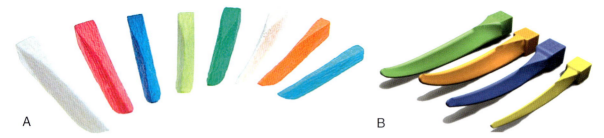

FIG. 8.21 Wedges. **(A)** Wooden anatomic wedges. **(B)** Plastic contoured wedges. (B, Courtesy Garrison Dental Solutions, Spring Lake, Michigan.)

> ### KEY POINTS
> **MATRIX BANDS**
> - Matrix systems consist of metal or plastic bands, wooden or plastic wedges and often a band holder or pressure ring.
> - Purpose of the band is to contain the composite and form natural tooth contours and proximal contacts.
> - The band may be circumferential or sectional.
> - A well-placed band will cover and seal the gingival margin of the proximal box, establish contact with the adjacent tooth, and shape tooth contours.
> - A well-placed wedge will press the band against and seal the gingival margin.
> - Create slight separation of the teeth and not distort the band.

LIGHT-CURING

Light-cured composite resins must receive the correct amount of light energy at the right exposure time and the right wavelength in order for them to polymerize completely. If the composite resin does not receive this correct curing combination, then it will have poorer physical properties and will not hold up as well clinically. The light source comes from a light-curing unit that may be built into the dental unit or free standing. Free-standing units have a handheld light guide (also called a wand) attached to a base by a cord or may detach from a recharging base and contain a battery pack.

Light Factors Affecting the Cure
The following are factors that can adversely affect the cure of a restoration:
- Short curing times
- Inadequate light output
- The wrong wavelength of light
- An incorrectly positioned light guide
- Chipped or damaged light guide
- Debris (bonding agent, composite) stuck to tip of light guide
- Plastic barrier for infection control over light guide tip (especially the seam)

Surveys of dental offices have found that many of the light-curing units had a reduced output of light energy. The light source may weaken in intensity with time and should be checked periodically with a radiometer (a meter that measures light output) (Fig. 8.22).

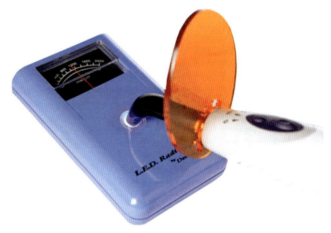

FIG. 8.22 Radiometer used to test the output of the curing light. (Courtesy Kerr Dental.)

Composites that are not completely cured may result in the following:
- Poor physical properties, such as rapid wear and poor strength
- Restoration with a short life span due to breakdown of margins
- Recurrent caries
- Discoloration of the composite

> **Clinical Tip**
> Periodically check the output of the curing light with a radiometer to make sure it has not diminished. Inadequate output will adversely affect the composite restoration.

Position of the Light Guide
The technique used to light-cure composite resin may also affect the amount of light that reaches the restoration. Ideally, the light guide should be held about 1 mm away initially and then almost in contact after a second or two. The tip of the light guide should be positioned at 90 degrees to the composite surface so the light shines directly on the composite. However, it is not always possible to position the guide at this angle or close to the composite surface. The shape and size of the light guide may be a limiting factor in the ability to position the tip ideally. When restoring molars in patients who cannot open fully or if matrix bands are

in the way, the closeness to the restoration and the light guide angulation may be compromised.

Curing in Proximal Box. A proximal box of a class II preparation may be 6 to 7 mm deep. When initiating cure from the occlusal surface, most light guides cannot reach the bottom of the box, and therefore the tip will be several millimeters away from the increment of composite on the gingival floor. It is thought that the high level of recurrent caries (much higher than with amalgam) seen at the gingival margin of the proximal box in a class II composite may be due, in part, to incomplete curing of the composite or bonding agent at the bottom of the box.

To address this issue:
- Increase the curing time
- Cure composite in the proximal box from the facial and lingual sides after the matrix band is removed. Anterior class III composites should also be cured from both facial and lingual surfaces.

Types of Light-Curing Units. Light-curing units are of four different types:
- Quartz-tungsten-halogen (*halogen*, as they are commonly called)
- Light-emitting diode (LED)
- Argon laser
- Plasma arc curing (PAC)

Light-Emitting Diode. Currently LED curing lights are the most widely used. Simple LED curing units have the lowest intensity of light and do not generate heat. The diodes can last as long as 5000 hours, and rechargeable batteries ensure portability and convenience. LED units emit blue light (within the visible light range) at 450 to 490 nm in wavelength. The initiator in the composite absorbs light between 460 and 480 nm and sets off the setting reaction. Some LED units can generate an energy output of about 1000 mW/cm^2 (Fig. 8.23).

Halogen. Halogen lights were the most widely used until LED units were introduced. They are next to lowest in light intensity. The halogen light bulb delivers a blue light that ranges from 400 to 500 nm in wavelength. The halogen bulb generates heat so an internal fan is built into the unit. The bulb lasts about 100 hours but deteriorates over time; the intensity therefore needs to be checked periodically with a radiometer to make sure it will provide an adequate cure. The bulb output should be 400 to 800 mW/cm^2. If it drops below 300 mW/cm^2, it should be replaced.

> **Clinical Tip**
>
> To test the halogen curing light for heat output, put the light tip on your fingernail and turn on the light for 20 seconds. If you can feel your nail getting hot, then your unit produces enough heat to cause some pulpal sensitivity in deep preparations. Use a stream of cool air on the composite during curing to help reduce the heat delivered to the tooth.

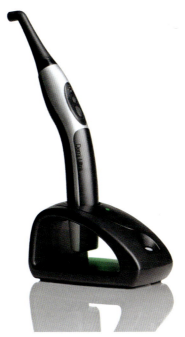

FIG. 8.23 Light-emitting diode wand-type recharging curing light. (Demi Ultra, Courtesy Kavo Kerr Group, Charlotte, North Carolina.)

Rapid Curing. PAC and argon laser lights are not widely used, but they provide the fastest cure. They also transmit heat to the composite and the tooth. Rapid curing greatly speeds up the procedure because conventional curing of many small increments each for 20 to 40 seconds increases the total time required. Rapid curing of increments of composite greater than 3 mm may not cure to the bottom of the increment because the light is scattered and absorbed and the intensity greatly diminishes. Thus additional curing time will be needed to achieve a complete cure beyond 3 mm as with bulk-fill composites.

Match the Curing Light to the Composite

Composites that use camphorquinone (CQ) as the photoinitiator are usually well matched with the curing units. However, some composites use different photoinitiators. The narrow light wave spectrum of argon lasers (490 nm) and some LED units (450–490 nm) may be a mismatch for these non–CQ-initiated composites, so they will not cure completely. Broadband LED units that have a broad light spectrum and a higher intensity are better to use to correct this problem. Halogen lights also have a broad light spectrum (400–500 nm) and will cure all of the current composites. Typical curing times for LED and halogen lights for thin layers are 20 to 40 seconds for each 2-mm increment. The intensity of the light diminishes rapidly the farther away the composite is from the tip of the light guide.

Factors requiring longer curing times for composite resins:

- Increments thicker than 2 mm (or 4 mm for bulk-fill composites)
- Very light shades for whitened teeth
- Opaque shades
- Darker shades
- Heavily filled composites (many small filler particles scatter the light)
- Composites located farther from the light tip than ideal (e.g., the bottom of a proximal box)

Areas of composite that lie just outside the borders of the light guide tip (typically 8 mm in diameter) should be cured separately. Wider tips are available and may be useful when curing broad areas such as occlusal composites or sealants or anterior veneers. The wider the tip, the more divergent the light beam will be, so longer curing times may be needed. Some manufacturers provide narrow diameter tips for reaching into proximal box preparations or other tight spaces.

The light guide on the curing unit is often glass, glass encased in metal, or a type of plastic. Some curing units are in the configuration of a wand; others are in the shape of a gun. Many units have the capability of being used remotely rather than being plugged into an electrical outlet, because they have rechargeable batteries.

Do You Recall?
What factors would be considered when determining how long to cure each increment of composite?

Desirable Features for Your Curing Light:

- Easy to use
- Simple infection control procedures
- Broad spectrum output to cure all composites
- High output for effective polymerization
- Has a radiometer to test output
- Wide curing tip angled at 90 degrees with short height for access in the posterior
- Durable

Eye Protection

The blue light emitted from a curing unit can be damaging to the retina of the eye. Curing units with high-intensity light output increase the risk for damage if precautions are not taken. A prolonged blast of blue light directly into the eye can cause immediate and irreversible damage to the retina. Repeated low-level exposure over time can accelerate aging of the retina and contribute to macular degeneration. Protective glasses with filters that block the blue light should be worn by those in the operatory—the operator, auxiliary, and patient. Some offices use an orange filter shield that is held between the operator and the light. Some units have a filter that attaches to the light guide (see Fig. 8.22). Looking directly at the light, even briefly, should be avoided.

Infection Control Methods. In many offices, the light guide and handle (or the entire unit, depending on the type) are covered with a disposable barrier, such as a clear plastic cover. The cover will also prevent bonding agent, composite resin, blood, and other debris from sticking to the tip of the guide. The ideal unit is one with a removable light guide that can be autoclaved and has smooth surfaces that can be wiped down with disinfectant. Autoclaving may cause some residue to accumulate on the tip of the light guide, but it can be polished off. Some disinfecting solutions may cause clouding of glass-fibered light guides and can discolor the plastic casing of the unit. Check with the manufacturer for the recommended disinfectant.

Guidelines for Light Curing

- Provide eye protection to those exposed to the light.
- Position the patient so as to provide best access for the light to the restoration.
- Check the light guide tip for damage or debris.
- Use curing times and output modes recommended by the manufacturer.
- Err on the side of using longer curing times than shorter.
- Direct the light at 90 degrees to the composite surface.
- Start curing with the tip about 1 mm from the composite surface and move closer after the surface has cured.
- Use longer curing times when the tip is farther away from the composite.
- When close access to the composite is limited (as with a class II proximal box), supplement with curing from buccal and lingual sides after the matrix is removed.
- With high-intensity curing units and extended exposure times, blow an air stream over the tooth to prevent overheating. Pause for a couple of seconds between curing cycles.

Data from Ferracane JL, Watts DC, Ernst C-P, et al: Effective use of dental curing lights: A guide for the dental practitioner. *ADA Professional Prod Rev*, 8:2–13, 2013.

Caution
Do not look directly at the light when curing materials. Stabilize the light tip using finger rests before you look away from the light to prevent it from drifting away from the restoration.
Use a light shield or filtering eyewear to protect the eyes. Have the patient close their eyes, or provide filtering eyewear.

Do You Recall?
Why should you avoid looking at the curing light beam?

> **KEY POINTS**
>
> **COMPOSITE CURING**
> Most of the composites used in restorative dentistry are light cured or dual cured.
>   Factors affecting the cure:
> - Inadequate light output
> - Incorrect position of the light guide—should be at 90-degree angle to composite and close
> - Inadequate curing time
> - Wavelength of light is incompatible with the type of composite used
>   Types of curing lights:
> - Quartz-tungsten-halogen
> - Light-emitting diode (LED)
> - Argon laser
> - Plasma arc curing
>   Typical curing times for halogen and LED lights for a 2-mm increment layer is 20 to 40 seconds.
>   Use longer curing times for:
> - Thicker increments
> - Dark shades
> - Opaque shades
> - Very light shades used for whitened teeth
> - Bulk-fill composite
> - Heavily filled composite
>   Precautions:
> - Avoid looking at the light
> - Provide eye protection for patient, operator, and assistant
> - Check for damaged or dirty light tip
> - Blow air over the tooth to prevent overheating when using high-intensity lights or long curing times

FINISHING AND POLISHING COMPOSITES

Finishing is the process used to correct irregularities in contour, remove excess material, and smooth the margins and external surfaces of the composite restoration. Polishing takes the process a step further by removing scratches using a step-wise application of sequentially finer abrasives to produce a glossy, very smooth surface. The smooth surfaces produced with polishing resist plaque retention and make cleaning with floss and a brush much simpler (see Chapter 17, for clinical techniques).

> **Clinical Tip**
>
> The finishing process will be much easier if care is taken during composite placement to carefully develop contours and not grossly overfill the cavity preparation.

WHY COMPOSITES FAIL

Composite resin has many applications in restorative dentistry. It is a versatile and very esthetic material, but it must be handled properly to maximize its longevity in the harsh environment of the mouth.

It has been estimated that 60% of all operative dentistry work done is to replace failing restorations. Studies have shown that amalgam restorations outlast composite restorations in similar applications. Composite restorations are more technique sensitive than amalgam restorations. However, composite resins have gained in popularity for posterior applications because patients demand esthetic restorations, and they have concerns about metals, especially mercury.

The average life span for composite resin restorations (both anterior and posterior) is 5.7 years. Two of the most common reasons for failure of light-cured composites are:
1. Fracture of the restoration
2. Recurrent caries

Composites are also replaced because of excessive wear, breakdown and leakage at the margins, discoloration, and fracture of the tooth. Patient factors such as poor diet, poor oral hygiene, and bruxism can contribute to recurrent caries and fracture but also operator errors are important causes. Operator errors include poor cavity preparation, inadequate isolation, over- or underetching, improper rinsing and drying of the tooth, poor incremental placement techniques, open proximal contacts, overheating the pulp, and inadequate curing of the bonding agent or composite resin (Procedure 8.1).

COMPOSITE REPAIR

Many clinicians who practice minimally invasive dentistry will attempt to repair existing composites rather than replace them when there are only minor defects at the margins or small areas of chipping. Usually, these are larger composites that are otherwise in good condition. There are no long-term clinical trials that indicate how effective the repair of an existing composite is in the oral environment. However, studies with 2- to 3-year follow-up show good success rates with repair of margins.

INDIRECT-PLACEMENT COMPOSITE RESINS

Indirect-placement esthetic materials are tooth-colored materials that are constructed outside of the mouth (chairside or in the laboratory) and then cemented in place. Composites can be used for indirect methods as well as direct. Some indirect-placement composite restorations are fabricated on a die (replica of the prepared tooth) and others are designed and milled from a block of composite material using CAD/CAM (computer-assisted design/computer-assisted machining) technology (see Chapter 10). The finished restoration is tried in the mouth, adjusted, and bonded into place with a bonding agent and resin cement (Fig. 8.24). Indirect materials were developed to try to eliminate the problems associated with polymerization shrinkage, such as marginal leakage, posttreatment sensitivity, and recurrent caries, and to reduce the wear seen with direct composites.

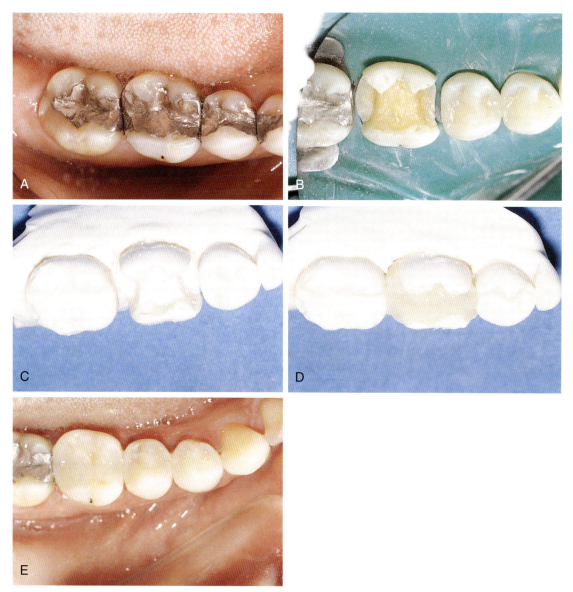

FIG. 8.24 Indirect composite techniques. **(A)** Pretreatment mesio-occluso-distal (MOD) amalgam restoration in the lower first molar. **(B)** Tooth prepared for MOD composite inlay. **(C)** Die of the preparation from an impression. **(D)** Composite inlay prepared outside of the mouth. **(E)** Composite inlay after cementation with a resin cement. (Courtesy Alton Lacy, University of California School of Dentistry, San Francisco, California.)

KEY POINTS

Indirect composites are made from conventional impressions or digital impressions:
- On a die in the laboratory
- By CAD/CAM technology
  Advantages:
- Polymerization shrinkage of composite occurs outside the mouth.
- Composite has a more complete cure when processed under heat and pressure.
- Contours and proximal contacts can be more accurately placed.

SUMMARY

Composite resins are very popular direct-placement esthetic materials. They have a wide variety of uses in both the anterior and posterior parts of the mouth. Composites are esthetically pleasing and durable restorative materials that are rapidly replacing amalgam as the material of choice in posterior teeth. They have applications in all classes of cavity preparations and many cosmetic applications. They can be used to close anterior diastemas as a conservative alternative to porcelain veneers. Indirect composites also have applications where reduced shrinkage and added strength can be achieved by processing the material in the laboratory or by using preprocessed composite blocks for CAD/CAM technology.

INSTRUCTIONAL VIDEOS

See the Evolve Resources site for a variety of educational videos that reinforce the material covered in this chapter.

Procedure 8.1 Placement of Class II Composite Resin Restoration

See Evolve site for Competency Sheet.

Consider the following with this procedure: *Safety glasses are recommended for the patient, PPE is required for the operator, ensure appropriate safety protocols are followed, and check local state guidelines before performing this procedure.*

EQUIPMENT/SUPPLIES (FIG. 8.25)

- Rubber dam setup
- Curing light and light shield
- Composite placement instruments
- Light-cured nanohybrid composite resin
- Bonding agent and finishing glaze
- Mixing wells or Dappen dish
- Finishing burs, diamonds, disks
- Articulating paper in paper forceps
- Local and topical anesthesia setup
- High-volume evacuator tip
- High- and low-speed handpieces
- Shade guide
- Etchant and applicator
- Matrix system and wedges
- Polishing points, cups, paste

PROCEDURE STEPS

1. Apply topical anesthetic. Local anesthetic is administered.

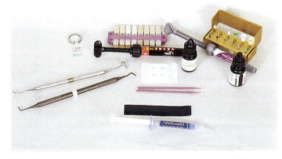

FIG. 8.25 Equipment/Supplies required for placement of Class II Composite Restorations.

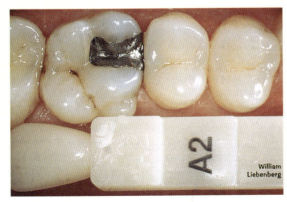

FIG. 8.26 Example of composite shade matching. Courtesy Dr. William Liebenberg, North Vancouver, BC, Canada.

2. Take a composite shade. Hold the shade guide close to the patient's mouth and select two or three shade tabs that are close to the patient's tooth color. Moisten and check each tab individually against the tooth under room light (and natural light, if possible) (Fig. 8.26). Verify the shade by taking a small amount of composite in the closest shade and light-curing it on the tooth for 20 seconds.

   NOTE: Shade is taken before the rubber dam is applied because the color of the dam might interfere with taking an accurate shade, and the teeth might dry out under the dam and appear lighter. Lipstick should be removed, and brightly colored clothing should be covered with a pale blue or gray patient bib to prevent the colors from influencing the perceived shade.

3. Apply the rubber dam.

   NOTE: Cotton roll isolation can be used, but a rubber dam provides more reliable isolation. Moisture from the breath can affect the bond adversely.

4. Rinse and dry the cavity prepared by the dentist.

5. Apply a sectional matrix, wedge, and pressure ring (Fig. 8.27).

   NOTE: A Tofflemire matrix can be used, but it is much more difficult to obtain tight contact when both mesial and distal interproximal spaces have matrix band in them at the same time. The wedge helps close the matrix band at the gingival margin to prevent overhang of composite, and it helps separate the teeth to make up for the thickness of the matrix band so that firm contact with the adjacent tooth can be established. The pressure ring helps adapt the matrix against the facial and lingual surfaces of the tooth and helps separate the teeth slightly.

6. Apply etchant to enamel first for 10 to 20 seconds, and then apply it to dentin for 10 seconds (Fig. 8.28).

   NOTE: Etching dentin for longer than 10 seconds will overetch it and contribute to weaker bond strength and postoperative sensitivity by opening the tubules

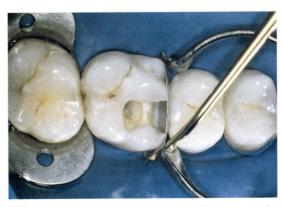

FIG. 8.27 Class II preparation with sectional matrix, wedge, and pressure ring. Courtesy William Liebenberg, North Vancouver, BC, Canada.

Continued

Procedure 8.1   Placement of Class II Composite Resin Restoration—cont'd

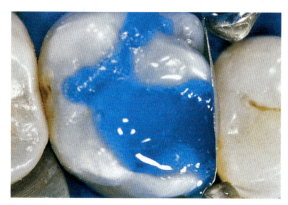

FIG. 8.28 Etchant applied to the tooth surfaces. Courtesy William Liebenberg, North Vancouver, BC, Canada.

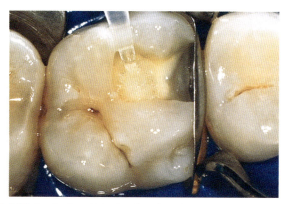

FIG. 8.29 Application of dentin primer/bonding resin with a brush applicator. Courtesy William Liebenberg, North Vancouver, BC, Canada.

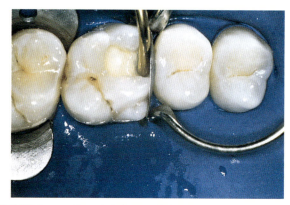

FIG. 8.30 Composite resin being applied in small increments. Courtesy William Liebenberg, North Vancouver, BC, Canada.

excessively. A self-etching bonding system could be used instead, and no rinsing would be needed (see Chapter 7).

7. Rinse thoroughly and dry lightly so that the dentin remains slightly moist (glistening but no pooling of water).
NOTE: Drying the dentin will cause collapse of the collagen fibrils and interference with penetration of the dentin primer into the tubules and etched dentin surface (see Chapter 7).
8. Apply dentin primer/bonding resin with a brush applicator as directed by the manufacturer (dentist's choice of one- or two-bottle bonding materials) and thin with a gentle stream of air (Fig. 8.29).
NOTE: See Chapter 7 for one- and two-bottle dentin primers and bonding resins. When the dentin primer and bonding resin are applied in separate steps, the dentin primer is usually light-cured for 10 to 20 seconds before placement of the bonding resin. Some dentists prefer to use a base or liner on the dentin before acid etching.
9. Dry gently and light-cure for 20 seconds.
NOTE: Drying at this step removes water and volatile solvents from the resin.

10. Apply composite resin in small increments, starting with the proximal box (Fig. 8.30). Each increment should be no more than 2 mm thick and light-cured for 20 to 40 seconds.
NOTE: Small increments are used to minimize the effects of polymerization shrinkage and to allow the light to cure the increment all the way through. Dark or opaque shades are more difficult for the light to penetrate and require longer curing times. Increase the curing time when the light probe is more than 1 mm from the composite. Some curing lights may have an initial low setting that ramps up to a high intensity to minimize shrinkage and stress within the material. Some very high-intensity curing lights require less curing time. Manufacturers' recommendations should be followed.
11. Remove the pressure ring, wedge, and matrix band after the cavity preparation is slightly overfilled with composite and cured. Cure the proximal box for an additional 20 to 40 seconds from the facial and the lingual sides. Contour the occlusal surface and remove excess material with finishing diamond and carbide burs. Disks and interproximal finishing strips are used on the proximal surfaces (Fig. 8.31). Check the contact area with floss to ensure solid contact and no overhang at the gingival margin.
NOTE: The composite in the proximal box should be cured again from the facial and lingual sides after removal of the matrix and wedge, because they may have partially blocked light transmission to the floor of the box, causing an incomplete cure of the composite.
12. Remove the rubber dam. Check occlusal contacts with articulating paper and adjust.
NOTE: A high restoration can cause a sore tooth by stressing the periodontal ligament, or a tooth that is temperature sensitive.
13. Polish surfaces with polishing points, cups, and brushes at low speed. A polishing paste can be used to produce a highly polished surface (Fig. 8.32).

Procedure 8.1 Placement of Class II Composite Resin Restoration—cont'd

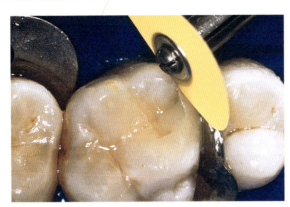

FIG. 8.31 Example of flexible disks utilized to contour proximal surfaces. Courtesy William Liebenberg, North Vancouver, BC, Canada.

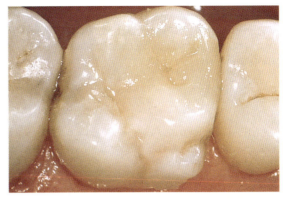

FIG. 8.32 Highly polished surface of a composite restoration. Courtesy Dr. William Liebenberg, North Vancouver, BC, Canada.

NOTE: Some operators prefer to apply a finishing glaze to the composite. A finishing glaze is an unfilled resin that bonds to the composite resin. Its purpose is to reseal the margins if polymerization shrinkage has caused the composite to pull away from the enamel margin, and it fills in any small voids in the surface that contribute to wear and staining. When the glaze is used, the tooth is isolated with cotton rolls, and the composite and adjacent enamel are etched for 10 seconds, rinsed, and dried. A brush is used to apply a very thin layer of glaze so as not to interfere with the occlusion. It is light cured for 20 seconds.

Review and Discussion

Review Questions

Select the one correct response for each of the following multiple-choice questions.

1. The major components of composite dental materials include all of the following *except* one. Which one is this exception?
   a. Bonding agent
   b. Resin matrix
   c. Coupling agent
   d. Fillers
2. Composite resins are often classified according to their:
   a. Strength
   b. Polishability
   c. Resin content
   d. Filler particle size
3. The shortcomings of flowable composites as compared with more viscous microhybrid composites include all of the following *except* one. Which one is this exception?
   a. They are weaker.
   b. They wear faster.
   c. They shrink more when polymerized.
   d. They are more difficult to polish.
4. What is the purpose of a silane coupling agent for composite resins?
   a. To improve the bond between the filler particles and the resin matrix
   b. To help the composite retain its color
   c. To reduce the oxygen-inhibited layer
   d. To help the various resin layers stick together
5. The curing light requires repair if:
   a. It causes a slower set of a dark-color composite.
   b. It has not been tested.
   c. A 2-mm-thick piece of composite does not cure through the bottom at the recommended exposure time.
   d. The light appears blue.
6. Polymerization shrinkage of a composite:
   a. Is cause for alarm
   b. Is greater than 10% of the volume
   c. Can be minimized by placing and curing a series of small increments
   d. Has no effect on the final restoration
7. Fillers are composed of all of the following *except* one. Which one is this exception?
   a. Quartz
   b. Resin
   c. Silica
   d. Glass
8. Which one of the following statements about a coupling agent is *false*?
   a. It minimizes the loss of filler particles.
   b. It reduces wear.
   c. It prevents filler from sticking to the resin.
   d. It is made of silane.
9. All of the following will *increase* the wear of a composite restoration *except* one. Which one is this exception?
   a. Use of large filler particles
   b. Incompletely curing the composite

Continued

Review and Discussion—cont'd

    c. Use of small amount of filler particles
    d. Saliva contamination of the etched enamel

10. Which one of the following types of composites is the weakest and should not be used in stress-bearing tooth surfaces?
    a. Hybrid
    b. Microfill
    c. Nanofill
    d. Nanohybrid

11. Which one of the following composites has the lowest viscosity and can be delivered from a syringe directly into a cavity preparation?
    a. Microcomposite
    b. Nanocomposite
    c. Flowable composite
    d. Nanohybrid composite

12. Heavily filling the resin matrix with nanosized fillers particles will *reduce* which one of the following?
    a. Curing time
    b. Strength of the material
    c. The esthetics
    d. Polymerization shrinkage

13. Which one of the following composites is most difficult to polish to a high shine?
    a. Macrofill
    b. Microhybrid
    c. Nanohybrid
    d. Hybrid

14. Which one of the following types of composites generally will shrink the most when polymerized?
    a. Bulk-fill composite
    b. Microhybrid
    c. Flowable composite
    d. Nanocomposite

15. What is the major shortcoming of chemical cured composites?
    a. They are the weakest of the composites.
    b. They cannot be polished.
    c. They generate excessive heat when they cure.
    d. They have limited working time.

16. Which one of the following is a drawback of bulk-fill composites?
    a. Difficult to cure a 4-mm increment to its entire thickness
    b. Excessive polymerization shrinkage
    c. Color is too opaque
    d. Weaker than other posterior composites

17. Common effects of polymerization shrinkage of composites may include all of the following *except* one. Which one is this exception?
    a. Microleakage
    b. Death of the pulp
    c. Microcracking of enamel causing white lines around the margins
    d. Postoperative sensitivity

18. Methods used to minimize polymerization shrinkage include all of the following *except* one. Which one is this exception?
    a. Cure the composite rapidly with a high-intensity light
    b. Use prepolymerized filler clusters
    c. Use composite with a high filler content
    d. Place composite using small increments

19. All of the following circumstances may require a longer curing time for a composite *except* one. Which one is this exception?
    a. Use of an opaque shade
    b. Use of increments of composite greater than 2 mm
    c. Placement of the curing light tip 6 to 8 mm from the composite
    d. Composite placed in a class III preparation on no. 8 mesial

20. What allows a new increment of composite to stick to the previously cured increment?
    a. Mechanical retention
    b. Chemical resin-to-resin bond
    c. Addition of a bonding agent to the cured increment
    d. The silane coupling agent

21. The function of the wedge placed interproximally with a class II preparation includes all of the following *except* one. Which one is this exception?
    a. Stop bleeding
    b. Create slight separation of the teeth
    c. Seal the matrix band against the tooth at the gingival margin
    d. Protect the gingival papilla during cavity preparation

For answers to Review Questions, see the Appendix.

Case-Based Discussion Topics

1. A 24-year-old aspiring actor comes to the dental office seeking replacement of occlusal amalgams in the mandibular molars because they are visible when speaking and singing. The patient is unaware of bruxing.
   From among the esthetic materials discussed in this chapter, which ones have properties that would make them suitable for use in this situation? Which ones are more suitable for anterior class III or V cavities?

2. A 42-year-old elementary school teacher had a class II MO composite on tooth 30 placed 8 months ago. At a recent cleaning appointment, the dental hygienist noted staining at the gingival margin of the composite at the proximal box.
   What are some possible reasons for the staining? What measures could be taken in the future to avoid this problem in other class II composites?

3. A 43-year-old nurse comes to the office complaining of tooth sensitivity to air, cold, and sweets. Examination reveals several deep, noncarious, cervical lesions caused primarily by heavy tooth brushing with stiff bristles. No dental caries is present.
   Considering that resistance to wear is an important physical property, are lightly filled, flowable composites suitable materials? Why or why not? What other materials could be used successfully in this situation?

4. An 18-year-old volleyball player was hit in the mouth with an elbow by a teammate. Tooth 9 was fractured at the mesioincisal edge, creating a 4 mm by 4 mm loss of tooth structure. The patient is being seen on an emergency basis, and the dentist asked you to set up the operatory.
   Which types of composites would work well for this situation? Why? Which type of composite should be avoided? Why?

BIBLIOGRAPHY

Bird D, Robinson D: *Restorative and esthetic dental materials*. In *Modern Dental Assisting*, ed 13, St. Louis, 2021, Elsevier.

Chen M-H: Update on dental nanocomposites, *J Dent Res* 89(6):549–560, 2010.

Choi KK, Condon JR, Ferracane JL: The effects of adhesive thickness on polymerization contraction stress of composite, *J Dent Res* 79(3):812–817, 2000.

Christensen GJ: Does your curing light have the most desirable characteristics? *Clinicians Report* 10(2), 2017. Spring.

Dietz W, Montag R, Kraft U, et al: Longitudinal micromorphological 15-year results of posterior composite restorations using three-dimensional scanning electron microscopy, *J Dent* 42(8):959–969, 2014.

Ferracane JL: *Dental Composites in Materials in Dentistry*, ed 2, Philadelphia, 2001, Lippincott Williams & Wilkins.

Ferracane JL, Watts DC, Ernst CP, et al: Effective use of dental curing lights: A guide for the dental practitioner, *ADA Professional Prod Rev* 8:2–12, 2013.

Glazer HS, Lowe R, Strassler HE: Rubberized-urethane composite for provisional restorations, *Inside Dentistry* 8(6):78–82, 2012.

Labella R, Lambrechts P, Van Meerbeek B, et al: Polymerization shrinkage and elasticity of flowable composites and filled adhesives, *Dent Mater* 15:128, 1999.

Leinfelder KF, Bayne SC, Swift EJ: Packable composites: overview and technical considerations, *J Esthet Dent* 11(5):234–249, 1999.

Marshall GW, Marshall SJ, Bayne SC: Restorative dental materials: scanning electron microscopy and x-ray microanalysis, *Scanning Microsc* 2(4):2007–2028, 1988.

Mitra SB, Wu D, Holmes BN: An application of nanotechnology in advanced dental materials, *J Am Dent Assoc* 134:1382, 2003.

Mousavinasab SM: Biocompatibility of composite resins, *Dental Res J* 8:S21–S29, 2011.

Powers JM, Wataha JC: *Direct esthetic restorative materials*. In *Dental Materials: Foundations and Applications*, ed 11, St. Louis, 2017, Elsevier.

Price RB, Ehrnford L, Andreou p, et al: Comparison of quartz-tungsten-halogen, light-emitting diode and plasma arc curing lights, *J Adhes Dent* 5:193, 2003.

Radz GM: Direct composite resins, *Inside Dentistry* 7(7):108–114, 2011.

Ritter AV, Boushell LW, Walter R: *Biomaterials*. In *Sturdevant's Art and Science of Operative Dentistry*, ed 7, St. Louis, 2019, Elsevier.

Sakaguchi R, Ferracane J, Powers J: *Restorative materials— resin composites and polymers*. In *Craig's Restorative Dental Materials*, ed 14, St. Louis, 2019, Mosby.

Shah P: *Composite roundup: the basics of bulk fill*. In *Dental Products Report*, 2013.

Shen C, Rawls HR, Esquivel-Upshaw JF: *Resin-base composites*. In *Phillips' Science of Dental Materials*, ed 13, St. Louis, 2022, Elsevier.

van Dijken JW, Pallesen U: Posterior bulk-filled resin composite restorations: a 5-year randomized controlled clinical study, *J Dent Res* 51:29–35, 2016.

9 Glass Ionomers, Compomers, and Bioactive Materials

http://evolve.elsevier.com/Eakle/materials/

Chapter Objectives

On completion of this chapter, the student should be able to:
1. Describe the composition of glass ionomer cement restorative materials.
2. Explain the uses of glass ionomer cement restorative materials and their advantages and disadvantages.
3. Explain the effects of fluoride-releasing, resin-modified glass ionomer restorations in the prevention of recurrent caries.
4. List the two major components of compomers.
5. Describe the uses for compomers.
6. Compare the clinical applications of composite resin restorative materials with glass ionomer cement restorative materials
7. Describe what bioactive dental materials are and what they are used for.

KEY TERMS

Glass Ionomer Cement a tooth-colored, self-adhesive, fluoride-releasing material used mainly for fillings or cementing crowns and bridges.

Resin-Modified (or Hybrid) Glass Ionomer a glass ionomer to which resin has been added to improve its physical properties

Nano-Ionomers glass ionomers that contain nanosized filler particles to enhance their physical properties

Compomer composite resin that has polyacid, fluoride-releasing groups added

Bioactive Dental Materials materials that interact with living tissue and are used to remineralize and repair dentin

Glass ionomer cements and compomers, like composite resins, are esthetic, direct-placement restorative materials. Glass ionomer cement restorative materials are used mainly for restoration of root caries and root abrasion. In the 1990s resin was added to glass ionomer cement to improve upon its properties such as strength, wear resistance, and esthetics. In 1995 compomers were developed to provide a blend of the handling and polishing properties of composite resins and the fluoride release of glass ionomer. Bioactive materials have also been developed that can be used to remineralize and repair dentin. The dental auxiliary should be familiar with these materials so they can either assist in placement or avoid damaging or displacement when cleaning the teeth.

GLASS IONOMER CEMENTS

Glass ionomer cements are esthetic, self-adhesive restorative materials with a variety of uses.

Glass ionomer cements are categorized into two main forms:
- Conventional glass ionomers
- Resin-modified glass ionomers (also called hybrid ionomers)

CONVENTIONAL GLASS IONOMER CEMENTS

Glass ionomer cements (GICs) were introduced in the early 1970s by Wilson and Kent. GICs are tooth-colored, self-cured, fluoride-releasing materials that bond to tooth structure directly without a bonding agent. They are made by mixing an acid (water-soluble polyacrylic acid) with a base (fluoroaluminosilicate glass powder). A reaction occurs in which the acid is neutralized by the base and fluoride is released. The mix has an initial set in about 3 to 4 minutes, but the acid-base reaction continues in the hardened mass for about 24 hours.

Several GIC materials have been developed and classified for use in dentistry. The four most common classes of the nine classes available are listed here:

Type I: Luting (cementation) agents
Type II: Restorative materials
Type III: Liners and bases for cavity preparations
Type IV: Fissure sealant

The materials in these four types are similar in chemical composition, but the size of the powder particles and the ratios of powder and liquid are different.

PHYSICAL AND MECHANICAL PROPERTIES OF GLASS IONOMER CEMENT

- Biocompatibility
  - Tolerated well by surrounding soft tissues
  - Kind to the pulp
- Bond to enamel and dentin
  - Bond directly to enamel and dentin
  - The only restorative materials that form an ionic (chemical) bond to calcium in the tooth
  - Does not require a bonding agent
- Setting shrinkage
  - Shrink about 2% to 3%
  - Gradual set minimizes the formation of internal stress
  - Absorb water over time; this helps to offset shrinkage and minimizes leakage
- Bond strength
  - Bond strength to the tooth is about one-fourth that of composite
  - But adequate in non-stressed areas of the mouth
- Microleakage
  - Seal to the tooth is superior on dentin compared with composite
  - Microleakage is minimized
- Fluoride release
  - Initially releases high level of fluoride for a few days
  - Then fluoride falls to low levels
  - Fluoride from in-office applications, fluoride rinses, or fluoride toothpaste can be absorbed and re-released gradually
  - Repeated release of fluoride helps to prevent recurrent caries around the restoration
- Solubility
  - Highly soluble and sensitivity to moisture uptake or loss during the first 24 hours
  - Cover with protective varnish (or Vaseline)
  - Prone to crack if dried too much during the first 24 hours (Fig. 9.1)
- Thermal expansion and contraction
  - Similar to tooth structure
- Modulus of elasticity
  - Stiffness is comparable to dentin
- Thermal protection
  - Good insulators against temperature extremes
- Compressive and tensile strength
  - Moderately high compressive strength
  - Low tensile strength
  - Brittle in thin sections
  - Should not be used in stress-bearing areas such as occlusal surfaces and incisal edges
- Wear resistance
  - Wear faster than composite resins
  - Surface gets rougher over time
  - Cannot be polished as smooth as composites
- Radiopacity
  - More radiopaque than dentin
- Color
  - More opaque than composite

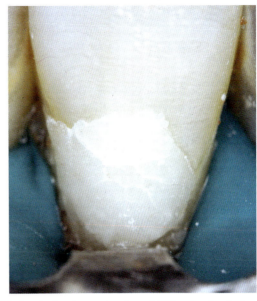

FIG. 9.1 Cracked and crazed surface of GIC restoration that was not protected from drying during setting. (Courtesy Dr. Saulo Geradeli)

Do You Recall?

Why do glass ionomer cement restorations not need a bonding agent?

USES FOR GLASS IONOMER CEMENTS

Luting Cements

(GIC as a luting cement is discussed in detail in Chapter 16.) Glass ionomer luting cements were once very popular because they are pulpally kind, bond to tooth structure, release fluoride, and have a low film thickness, so crowns can be seated easily. Their use has decreased since the introduction of hybrid ionomer cements and resin cements that are stronger and less soluble.

The stronger hybrid ionomer cements are also used to cement orthodontic brackets. They have the advantage over resin cements of releasing fluoride into the surrounding enamel that helps to prevent decalcification, seen as white lines around brackets or bands from poor oral hygiene.

Restorative Materials

Glass ionomer restoratives are used in non–stress-bearing areas because they are weak in tensile strength and are not as wear resistant as composites.

Root Caries. GICs are used for restoration of root caries because they bond and seal to the root better than composites and act as a reservoir to release fluoride to resist recurrent caries.

Root Abrasion/Erosion. GICs are useful for restoration of noncarious cervical lesions (such as toothbrush abrasion and acid erosion), because they can be placed conservatively without the need to cut away sound tooth structure to create retentive cavity preparations, as is necessary with amalgam. Studies show that they are better retained than composites in class V preparations.

Proximal Surface Caries. GICs can be used in anterior class III cavities when color match is not an issue. They can also be used on posterior proximal caries that can be accessed from the facial or lingual approach.

Pediatric Dentistry Uses. GICs are widely used in pediatric dentistry for restoration of dental caries. Their ease of use, fluoride release and bond to the tooth make them the material of choice for primary teeth, especially since mercury-containing amalgam is no longer recommended for use in children.

Encapsulated Glass Ionomer Cement Preferred. Single-use capsules of GIC are desirable because powder-to-liquid ratios can be better controlled. Handling and cleanup is simplified. Mixing is done in a triturator and provides a consistent mix with less trapped air than is seen with hand-mixing. The mixed material can also be dispensed directly into the cavity from the capsule, which has a dispensing tip attached (Fig. 9.2). Infection control is simplified since the capsule is used on only one patient and then thrown away.

Cermets. In the 1980s, GIC restoratives called *cermets* were developed to improve on the properties of GIC. These products have silver particles added to improve their wear resistance and strength. However, the gain in strength is still inadequate to use them in stress-bearing areas. They are dark gray in color, so they are used in locations where esthetics is not a concern. Resin-modified GICs have, for the most part, replaced them.

Liners and Bases.

Liners. Glass ionomer liners are materials used to cover dentin for pulpal protection from chemicals found in other restorative materials or acid etchants. With their low powder content, they are more fluid when mixed and, therefore, easier to spread over the dentin. They are applied in thin layers that are relatively weak.

Bases. Glass ionomer bases are used to rebuild missing dentin within the cavity preparation and provide thermal protection for the pulp, especially with

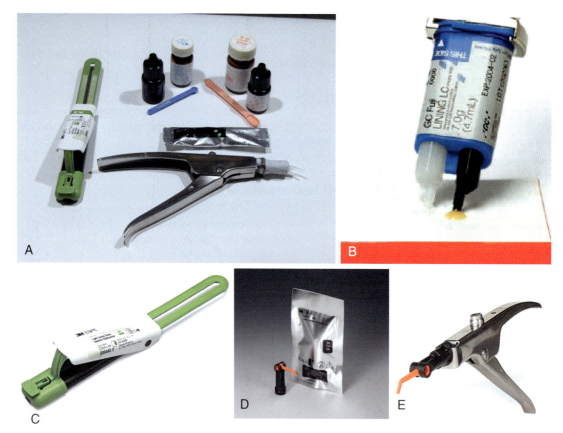

FIG. 9.2 Delivery systems for glass ionomer cements (regular and resin-modified). **(A)** Glass ionomer may be supplied as powder and liquid in containers with powder measuring spoons (liner and luting at *top left* and *right*, respectively) or as powder and liquid premeasured in capsules. The encapsulated material is mixed in a triturator and delivered by a gun dispenser *(bottom).* **(B)** Paste-paste resin-modified GIC dispenser. **(C)** Glass ionomer may also come in a paste-paste system with a dispenser that distributes the proper proportions. **(D)** Packaging of single-unit automix capsule for two-paste resin-modified GIC. **(E)** Two-paste capsule activated and in delivery gun with dispensing nozzle extended. (B–E, From Sakaguchi RL, Powers JM. *Craig's Restorative Dental Materials.* 13th ed. Elsevier; 2012.)

metal restorations such as amalgam. They are placed in thicker layers than liners. They have a higher powder content, making the mix thicker, and they are stronger.

Lamination or "Sandwich" Technique. On occasion, glass ionomer is used in combination with another restorative material to gain the best properties of each material. In 1985 John McLean described a lamination technique (called the "sandwich" technique) with GIC and composite resin. It is most commonly used when the proximal box of a deep class II cavity preparation has the gingival floor located on the root rather than enamel. GIC is placed as the first layer on the gingival floor of the proximal box. Glass ionomer can obtain a better seal to the root than composite and additionally will act as a fluoride reservoir releasing fluoride into the surrounding root surface to resist recurrent caries. Composite resin is used to complete the restoration (Fig. 9.3).

Glass Ionomer Cement as Fissure Sealant. Pits and fissures in newly erupted teeth are highly susceptible to caries. Glass ionomer cements have been used to seal the pits and fissures because of their fluoride release and fluoride reservoir action. Some GICs have been formulated with very high fluoride content (about six times as much as regular GIC). Studies have shown that GICs are not retained as well as resin sealants. Even a thin mix of GIC does not penetrate narrow fissures as well as resin sealants. Additionally, they wear and chip readily. However, those who advocate the use of GIC suggest that it will provide fluoride to the newly erupted tooth surface and make it more resistant to future caries, even if they are lost in a year or so.

Caries Control. Provisional (temporary) restorations
High-fluoride-containing materials and high-viscosity materials are also used as provisional restorations in caries-active patients. These patients often have numerous carious lesions that are placed in provisional restorations, while dietary and hygiene measures are learned by the patient before final restorations are placed.

Atraumatic Restorative Treatment. In developing countries with rural villages or in areas of high poverty in the United States where dental treatment is not available, dental caries often go untreated. Serious and painful abscesses can occur and teeth can be lost. The atraumatic restorative treatment technique allows nondentists to help stop or slow down the progression of open carious lesions without the use of dental drills. Personnel rendering treatment dig out as much decay as they can from frank open cavities with whatever instruments they have. This action removes a lot of the dentin infected with decay-causing bacteria. Next, they mix specially formulated fast-setting, reinforced, high-viscosity GIC. The mix is rolled between the fingers into a ball and pressed by hand into the cavity. The patient bites down, while the material is still soft, to establish the occlusion. Excess material is wiped away. Although a less-than-ideal procedure, it helps to maintain teeth when no other options are available.

  Do You Recall?

Why are encapsulated GICs so popular for restorations?

Glass Ionomer Cements

ADVANTAGES
- Chemically bond to enamel and dentin
- Release fluoride
- Take up fluoride to act as a fluoride reservoir
- Reduced microleakage on dentin
- Reduced postoperative sensitivity
- Biocompatible
- Expand and contract similar to tooth structure

DISADVANTAGES
- High wear rate
- Too weak for stress-bearing restorations
- Less esthetic (more opaque) than composites
- Cannot polish as well as composite—rough surface
- Initially sensitive to water loss or uptake

RESIN-MODIFIED (HYBRID) IONOMERS

To improve on the physical properties of glass ionomers, resin (2-hydroxyethyl methacrylate) has been added. These materials are called **resin-modified (or hybrid) glass ionomers** because they are a blend of resin and glass ionomer.

Resin-modified glass ionomers (RMGICs) are used for many of the same applications as regular glass ionomers and are favored because of their superior properties.

PROPERTIES

RMGICs have some properties of composites and many of the properties of glass ionomers. Resin makes

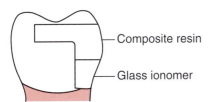

FIG. 9.3 Sandwich technique with glass ionomer "sandwiched" between the tooth and composite restoration. Glass ionomer (GI) is "sandwiched" between the tooth and composite. GI seals better on the root while composite is more wear resistant and esthetically pleasing.

them stronger, more esthetic, more polishable, and more wear resistant. They are more esthetic than conventional GIC because they are not as opaque. Once the resin polymerizes, it protects the glass ionomer component from exposure to moisture and drying while the acid-base reaction goes to completion. The polymerized resin makes the RMGIC less soluble and gives it early strength. RMGICs can be finished immediately after placement. They release fluoride, absorb fluoride from fluoride products, and act as a fluoride reservoir like conventional GICs. Their thermal expansion and contraction is similar to tooth structure. They are radiopaque on x-rays.

CURING MODES

RMGICs are available as light-cured materials. Light polymerization of the resin component occurs in a similar fashion to composite resins. Most of these materials also have a chemical cure of the resin in the absence of light, as well as the acid-base reaction of the glass ionomer cement. The chemical cure allows for final curing in locations where light cannot reach, but it takes longer to cure than when light activated. For example, if caries that extended under the margin of a gold crown were repaired with RMGIC, the portion of the RMGIC under the margin would not be reached by the curing light. The gold blocks the light, but the RMGIC would chemically cure in a few minutes.

USE FOR PEDIATRIC DENTISTRY

RMGIC restorative materials have the same applications in pediatric dentistry as conventional GICs, but they are more popular because of their superior properties and fast set with light curing. (Clinicians do not want to wait for a conventional GIC to set in a squirming child.)

OTHER USES

Like conventional GICs, RMGICs are very useful for restoring root caries and root abrasion or acid erosion lesions (Fig. 9.4). RMGICs are preferred because they are more esthetic and can be finished right away.

RMGIC is formulated for use as lining cement and luting cement as well.

NANO-IONOMERS

Nanoparticle technology has been applied to RMGICs to improve their physical properties. These **nano-ionomers**, or nano-GICs, were first introduced in 2007. The filler particles are nanosized, silane-treated particles and nanoclusters similar to those found in nanocomposites. They match tooth colors better, are more wear resistance, and have improved polishability. They are also dual cured.

The nano-ionomer was first introduced as a two-paste system with a dual-chamber cartridge. The two pastes are extruded onto a pad and hand-spatulated. Another version is packaged as a premeasured two-paste system in an automixing capsule, and the mixed material can be dispensed directly into the cavity preparation through a nozzle attached to the capsule.

Dispensing systems for resin-modified glass ionomers can be seen in Fig. 9.2.

 Do You Recall?

What benefits were gained by adding resin to GIC?

CLINICAL APPLICATION OF GLASS IONOMER CEMENTS

Packaging and Mixing

GICs are supplied in three ways: (1) hand-mixed powder and liquid, (2) encapsulated powder and liquid, and (3) two-paste cartridges (see Fig. 9.2).
1. With the powder-liquid system a scoop provided by the manufacturer is used to measure the powder. Typically, one or two drops of liquid (amount according to manufacturer) are used per scoop. The powder and liquid are hand-mixed quickly (usually less than

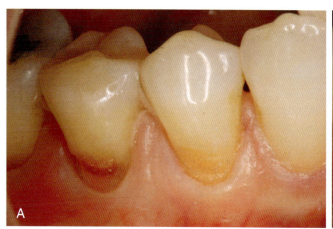
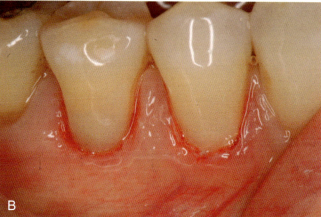

FIG. 9.4 Restoration of root surface lesion: **(A)** abrasion/erosion lesion on mandibular second premolar. **(B)** Lesion was restored with resin-modified glass ionomer cement. (Courtesy Dr. Thomas J. Hilton, Portland, Oregon.)

30 seconds) at chairside on a paper pad, and delivered on an instrument into the cavity preparation.
2. GIC also comes in single-use capsules with premeasured powder and liquid. The capsule is activated by depressing a button on the capsule that ruptures a membrane that separates the powder from the liquid. The capsule is placed in a triturator and is mixed at speeds and times recommended by the manufacturer. The capsule is then inserted into a gun-type applicator, and the mixed GIC is delivered into the cavity preparation through a nozzle on the capsule.
3. With the paste-paste system, each paste is contained in one of two chambers on the cartridge. Pressing a lever on the cartridge dispenses equal portions of the pastes onto a paper pad. They are quickly mixed together and applied to the cavity preparation. Very fine glass powder is used in the pastes to provide a creamy consistency when mixed. A variation of the paste-paste system uses an automixing tip on the cartridge to deliver the mixed pastes directly into the cavity preparation with a fine nozzle.

GICs are manufactured in a variety of shades but not in the wide selection available with composites.

Placement and Manipulation

Before placing GIC, cutting debris (*smear layer*—see Chapter 7) on cavity preparation surfaces must be removed for GIC to chemically bond to the tooth. To remove only the smear layer and not the calcium in the surface of the preparation, a weak acid (usually 10% polyacrylic acid) is applied for 10 seconds, and then rinsed and lightly dried. Phosphoric acid used to etch the tooth for composite procedures should not be used on dentin. It is too aggressive and removes not only the smear layer but also removes calcium from the dentin surface, exposing collagen. The GIC cannot bond to the collagen, and therefore no bond or only a weak bond is formed. Without a bond, the restoration may leak or have postoperative sensitivity.

GIC can be placed in bulk and manipulated with an instrument to slightly overfill the cavity preparation. It can be contoured somewhat with a plastic instrument or with a cervical matrix for a Class V preparation. Unlike composite, GIC is not very viscous and cannot be readily shaped before it sets. Overfilling the cavity preparation provides enough excess material to allow for contouring and finishing of the restoration.

It is important when placing the GIC or RMGIC to stop manipulating it when the initial gel stage begins. The gel stage can be identified by a loss of shininess of the material and an increase in viscosity. Working time varies from 1.5 to 3 minutes, depending on the manufacturer and whether or not the material is regular or fast set. Even light-cured RMGIC starts to gel in less than 3 minutes in the oral cavity when not exposed to the curing light.

Finishing and Polishing

Approximately 5 minutes after the initial set, most current formulations of conventional GICs can be contoured and finished with carbide or diamond finishing burs or abrasive disks under water spray. A smooth surface can be achieved with abrasive-impregnated rubber polishing points or disk. Some clinicians like to follow that with fine-grit polishing paste. Light-cured RMGICs can be finished right away.

It is best to apply a protective varnish that is usually furnished with the material or to coat it with an unfilled resin surface sealer. Even though the material has gone to its initial set, an acid-base reaction still occurs for several hours within the material. The coating protects it from excessive uptake of moisture from the saliva or from drying if the restoration remains isolated for a while.

Glass ionomer cements have grown in popularity as their handling characteristics, esthetics, and ease of use have improved.

Do You Recall?

When using conventional or resin-modified glass ionomer cement, when should it no longer be manipulated?

Clinical Tip

Before applying glass ionomer cement to a cavity preparation, remove the smear layer that forms when a preparation is cut. Use a conditioner (typically 10% polyacrylic acid) for 10 seconds on enamel and dentin. Rinse and lightly dry. The clean surface will allow the glass ionomer to bond to the calcium in the tooth surface. Do *not* use phosphoric acid on dentin. It will remove the calcium from the surface and expose collagen. GIC cannot bond to collagen.

KEY POINTS

GLASS IONOMER CEMENTS

Glass ionomer cements are versatile dental materials with the following uses:
- Luting cements
- Restorative materials
- Liners and bases
- Fissure sealants

Favorable features include:
- Biocompatible
- Release fluoride and act as a fluoride reservoir
- Chemically bonded directly to enamel and dentin
- Provide a good seal of the restoration reducing microleakage
- Being ideal for root caries
- Being popular for restorations in pediatric dentistry.

Drawbacks include:
- Being too weak to use in stress-bearing parts of the mouth
- Wearing faster than composites or amalgams

> **KEY POINTS—cont'd**
> - After initial set, they are adversely affected by early exposure to moisture or drying
> - Although tooth colored, they are more opaque and not as esthetic as composites.
>
> Resin-modified GICs: Adding resin improved the following:
> - Increased strength
> - Not as sensitive to water uptake or drying
> - More esthetic
> - Light-cure with chemical cure as well
> - Immediate finishing
> - Improved esthetics and polish, especially with nanofillers.

COMPOMERS

Compomers are esthetic restorative materials that came on the market in the 1990s. They are essentially composite resins that have been modified with polyacid. They contain filled composite and an acid-base reaction as with glass ionomers; hence the name *compomers*. The idea was to join the good qualities of composite (namely strength, wear resistance, esthetics, and polishability) with the fluoride release of glass ionomer. Light-activated chemicals are included to make the compomers light cured. The fillers (about 45%–65% filled by volume) are glasses similar to those used in composites, along with some fluoride-releasing silicate glasses, ranging in size from 0.8 to 5.0 μm.

FLUORIDE RELEASE

Fluoride release from compomers is not comparable to that from glass ionomers. Likewise, there is little or no recharging of the compomer with fluoride products, as with glass ionomers. The fluoride released from compomers is about 10% of that with glass ionomers. So, they are not likely to demonstrate a significant caries-fighting effect.

PACKAGING

Compomers for restorations are available as a light-cured single paste that is packaged in single-use compules or screw-type syringes or in a flowable form much like flowable composites (see Fig. 9.5).

Compomers are made for luting as well and are manufactured as a powder and liquid or as a two-paste dual cartridge with automixing capability. Luting agents may be chemical cured, light cured, or dual cured.

SETTING REACTION

The setting reaction in restorative compomers occurs in two phases. Phase 1 is similar to that of the light-activated composite resins and forms a resin network encompassing the fillers. This causes the material to harden in the cavity preparation. Phase 2 is an acid-base reaction that occurs more slowly over several days as the restoration absorbs water.

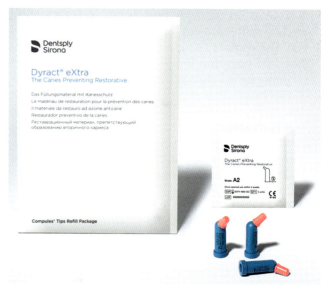

FIG. 9.5 Compomer restorative material. Dyract eXtra (Dentsply Sirona) in compules. (Courtesy Dentsply Sirona.)

BONDING

Compomers do not bond to tooth structure as glass ionomers do. A bonding adhesive is indicated during placement of compomers. The bond strength to dentin is about the same as that of an RMGI. The bonding agents will reduce the chances of fluoride leaching from the material into the dentin.

USES

They can be used in most situations where a microfilled composite would be used; that is, mostly for low stress–bearing class III and V restorations. For pediatric dentistry, they can be used for small, well-protected (from biting stresses) Class I and II restorations on primary teeth.

PLACEMENT AND FINISHING

They are easy to handle and are placed in 2 mm increments just as for composites. Finishing and polishing also are the same as for composites. No varnish or coating is needed after setting as with glass ionomers.

PROPERTIES

See Table 9.1 for a comparison of the properties of compomers, glass ionomers, and composites.

GIOMERS

Giomers are a subset of compomers. The name "giomer" is derived from the words "glass ionomer" and "composite," as these materials have some of the desirable properties of each. Giomers release fluoride but less of it and at a slower rate than glass ionomers. Unlike regular compomers, they can be recharged with fluoride from toothpaste or mouth rinse to act as a fluoride reservoir. They obtain their fluoride from fillers

TABLE 9.1 Comparison of Properties of Direct Esthetic Restorative Materials

MATERIAL	COLOR MATCH	BONDING AGENT NEEDED	FLUORIDE RELEASE	WEAR RATE	POLISHABILITY	COMPRESSIVE STRENGTH	FLEXURAL STRENGTH
Glass ionomer	Low	No	High	High	Low	Low	Low
Resin-modified ionomer	Medium	No	Medium	Medium	Medium	Medium	Medium
Compomer	Medium-high	Yes	Low	Medium	High	Medium	Medium
Microfill composite	High	Yes	No	High	High	Medium	Medium
Microhybrid composite	High	Yes	No	Low	High	High	High

Adapted from Craig RG, Powers JM, Wataha JC. *Dental Materials: Properties and Manipulation.* 7th ed. Mosby; 2000.

that are a product of grinding up glass ionomer that has set already. It is the pre-set glass ionomer fillers that differentiate giomers from regular compomers. The filled resin component provides good handling properties, esthetics, and polishability. Like composites and regular compomers, they are light cured and require the use of a bonding agent. Ionomers are packaged in single-paste compules or syringes or as directly delivered flowables (including a bulk-fill flowable). They are used for the same restorative procedures as regular compomers.

BIOACTIVE DENTAL MATERIALS

Bioactive materials interact with living tissues and initiate repair or regeneration in these tissues. One of the first bioactive materials was a bone grafting material, which formed chemical bonds with bone. For dental purposes, it binds to dentin surfaces and blocks dentinal tubules. In dentistry, the term *bioactivity* has come to mean the ability of a material to form apatite-like substance on its surface when exposed to saliva or other bodily fluids, as in the case of bone stimulating graft materials. (Hydroxyapatite is the mineral component of enamel and dentin.)

The dental biomaterials with this apatite-forming ability used in clinical applications fit into two groups: (1) calcium silicates and (2) calcium aluminates. When powders of these materials are mixed with water, they undergo an acid-base reaction that ends in an alkaline pH when set. The higher pH tends to stimulate more bioactivity. Calcium aluminate-based and calcium silicate-based cements have been shown to have some degree of bonding to dentin.

PHYSICAL PROPERTIES

Their physical strength and other properties are similar to conventional glass ionomer cement.

USES

Bioactive dental cements were introduced in the mid-1990s for root sealing and repair.

Bioactive cements also have been used as liners and pulp capping materials, bases, and luting cements to remineralize and stimulate repair of dentin. For endodontics, there are root canal sealers and root repair materials (such as mineral trioxide aggregate that is similar in composition to Portland cement).

Bioactive materials have been added to resins to promote bioactivity. One product is a bulk-fill, bioactive composite that seals dentin and stimulates apatite formation.

KEY POINTS

COMPOMERS AND BIOACTIVE MATERIALS

Compomers
- They have components of both composite and GIC.
- They are closer to composites since their fluoride release is minimal and they do not recharge when exposed to fluoride products.
- They require a bonding agent to bond to the tooth structure.
- They are stronger, more wear resistant, esthetic, and polishable than GIC.
- Their setting reaction has the light activation of composite, but also has an acid-base reaction of GIC.
- They are used in low stress applications, such as Cl III or V cavities, or small, protected Cl I and II cavities on primary teeth.

Bioactive Materials
- They create an apatite mineral similar to the tooth structure on the dentin surface so they are used as a reparative material to remineralize or repair dentin.
- Applications include liners, pulp capping, bases, luting cements, and root repair.
- Their physical properties are similar to GIC.

SUMMARY

Glass ionomer cement restorative materials are not as esthetically pleasing and strong as composite resin and cannot be polished to a high shine, but they offer the advantages of releasing fluoride, bonding directly to the tooth without a bonding agent and providing a better seal to the root structure. They have wide applications in pediatric dentistry and for restoration of root caries in the elderly. Compomers are materials that are closer to composites than to glass ionomers, but do not have the best qualities of either material. Like giomers, they are not widely used. Bioactive materials with the capability to repair and remineralize damaged dentin show much promise.

Review and Discussion

Review Questions

Select the one correct response for each of the following multiple-choice questions.

1. One of the advantages of glass ionomer compared to composite is:
   a. The ability to finish it immediately
   b. That it has higher strength than composite because of the glass fillers
   c. That it uses the same bonding agents as composites
   d. That it has been shown to release fluoride

2. Which one of the following statements about glass ionomer cement (GIC) is *false*?
   a. GIC chemically bonds to calcium in the tooth.
   b. GIC releases fluoride.
   c. GIC is more esthetic than a microfill composite.
   d. GIC reduces microleakage at margins of a restoration on the root.

3. Resin-modified (hybrid) glass ionomers have all of the following advantages over conventional glass ionomers, *except* one. Which one is this *exception*?
   a. Stronger
   b. Less sensitive to moisture when set
   c. Can be finished at the same appointment
   d. Contain quartz fillers like some composites

4. In order for glass ionomer to bond to the tooth, which one of the following things must be done?
   a. The smear layer must be removed
   b. A bonding resin must be applied and cured
   c. The tooth must be rinsed thoroughly with a strong water and air spray
   d. The enamel and dentin must be etched with phosphoric acid for 20 seconds

5. Glass ionomer cement is indicated for use in all of the following *except* one. Which one is the exception?
   a. Restoration of root caries
   b. An MOD restoration in an adult
   c. Cementing a crown
   d. A cavity liner

6. Nano-ionomers have all of the following properties *except* one. Which one is this *exception*?
   a. Improved esthetics
   b. Increased wear resistance
   c. Improved polish
   d. Greater strength than nanocomposites

7. Which one of the following statements about compomers is true?
   a. Compomers act as a fluoride reservoir, just like GICs.
   b. Compomers polish better than GICs.
   c. Compomers are less esthetic than GICs.
   d. Compomers wear faster than GICs.

8. Which one of the flowing statements about compomer restorative materials is true?
   a. Release as much fluoride as GICs
   b. Are only self-curing
   c. Are closer to composite resins in their makeup than to GICs
   d. Are like GICs in that they do not require a separate bonding agent

9. Which one of the following materials is not light-cured?
   a. Conventional glass ionomer cement
   b. Compomer
   c. Microhybrid composite
   d. Resin-modified glass ionomer cement

10. Which one of the following is not a use for bioactive dental materials?
    a. Crown buildup
    b. Repair of dentin
    c. Pulp capping
    d. Root repair

Case-Based Discussion Topics

1. A 75-year-old retired plumber who is taking medication to control blood pressure is found on examination to have a dry mouth and numerous root caries.

Which types of direct-placement esthetic materials discussed in this chapter would have the greatest advantage for restoring root caries? Why? How do these materials bond to the tooth structure?

2. A 57-year-old secretary comes to the dental office for a periodic examination and prophylaxis. The patient has maxillary anterior composite veneers and Class V glass ionomers on the maxillary premolars.

What must the dental auxiliary be concerned about when treating patients who have esthetic composite and glass ionomer restorations present in their mouths?

BIBLIOGRAPHY

Donly KJ, Segura A, Weffel JS: Evaluating the effects of fluoride-releasing dental materials, *J Am Dent Assoc* 130:819, 1999.

Jefferies SR: Bioactive dental materials: composition, properties and indications for a new class of restorative materials, *Inside Dent* 12(2), 2016.

Mount GJ, Hume WR: Glass-ionomer materials, composite resins, and rigid materials used in tooth restoration. In *Preservation and restoration of tooth structure*, Philadelphia, 1998, Mosby.

Nagaraja UP, Kishore G: Glass ionomer cement—the different generations, *Trends Biomater Artif Organs* 18:158–165, 2005.

Powers JM, Wataha JC: Direct esthetic restorative materials. In *Dental materials: foundations and applications,* ed 11, St. Louis, 2017, Elsevier.

Sagaguchi R, Ferracane J, Powers J: Preventive and intermediary materials. In *Craig's restorative dental materials*, ed 14, St. Louis, 2019, Elsevier.

Shen C, Rawls HR, Esquivel-Upshaw JF: Dental Cements. In *Phillips' science of dental materials,* ed 13, St. Louis, 2022, Elsevier.

Sidhu SK, Nicholson JW: A review of glass-ionomer cements for clinical dentistry, *J Funct Biomater Sept* 7(3):16, 2016.

Wilson AD, Kent BE: A new translucent cement for dentistry: the glass ionomer cement, *Br Dent J* 132:133–135, 1972.

10 Dental Ceramics

http://evolve.elsevier.com/Eakle/materials/

Chapter Objectives

On completion of this chapter, the student should be able to:

1. Discuss the attributes and shortcomings of dental porcelains.
2. Compare the clinical applications of restorations made from porcelain with those made from lithium disilicate.
3. Explain why crowns made from zirconia can be used to restore molars.
4. Describe the methods used to process ceramic restorations.
5. Present a rationale for the selection of ceramic materials for restorations used in the anterior and posterior parts of the mouth.
6. Describe how porcelain bonds to metal for porcelain-fused-to-metal crowns.
7. Identify common causes for failure of ceramic restorations.
8. Compare the relative strengths of feldspathic porcelain, lithium disilicate, and zirconium.
9. Explain how CAD/CAM technology is used to fabricate a ceramic crown.
10. List the clinical applications for all-ceramic restorations.
11. Assist the dentist in cementing an all-ceramic crown or veneers.
12. Properly prepare the conditions in the operatory for shade taking and assist the dentist in obtaining a shade.

KEY TERMS

Ceramics materials composed of inorganic metal oxide compounds, including porcelain and similar ceramic materials that require baking at high temperatures to fuse small particles together

Crown an indirect restoration that covers all or part of the crown of a tooth (extracoronal) and is composed of metal, ceramic, or a combination of the two. It can also cover an implant

Fixed Bridge a dental prosthesis that replaces one or more missing teeth and is cemented to adjacent natural teeth or implants. It is composed of the same materials as crowns

Inlay an indirect restoration composed of ceramic, composite resin, or metal that is fitted to a cavity preparation that is within the crown of a tooth (intracoronal)

Onlay restoration that is similar to an inlay but covers or replaces one or more cusps

Veneer thin layer of ceramic or composite resin that is bonded to the facial surfaces of teeth to improve their color, shape, size, or length

Glass-Based Ceramics ceramic materials with a silica (glass) matrix with or without fillers such as leucite or lithium disilicate

Nonglass-Based Ceramics crystalline-based ceramics without a glass matrix

All-Ceramic Restoration ceramic restoration with no metal core

Porcelain a tooth-colored ceramic material composed of crystals of feldspar, alumina, and silica that are fused together at high temperatures to form a hard, uniform, glasslike material

Flexural Strength the ability to withstand bending forces without fracturing

Sintering fusion of ceramic particles at their borders by heating them to the point that they just start to melt

Lithium Disilicate Ceramics glass-based ceramics with lithium disilicate fillers to enhance physical and mechanical properties, especially flexural strength

Zirconia a nonglass polycrystalline ceramic that is the strongest ceramic used in dentistry

Fracture Toughness material's ability to resist fracture from crack propagation

Slip-Casting process whereby ceramic powder is mixed with a water-based liquid to form a mass or slip. The slip is pressed into a form and baked at high temperature

Heat Pressing pressing molten ceramic material into a mold at high temperature and pressure

CAD/CAM computer-assisted design/computer-assisted machining that uses a scanning device to capture an image of the preparation and is integrated with computer software to design and a milling device to cut restorations from blocks of restorative dental material

Porcelain-Fused-to-Metal Restoration restoration that has a metal core over which porcelain is fused at high temperature. Also called porcelain-bonded-to-metal (PBM)

Ceramic materials are used for a variety of restorations, such as crowns, fixed bridges, inlays, onlays, and veneers. Advances in ceramic materials and techniques have assisted the dental team in delivering the esthetic results that patients demand. The dental team must keep current with the rapid changes that occur in materials and techniques. Good listening skills are needed to determine the types of esthetic services the patient is requesting, so that the dental team and the patient are working together toward the same goal. Dental auxiliary are important members of the dental team that must understand the properties of these materials so they can help the dentist to assess the performance of the restorations and alert the dentist when they perceive that a restoration may be failing. The dental auxiliary needs to be familiar with the physical properties of materials so that they do not damage the restorations during coronal polishing and preventive procedures. Dental assistants need to know the handling characteristics of esthetic materials, so that they can either assist the dentist in their placement or perform steps in their placement as permitted by state dental practice acts. In addition, they will be called on to assist in shade taking for the restorations.

This chapter describes the physical and mechanical properties, processing methods including computer-assisted design/computer-assisted machining (CAD/CAM) technology, clinical applications, attributes, and shortcomings of esthetic ceramic materials. The rationale for the selection of ceramic materials for various clinical applications is presented. The principles for adjusting, finishing, polishing, and cementation of ceramic restorations are reviewed. Guidelines for selection of the shade of these materials to obtain satisfactory cosmetic results are also discussed.

DENTAL CERAMICS

The general term ceramics is used to describe porcelain and a variety of materials that are similar in appearance to porcelain but vary in their composition, mode of fabrication, and physical and mechanical properties.

A BRIEF HISTORY OF DENTAL CERAMICS

Amalgam and gold were the main restorative materials until ceramics were introduced into dentistry over 100 years ago. Ceramics were first used for the fabrication of denture teeth, and then in the 1900s Charles Land introduced crowns and inlays fabricated entirely from porcelain. Land's porcelain crowns were very esthetic, but the porcelains of the time were brittle and tended to crack when used in high-function areas of the mouth. In the late 1950s porcelain was fused to a metal core to make esthetic crowns much stronger. In Europe in the 1970s the first computer-aided design/computer-aided manufacturing (CAD/CAM) system was developed using ceramic blocks to produce inlays and onlays. In 1987 the first chairside CAD/CAM system (CEREC 1, Siemens Dental) was introduced. Also in the 1980s the introduction of a castable glass-based ceramic launched numerous innovations in ceramic processing.

Within the past three decades, all-ceramic materials have been introduced that are much stronger than the original porcelains, and with some improvements in esthetics. As a result, the use of all-ceramic restorations has dramatically increased while the use of the less esthetic porcelain-fused-to-metal (PFM) crowns has decreased.

ADVANTAGES AND DISADVANTAGES OF CERAMIC RESTORATIONS

Esthetic restorations can be made from composite resin, ceramic with a metal substructure (core), or entirely ceramic.

Advantages

The primary advantages of all-ceramic restorations over composite resin, glass ionomer cement, or amalgam include:
- Esthetics
- Biocompatibility
- Wear resistance under function
- Color stability
- Stain resistance
- Ability to precisely place contacts and contours of the restorations

Disadvantages

Disadvantages of all-ceramic restorations include:
- Brittleness (can lead to fracture)
- Wear of the opposing enamel or restorations
- Difficulty or inability to repair the restoration in the mouth
- Need for two appointments (except for chairside CAD/CAM restorations)
- Difficulty polishing them in the mouth

CLASSIFICATION OF DENTAL CERAMICS

Dental ceramics can be classified in a variety of ways based on their:
- Composition
- Processing method
- Fusing temperature
- Microstructure
- Translucency
- Fracture resistance
- Abrasiveness

GLASS AND NONGLASS CERAMICS

To simplify the understanding of dental ceramics they will be classified in this chapter into two broad categories according to their composition: glass-based and nonglass-based materials.
- Glass-based ceramics have silica as a main component and have a glassy matrix. They include feldspathic porcelains, leucite-reinforced ceramics, and lithium disilicate ceramics. They are more esthetic than nonglass-based ceramics.

- **Nonglass-based ceramics** are crystalline in nature and composed of simple or complex oxides with no glassy matrix. They include alumina and zirconia. They are the strongest of the ceramics.

GLASS-BASED CERAMICS

PORCELAIN

Porcelain is a term that has been used in dentistry for many years to describe glasslike tooth-colored dental materials. Some people use the term interchangeably with ceramics, but porcelain is actually a subgroup of ceramic materials composed of feldspar (mineral that provides luster to porcelain), silica or quartz (glasslike minerals), and kaolin (a type of clay). Ceramic materials that are high in glass content are very esthetic, because their optical properties mimic those of enamel and dentin. However, they are brittle and more prone to fracture than low-glass, reinforced glass, or nonglass ceramics. Their flexural strength is no more than 20% of that of the strongest nonglass ceramics.

Feldspathic Porcelain

Until advances in ceramic materials were made over the past four decades, the dental ceramic material most commonly used was feldspathic porcelain manufactured from fine crystalline powders of alumina, feldspar, and silica oxide (or quartz). As the powder is heated to certain critical temperatures, the porcelain particles are fused together (a process called sintering) at their points of contact to form a type of glass (Fig. 10.1).

Feldspathic porcelain is the oldest of the porcelains used in dentistry (introduced in the early 1900s). It is the most esthetic but the weakest of the ceramic materials in use.

Alumina Porcelain

Alumina porcelain was developed to enhance (about double) the fracture resistance compared with conventional feldspathic porcelain. It is also a glassy type of porcelain that is about half aluminum oxide by weight in a melted glass (silica) matrix.

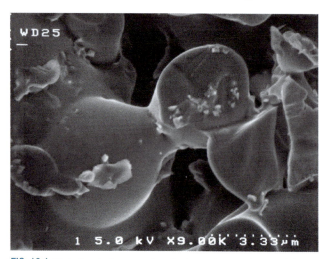

FIG. 10.1 Sintering. In the scanning electron micrograph, porcelain particles can be seen that have partly melted at high temperature and fused at their points of contact. This is sintering. (From Rosenstiel SF, Land MF. *Contemporary Fixed Prosthodontics*. 5th ed. Elsevier; 2016.)

Uses of Porcelain

Porcelain is manufactured in a variety of colors. The different colors (called shades) are produced by the addition of metal oxides to create different shades to match the teeth. The laboratory technician selects powders based on the shade prescription provided by the dentist. These porcelains were initially used for all-porcelain crowns. These crowns were very esthetically pleasing but had a high fracture rate.

At present, the feldspathic porcelains have a variety of uses. They are used to cover (or veneer) a metal core to fabricate PFM crowns and to veneer high-strength ceramic cores such as zirconia. They are also used for very esthetic anterior veneers that can be rather thin, allowing for conservative preparations. Porcelain veneers are most successful when they are bonded to enamel. Enamel is rigid and provides a firm support and a strong bond. Dentin, however, is not as rigid and bonds to it are weaker. When under function or a sudden heavy load is applied (e.g., biting on a fork), the bond between the veneer and the dentin can fail or the porcelain can break. If dentin is the main support for the veneer, then a stronger esthetic material should be selected.

Fusing Temperatures

Porcelains can be classified according to their fusing temperature:
- High fusing (2360°F–2500°F): used mostly for denture teeth
- Medium fusing (2000°F–2300°F): used for some all-ceramic restorations
- Low fusing (1600°F–1950°F): used for veneering metal in PFM crowns and to fabricate some all-ceramic restorations.

Reinforced Glass-Based Ceramics

Because porcelains are prone to fracture, stronger ceramic materials were developed. The most common of these stronger glass-based ceramics are leucite-reinforced ceramics and lithium disilicate ceramics. Reinforcing the material with leucite crystals or lithium oxide has more than tripled their fracture resistance.

Lithium Disilicate

Lithium disilicate ceramic is composed of quartz, lithium dioxide, alumina, phosphor oxide, potassium oxide, and small amounts of other components. The resulting glass ceramic has high strength, good marginal integrity, and biocompatibility and, unlike porcelain, can be used in both the anterior and posterior parts of the mouth. It is a very esthetic material because of its high translucency.

Because of its favorable properties, lithium disilicate ceramic has become very popular for veneers and esthetic anterior and posterior crowns. It has high flexural strength and can be used for short-span fixed bridges if not subjected to excessive forces, as with people who grind their teeth. It is manufactured in a variety of shades and comes as ingots for the heat-pressed technique or as ceramic blocks for CAD/CAM milling.

Cementation. As with the other glass-based materials, restorations made from lithium disilicate should be bonded to the tooth with resin cement for maximum strength.

Survival Rates for Glass-Based Ceramics

Glass-based ceramic inlays, onlays, and veneers have a 5-year survival rate of 93% to 98% and a 10-year rate of 64% to 95%. When used for full crowns limited to the anterior part of the mouth, the survival rate is also high for reinforced glass materials. These materials owe their high success rate to their inherent strength and the fact that they can be bonded to enamel and dentin for support.

 Do You Recall?

What are some of the advantages of lithium disilicate over feldspathic porcelain for dental restorations?

NONGLASS-BASED CERAMICS

Nonglass-based ceramics are crystalline-based with no glass matrix and are composed of oxides of alumina and/or zirconia with minor amounts of other components to improve their properties.

ALUMINA

A nonglass material with a crystalline matrix (composed of alumina) was developed as an alternative to the PFM crown. It was the first all-ceramic material that could be used for both anterior and posterior crowns and anterior short-span bridges. Alumina has a very high flexural strength, about three times that of glass-based materials. It is less translucent, and therefore it is less vital looking. Alumina ceramic systems have been replaced for the most part by zirconia and lithium disilicate because of their higher failure rate when used for molar crowns.

ZIRCONIA

Zirconia (zirconium oxide) ceramics are the strongest ceramic materials currently used in dentistry. They have the highest flexural strength (Table 10.1) and fracture toughness, at least twice as strong as alumina-based ceramics. As with lithium disilicate, they can be heat pressed or machined. Zirconia can be used in the anterior and posterior parts of the mouth for single-unit crowns or as cores for three-unit bridges.

Cementation

Because of their high strength, zirconia crowns can be cemented with conventional cements or bonded with resin cements.

Improving the Esthetics of Zirconia

Zirconia is a much more opaque ceramic than lithium disilicate ceramic. To achieve better esthetics, a layer of veneering porcelain can be added to a zirconium core (Fig. 10.2). If the crown fractures, it is usually caused by a fracture of the porcelain veneer or a separation of the porcelain from the zirconia. A more recent development is high-translucency zirconia, which can be used as an all-zirconia crown without the need for porcelain layering in many posterior applications.

PHYSICAL AND MECHANICAL PROPERTIES

FLEXURAL STRENGTH

Flexural strength is the ability of a material to resist bending under a load. However, ceramic materials tend to be stiff and brittle and do not bend well. The ceramic materials that can resist bending forces have good flexural strength.

Glass-based ceramic materials such as porcelains have relatively low flexural strength. Lithium disilicate has the highest flexural strength of these glassy materials. Nonglass-based ceramic materials have very high flexural strengths. Zirconia has the highest flexural strength of the crystalline materials and also has the highest fracture toughness. See Table 10.1 for a comparison of ceramic materials strength.

Table 10.1 Strength of Various Types of All-Ceramics

CERAMIC TYPE	ESTHETICS	FLEXURAL STRENGTH (MPA)[a]	FRACTURE TOUGHNESS (MPA · M$^{0.5}$)
Feldspathic porcelain	Very high	120–130	0.78
Leucite-reinforced glass ceramic	High	104–160	1.2–2.4
Lithium disilicate glass ceramic	Moderately high	262–306	3.0
Glass-infiltrated alumina	Moderate-to-low	340–700	3.2–4.4
Zirconia	Moderate-to-low unless veneered with more esthetic material	800–1300	4.0–6.3

[a]Approximate, depending on processing. 1 MPa = 145 psi (pounds per square inch).

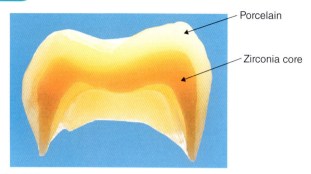

FIG. 10.2 Cross-section of a veneered crown. Opaque zirconia core has been veneered with more translucent porcelain to improve esthetics. (From Shen C, Rawls HR. *Phillip's Science of Dental Materials.* 13th ed. Elsevier; 2022.)

THERMAL PROPERTIES

Ceramic materials act as insulators because they do not conduct heat or cold readily, as do metallic restorations. However, they will expand or contract when subjected to temperature changes. The degree to which they expand or contract is called the *coefficient of thermal expansion* (CTE). The higher the CTE, the more the ceramic expands or contracts with temperature changes. This change in dimension is not critically important with a restoration made from a single material. However, when two ceramic materials are used jointly in a restoration, as with a porcelain veneer with a zirconia core or porcelain bonded to a metal core (as with a PFM crown), the two materials must have compatible CTEs. Otherwise, the veneering ceramic material may fracture.

OPTICAL PROPERTIES

Transparency
Transparent materials allow light to pass through in an unaltered path, that is, window glass (see Fig. 10.3). Since transparent materials do not resemble the tooth structure, there is little need for them in dentistry.

Translucency
Translucent materials allow light to pass through the surface and into the body of the material; some of the light is reflected back out. Glass-based ceramic materials are more translucent than nonglass ceramics and, as a result, mimic enamel better.

Reflectance
The surface of a ceramic material may reflect light that hits it. How much light is reflected is influenced by the surface texture and polish and the basic structure of the ceramic material. The portion of the light that is not reflected passes into the ceramic and is either absorbed or passes through it.

Opacity
Opaque ceramic materials do not allow light to pass through them. The light is absorbed or reflected.

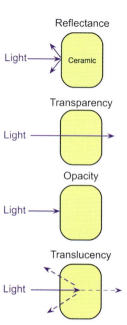

FIG. 10.3 Optical properties. (From Powers JM, Wataha JC. *Dental Materials: Properties and Manipulation.* 11th ed. Elsevier; 2017.)

Nonglass ceramic materials are the most opaque. These materials are the least esthetic of the ceramic materials.

Vitality
Glass-based ceramic crowns have a more lifelike appearance (sometimes called *vitality*) than PFM crowns. They appear similar to natural teeth or vital because
- They are *fluorescent*.
  - Emit light in the visible wave spectrum when ultraviolet light hits them.
- They are *opalescent*.
  - Take on a slight bluish tinge when light reflects off of them and a slight orange-yellow tinge when light passes through them.

BIOCOMPATIBILITY

Ceramic materials are considered to be among the most biocompatible of the restorative dental materials. Clinical studies have not shown an adverse tissue response to these materials. Glass-based ceramic materials will leach some components in minute amounts over time; much less so than alloys or resins. Lithium disilicate shows some initial toxicity in cell cultures that fades with time. Nonglass ceramics have shown no toxicity to date, and zirconia has been successfully used for dental implant fixtures.

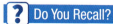 **Do You Recall?**

What is the major advantage for using zirconia for dental restorations and what is its main shortcoming?

> **KEY POINTS**
>
> **GLASS AND NONGLASS CERAMICS**
> Glass-based ceramics:
> - Most esthetic.
> - Mimic the optical properties of enamel and dentin.
> - But have low flexural strength, especially porcelain.
> - Lithium disilicate is the strongest of the glass-based ceramics.
>
> Nonglass ceramics:
> - Less esthetic, more opaque.
> - Very high flexural strength.
> - Zirconia is the strongest of the nonglass ceramics.
> - Zirconia is often veneered with porcelain to make it more esthetic.

CERAMIC PROCESSING TECHNIQUES

All-ceramic restorations can be made by four different techniques depending on the type of ceramic material that will be used.

- **Sintering**: Ceramic particles are heated until they start to melt and fuse to adjacent particles at their borders (Fig. 10.1). To achieve the desired color match, stains (color pigments) are added and fused in a ceramic oven.
- **Slip-casting**: A mixture of ceramic powder and a water-based liquid called a slip is pressed onto a porous die and fired at high temperature to create a ceramic core. The core is infused with molten glass ceramic to form a dense, strong core to which porcelain is added to develop the desired color and contours.
- **Heat pressing**: A pressable ceramic ingot of the desired shade is heated at a high temperature until it becomes a thick liquid and is pressed into a mold of the restoration shape.
- **Computer-aided machining**: A computer software program designs the restoration from digital images (optical impression) of the prepared tooth. A block of ceramic material of the desired shade is put in a milling machine. The computer program instructs the milling machine to cut the restoration out of the ceramic block.

CAD/CAM TECHNOLOGY

Advances in technology over the past three decades have led to the development of sophisticated computer-aided design and computer-aided machining (CAD/CAM) for general industry and dental applications. Initially, CAD/CAM technology in dentistry was used solely for crown and bridge restorations.

Preformed ceramics or resin ceramic blocks or disks are used to fabricate a variety of restorations including inlays, onlays, veneers, crowns, and bridges. As the technology has advanced and full arch scanners have become available, many other applications have emerged, including surgical guides, custom implant abutments, orthodontic aligners, custom braces, orthodontic appliances, and complete and partial dentures.

BASIC COMPONENTS OF CAD/CAM SYSTEMS

CAD/CAM systems have three basic components:
1. An optical scanner
2. A computer with design software
3. A milling device (Fig. 10.4)

Scanning

The optical scanner can make "impressions" (digital images) of tooth preparations, opposing teeth, and the occlusal relationship (bite) that are integrated with computer software (for details on digital impressions, see Chapter 5).

Design

The computer software then designs the restoration to fit the preparation, establishes proper contours and contacts, and shapes the restoration to fit the opposing occlusion. Improvements in the software permit the operator to view the designed restoration in three dimensions and rotate it in all directions so that each aspect can be inspected. The dentist or dental auxiliary can modify the design as needed, using the design tools provided.

Milling

The design is fed into a computer-controlled machine that uses diamond instruments to mill (cut and shape) an all-ceramic restoration from a block of ceramic material (Fig. 10.5).

CAD/CAM RESTORATIONS

CAD/CAM technology can be used to produce monolithic (all the same material) single-unit inlays, onlays, crowns, and veneers. In addition, it can be used to make ceramic cores for crowns and bridges that are subsequently veneered with porcelain or other ceramic material. A few manufacturers have developed multicolored blocks with layers that mimic enamel and dentin. Provisional (temporary) restorations can be fabricated from acrylic blocks. Implant abutments and metal partial denture frameworks can also be milled.

Properly designed restorations made with the use of CAD/CAM technology require fewer remakes; shorter seating time and adjustments; and better contours, contacts, and occlusion. Restorations have good marginal integrity which falls within the 50-μm parameter established by the American Dental Association.

CERAMIC CAD/CAM MATERIALS

Ceramic blocks made for CAD/CAM use have been produced under well-controlled conditions so that they are uniformly dense with no porosity. Porosities are weak points in the material that lead to the development of small cracks that propagate and eventually cause fracture of the restoration. Preproduced blocks eliminate the variations and errors that can occur with conventional laboratory procedures. Blocks contain bar codes that indicate the density of each block so

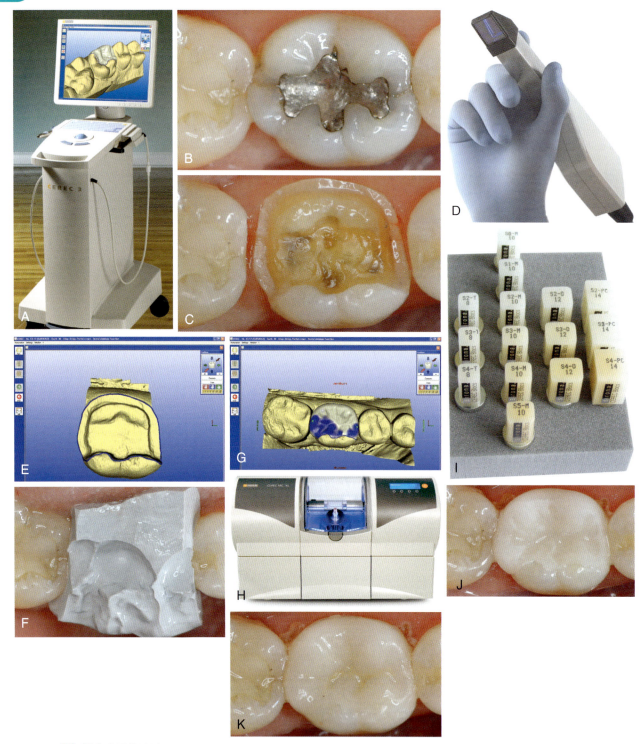

FIG. 10.4 CAD/CAM (computer-aided design and computer-aided machining) in-office system for making all-ceramic restorations: **(A)** CAD/CAM control unit with attached digital camera. **(B)** Cracked lower first molar. **(C)** Cracked molar prepared for a ceramic onlay. **(D)** Camera captures and stores images of the prepared molar and the bite relationship. **(E)** The image of the molar and the margins marked in blue. **(F)** Bite registration placed over the prepared molar. Its image will be captured, and computer software will configure the occlusal relationship with the ceramic onlay. **(G)** Computer-generated occlusal contacts (blue) made from the bite registration. **(H)** Milling unit directed by design software on how to sculpt the onlay from a ceramic block of the selected shade. **(I)** Ceramic blocks in a variety of shades and sizes. **(J)** Unpolished ceramic onlay tried on the molar for fit. **(K)** Ceramic onlay after polishing and cementing. (Courtesy Dentsply Sirona and Todd Ehrlich (private practice in Bee Cave, Texas) for clinical photographs.)

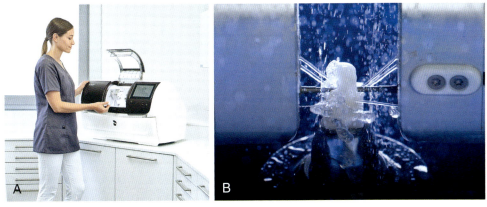

FIG. 10.5 Milling the restoration: **(A)** Ceramic block is placed in the milling machine. **(B)** Diamond instruments mill the restoration from the block according to the design feed from the computer software. (CEREC MC XL, Courtesy Dentsply Sirona.)

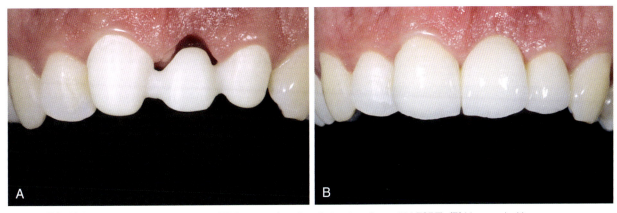

FIG. 10.6 Ceramic bridge teeth 8–10: **(A)** Opaque zirconia substructure (Lava, 3M ESPE). **(B)** Veneered with more translucent ceramic for esthetics. (Courtesy 3M ESPE and Bonatz V.)

calculations can be made by the computer software to allow for shrinkage that occurs when the restoration is given its final oven firing.

Blocks of the appropriate materials can be used to generate inlays, onlays, crowns, fixed bridges, veneers, and implant abutments. In general, monolithic restorations are stronger than veneered restorations (a core of one material and a veneer of another material). Veneered restorations have the potential to chip or separate at the junction of the veneer material and the core material (called delamination).

Glass-Based and Nonglass CAD/CAM Materials

Machinable glass-based ceramic materials are available in monochromatic or multicolored layers blocks with low and high translucency. Most nonglass ceramic blocks tend to be opaque, but newer materials have higher translucency, reducing the need to produce a core and then veneer it with a more esthetic material (as seen in Fig. 10.6). Their physical and mechanical properties are similar to non-CAD/CAM glass-based and nonglass ceramics.

Processing the Material

Milling the Blocks. Blocks of hard, fully sintered, high-strength materials, such as lithium disilicate or zirconia, are difficult and time-consuming to mill. Milling them can quickly wear out the milling tools and create residual flaws at the surface. To make milling the block easier, they are not processed (sintered) completely until after they are milled. This makes the material somewhat softer. Some milling units can cut out a full crown in approximately 5 minutes. Some lithium disilicate blocks appear purple when they are only partially sintered (Fig. 10.7) and turn tooth-colored after final processing.

Firing the Blocks. Once milling is complete, the restorations are fired in a ceramic oven to fully sinter them and transform them to the selected color (Fig. 10.8).

Stains and Glazes. Color modifiers called stains contain metal oxides. They are used on the surface to characterize a restoration by mimicking imperfections seen in the natural tooth such as:
- White spots.
- Fine crack lines.
- Stains in occlusal grooves.
- Other imperfections in the natural dentition.
- Also to improve the color of the restoration when a preformed block does not provide an exact color match.

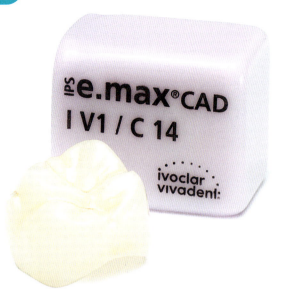

FIG. 10.7 (Top to bottom) Partially sintered block (*purple*) of lithium disilicate ceramic, and fully sintered glazed crown. Courtesy Ivoclar Vivadent (IPS e.max CAD.)

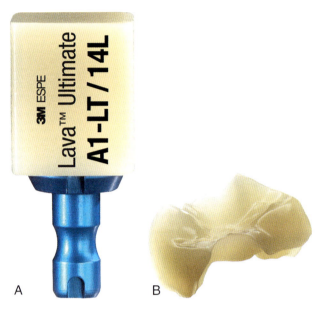

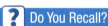

FIG. 10.9 Hybrid resin nanoceramic: **(A)** CAD/CAM block. **(B)** Completed onlay. (Lava Ultimate, Courtesy 3M ESPE.)

spray-on glaze, which is fused to the restoration in a ceramic oven.

> **? Do You Recall?**
>
> After partially sintered CAD/CAM ceramic blocks are milled, what is the next step to make them fully sintered and usable for a restoration?

Hybrid Resin Ceramics

Hybrid resin nanoceramic materials (Fig. 10.9) combine composite resin and nano-sized ceramic filler particles. They are easy to mill and polish to a high shine and do not need to be oven fired. Hybrid resin nanoceramic materials produce tough, durable restorations that are not abrasive to the opposing teeth. They are available in several common shades consisting of high and low translucency options. They are stain and wear resistant and color stable. They are indicated for single-unit anterior and posterior crowns, inlays, onlays, and veneers.

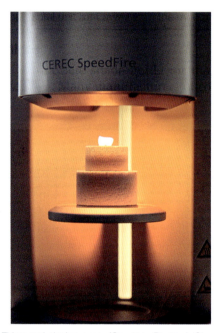

FIG. 10.8 Firing and glazing oven. (Courtesy Dentsply Sirona, CEREC SpeedFire ceramic oven.)

A glaze provides a glossy, enamel-like surface. Stains and glazes are applied in thin layers on the surface of the restoration and fired at the time of final sintering. They are heated in a ceramic oven to a point that allows them to fuse with the ceramic restoration.

Polishing the Restoration. After the fit is verified, the restoration is finished and polished. Abrasive rubber wheels and points can be used and a high gloss achieved with diamond paste on bristle brushes. Instead of polishing, some clinicians prefer to apply a

SUMMARY OF CAD/CAM STEPS FOR PRODUCING A RESTORATION

- Complete the preparation using principles for all-ceramic restorations.
- Use the optical scanner to obtain an image of the preparation. Some scanners require coating the preparation with a powder to enhance scanning accuracy.
- Use the computer software to design the restoration: mark margins and establish restoration contours on the computer screen.

- Use the software to simulate the bite in side-to-side movement.
- Select block of the correct shade of the ceramic material and place it in the milling machine.
- Program the milling machine for the material being used and activate the machine.
- If the milled restoration was partially sintered, it will need to be fired to complete the sintering process.
- Characterization with surface stains can be accomplished while applying the glaze.
- Try in the completed restoration and polish as needed.
- Cement the restoration after etching internally and applying silane (zirconia should not be etched or silanated; it has special primers).
- Check and adjust the occlusion as needed after cementation.

CLINICAL APPLICATIONS FOR CERAMIC MATERIALS

Ceramic materials such as lithium disilicate and zirconia are much stronger than porcelain and have replaced their use in many clinical applications. They are strong enough to be used in the posterior part of the mouth in many (but not all) individuals. People who grind their teeth apply greater stress to ceramic materials and are at greater risk of fracturing it. However, some patients are willing to accept the risk of fracture to achieve the high esthetics of all-ceramic crowns. It is very important that patients be made fully aware of the fracture risks of using porcelain or other ceramics so they can make informed decisions about their care. When the patient has multiple ceramic restorations, use of an occlusal guard to reduce fracture risk is recommended. Many offices use informed consent forms to explain the pros and cons of treatment and patients must sign the form before esthetic treatments are started. Although the dentist has the final responsibility, the dental auxiliary may be called on to inform the patient about the pros and cons of various dental materials.

RATIONALE FOR THE SELECTION OF CERAMIC MATERIALS

Different types of ceramic materials have different physical properties and esthetics and therefore are not universal in their applications. See Table 10.2 for indications and contraindications for the various ceramic materials.

CERAMIC VENEERS

Veneers are thin layers (like press-on nails) of esthetic ceramic materials that are used to improve the appearance of the teeth. They are bonded to the fronts of the teeth, most often anterior teeth and premolars. They can be used to:
- Lighten the color of teeth
- Cover stains
- Repair chips or other defects
- Lengthen worn teeth
- Increase the size of small teeth
- Close spaces (diastemas)
- Reshape crooked teeth so that they look as though they are in proper alignment

The most commonly used materials are glass-based ceramics. They are made of:
- Traditional feldspathic porcelain
- Pressed ceramics
- CAM ceramics
- Such as lithium disilicate

Clinical Consideration for Veneers

Veneers can be made relatively thin and require a minimal reduction of the enamel by 0.5 mm on the facial and at least 1.0 mm at the incisal edge. Esthetic demands might require greater reduction to correct overlapping teeth or to hide dark teeth or discolorations.

Masking Dark Teeth. Porcelain veneers can be made to be slightly translucent to let the color of the underlying tooth come through, or more opaque to hide the color of a darker natural tooth. Dark teeth are more

Table 10.2 Indications and Contraindications for Use of Various Types of Ceramics

CERAMIC TYPE	MAIN USES	OTHER USES	CONTRAINDICATIONS
Feldspathic porcelain	PFM ceramics Anterior veneers	Single surface inlays in low-stress sites	Inlays, onlays, crowns, bridges (except as metal ceramic veneers)
Leucite-reinforced glass ceramic	Anterior use for single crowns or veneers	Low-stress inlays and crowns in premolars	Bridges High stress: Bruxers
Lithium disilicate glass ceramic	Anterior and premolar crowns Anterior bridges	Anterior veneers Bridges no farther back than premolars	High stress: Bruxers Bridges involving molars
Glass-infiltrated alumina or zirconia	Posterior crowns Bridge substructure to 3 units	Anterior bridge substructure to 3 units	Translucent anterior applications: Veneers and crowns
Zirconia with or without veneering ceramic	Posterior crowns and bridges Posterior bridge substructure	Implant abutments in the smile zone	Where high translucency is needed: Anterior veneers, crowns, or bridges Bruxers

PFM, Porcelain-fused-to-metal.
Adapted from Anusavice KJ, Shen C, Rawls HR. Dental ceramics. In: *Phillips' Science of Dental Materials.* 12th ed. Saunders; 2013.

challenging to cover with veneers and still achieve an esthetic result. Adding some opaque porcelain (up to approximately 15%) helps to hide the darkness, but too much opaqueness will cause a loss of the vitality. On occasion, whitening of dark teeth may be attempted first to reduce the darkness before veneers are placed. On occasion, all-ceramic crowns might be a better option for improving the appearance of very dark teeth and still achieving an optimal esthetic effect.

Try-in of Veneers. Veneers are tried on the teeth, using water or a try-in gel on the surfaces that contact the teeth. The gel is a water-soluble material that occupies the air space between the veneer and the tooth surface. Without the water or gel, light transmitted through the veneer would be scattered by the air space, altering the appearance of the veneer. The gels can be clear or slightly shaded to correspond to shades of bonding resins.

Veneers Are Fragile. Before being bonded to the teeth, the ceramic veneers are somewhat fragile because they are very thin. The veneer must be handled with care when they are tried on the teeth to confirm the fit or to adjust the contact areas. They might crack if too much pressure is applied to them. Once bonded, the veneer gains support from the underlying tooth structure and greatly increase in strength.

> ❗ **Caution**
> Handle veneers carefully! They are very fragile until bonded!

Cementation of Veneers. Veneers are bonded to the teeth with resin cement, using the acid-etch technique and a resin bonding agent (Fig. 10.10). Resin cements come in a variety of colors, including a clear resin. If needed, a resin color can be selected to slightly alter the final appearance of the veneer to help mask the color of the underlying tooth.

Preparing the Porcelain Surface. To get the resin to stick to the porcelain, the internal surface of the veneer is roughened by etching it with hydrofluoric acid. A saline coupling agent is added to the etched porcelain surface to enhance the bond and form a chemical union between the porcelain and the resin cement (see Table 10.3 for a summary of how to bond to ceramic surfaces).

Seating the Veneer. Once the tooth surface and the internal veneer surface have been properly prepared, the resin cement is placed on the veneer and it is carefully seated while an attempt is made to avoid trapping air. The veneer is lightly vibrated with an instrument or finger to fully seat it and dislodge any entrapped air bubbles.

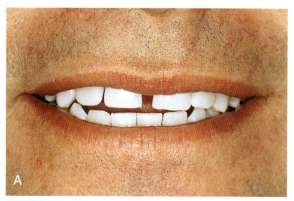
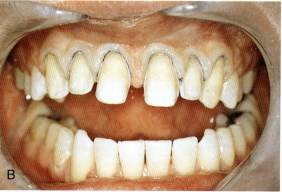
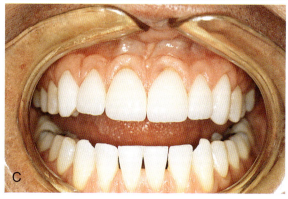

FIG. 10.10 Placement of porcelain veneers to correct a large space between the teeth (diastema): **(A)** Pretreatment photograph showing large midline diastema. **(B)** Maxillary anterior teeth prepared for veneers. Retraction cord is in place. **(C)** After cementation of veneers with resin cement. (Courtesy Dentsply International, York, Pennsylvania.)

Removing Excess Cement. Excess cement can be removed from the margins at this stage with small microbrushes. Alternatively, the curing light can be waved over the surface for 3 or 4 seconds to cause the resin to slightly gel but not fully cure. The gelled excess resin can then easily be removed with an explorer or thin scaler.

Finishing and Polishing. Some additional finishing and polishing might be required. Various techniques are available for this last step:
- Using combinations of finishing strips and disks
- Carbide and diamond finishing rotary instruments
- Rubber polishing points or diamond polishing pastes

TABLE 10.3 Bonding to Common All-Ceramic Restorations: A Summary

PROCEDURE STEPS	FELDSPATHIC PORCELAIN	LITHIUM DISILICATE	ZIRCONIA
Etch ceramic	Hydrofluoric acid 60 s	Hydrofluoric acid 60 s	No etch. Sandblast to roughen
Rinse	Yes	Yes	No
Silane	Yes (unless universal adhesive contains silane)	Yes (unless universal adhesive contains silane)	No, if universal adhesive contains silane
Bonding agent	Apply etch-and-rinse adhesives	Apply etch-and-rinse adhesives	Apply special primer and universal adhesive
Cement	Light- or dual-cured resin cement	Light- or dual-cured resin or self-adhesive resin cement	Self-adhesive resin cement; resin-modified glass ionomer; or special primer, universal bonding agent, and resin cement

Adapted from Farah JW, Power JM. Bonding agents—2008. *The Dental Advisor.* 2008;25:1–9.

 Do You Recall?

Which is the better substrate to bond veneers to, enamel or dentin? Why?

CERAMIC INLAYS, ONLAYS, FIXED BRIDGES

Ceramic inlays, onlays, and fixed bridges are placed in the functional areas of the mouth, and therefore strength is an important factor. Feldspathic porcelains are not the materials of choice for restorations in the posterior of the mouth because they are too weak. Heat-pressed materials are commonly used, but CAD/CAM-produced zirconium materials are gaining in popularity because of their high strength.

 Clinical Tip

Ultrasonic scalers, if improperly applied, can chip and graze margins of esthetic materials.

FINISHING AND POLISHING CERAMIC RESTORATIONS

An important factor in wear of the opposing dentition by ceramic restorations is the smoothness of the ceramic surface. Modern ceramic materials, such as lithium disilicate and zirconia ceramics, are less abrasive than porcelain and can be polished smoother. Once the occlusal surface of a restoration has been adjusted with a diamond bur, the roughness of the surface can be very abrasive to the opposing enamel or restorative material. It is imperative to reestablish the surface smoothness through careful finishing and polishing techniques.

Coarse diamond burs should not be used to adjust the surface because the larger diamond particles leave a rougher surface that is more difficult to re-polish, and they tend to generate heat that can damage the ceramic. Fine diamond burs are recommended.

Principles of Finishing and Polishing Ceramics

Some basic principles of finishing and polishing dental ceramic materials should be followed:
- First, heavy pressure should be avoided; use a light touch.
- Second, low speed should be used with water spray. Following both of these principles will minimize the generation of heat and damage to the surface and beneath it.

Sequential Finishing and Polishing. When trying to achieve a smooth surface, it is important to follow a proper sequence progressing from coarser to fine and yet finer abrasive finishing and polishing instruments. Steps cannot be skipped. Larger scratches must be sequentially reduced to smaller and smaller scratches until they are no longer perceptible. Several manufacturers have developed special finishing and polishing instruments designed for use with porcelains, lithium disilicate, or zirconia.

Use of Polishing Pastes. Polishing pastes contain very fine abrasives to create a highly smooth surface after the use of polishing instruments. Pastes containing aluminum oxide are safe to use on porcelain. If the objective is to produce a high shine or luster, a diamond polishing paste should be used. As with most products, follow the manufacturer's recommendations for which pastes to use on the various ceramic materials.

 Clinical Tip

Generation of heat during adjustment, finishing, and polishing of ceramics can cause damage that may progress to fracture of the restoration. Use rotary instruments at low speed with water spray and light pressure.

CEMENTATION OF ALL-CERAMIC RESTORATIONS

All of the glass-based ceramic materials (porcelain, leucite-reinforced ceramic, and lithium disilicate ceramic) should be bonded to the teeth with resin cement. Bonding them to a rigid substrate greatly enhances their resistance to fracture.

Try-in of Restoration

The delivery of ceramic restorations begins with good isolation. Use of the rubber dam is ideal but not always practical, so alternatives such as absorbent pads and cotton rolls may be used. Next, the provisional restoration is removed, bits of adherent cement are picked off with an explorer or other instrument, and the prepared tooth surfaces are cleaned with pumice and water on rubber cups or brushes and then rinsed and dried.

The restoration is tried in and interproximal contacts are adjusted. As for veneers, translucent ceramic restorations are tried in using a water-soluble try-in paste, glycerin, or K-Y Jelly is used to verify the color and to determine the color of resin cement to use. For zirconia and alumina restorations, their opaqueness hides the color of the underlying tooth.

For weaker materials such as porcelain or leucite-reinforced ceramics, the occlusion should not be checked in the mouth until after cementation because they might crack. The occlusion is checked on the mounted dies before cementation (unless processed by CAD/CAM, for which there are no physical dies).

Preparing the Restoration

Glass-Based Ceramics. If the laboratory has not already etched the internal surface (intaglio) of the restoration, then apply 10% hydrofluoric acid for 1 minute, and then rinse and dry. A silane coupling agent is applied to the etched surface for 60 seconds, and then air-dried (Procedure 10.1).

Nonglass Ceramics. Because of their high strength, zirconia crowns can be cemented with conventional cements or bonded with resin cements. Zirconia restorations are not etched before cementation. They do not respond to acid etchants like glass-based ceramics, and attempts at etching might produce a powdery residue on the interior of the crown that is difficult to remove and may interfere with bonding. These restorations can be sandblasted internally to provide a roughened surface for bonding. Zirconia ceramic materials do not need silane treatment but may be treated with special primers with acidic adhesive monomers to improve the bond with resin cement.

The protocol for bonding zirconia has three steps:
1. sandblasting the interior
2. applying primer
3. bonding with adhesive resin cement

Preparing the Tooth

The prepared tooth surfaces are wiped with a wet cotton pellet to remove any remnants of try-in materials. If any bleeding has occurred, the tissue can be infiltrated with local anesthetic with epinephrine to constrict the capillaries, or a hemostatic agent can be used.

Next, the tooth surface (enamel, dentin, or both) is conditioned according to the manufacturer's instructions for the bonding materials being used. A bonding agent is applied to establish a resin-infused surface for bonding with resin cement. An alternative to the etch-and-rinse bonding agent is a self-etch bonding agent that eliminates the need for phosphoric acid etching (see Chapter 7).

Cementation of the Restoration

Resin cement systems commonly used with ceramic restorations are dual cured, so if the light from the curing unit is unable to reach all of the cement, it will cure chemically on its own.

Cement Application. The resin cement is mixed and applied to the internal part of the restoration. Use enough to coat all of the walls of the restoration and the margins. Do not overfill a crown because the hydraulic pressure created by excess cement trying to escape when seating the crown may prevent the restoration from seating completely.

Removal of Excess Cement. Wipe away excess cement with a microbrush. Use the curing light for about 3 seconds over the area of the margins to cause the resin to gel but not set completely. This is called tack curing and will facilitate easy removal of any remaining excess cement.

Remove excess cement with an explorer or another hand instrument. After the excess cement is removed, cure for 60 seconds (halogen light) or less with high-intensity lights. With opaque restorations of zirconia the light may be ineffective for reaching cement under the restoration, but the chemical-cure component of the cement will allow it to set in a couple of minutes.

 Do You Recall?

What is the difference between glass-based and nonglass-based ceramic restorations in their surface preparation for bonding?

MAINTENANCE OF ALL-CERAMIC RESTORATIONS

The patient should be given home care instructions for proper brushing and flossing around ceramic restorations. For bridges, additional hygiene aids, such as floss threaders, interproximal brushes, or superfloss, may be recommended. Patients should be advised against biting on hard objects or food. At periodic recall appointments, recheck the occlusion for heavy contact points, review the gingival health, and make sure no excess cement remains.

Precautions

Care should be taken when working around ceramic restorations. It is important for the clinician to identify the junction of the tooth and the margins of any of the ceramic restorations when removing excess cement or when doing scaling or root-planing procedures. The hand scaler or ultrasonic tip used at high settings may cause chipping of the margins if the clinician is not careful. However, properly fabricated and adjusted ceramic restorations should present minimal problems for the clinician performing these procedures. If significant overhang or catching of the margins is noted, the auxiliary should alert the dentist, who may correct them or prescribe replacements.

When providing in-office fluoride treatments to adults with ceramic restorations, the auxiliary needs to select a fluoride product that is not acidic. Acidulated fluoride products can etch ceramic surfaces. Likewise, when doing bonding procedures on adjacent teeth, avoid allowing etching gels to touch the ceramics, because they will roughen the surface. Ultrasonic scalers should be used with care around ceramic restorations so as not to induce heat damage or initiate microcracks at the margins. Patients who grind their teeth or have edge-to-edge bites should be provided with occlusal guards to help protect anterior ceramic crowns and veneers.

Caution
Avoid acid etchants and acidic fluorides on ceramic restorations. They will roughen the surface of the ceramic.

PORCELAIN-FUSED-TO-METAL RESTORATIONS

Before strong, esthetic ceramics were developed, the most commonly used esthetic restorations in crown and bridge procedures were combinations of porcelain and metal. The main advantages of the combination of porcelain and metal are the strength and durability provided by the fusion (bond) between oxides on the metal internal core and the esthetic external porcelain covering (porcelain-fused-to-metal restorations) at high temperature. The restorations are strong enough to be used as single-unit crowns or multiunit bridges in both the anterior and posterior parts of the mouth. The survival rate at 5 years for porcelain-metal restorations is about 94%.

Application of Porcelain to the Metal Core

The method for layering porcelain on a metal core is similar to that for a ceramic core or for building up porcelain on a die (replica of the prepared tooth). Low-fusing porcelain is used most often for bonding to metal. These restorations are referred to as porcelain-fused-to-metal (PFM) or porcelain-bonded-to-metal (PBM) restorations. The metals that are used as the core for PFM/PBM crowns are alloys of specific metals that will form an oxide layer as the metal is heated (see Chapter 12).

Trying to hide the metal core with porcelain can present some esthetic challenges. A color of porcelain is selected that corresponds to the color or shade that matches the patient's dentition. The porcelain comes as a powder that is mixed into a paste with deionized water or a water-based liquid, or may be in a paste form already.

The first layer of porcelain applied to the metal is opaque porcelain to help hide the metal oxide and is the main color used for the crown (Fig. 10.11). The oxidized metal and porcelain are heated under a vacuum to remove air and increase density at temperatures ranging from 1598°F to 2498°F, depending on the type of porcelain used. The porcelain particles melt at their borders and fuse together (sintering) and also wet the metal oxides. The oxides and porcelain chemically fuse together and mechanically interlock. Sintering results in shrinkage of the porcelain mass by about 25% to 40%.

Additional layers of porcelain called body and incisal porcelains are built up to simulate dentin and enamel colors and translucency (Fig. 10.12). The incisal porcelain is more translucent, so the body color shows through readily and has a greater influence on the final appearance.

The layers of porcelain are heated (fired) in an oven until they fuse to each other and to the underlying opaque porcelain.

Firing Porcelain

A programmable porcelain oven is used to gradually raise the temperature of the porcelain and metal. If the temperature is increased too quickly, water in the wet porcelain mass will form steam which can blow the condensed mass of porcelain apart. The porcelain is first heated to approximately 1650°F to partially fuse (sinter) the particles (see Fig. 10.1). As the glass matrix softens, it flows and reduces porosities.

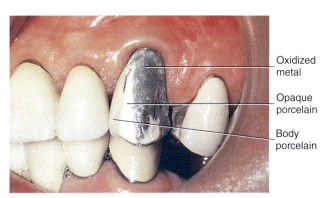

FIG. 10.11 Porcelain failure with porcelain-fused-to-metal crown. The metal is exposed, as is a portion of the opaque layer of porcelain used to hide the dark metal. (Courtesy Dr. Steve Eakle, University of California, San Francisco.).

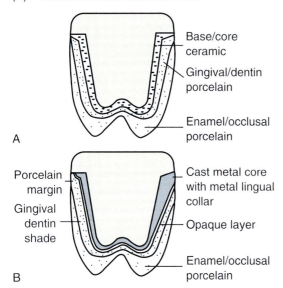

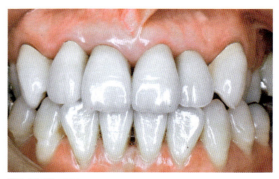

FIG. 10.12 Section through **(A)** an all-ceramic crown and **(B)** a porcelain-bonded-to-metal crown, showing the layers of porcelain and the metal substructure of the crown.

FIG. 10.13 PFM crowns 6 to 11 with glazed surfaces that resemble the luster of the natural teeth in the lower anterior. (From Rosenstiel SF, Land MF. *Contemporary Fixed Prosthodontics*. 5th ed. Elsevier; 2016.)

Next, the porcelain is fired at high temperature and vacuum. If it is held at firing temperature too long, the glass will slump and the restoration will lose its shape. It is important to use the correct time and temperature for the firing cycle as an inadequate or too great a temperature can greatly reduce the flexural strength of the restoration. Additionally, the development of translucency occurs only after firing at the proper temperature and time. After firing has been completed, the resulting restoration will have shrunk about 25% because of the fusion of the porcelain particles.

Glazing
After final contouring of the crown, another firing maintaining the temperature at the fusing temperature for a while will produce a surface glaze. The surface layer of porcelain will heat first, allowing it to melt and run together, producing a dense, shiny, smooth surface (Fig. 10.13).

Color Modification
Stains are used with veneering porcelain for the same purposes as for all-ceramic restorations, that is, they can characterize the restoration and improve color matching.

Re-polishing
The porcelain surface, once it has been fused under temperature, is very hard and smooth. When porcelain or PFM restorations are delivered, the proximal contacts or occlusal surfaces often must be adjusted. These restorations could be returned to the laboratory to be re-glazed before cementing. Because this is seldom practical, various abrasives have been developed for polishing the porcelain surface after adjustment.

Porcelain Failures
Most porcelain failures result from small cracks in the porcelain that develop when the porcelain is put under occlusal loading, and they spread over time until the porcelain gives way. Other modes of failure are caused by problems related to the chemical bond between the porcelain and the metal oxides. The oxide layer may be too thick or inadequate in quantity and quality, leading to failure at the interface of the porcelain and metal. It is important that the coefficients of thermal expansion of the porcelain and the metal be compatible. The best arrangement is for the porcelain to have slightly less thermal expansion than the metal. This will keep it from cracking at the metal-porcelain interface and will reduce the chance of failure (see Fig. 10.11).

 KEY POINTS

PFM RESTORATIONS
1. Restoration consists of porcelain fused to oxide layer on a metal core
2. Porcelain layering:
   - Opaque layer to hide the dark metal
   - Body layer to simulate dentin
   - Incisal layer to simulate translucency of enamel
3. Porcelain layers fired in porcelain oven at high temperature to fuse particles together and with metal oxides
4. Color modifiers—stains applied to alter color or mimic stained grooves or white spots
5. PFM uses in anterior and posterior parts of mouth:
   - Single-unit crowns
   - Multiunit bridges
6. Reasons for PFM fracture:
   - Cracks in porcelain from single heavy load or repeated loads
   - Poor bond of porcelain to metal from inadequate oxide layer
   - Incompatibility of thermal expansion between metal and porcelain

> **? Do You Recall?**
>
> With PFM crowns, how does the porcelain adhere to the metal core?

SHADE TAKING

The auxiliary may be asked to assist the dentist in obtaining the appropriate shade for a restorative procedure. An inappropriate shade selection will result in a mismatch to the patient's dentition. Usually the restoration will need to be returned to the dental laboratory for a remake or for reapplication of porcelain. This is disappointing for all involved and usually results in an additional laboratory fee and the in-office expense of an additional appointment and an inconvenience for the patient. Therefore it is important for all clinical members of the dental team to have an understanding of what goes into the perception of color, how to accurately match the variety of shades within a single tooth, and how to communicate this to the dental technician.

INVOLVING THE DENTAL AUXILIARY AND THE PATIENT

Having the doctor, auxiliary, and patient working together to determine the shade often gets a result all can be happy with.

The dental auxiliary can get the dental office environment and the patient ready for taking the shade. This is done in the same manner as when taking a shade for composites (see Chapter 8).

Shade Guides for Ceramics

The most popular shade guides are the VITA Lumin system (VITAPAN Classical or VITA 3D-Master; VITA North America) (Fig. 10.14) and Chromascop (Ivoclar Vivadent). The shades in the VITA guide are as follows:
- A shades are reddish-brown.
- B shades are reddish-yellow.
- C shades are gray.
- D shades are reddish-gray.
- A3 and D3 are similar in color, but A3 is brighter than D3.

As teeth darken with age, patients who were once in the A shade range may transition into the D shades.

A typical shade tab is composed of several colors arranged to simulate a natural tooth. An opaque color is used as a backing on the tab for the color of the body of the tooth crown and the color of the root (also called the neck) but does not include the incisal portion that is typically translucent (Fig. 10.15).

STEPS FOR CERAMIC SHADE TAKING

In general, the shade should be taken before the tooth is isolated or prepared. The following steps should be used when taking the shade of the teeth:
- Use natural light when possible
- Use cheek retractors for an unobstructed view of the teeth
- Raise the patient to view the teeth at eye level to use the color-sensitive part of the retina
- Wet the shade tab and the teeth to remove surface texture differences
- Place the shade tab in the same plane as the teeth, not in front or behind

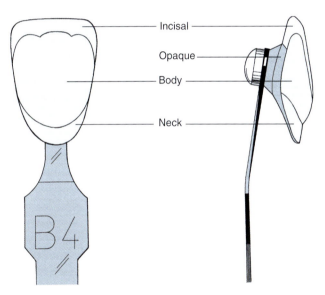

FIG. 10.15 Color arrangements in a typical porcelain shade tab. (From Rosenstiel SF, Land MF. *Contemporary Fixed Prosthodontics.* 5th ed. Elsevier; 2016.)

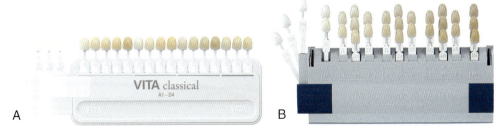

FIG. 10.14 Two popular commercial shade guides that use different methods for selecting the shade: **(A)** VITA Classical A1-D4 with whitening shades. **(B)** VITA Toothguide 3D-Master groups colors by value (light to dark). (Courtesy VITA North America, Yorba Linda, California.)

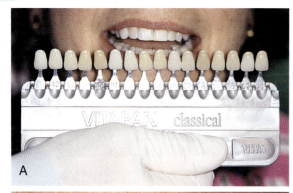

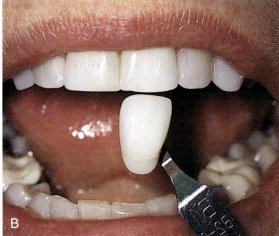

FIG. 10.16 Shade taking for ceramic restorations: **(A)** Shade guide placed near the mouth to select the basic color (hue). **(B)** The shade tab in the right color is compared with the teeth to be matched; select the color with the proper value (darkness or brightness) and chroma (intensity of color).

- View the teeth and tab for no more than 5 seconds at a time
- Rest the eyes between viewings by staring at a neutral gray color
- Pick the best three shade tabs quickly
- With the input of patient, doctor, and assistant, select the best of the three
- If possible, use photography to aid the lab technician. Place the shade tab next to the teeth in the photo
- Note tooth factors the lab will need to characterize (see Characterizing the Shade below)

The patient, dentist, and auxiliary should view the tabs and rank them as to the closest match for color intensity and lightness or darkness. It is often necessary to take separate shades for the cervical portion of the tooth, for the occlusal surfaces of posterior teeth, and for the incisal edges of anterior teeth (Fig. 10.16).

Characterizing the Shade

Surface Luster and Texture. In addition to the shade, the surface luster and texture should be noted. Luster is the degree to which the surface appears shiny and reflects light. The enamel surface has slight convexities and concavities that create texture. Textured teeth tend to scatter light. As a person ages, the slight convexities and concavities become smoother from wear and reflect light differently than highly textured teeth. The laboratory technician can add surface glazes to ceramic to create a shiny surface and can add texture to scatter light.

Translucency/Opacity. The amount of translucency of the enamel and its location (e.g., incisal edge) should also be communicated to the laboratory. The laboratory technician may need to place layers of opaque porcelain to mask darkly colored dentin when fabricating all-ceramic restorations. The opacity will cause of loss of vitality in the restoration. The technician may need to produce the perception of translucency by using color modifiers to tint the porcelain (e.g., blue tints may produce a hint of translucency).

Other Tooth Characteristics. Teeth may have opaque white spots or lines, stained cracks, wear facets, and other characteristics that should be conveyed to the laboratory if the patient is trying to match existing teeth. The process of incorporating into the restoration texture, translucency, opacity, and the many other tooth features is called characterization.

Shade Mapping. A written description and drawing of the shade distribution (called shade mapping) and location of translucency and any special characterizations, surface texture, and luster should be sent to the laboratory to help guide the technician.

Digital Photography. Often it is helpful to the technician if a digital photograph of the teeth is transmitted. If photography is used, the shade tab should be included in the picture because some photographs will be a little more red or blue than the actual color. The bright operatory light should not be used to illuminate the patient's mouth, as this will cause the recorded image to appear lighter. The shade tab should be in the same plane as the tooth to be matched, so that it will be in the same focus as the teeth; that is, it should not be in front of the teeth or outside of the mouth and will have the same illumination as the teeth when flash photography is used.

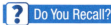 **Do You Recall?**

What factors need to be considered when preparing the operatory and the patient for shade taking?

Custom Shade Matching. On occasion, some teeth are not a close match to the shade tabs. This requires that the technician see the teeth to custom blend different shades of porcelain or use surface stains to match the color. The patient may be sent to the laboratory, or the technician may come to the operatory for this "custom" shade taking. This is particularly true for whitened teeth. Whitened colors of teeth may not match existing shade guides. So, shade guides with whitening shades that are extra light (low chroma and high value) should be used. Even with these whitening shades, it may be difficult to match the color of whitened teeth.

Dentin Shade Matching for All-Ceramic Restorations

Some all-ceramic restorations are relatively translucent. A special shade guide for dentin color is used to help the technician in the fabrication of a crown (Fig. 10.17). Cosmetically, it might be important to hide dark dentin with opaque ceramic colors to achieve a lighter color in the restoration. The final shade of the all-ceramic restoration is influenced by:

1. The shade of the ceramic coping (substructure for a crown or framework for a bridge)
2. The veneering porcelain or ceramic
3. The shade of the prepared tooth
4. The shade of the luting material (conventional cement or bonded resin)

DEVICES FOR TAKING THE SHADE

Because of the complexity involved in achieving a good shade match of a ceramic material to the natural tooth, a number of devices have been introduced that help in obtaining an accurate reading of the shade of the teeth. These devices use optical readers (spectrophotometers) to determine the correct shade (Fig. 10.18).

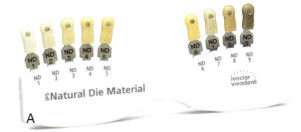
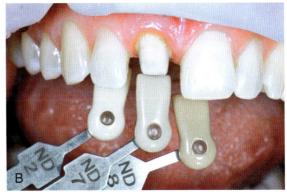

Fig. 10.17 Shade guide for taking dentin shades: **(A)** dentin shade guide and **(B)** dentin shade tabs used to match dentin from the prepared tooth. (From Rosenstiel SF, Land MF. *Contemporary Fixed Prosthodontics*. 5th ed. Elsevier; 2016.)

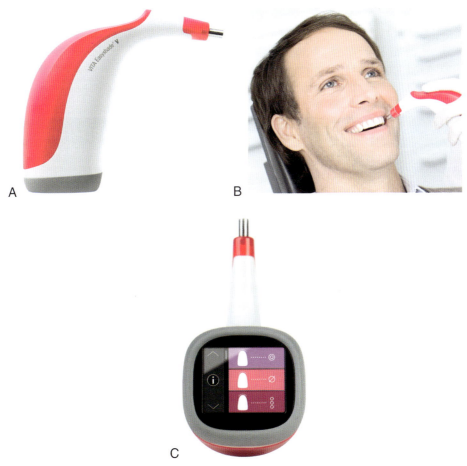

FIG. 10.18 Shade-taking device: **(A)** Optical shade reader (Easyshade V). **(B)** Device used to take the shade. **(C)** Digital display of the shade captured by the device. (Courtesy VITA North America, Yorba Linda, California.)

Having the information captured by an optical device removes the subjectivity of the individual trying to interpret the shade and trying to describe the shade to the dental laboratory technician. This eliminates the extraneous light sources and conflicting colors in the room or on the patient that confuse the human eye's perception of color. One such device, the VITA Easyshade V (Vident/VITA), can match the shade it records with the company's popular brand of VITA porcelains. These devices can provide a map or layout of the subtle variations in shade within a given tooth. With proper training, the dental assistant or hygienist can operate the device and acquire the shade. This increases office efficiency and consistency of shade matching. The accuracy of the shade taken by these devices can potentially save time and expense associated with sending the crown back to the laboratory to correct a mismatched color.

Advances in technology are making communication with the laboratory simpler and more accurate.

SUMMARY

A wide variety of tooth-colored ceramic materials are available to the dental team to restore a patient's dentition. They can be glass-based or nonglass-based ceramics. In general, glass-based ceramics are more esthetic but not as strong as nonglassed-based ceramics. Patients demand high-quality restorations with a close match to their existing teeth, or in some cases, they demand restorations that produce a lighter, youthful smile.

CAD/CAM technology is providing new avenues for the dental team to provide esthetic dentistry, making many procedures faster and easier on patients.

It is important that all members of the dental team understand the handling characteristics, physical properties, and potential shortcomings of these materials. Before working in the patient's mouth, it is wise to review the dental charting section of the patient's record or perform a brief oral inspection to detect the presence of esthetic restorations.

The selection and use of proper polishing and scaling devices are an important consideration for the hygienist and assistant when working around these restorations. Additionally, it is important to keep in mind that the surfaces of these esthetic restorations can be dulled by the use of acidulated fluoride solutions and gels and phosphoric acid etchants for bonding. Certain coarse abrasives used for coronal polishing can also adversely affect the surface luster of porcelain.

As new esthetic materials are adopted in the practice, it is important to become familiar with their handling characteristics, physical properties, uses, and precautions.

INSTRUCTIONAL VIDEOS

See the Evolve Resources site for a variety of educational videos that reinforce the material covered in this chapter.

Procedure 10.1 Surface Treatment for Bonding Glass-Based Ceramic Restorations

See Evolve site for Competency Sheet.

Consider the following with this procedure: safety glasses are recommended for the patient, personal protective equipment is required for the operator, ensure appropriate safety protocols are followed, and check your local state guidelines before performing this procedure.

EQUIPMENT/SUPPLIES (FIG. 10.19)

- High- and low-speed handpieces with prophy attachment
- Dappen dish with flour of pumice and rubber prophy cup
- Isopropyl alcohol or acetone, hydrofluoric acid, silane, enamel and dentin bonding resin
- 37% phosphoric acid, resin luting cement, curing light

PROCEDURE STEPS

1. Isolate area to be bonded and clean the tooth with slurry of flour of pumice. Try in ceramic restoration for fit.

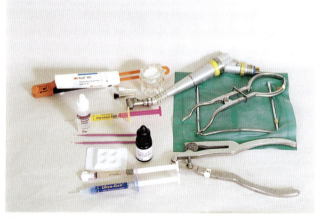

FIG. 10.19 Equipment and supplies for the procedure.

Pumice removes any plaque or pellicle that might interfere with etching and bonding.

NOTE: Isolation is necessary to prevent moisture contamination of the surfaces during bonding.

Continued

Procedure 10.1 Surface Treatment for Bonding Glass-Based Ceramic Restorations—cont'd

2. Clean the internal surface of the ceramic with alcohol or acetone to remove salivary contaminants from the try-in.
3. Apply 10% hydrofluoric acid to the cavity side of the ceramic for 1 minute to etch it.
4. Rinse with water for 10 seconds and air-dry (Fig. 10.20).
5. Apply silane to etched ceramic for 60 seconds, and then air-dry to remove alcohol solvents.

   Some ceramics may require special primers for bonding. Check the manufacturer's recommendation.
   NOTE: Silane allows bonding of resins to the treated ceramic surface.
6. Apply bonding resin to ceramic, but do not light cure it.
   NOTE: The thickness of the bonding resin may prevent proper seating of the restoration if cured at this stage.
7. Etch the tooth surfaces to be bonded with 37% phosphoric acid: 20 seconds for enamel and 10 seconds for dentin.
8. Rinse with water for 10 seconds.
   NOTE: If the surface is enamel only, dry thoroughly. If dentin is to be bonded, leave both enamel and dentin slightly moist. Trying to dry the enamel may overdry the dentin.
9. Apply enamel-dentin bonding resin (Fig. 10.21). Blow the bonding resin thin with air.
   NOTE: Do not allow it to pool in the preparation or it will interfere with seating of the restoration.
10. Light cure for 20 seconds.
11. Apply resin cement to the restoration and seat it firmly (Fig. 10.22).
12. Remove gross excess cement and then light cure for 3 seconds to cause the resin to partially set. Remove the remaining excess resin (Fig. 10.23).
    Note: With high-intensity curing lights, just wave the light over the restoration for 1 to 2 seconds. Otherwise, the resin cement may set too firmly.
13. Light cure for 40 to 60 seconds or longer if needed for final set.
    NOTE: Self-cured or dual-cured resins are used for cementation of inlays, onlays, or crowns because the thickness of the restoration prevents adequate penetration of the light. With thin veneers, a light-cured resin can be used. Some high-speed curing lights with high light intensity might alter these recommended curing times. Check manufacturer's recommendations.

Courtesy Alton Lacy, University of California School of Dentistry, San Francisco, California

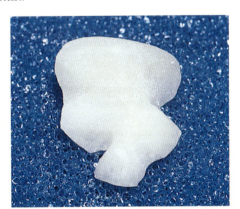

FIG. 10.20 Ceramic inlay after acid etching of interior surface in preparation for bonding.

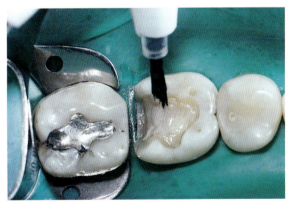

FIG. 10.22 After etch and rinse, a bonding resin is applied to the cavity preparation.

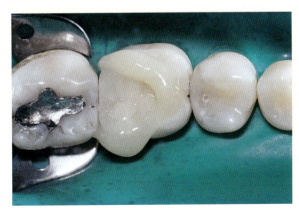

FIG. 10.21 The cavity-side of the ceramic restoration is prepared for bonding it to the tooth.

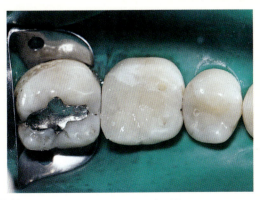

FIG. 10.23 Completed ceramic inlay tooth #19.

Review and Discussion

Review Questions

Select the one correct response for each of the following multiple-choice questions.

1. Feldspathic porcelain restorations have:
    a. Great stain resistance
    b. Low wear resistance
    c. High strength
    d. Easy reparability
2. Porcelain bonds to metal by which one of the following mechanisms?
    a. Micromechanical retention much like resin bonded to etched enamel
    b. Penetration through the surface of the metal
    c. Fusion with oxides on the surface of the metal
    d. Shrinkage when fired so that it locks onto the metal
3. What is the main advantage of all-ceramic crowns over porcelain-bonded-to-metal crowns?
    a. Their superior esthetics
    b. Their strength
    c. Their ease of cementation
    d. The ease of taking shades
4. What is the main drawback of feldspathic porcelain for all-porcelain crowns?
    a. Their tendency to fracture
    b. Their opacity
    c. The difficulty involved in making them
    d. That shrinkage when fired makes them difficult to fit to the prepared tooth
5. An in-office CAD/CAM system for ceramic restorations provides all of the following advantages *except* one. Which one?
    a. The restoration does not have to be fabricated in an outside laboratory.
    b. A provisional crown is not needed.
    c. The procedure can be completed in one visit.
    d. Local anesthesia is not needed.
6. What is the basic color of the tooth called?
    a. Base shade
    b. True value
    c. Chroma
    d. Hue
7. All of the following should be avoided when taking the shade of a tooth *except* one. Which one?
    a. Lipstick on the patient
    b. Brightly colored clothing
    c. Dirty teeth (covered with plaque)
    d. Neutral wall colors in the room
8. All of the following materials should be avoided around ceramic restorations *except* one. Which one?
    a. Acidulated topical fluoride products
    b. Alginate impression material
    c. Coarse prophy paste
    d. Acid etchant
9. The impression for a CAD/CAM crown typically is:
    a. Done with alginate
    b. Done with polyvinylsiloxane impression material
    c. Done with polyether impression material
    d. Done by capturing an image of the prepared tooth with an optical scanner
10. When preparing a porcelain-fused-to-metal crown, the technician applies feldspathic porcelain in layers to the metal coping. What is the initial layer?
    a. Translucent porcelain to mimic enamel
    b. Body porcelain to mimic dentin
    c. Opaque porcelain to hide the oxidized metal
11. On occasion, special porcelain stains are used on the surface of the porcelain. These stains contain metal oxides and are used to:
    a. Create a shiny, smooth surface
    b. Mimic white spots or fine crack lines to resemble adjacent teeth
    c. Hide flaws created in the porcelain by firing it at high temperatures
12. Which one of the following statements about porcelain veneers is *false*?
    a. Porcelain veneers are more durable than composite veneers.
    b. Porcelain veneers are usually cemented with zinc phosphate or glass ionomer cement.
    c. It is difficult to mask a darkly colored tooth with a porcelain veneer.
    d. Porcelain veneers must be handled carefully when one is trying them on because they are very fragile until bonded to the tooth.
13. When assisting the dentist with taking the shade of a tooth, the dental assistant should:
    a. Dry the teeth thoroughly
    b. Shine the operatory light directly on the teeth
    c. Cover brightly colored clothing with a pastel, neutral-colored bib
    d. Stare at the tooth and shade guide intensely for at least 30 seconds to let the eyes adjust to the colors
14. Which one of the following ceramic materials is the strongest and most fracture resistant?
    a. Leucite-reinforced porcelain
    b. Zirconia
    c. Feldspathic porcelain
    d. Lithium disilicate
15. Which one of the following ceramic materials is the most opaque and, therefore, the least esthetic?
    a. Feldspathic porcelain
    b. Lithium disilicate
    c. Zirconia
    d. Leucite-reinforced porcelain
16. For anterior ceramic restorations, the ceramic material used at the incisal edge tends to be which one of the following?
    a. Opaque
    b. Highly reflectant
    c. Translucent
    d. Transparent
17. The lightness or darkness of a color is referred to as which one of the following?
    a. Chroma
    b. Value
    c. Hue
    d. Radiance

Review and Discussion—cont'd

18. Which of the following ceramic materials is not etched by hydrofluoric acid in preparation for cementation but may be sandblasted internally instead?
    a. Zirconia
    b. Lithium disilicate
    c. Feldspathic porcelain
    d. Leucite-reinforced porcelain
19. Porcelain veneers are bonded to the tooth with resin cement. This provides the opportunity to do all of the following *except* one. Which one?
    a. Increase the strength of the restoration
    b. Increase the retention of the restoration
    c. Slightly modify the shade of the cemented restoration with a colored resin cement
    d. Whiten the tooth with the acid etchant
20. All of the following considerations should be applied when finishing or polishing a ceramic material *except* one. Which one?
    a. Use slow speed
    b. Use a coarse diamond bur for adjustments
    c. Use light pressure
    d. Progress from medium abrasives to finer ones
21. All of the following are processing methods for ceramic materials, *except* one. Which one?
    a. Sintering
    b. Heat pressing
    c. Cold curing
    d. CAD/CAM
22. When taking photographs of the teeth to send to the dental laboratory to help convey the correct shade, what is the proper location for the shade tab in the photograph?
    a. Outside of the mouth
    b. Inside the mouth and in front of the teeth
    c. In the same plane as the tooth being matched
    d. None of the above (the shade tab does not have to be included in the photograph)

For answers to Review Questions, see the Appendix.

Case-Based Discussion Topics

1. A 57-year-old secretary comes to the dental office for a periodic examination and prophylaxis. There are composite veneers present on the maxillary anteriors and all-ceramic crowns on the mandibular incisors. *Describe the factors that might contribute to chipping of the ceramic restorations. What must the dental auxiliary be concerned about when treating patients who have esthetic composite and ceramic restorations present in their mouth?*
2. An active 80-year-old patient comes to the dental office for preparation of the maxillary anterior and premolar teeth for porcelain veneers. The patient wants to lighten the teeth but wants to keep the same color (hue). At the time of the appointment, the patient is wearing brightly colored clothing and lipstick. *What steps can the dental auxiliary perform to help in the initial shade taking? Under what lighting conditions should the shade be taken?*
3. A 60-year-old postal worker was hit in the mouth by a falling package in the warehouse. The mesio-incisal edge of a porcelain-fused-to-metal crown on tooth 8 was fractured. The patient has asked to have the crown replaced with a more esthetic material. *What ceramic materials could be used in this location? What must the patient be told regarding the risks of fracture of the various ceramic materials?*
4. A 30-year-old business executive has several large occlusal amalgam restorations on the lower molars and premolars that are visible when speaking. The patient frequently gives presentations to small groups and would like to eliminate the dark restorations. Additionally, the patient grinds their teeth during sleep and clenches during the day. *What materials could be used to satisfy the patient's esthetic needs? Of the ceramic materials, which would be most likely to fracture in the mouth and which would be most likely to survive bruxing?*
5. A 25-year-old fashion model has large mesial and distal class III composites on tooth 8, which have turned brown; the composites are visible when smiling. The patient wants to get rid of the composites and the discoloration. The dentist has recommended a porcelain-fused-to-metal crown. The fashion model wants an all-ceramic crown to maximize the esthetics. *What are the pros and cons of each type of crown for this application? If an all-ceramic crown is done, what type of ceramic material is best for this application? Should the crown be bonded or just cemented? Why?*

BIBLIOGRAPHY

Ferracane JL: *Materials for inlays, onlays, crowns and bridges.* In *Materials in dentistry,* ed 2, Baltimore, 2001, Lippincott Williams & Wilkins.

Giordano R: Materials for chairside CAD/CAM-produced restorations, *J Am Dent Assoc* 137:14S–21S, 2006.

Kois JC, Chaiyabutr Y: Intraoral occlusal adjustment and polishing for modern ceramic materials, *Inside Dentistry* 11(3), 2015.

McLean JW, Hughes TH: The reinforcement of dental porcelain with ceramic oxides, *Br Dent J* 119:251–267, 1965.

McLaren EA: CAD/CAM dental technology: a perspective on its evolution and status, *Compendium* 32(4), 2011.

McLaren EA, Whiteman YY: Ceramics: rationale for material selection, *Inside Dentistry*: 38–50, 2012.

Poticny DJ, Klim J: CAD/CAM in-office technology: innovations after 25 years of predictable, esthetic outcomes, *JADA* 141(Suppl 6):5S–9S, 2010.

Powers JM, Farah JW, O'Keefe KL, et al: Guide to all-ceramic bonding, *Dent Advisor* 29(4), 2012.

Powers JM, Wataha JC: *Dental ceramics.* In *Dental materials: foundations and applications,* ed 11, St. Louis, 2017, Elsevier.

Ritter AV, Boushell LW, Walter R: *Additional conservative esthetic procedures.* In *Sturdevant's art and science of operative dentistry,* ed 7, St. Louis, 2019, Elsevier.

Rosenstiel SF, Land MF, Walter RD: Ceramic restorations. *Contemporary fixed prosthodontics,* ed 6, Philadelphia, 2023, Elsevier.

Sakaguchi RL, Ferracane J, Powers JM: *Restorative materials: ceramics. Craig's restorative dental materials,* ed 14, St. Louis, 2019, Elsevier.

Santos MJ, Costa MD, Rubo JH, et al: Current all-ceramic systems in dentistry: a review, *Compend Contin Educ Dent* 36(1):31–37, 2015.

Shen C, Rawls HR, Esquivel-Upshaw JF: *Ceramic-based Materials.* In *Phillips' science of dental materials,* ed 13, St. Louis, 2022, Elsevier.

Sorensen JA: Finishing and polishing with modern ceramic systems. *Inside, Dentistry* 9:10–16, 2013.

Trost L, Stines S, Burt L: Making informed decisions about incorporating a CAD/CAM system into dental practice, *J Am Dent Assoc* 137:32S–36S, 2006.

Warreth A, Elkareimi Y: All-ceramic restorations: a review of the literature, *Saudi Dent J* 32(8):365–372, 2020 Dec.

Dental Amalgam

11

http://evolve.elsevier.com/Eakle/materials/

Chapter Objectives

On completion of this chapter, the student should be able to:

1. List the main components of dental amalgam.
2. Describe the particle shapes in lathe-cut, admix, and spherical alloys, and discuss their effects on the condensation resistance of freshly mixed amalgam.
3. Identify, corrosion, and tarnish.
4. Compare the strength of amalgam with that of composite resin or glass ionomer cement.
5. Discuss the effect of mixing time on the strength and manipulation of amalgam.
6. Discuss the advantages and disadvantages of amalgam as a restorative material.
7. Discuss the safety of amalgam as a restorative material.
8. Perform safe mercury hygiene practices in the dental office.
9. Collect and process amalgam scrap for recycling.
10. Select an appropriate size of matrix band for a class II amalgam preparation.
11. Assemble a Tofflemire band in its retainer.
12. Evaluate a class II amalgam matrix setup for meeting proper placement criteria.
13. Assist with or place (as allowed by state law) amalgam in a class II cavity preparation.

KEY TERMS

Alloy a mixture of two or more metals

Amalgamation reaction that occurs when silver-based alloy is mixed with mercury to form an amalgam

Dental Amalgam metallic restorative material composed of silver-based alloy mixed with mercury

Lathe-Cut Alloy irregularly shaped particles formed by shaving fine particles from an alloy ingot

Spherical Alloy small spheres of alloy particles produced by spraying a fine mist of liquid alloy into an inert gas environment

Admixed Alloy mixture of lathe-cut and spherical alloys

Delayed Expansion expansion of amalgam containing zinc when it is contaminated with moisture (e.g., saliva) during condensation. Inside the amalgam hydrogen gas develops from the interaction of water and zinc, and it creates an outward pressure that causes creep to occur

Creep gradual change in the shape of a restoration usually caused by compression from occlusion or adjacent teeth and can cause amalgam to bulge out of the cavity preparation

Tarnish oxidation affecting a thin layer of a metal at its surface that does not change the metal's mechanical properties

Corrosion breakdown of a metal by chemical or electrochemical reaction with substances in the environment such as water or air. It negatively impacts the properties of amalgam

Triturator or Amalgamator mechanical device used to mix silver-based alloy particles with mercury to produce amalgam

Condensation the act of pressing amalgam mix into a cavity preparation with instruments to produce a dense mass

Burnishing after the amalgam mix is placed, an instrument is used to further condense and smooth the amalgam surface

Amalgam Separator a device that collects amalgam particles and mercury from evacuation systems that might otherwise escape into the wastewater and therefore enter the environment

---

Dental amalgam has been in use as a restorative material for more than 180 years. Dental amalgam is a combination of metals also known as an amalgamation of metals, mostly silver alloy powders and mercury. It is easy to manipulate, has good clinical durability, and is low cost. However, its use has been gradually diminishing in many countries as patients demand more esthetic materials, such as composite resin and ceramic restorations, which have continually improved in their physical properties and handling characteristics. In addition, health and environmental concerns have been raised due to the mercury content of the amalgam causing some countries to move away from its use.

It is essential that oral health practitioners have an understanding of the characteristics of the various amalgam alloys, so they can correctly select, mix, place, and carve them. In addition, knowledge of safe mercury hygiene measures is important for health and safety reasons. Dental auxiliary will be asked questions by patients regarding the mercury content of amalgams and the health risks. Patients need to be provided with accurate information about this issue. Some states mandate patients be provided with a dental materials fact sheet listing pros and cons of the materials. This chapter covers the properties and handling of amalgam and mercury hygiene.

DENTAL AMALGAM

Amalgam has been studied and tested more than any other restorative material. Although composite resins are being requested by patients with increasing frequency for posterior restorations, amalgam is still a widely used direct-placement material for the posterior region of the mouth. No other direct restorative material has the durability, ease of handling, and good physical characteristics of amalgam. Its wear resistance and compressive strength are superior to composite resin and glass ionomer cement.

ALLOYS USED IN DENTAL AMALGAM

An alloy is a mixture of two or more metals. The alloy used to produce dental amalgam is composed predominantly of silver but also contains copper and tin. A variety of other metals, such as palladium, indium, or zinc, may be added in much smaller quantities to produce specific properties in the alloy. When the silver-based alloy particles are mixed with mercury, the reaction that occurs is called amalgamation and the material that is produced is a strong, hard, durable material called dental amalgam.

SILVER-BASED AMALGAM ALLOY PARTICLES

Silver-based amalgam alloys are classified as irregular, spherical, or admixed according to the shape of the particles in the powder (Fig. 11.1). Each of these particle shapes contributes certain handling characteristics to the amalgam, and to some degree the amalgam type is selected by the dentist according to these characteristics. See Table 11.1 which details alloy particle shapes.

Composition of Amalgam Alloys

Dental alloys for amalgam are composed mainly of silver and tin. Copper is added to replace some of the silver to lessen the brittleness. Alloys can be grouped or classified by their copper content. Modern dental alloys are considered to be high in copper content (13% to 30%) compared with their predecessors, see Table 11.2.

Manufacturers can change how amalgam handles by varying the components of the alloy and by varying

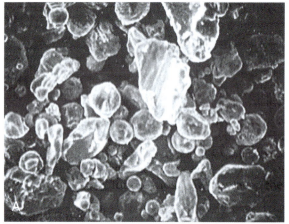

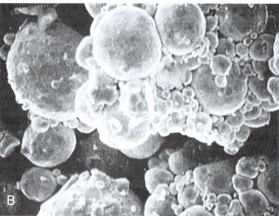

FIG. 11.1 (A) Scanning electron micrograph (SEM) of admixed alloy showing a mixture of irregularly shaped particles and spherical particles. **(B)** SEM of spherical alloy with spherical particles of various sizes. (Courtesy Grayson W. Marshall, University of California School of Dentistry, San Francisco, California.)

the shape, size, and distribution of the sizes of particles. The manufacturer, too, can control how fast the amalgam sets by various treatments of the alloy particles, such as heat-treating them or removing oxides from their surface. The dentist, then, can select alloys with slower or faster setting times depending on the intended application.

SETTING TRANSFORMATION (AMALGAMATION)

When the alloy in powder form is mixed with liquid mercury, a chemical reaction occurs. The chemical reaction:
- Starts at the surface of the alloy
  - The size and shape of the alloy particles will affect the setting process
- The alloy particles dissolve into the mercury
  - When no more metal can dissolve into the mercury, a mixture of metallic compounds begins to crystallize in the mercury (a process called amalgamation) and continues until the liquid mercury is used up
  - All of the alloy particles are not dissolved before the mercury is used up
  - The remaining particles in the core of the amalgam are held together by compounds of mercury with silver and tin (acting as a matrix) making up about half of the amalgam volume

Table 11.1 Alloy Particle Shapes

PARTICLE SHAPE	PARTICLE SIZE	PARTICLE FABRICATION
Lathe-cut Alloy	10–70 μm in width and 60–120 μm in length	Formed by shaving fine particles off a heat-treated ingot of the alloy with a cutting machine called a *lathe*. The particles are sifted to separate them into fine and ultrafine particles.
Spherical Alloy	2–43 μm	Produced by spraying (atomizing) a mist of molten alloy into an inert gas. Small spherical particles are formed as the atomized droplets cool. The spherical particles are heat-treated and washed in acid to remove surface contaminants.
Admixed Alloy		Admixed particles consist of a mixture of lathe-cut and spherical particles

Table 11.2 Main Components of Amalgam Alloy

COMPONENT	FUNCTION	OTHER EFFECTS	HIGH-COPPER ALLOY, %	LOW-COPPER ALLOY, %
Silver (Ag)	Increases strength Increases durability Decreases creep	Decreases setting time Tarnishes easily	40–70	68–72
Tin (Sn)	Improves physical properties when compounded with silver	Reduces setting expansion Increases setting time	12–30	28–36
Copper (Cu)	Increases strength Increases hardness Reduces corrosion	Increases setting expansion- Decreases creep	13–30	4–6
Zinc (Zn)	Reduces oxidation of other metals	Causes delayed expansion with moisture contamination	0–1	0–2

Table 11.3 Amalgam Setting Reactions

Phase one	Phase two	Phase three
Gamma phase (γ)	Gamma-1 phase (γ_1)	Gamma-2 phase (γ_2)
Silver alloy phase	Consisting of mercury reacting with the silver	Reaction of mercury with tin
Strongest phase	Strong and corrosion resistant, although not as resistant as the gamma phase	Weak
Has the least corrosion		Corrodes readily

- These particles contribute to the strength and corrosion resistance of the amalgam
- The freshly mixed amalgam has a putty-like consistency that can be packed into the cavity preparation
- Over the next several minutes, the free mercury is used up in the crystal formation and the mix gradually becomes firmer
  - During the first part of this firming phase, the amalgam can be carved (during the working time or time available to manipulate the amalgam) to the anatomic shape of the tooth
- Once the amalgam reaches its initial set, it can no longer be carved and is firm but is not fully reacted
  - It is relatively brittle at this point, and the patient is advised not to bite on it for several hours
  - Many of the high-copper spherical amalgams gain approximately 50% of their compressive strength in the first hour, but it takes up to 24 hours for most amalgams to gain their maximum strength
- Once fully set, they are hard, strong, durable restorations

Setting Reactions

The chemical reaction that occurs when the alloy and mercury are mixed has three phases. See setting reaction Table 11.3. Tin is used in amalgam to control the rate of set. Both silver and tin dissolve into the liquid mercury until the solution becomes saturated with them, and they also absorb mercury. Newly formed particles begin to precipitate (crystallize) out of the mercury until there is no more mercury left to react. This process may take up to 24 hours for final set. Low-copper amalgams had much more corrosion because of the chemical reaction of tin and mercury. High-copper amalgams are superior in their clinical performance, displaying reduced corrosion and tarnish, higher compressive strength, less dimensional change, and better integrity of margins than low-copper amalgams. See Table 11.4 for some of the properties of high-copper amalgam.

PROPERTIES OF AMALGAM

The American National Standards Institute/American Dental Association (ANSI/ADA) Standard No. 1 for

Amalgam has set maximum values for dimensional change and creep and minimum values for compressive strength as a measure of amalgam quality (see Table 11.5).

Strength

Amalgam is among the strongest of the directly placed restorative materials. Its compressive strength is similar to tooth structure. It has the ability to resist the strong forces of the bite repeatedly over many years when properly placed. Amalgams are relatively weak in tension and shear. All amalgams are considered to be brittle. Therefore they require adequate bulk to resist breaking. If the cavity preparation is too shallow or the occlusal morphology of the restoration is carved too deeply, the restoration is more likely to fracture. Thin excesses of amalgam left over the cavosurface margins lack strength and chip away over time, creating an irregular margin that tends to collect plaque and contribute to recurrent caries. Excessive forces from bruxing, such as chewing on ice or biting on a popcorn kernel, can cause a fracture of the amalgam.

The strength of the amalgam can be affected by the speed and duration of trituration. Under- or over-triturating the amalgam mix and a mix that is too wet or dry can decrease the strength of the amalgam. Likewise, the amount of mercury used in the mix can affect strength. A mix that is poorly condensed into the cavity preparation can result in voids that weaken the final restoration.

Dimensional Change

Ideally, the dimensions of a newly placed amalgam should not change. If amalgam contracts excessively, it will open gaps at the margins between the tooth and the restoration, contributing to leakage of fluids and bacteria to cause sensitivity. If the amalgam expands excessively, it can put pressure on the cusps and cause pain with biting pressure or may result in fracture of the cusps. Some expansion and contraction is expected to occur during the setting reaction of the amalgam. It is the net effect of these two processes that is important. The composition of the alloy particles, the ratio of the mercury to alloy powder by weight, and salivary/moisture contamination are other factors that contribute to dimensional changes. Low-copper amalgams containing zinc are prone to expansion over time if they are exposed to moisture during placement. This gradual expansion after placement is called **delayed expansion** (Fig. 11.2). Delayed expansion can cause the restoration to expand beyond the cavity walls, causing cracking in the adjacent enamel. Most high-copper amalgams do not contain zinc or have very small amounts, and they contract slightly by the time they set because of smaller alloy particle size and the use of less mercury.

Creep

Creep in dental amalgams refers to the gradual change in shape of the restoration from compression by the opposing dentition during chewing or by pressure from adjacent teeth. High-copper alloys exhibit far less creep (less than 0.5%) and have superior marginal integrity.

Tarnish

Tarnish is an oxidation that attacks the surface of the amalgam and extends slightly below the surface. It results from contact with oxygen, chlorides, and sulfides in the mouth. Tarnish causes a dark, dull appearance, but it is not very destructive to the amalgam (Fig. 11.3). The rougher the surface, the more it tends to tarnish. Metals such as palladium are sometimes added to help reduce tarnish. Polishing of the restoration can also reduce tarnish. Polishing of amalgams is best done after the restoration has set for a period of 24 hours or longer. Controversy exists among dental educators and clinicians as to whether high-copper amalgams need

Table 11.4 Properties of High-Copper Amalgam

	ADMIX	SPHERICAL
Compressive strength ([a]MPa) 1 hour	110–220	260–315
1 day	400–440	450–500
Tensile strength (MPa) 1 day	43–50	49–64
Dimensional change at 24 hours (μm/cm)	−1.9 to −3	−5 to −8.8
Creep (%)	0.25–0.45	0.05–0.15

Approximate – values vary with each product.
[a]1 MPa = 145 psi (pounds per square inch)

Table 11.5 ANSI/ADA Standard No. 1 for Amalgam

PROPERTY	VALUE
Dimensional change	Maximum of 20 μm/cm
Creep	Maximum of 1%
Compressive strength	Minimum at 1 h: 80 MPa
	Minimum at 24 h: 300 MPa

ANSI/ADA, American National Standards Institute/American Dental Association; *MPa*, megapascals.

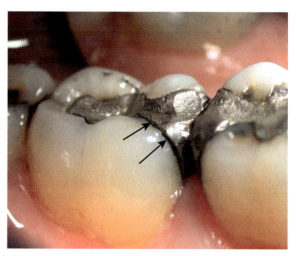

FIG. 11.2 Delayed expansion of amalgam. Margins of the restoration stand up from the tooth leaving a ledge. (Courtesy Dr. Steve Eakle, University of California, San Francisco, California.)

polishing as they tend to have a smoother surface after carving. Generation of excessive heat during polishing can cause a release of mercury from the silver-mercury phase resulting in a mercury-rich surface that will corrode more readily and deteriorate at the margins.

Do You Recall?

Why are high-copper amalgams superior to low-copper amalgams?

Corrosion

Corrosion can occur from a chemical reaction between the amalgam and substances in saliva or food, resulting in oxidation of the amalgam. It can also occur when two dissimilar metals interact in a solution containing electrolytes such as saliva. This oxidation is responsible for corrosion of the amalgam. Corrosion also takes place within the amalgam through interaction of its metal components. It weakens the amalgam over time, can stain the surrounding tooth structure as corrosion products enter the dentinal tubules, and can lead to deterioration of the margins (see Fig. 11.3). Corrosion can occur within an amalgam without the patient ever being aware of the process.

Galvanic Reaction. Clinically, a galvanic reaction may occur when a newly placed amalgam contacts another metal restoration such as a gold crown. This problem may persist until the amalgam completes its setting reactions, until oxides build up on one of the metals to stop the electrical current, or until the offending restoration is replaced with a nonconducting restoration.

Do You Recall?

Why a patient should be aware of a phenomenon known as galvanism when two different metals are present in the mouth?

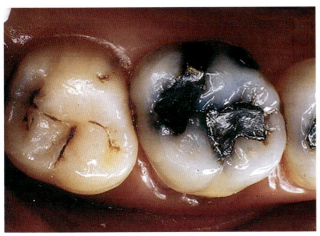

FIG. 11.3 Low-copper amalgam restoration showing surface tarnish, margin deterioration, and corrosion. Tooth has darkened as corrosion products from the amalgam have penetrated the dentinal tubules. (From Bird DL, Robinson DS: *Modern dental assisting*, ed. 13, St. Louis, 2021, Saunders.)

Thermal Conductivity

Amalgam, being a mix of metals, is a good conductor of heat and cold. In shallow cavity preparations, the thickness of the dentin remaining over the pulp is usually adequate to dissipate the heat or cold. However, in deeper cavity preparations or in teeth that were sensitive before the placement of the amalgam restoration, a base or liner should be used for the comfort of the patient.

APPLICATIONS FOR DENTAL AMALGAM

Amalgam is useful for:
- Small-to-moderate intracoronal restorations
- Posterior teeth
- Teeth where esthetics is not a concern
- Stress-bearing areas
- Large cavity preparations and replacing missing cusps when patients cannot afford crowns and onlays
- Foundations (buildups) for crowns
- Sealing a root apex after apical surgery
- Restoring a cavity where control of saliva and blood is difficult

Amalgams are the least technique sensitive of the direct placement restorative materials.

KEY POINTS

Main components: silver, mercury, copper, and tin
Properties: High copper amalgam is superior to low copper amalgam
1. Higher compressive strength.
2. Less corrosion and tarnish.
3. Less dimensional change.
4. Better integrity of restorations margins.

Do You Recall?

Why is a base required under an amalgam when the cavity preparation is close to the pulp chamber?

MATRIX SYSTEMS

A matrix for amalgam restorations usually consists of three components:
1. A flexible metal band that is placed around all or part of the tooth to temporarily form a wall to contain and shape the amalgam during placement
2. A device that helps to retain or hold the band in place
3. A wooden or plastic wedge that secures the band against the tooth and produces some separation of the two adjacent teeth.

USE OF MATRIX BANDS

A matrix band is used to help contain the amalgam during condensation in a class II preparation and helps to form the proximal contours and contacts of the restoration. Matrix bands are thin strips of material that encompass all (circumferential bands) or part (sectional bands) of the tooth. For amalgam the bands are typically composed of stainless steel.

Band thickness: Metal bands are available in thicknesses of.
- 0.001 inches (thinnest)
- 0.0015 inches
- 0.002 inches

Band height. The bands are made in various heights occlusogingivally (narrow and wide) to accommodate shorter or taller teeth (premolars, adult molars, and primary molars). The universal matrix band will adapt to most posterior teeth, but occasionally on taller teeth or teeth with deep gingival box forms the universal band will be too short to cover the entire cavity preparation. A band with extensions to cover deep mesial and distal box forms (called an extension band or a mesio-occluso-distal [MOD] band) is then selected (Fig. 11.4).

Shaping the band. If the metal band is flat as the conventional bands often are, then it must be shaped to form the proper contours of the final restoration. To shape the band, place it on a soft paper pad or a gauze square and at the location of the contact area begin rubbing a burnisher against the inner portion of the band until a smooth convexity is formed on the outside of the band (Fig. 11.5).

This will form the contact area when the amalgam is condensed into the box form of the class II cavity preparation. Bands that are 0.002 inch in thickness are easier to contour and hold their shape better when placed in the retainer. Bands are also available that are already contoured and need little or no adjustment (Fig. 11.6).

Matrix Band Retainers

Some bands require a retainer to hold the band in place and enables the operator to tighten the band around the tooth. The Tofflemire-type retainer is the most widely used. It comes in two designs: straight or contra-angled. A smaller version is available for use on primary teeth. The contra-angled retainer is useful when the retainer is placed on the lingual side of the teeth instead of the typical buccal placement and on posterior teeth where the straight retainer does not fit well.

Parts of the retainer: The retainer has four parts:
- A U-shaped head that has three slots for positioning the band.
- A locking vise with a sliding component that holds the band.
- A long, knurled knob that is turned to tighten the diameter of the band.
- A short knob that locks the band within the sliding component (Fig. 11.7).

Placing the Band in the Retainer

The band is slightly curved to allow a larger circumference on one edge and a smaller circumference on the other edge when the band is folded to form a loop (see Fig. 11.4). The edge with the smaller circumference is placed toward the gingiva because most teeth constrict toward the cervical. The edge with the wider circumference is oriented toward the occlusal side and is placed into the retainer. The ends of the band are placed into the slot of the locking vise, and then the loop of the band is positioned into the slot of the retainer head that orients it toward the tooth with the retainer on the buccal side of the tooth. The small locking knob is turned clockwise to secure the band in the retainer.

Placing the Band on the Tooth

- If the band loop has been constricted when putting the band in the retainer, use a mirror handle inside the loop to open it and round it out (Fig. 11.8).
- If the diameter of the loop is larger than needed to go around the tooth, then adjust the diameter by tightening the inner knob. Slide the matrix band around the tooth.
- If the band cannot pass through a tight contact area, try placing a wedge to slightly separate the teeth.
- The gingival edge of the band should be properly oriented and the open end of the retainer head should be positioned toward the gingiva (to allow it to be removed in an occlusal direction).
- Fully seat the band so that the gingival edge extends at least 0.5 mm beyond the gingival floor of the preparation and the occlusal edge extends approximately 1 mm above the marginal ridge of the adjacent tooth (assuming both teeth had marginal ridges at the same height before the preparation).
- If the universal band is short of the gingival floor of the proximal box, then the MOD extension band should be used.
- If the preparation involves only one proximal surface or only one proximal box is deep, then with scissors cut away the extension of the band that is not needed when the MOD band is in use (i.e., if the distal box is deep but not the mesial, then cut away the mesial extension level with the rest of the band), otherwise that unneeded extension may not let the band seat fully (Fig. 11.9).

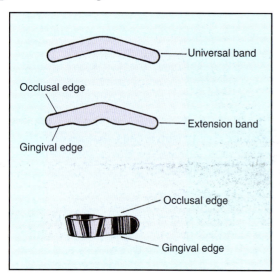

FIG. 11.4 Common types of posterior metal matrix bands for Tofflemire-type retainer. (From Bird DL, Robinson DS: *Modern dental assisting*, ed 13, St. Louis, 2021, Elsevier.)

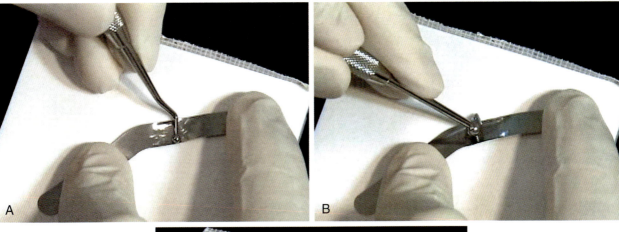

FIG. 11.5 Burnishing the matrix band: **(A)** A flat metal matrix band is burnished with a small burnisher on a paper pad to provide proper contours for the contact area. **(B)** A football burnisher forms the contours for mesial and distal contact areas. **(C)** Proper contours are present in the band. (Courtesy Aldridge Wilder, DDS from Ritter A, Boushell LW, Walter R: *Sturdevant's art & science of operative dentistry*, ed 7, St. Louis, 2019, Elsevier.)

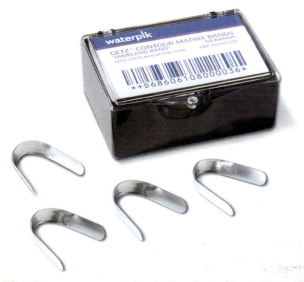

FIG. 11.6 Precontoured matrix bands. (Getz Contour Bands, Waterpik.)

Criteria for Matrix Band Placement for Class II Preparation

Criteria	Reason
1. Band approximately 1 mm above level of the marginal ridge	1. If band is higher, amalgam packed too high at the ridge is likely to fracture when removing the band
2. Band should not be lower than marginal ridge level	2. Amalgam packed over the top of the band will fracture when removing the band. Difficult to establish marginal ridge contours
3. External surface of band should be convex and establish contact with adjacent contact area	3. Establishes proper proximal contours and contact
4. Band firmly in contact with the gingival margin of box	4. Prevents overhang at gingival margin
5. Band well adapted at buccal and lingual margings of box	5. Reduces excess amalgam at buccal and lingual margins and makes carving easier

- While holding the band from the occlusal surface with a finger, tighten the band to the tooth by turning the long knob clockwise until the band is snug to the tooth.
- Check with an explorer to see that there is no gap at the gingival margin with the band.
- Next, use a plastic instrument or an interproximal burnisher to burnish the band against the adjacent tooth.

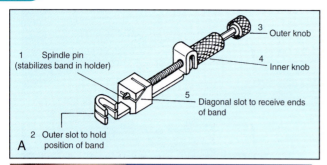
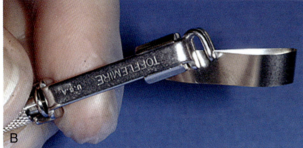
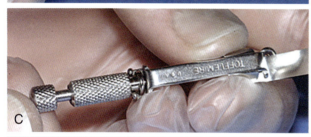
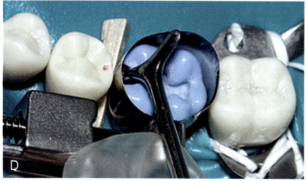

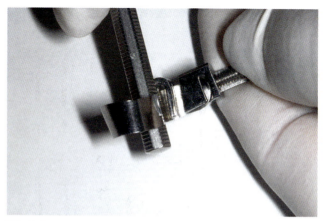

FIG. 11.8 Opening and rounding a constricted matrix band loop. (From Bird DL, Robinson DS: *Modern dental assisting*, ed 13, St. Louis, 2021, Elsevier.)

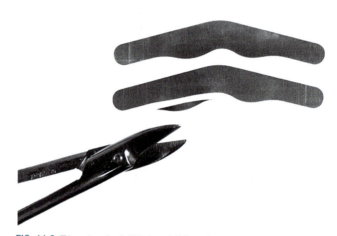

FIG. 11.9 Trimming the MOD band. When the matrix band extension is needed only on one proximal surface, the other extension is removed to allow full seating of the band. (From Ritter A, Boushell LW, Walter R: *Sturdevant's art & science of operative dentistry*, ed 7, St. Louis, 2019, Elsevier.)

FIG. 11.7 Use of the Tofflemire-type retainer: **(A)** Components of the retainer. **(B)** Metal band placed in guide slot and diagonal slot. The closed end of the guide slots is oriented toward the occlusal surface of the teeth, and the occlusal edge of the band is inserted first toward the closed end. **(C)** Tighten locking nut to secure band in the retainer. **(D)** Note that band has been angled through the left guide slot to be positioned on the buccal surface of the tooth. The band is tightened around the tooth by turning the inner knob clockwise. A wedge is inserted firmly into the lingual embrasure to create separation of the teeth and hold the band against the tooth gingivally. (A, From Bird DL, Robinson DS: *Modern dental assisting*, ed 13, St. Louis, 2021, Elsevier; B, From Darby ML, Walsh MM: *Dental hygiene: theory and practice*, ed 4, St. Louis, 2015, Elsevier; C, From Darby ML, Walsh MM: *Dental hygiene: theory and practice*, ed 3, St. Louis, 2010, Elsevier.)

The Wedge

The function of the wedge is to adapt the matrix tightly against the gingival margin of the preparation's proximal box and to produce some separation of the teeth to compensate for the thickness of the matrix band. Otherwise, when the band is removed, there would be a gap between the restoration and the adjacent tooth (called an open contact). Commercially made wedges are often triangular-shaped pieces of wood or plastic. Some clinicians prefer to use wedges made from round toothpicks.

Select a wedge that is large enough to fit the gingival embrasure space and will hold the band against the gingival margin of the box form without distorting the band (Fig. 11.10).

The wedge is usually inserted firmly into the gingival embrasure from the lingual side because this is typically the widest of the two embrasures. The wedge must be placed firmly to separate the teeth enough to make up for the thickness of the matrix band. If a circumferential band (encircles the tooth) is used, there are two thickness of matrix band (mesial and distal) to compensate for. So, the wedging pressure must be greater than when a sectional band (goes only on one proximal surface - see Chapter 8) is used. Some manufactured wedges are concave on their sides to accommodate the convexity of the tooth. If the cavity preparation includes both mesial and distal proximal boxes, then a wedge will be needed for each embrasure.

Once the wedge is in place, loosen the retainer by turning it counterclockwise one quarter turn. This will loosen the band slightly so it can be adapted to the adjacent contact area and will allow the condensed amalgam to push the band against the adjacent contact. Once the band is loosened, burnish it against the adjacent tooth with an interproximal burnisher or the back of a large spoon excavator.

Atypical Wedge Placement

The wedge may have to be placed in an unconventional way depending on a number of factors:
1. On occasion, the shape of the wedge is not compatible with the convex shape of the tooth. In this case, the wedge can be custom shaped by carving it with an amalgam knife or a scalpel.
2. If the wedge sits too high in the embrasure space, it may distort the matrix band, fail to seal the gingival margin, and cause concave proximal contours in the gingival aspect of the restoration (Fig. 11.11).
3. If the embrasure space is very large because the gingival tissue has receded, it will be difficult to secure the band against the gingival margin of the proximal box with a single wedge because it will be apical to the gingival margin. It may be necessary to place a second, smaller wedge on top of the first wedge.
4. If the cavity preparation has resulted in a very wide proximal box (from facial to lingual), it may be necessary to place two wedges, one from the facial and one from the lingual to ensure that the two gingival corners of the proximal box are sealed by the band.

> **Clinical Tip**
>
> The presence of a rubber dam may make wedge insertion more difficult as it tends to push the wedge back out. To lessen this problem, stretch the interseptal portion of the rubber dam in the opposite direction of wedge placement while inserting the wedge. After the wedge is fully seated, gently release the dam.

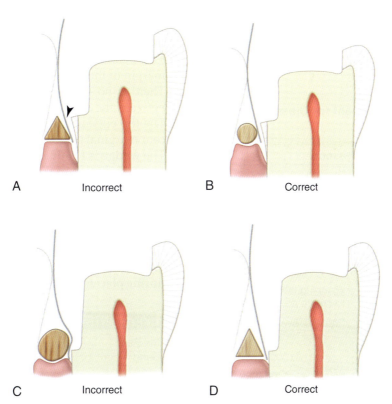

FIG. 11.10 Indications for use of a round toothpick wedge versus a triangular (i.e., anatomic) wedge: **(A)** Often the triangular wedge does not firmly support the matrix band against the gingival margin in conservative class II preparations *(arrowhead)*. **(B)** The round toothpick wedge is preferred for these preparations because its wedging action is nearer the gingival margin. **(C)** In class II preparations with deep gingival margins, the round toothpick wedge crimps the matrix band contour if it is placed occlusal to the gingival margin. **(D)** The triangular wedge is preferred with these preparations because its greatest width is at its base. (From Ritter A, Boushell LW, Walter R: *Sturdevant's art & science of operative dentistry*, ed 7, St. Louis, 2019, Elsevier.)

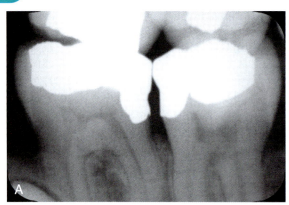
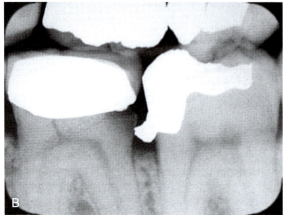

FIG. 11.11 Radiographs depicting poor proximal contours of the amalgams: **(A)** Caused by a wedge placed too far coronal to the gingival margin of the cavity preparation that distorted the matrix band. **(B)** Overhang of amalgam, caused by a wedge that was not firmly placed, was placed slightly above the gingival margin, or the band did not cover the deep gingival margin. (Courtesy Dentaljuce CPD Providers Ltd, https://www.dentaljuce.com/direct-restorations-wedges.)

Criteria for Wedge Placement for Class II Preparation

Criteria	Reason
1. Wedge firmly seated	1. To separate teeth enough to make up for thickness of band
2. Wedge holds matrix band against gingival margin of proximal box	2. Prevents amalgam overhang
3. Wedge is not located coronal to the gingival margin of proximal box	3. Prevents amalgam from escaping under the band to create an overhang
4. Wedge is not located too far apical to gingival margin of proximal box	4. Prevents overhang
5. Wedge does not deform the band contours	5. Allows proper anatomic proximal contours

Final Evaluation of the Matrix Before Condensation

Once the matrix band has been placed around the prepared tooth, the retainer appropriately tightened and the wedge snugly pressed into place, a final check is made of the matrix assembly before the preparation is filled with amalgam. Check for the following features (Fig. 11.12):

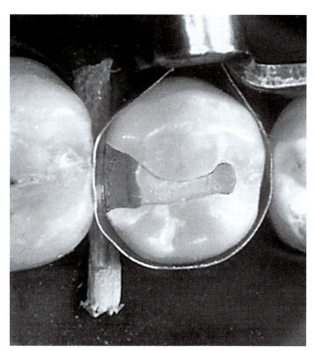

FIG. 11.12 Properly placed and wedged matrix band for class II cavity preparation. (From Ritter A, Boushell LW, Walter R: *Sturdevant's art & science of operative dentistry*, ed 7, St. Louis, 2019, Elsevier.)

1. The matrix band extends apical to the gingival margin of the proximal box by about 1 mm.
2. There is no gap between the band and the gingival margin of the box form.
3. There is no gingival tissue or rubber dam caught between the band and the tooth.
4. The top edge of the band extends beyond the adjacent marginal ridge by approximately 1 mm.
5. The wedge is firmly in place, so that it will produce some separation of the teeth.
6. The band is well adapted to the buccal and lingual walls of the proximal box.
7. The band is adapted to the adjacent tooth.
8. The wedge has not distorted the convexity of the band in the cervical area.
9. The band is stable so that it will not move around during placement and condensation of the amalgam.

KEY POINTS: Placement of Matrix Band and Wedge

Matrix Band
1. Band 1 mm above marginal ridge level, never lower than ridge.
2. External band surface is convex and in contact with adjacent tooth contact area.
3. Band in firm contact with gingival margin of proximal box and extends slightly apical to it.

Wedge
1. Seated firmly and large enough to separate the teeth slightly.

2. Holds matrix band against gingival margin of proximal box.
3. Base of wedge located properly, not coronal to or too far apical to gingival margin of proximal box.
4. Does not deform the band contours.

See Procedure 11.1 at chapter end for placement and carving of class II amalgam.

Retainerless Matrix Systems

Some matrix systems do not require a retainer. The AutoMatrix (Dentsply) and ReelMatrix (Garrison Dental) have a band formed into a circle with a coil-like loop at the end. A special tool is used to wind the coil and tighten the band (Fig. 11.13). Other bands include the copper T-band (Fig. 11.14) used in pediatric dentistry and custom spot welded bands that are formed to the teeth and then removed and spot welded to retain the loop.

SECTIONAL MATRIX SYSTEMS

Some systems use bands that do not go entirely around the tooth. These are called *sectional bands*. They are typically used with composite resin restorations, but can be used for class II or class III (distal of canines) amalgam preparations, particularly where only one proximal surface has been prepared (mesiocclusal or distocclusal).

 Do You Recall?

Why is a properly fitted matrix band essential for the success of a class II amalgam restoration?

MANIPULATION OF AMALGAM (SEE PROCEDURE 11.1)

High-copper alloys are mostly admix or spherical types (see Table 11.6 for a comparison of admix and spherical alloys). Low-copper alloys have inferior properties and are not used much.

DISPENSING OF ALLOY AND MERCURY

Amalgam must be handled properly through the entire manipulation and placement process if a restoration is to be successful. The preferred dispensing of alloy powder and mercury is done in commercially prepared capsules that contain factory-measured amounts of alloy and mercury separated from each other by a plastic membrane. The manufacturers determine the optimal ratio of alloy and mercury for their products based on testing of materials for their best properties.

Usually capsules are available with different quantities of materials depending on the size of the restoration. They are offered as:

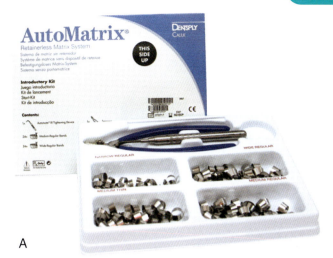
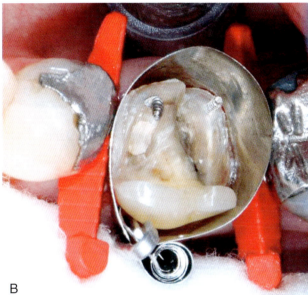

FIG. 11.13 Retainerless matrix systems use a tool to tighten the matrix band into a coil: **(A)** Automatrix Kit. **(B)** Coil is tightened with tool to tighten it against the tooth (Automatrix band). (A, Courtesy Dentsply Caulk; B, Courtesy Dentaljuce CPD Providers Ltd, https://www.dentaljuce.com/direct-restorations-wedges.)

- Single mix (also called one spill, containing 400 mg of alloy)
- Double mix (two spill, 600 mg)
- Triple mix (three spill, 800 mg)
- Larger mixes may be available depending on the manufacturer
- Capsules are color coded to indicate the quantity

With large preparations, several capsules may be needed.

TRITURATION

(See Procedure 11.1). The powder and mercury are mixed together in a mechanical device called a **triturator** (or **amalgamator**). The triturator has settings that allow adjustment in the speed and time of the mixing process depending on the spill and manufacturer's recommendations. Some capsules require activation

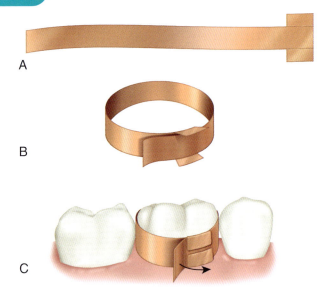

FIG. 11.14 Copper T-band used for primary molars: **(A)** T-band. **(B)** T-band prepared for placement. **(C)** T-band positioned around the tooth and tightened by folding the flaps. (Copyright Elsevier Collection.)

Table 11.6	High-Copper Amalgams: Admix and Spherical
ADMIX	**SPHERICAL**
Needs greater condensation pressure	Needs less condensation pressure
Adapts readily to cavity preparation	Requires both vertical and lateral condensation
Establishes contact readily	Requires heavier wedging to establish contact
Medium early strength	High early strength
Needs more mercury	Needs 10% less mercury
Longer working time	Faster set

before trituration to break the membrane and allow the alloy and mercury to mix. Other capsules are self-activating, meaning the membrane ruptures with the forces created by rapid movement of the triturator. While other capsules have a small plastic or metal rod called a pestle inside to aid in the mixing process. The proper setting times and speed are set on the triturator, the capsule is placed in the retaining arms (see Procedure 11.1; Fig. 11.21), and the device is activated. The retaining arms move back and forth rapidly to mix the powder and mercury, much like an automatic paint mixer.

A less frequently used form of alloy is a pellet that is placed into a reusable capsule with a pestle and mercury is added from a dispenser. The pestle pulverizes the pellet into a powder during mixing in the triturator. This older method of mixing the amalgam has declined in use because the capsules often leak mercury into the operatory during mixing, mixes are not as consistent, and the dispenser is a potential source of mercury spills.

> **Clinical Tip**
>
> Do not activate the capsule before you are ready to begin the mixing process. Activating the capsule and placing it in the triturator before completing the cavity preparation will allow the alloy powder to be partially wet by the mercury. When the mix is actually triturated a few minutes later, some of the reaction will have already started. The resulting amalgam will not have optimal properties and may have reduced working time. Self-activating capsules avoid this potential problem.

CONSEQUENCES OF IMPROPER HANDLING

Expansion, contraction, creep, and corrosion can be caused by improper manipulation, moisture contamination, over-trituration, and under-trituration.
- Under-triturated alloy has a dry, crumbly appearance; sets too quickly; and does not condense well.
  - It results in a weaker restoration because the components have not totally mixed, leaving a higher level of unreacted mercury and alloy particles.
- Over-triturated alloy is too wet and has low resistance to condensation.
  - It also results in an amalgam that sets too quickly because of the heat produced by prolonged mixing.
  - It results in a weaker restoration that will corrode more readily because it forms too many reaction products (silver-mercury and copper-tin).
- Properly triturated alloy has a satin appearance (Fig. 11.15) and produces the desired physical properties and resistance to condensation.

WORKING AND SETTING TIMES

After the amalgam has been mixed, the amount of time needed to place, condense, and carve the amalgam before it begins to harden is the working time. After the working time has been exceeded, the amalgam cannot be condensed or carved without causing problems in the material. Alloys are commercially available in fast-, regular-, and slow-set formulations. The amount of working time selected is by operator preference. A slower-set material may be desired if a very large restoration needs to be done and more time is needed to place and condense the material.

The setting time has two components: the initial setting time and the final setting time.
- The initial setting time is the time at which the amalgam reaches a predefined firmness in the setting process.
  - Usually, this is the time when the restoration can no longer be carved and the occlusion can be checked and adjusted without damaging the amalgam.
- The final setting time is the time when the setting reaction has been completed.
  - The final set usually occurs 12 to 24 hours after trituration depending on the type of alloy used.

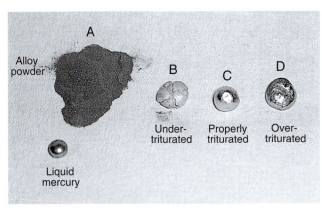

FIG. 11.15 (A) Alloy powder and mercury. (B) Under-triturated amalgam is dry and crumbly. (C) Properly triturated amalgam has a satin-like appearance. (D) Over-triturated amalgam appears too wet.

Do You Recall?

How can the initial set of an amalgam restoration be determined?

PLACEMENT AND CONDENSATION

See Procedure 11.1 for a detailed and illustrated description of how to mix, place, condense, and carve amalgam in a class II cavity preparation.

FINISHING AND POLISHING

Finishing and polishing (see Chapter 17) is best done 24 hours or more after the initial placement to allow crystallization within the amalgam to go to completion. The purpose of finishing is to make the amalgam flush with the cavosurface margins of the tooth, adjust the contours, and eliminate roughness. Finishing is usually accomplished with multi-fluted finishing burs or fine abrasive disks. Polishing further smooths the surface and creates a high shine. Many clinicians do not finish and polish their amalgam restorations, because:
1. It requires a second visit.
2. Modern amalgams are smoother after carving.
3. High-copper amalgams have low tarnish and corrosion.

Although not ideal, some clinicians choose to finish and polish at the time of placement. With their high early strength, spherical amalgams can be lightly polished after their initial set. Polishing should be done using a water coolant and a light touch to avoid generating heat that can potentially irritate the pulp and bring mercury to the surface. Typically, polishing agents such as silex or a slurry mix of fine pumice or abrasive-impregnated rubber polishers are used. When amalgam is polished early (after the initial set), a smooth satin surface is produced but a high shine cannot be achieved.

Advantages and Disadvantages of Amalgam

Advantages	Disadvantages
Can withstand high chewing forces	Not an esthetic material
Biocompatible	May require more tooth structure removal to retain the restoration
Useful when isolation is difficult	Cannot chew on it immediately after placement
Easy to manipulate	Possible temperature sensitivity after placement
Very durable and wear resistant	Possible galvanic reaction with other metals in the mouth
Relatively inexpensive	Requires mercury hygiene measures with scrap material
Alternative for cusp replacement when patient cannot afford a crown	Fills the cavity preparation but does not support the surrounding walls like a bonded composite or ceramic restoration
Strongest direct placement material for crown buildups (cores)	Cannot be used for buildup with all-ceramic restorations (gray color shows through)

Clinical Tip

Care should be taken when polishing amalgam to avoid generating heat. Heat greater than 60°C (140°F) causes mercury to come to the surface of the restoration, weakening the surface and margins; and pulpal irritation can occur. Do not polish an amalgam dry; use low speed and a light touch, particularly with abrasive rubber points and cups.

USE OF A CAVITY SEALER

For many years, a copal resin varnish was routinely placed in the cavity preparation before the amalgam was inserted (Fig. 11.16). The purpose of the varnish was to prevent microleakage at the amalgam margins and, thereby, reduce sensitivity. The copal resin tended to wash out with time. Corrosion products at the interface of the amalgam and the preparation over time greatly reduced the microleakage. With low-copper amalgams, corrosion occurred relatively quickly as the varnish began to disappear. However, with the introduction of high-copper amalgam, corrosion was greatly reduced and the amalgam shrank as it set. So, as the copal resin washed out, microleakage and resulting postoperative sensitivity was often seen. Some clinicians lined the dentin with calcium hydroxide to cover exposed dentin and act as a thermal insulator under the amalgam. Studies showed that calcium hydroxide also washed out over time (Fig. 11.17). Currently, many clinicians use bonding agents as sealers at the margins and over exposed dentin. These materials tend to hold up better over time than cavity varnish, and they can actually seal the dentinal tubules while cavity varnish merely placed a temporary cover over the tubules.

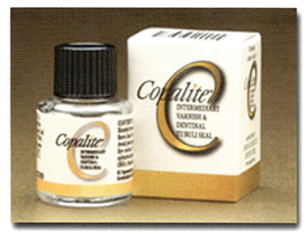

FIG. 11.16 Copal resin varnish for cavity sealing. (Copalite, Temrex Corporation.)

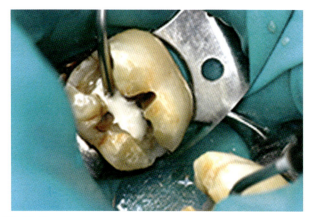

FIG. 11.17 Calcium hydroxide cavity liner for pulpal protection (Dycal, Dentsply Sirona). (From Rada RE: New options for restoring a deep carious lesion. *Dentistry Today*. Category: Dental Materials. Created: Monday, 18 March 2013 13:56.)

Bases and liners are used less frequently under amalgam than in the past, because the need for their use on a routine basis has not been established. They are applied mostly in deeper cavity preparations for thermal insulation and pulpal protection.

LONGEVITY OF AMALGAMS

High-copper amalgams in use today last longer than low-copper amalgams due to superior physical and mechanical properties (Table 11.7). High-copper amalgams are stronger, corrode less, creep less, and have better marginal integrity. Although there are many factors that go into how long amalgams last, the typical survival rate ranges from 7 to 15 years. However, some amalgams have been documented to last as long as 40 to 50 years, whereas some fail in just a few years.

Clinically, an amalgam restoration needs to be replaced when it is no longer functional. This means you can no longer chew on it, it is loose, part of it has fallen out, or part of the tooth has fractured away from the amalgam. Other reasons include defective margins, recurrent caries, voids or cracks in the amalgam, gross overhangs causing damage to the periodontium, or poor contours or contacts causing food impaction.

Many of the reasons for failure of the amalgam are caused by operator error, see accompanying box detailing why amalgams fail.

Occasionally after placement, a new amalgam may have postoperative sensitivity or pain. Some of the reasons for this are:
- Inadequate cooling of the tooth during preparation
- Leaking margins
- Incomplete caries removal
- Hyperocclusion
- Cracked tooth
- Galvanism

Table 11.7 Common High-Copper Amalgams

MANUFACTURER AND BRAND NAME	TYPE OF ALLOY	SET SPEEDS AVAILABLE
Dentsply		
Dispersalloy	Admix	Regular and Fast
Megalloy EZ	Spherical	Regular
Ivoclar Vivadent		
Valiant	Spherical	Regular
Valiant Ph.D.	Admix	Regular
Kerr Dental		
Contour	Admix	Regular and Fast
Tytin	Spherical	Slow and Regular
Tytin FC	Spherical	Regular and Fast

Why Amalgams Fail?

Reasons for Amalgam Failure

Poor Case Selection	Not a Good Place to Use Amalgam
Improper cavity design	Too deep, too shallow, inadequate extensions of the preparation, improper isthmus width, inadequate retention, cavosurface margins not 90 degrees
Improper manipulation	Over-trituration or under-trituration
Poor placement	Improper condensation leaving voids or porosity, using a mix that is too dry or wet
Improper carving	Too deep or too shallow, poor carving or finishing of margins leaving gross overhangs
Inadequate isolation	Contamination of the cavity preparation by blood and saliva
Improper use of matrix	Poor matrix selection, careless matrix placement and removal, poor contouring and wedging
Other factors	Too much force placed on the new restoration before it has gained full strength causing fracture, a restoration that is too high in occlusion, poor oral hygiene leading to recurrent caries

REPAIR OF AMALGAM

Using Amalgam

At times part of a large amalgam may fracture or have a minor defect. A decision involving the patient's informed consent may be made to repair the existing amalgam rather than replace it. To repair the amalgam a retentive preparation (possibly using mechanical interlocks, undercuts, grooves, and troughs) needs to be made in the existing amalgam and possibly the surrounding tooth structure. The prepared surfaces need to be rough but free of any cutting debris, blood, or saliva. Fresh amalgam is then condensed into the preparation against the roughened amalgam walls. The repair will not have the strength of unrepaired amalgam but if not under excessive occlusal loading may serve the patient well for a number of years.

BONDING AMALGAM

Bonding of amalgam was popular in the 1990s, but mixed research results have cast a shadow on its usefulness. This technique uses bonding methods similar to those used with composite resin (see Chapter 8).

ALLERGY TO AMALGAM

Allergy to components of amalgam is uncommon occurring in less than 1% of patients. A local hypersensitivity reaction is most typically encountered; more severe reactions with swelling, difficulty breathing, and anaphylaxis are extremely rare. Local contact dermatitis is usually seen as red or combined red and white lesions (resembling lichen planus and thus called lichenoid lesions) of the buccal mucosa (Fig. 11.18) or lateral border of the tongue in close proximity to the amalgam. On occasion, the gingiva surrounding a cervical amalgam may be affected as well. Usually, replacement of the amalgam restoration with an alternative material (such as composite, ceramic, or gold) will usually resolve the problem.

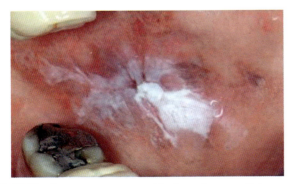

FIG. 11.18 Inflammatory response of the buccal mucosa (lichenoid lesion) to contact with an amalgam restoration in a sensitive patient. (From https://www.proprofs.com/flashcards/cardshowall.php?title=oral-path-exam-3.)

THE SAFETY OF DENTAL AMALGAM

The safety of amalgam has been called into question in recent years, but a study conducted by the National Institutes of Health from 1991 to 1993 concluded that amalgam is safe for human use. In addition, the US Public Health Service, the US Food and Drug Administration (FDA), the American Dental Association, the Centers for Disease Control and Prevention, and the World Health Organization all consider amalgam to be a safe material.

ADA STANCE ON DENTAL AMALGAM SAFETY

The amount of mercury that is released from a set amalgam is very small and has not been shown to be dangerous to patients. The amount of mercury released in vapor form from amalgam is about 1 to 2 micrograms (μg)/day, but the total exposure to the patient will depend on a number of factors, including the number and type of amalgam restorations and their size, frequency of chewing, and whether or not the patient grinds their teeth. The ADA has addressed health concerns about mercury in amalgam (see the ADA Council on Scientific Affairs [CSA] Statement on Dental Amalgam and the CSA Amalgam Safety Update, both of which can be accessed at the ADA website, www.ada.org), as has the FDA (see their Update/Review of Potential Adverse Health Risks Associated with Exposure to Mercury in Dental Amalgam, which can be accessed at www.fda.gov).

In 2004 a review of the scientific literature was conducted by the Life Sciences Research Office and funded by the National Institute of Dental and Craniofacial Research (National Institutes of Health) and the Center for Devices and Radiological Health (a branch of the FDA). Their report states that "The current data are insufficient to support an association between mercury release from dental amalgam and the various complaints that have been attributed to this restoration material. These complaints are broad and nonspecific compared to the well-defined set of effects that have been documented for occupational and accidental elemental mercury exposures. Individuals with dental amalgam–attributed complaints had neither elevated urinary mercury nor increased prevalence of hypersensitivity to dental amalgam or mercury when compared with controls."

CONCERNS ABOUT MERCURY EXPOSURE

Elemental mercury can pass through the gastrointestinal tract without being absorbed. It is mercury vapor that is of greatest health concern as it is absorbed by the lungs. Exposure to mercury vapor occurs during placement or removal of amalgam. Low levels of mercury vapor are released from the set amalgam under function (eating) or bruxing. Mercury can accumulate over time in certain body tissues such as the brain and kidneys. Low-level exposure creates no demonstrable problems. However, higher levels such as those experienced by workers who are exposed to the vapors at their jobs may experience signs and symptoms including headaches, irritability, fatigue, memory loss, or neurological signs.

Concerns about the safety of amalgam and the mercury it contains should be considered from three aspects:
1. Safety of the patient
2. Safety of the dental staff
3. Safety of the environment

Safety for Patients

Prudent oral health providers should limit the exposure of patients to mercury. Mercury can enter the body through ingestion, direct contact with the skin, and by inhalation of the vapor. Care should be taken when placing or removing amalgam restorations to prevent swallowing of amalgam particles or inhalation of mercury vapor. However, the mercury in swallowed particles is not absorbed well and typically excreted. Use of the rubber dam and high-volume evacuation will aid in minimizing both.

Mercury in the bloodstream of pregnant mothers can pass through the placental barrier to reach the developing fetus. It can also be passed in breast milk to nursing infants. The developing nervous system may be more sensitive to the mercury vapor. To be cautious, many countries throughout the world have banned the use of amalgam in pregnant females or young children.

Safety for Office Staff

In some dental offices, dentists and their staff have been found to have higher levels of mercury than the population in general. Precautions should be taken in the dental office to limit the exposure to the dental team. The Occupational Safety and Health Administration (OSHA) has set an acceptable level of exposure to mercury at $0.05\,mg/m^3$ for a 40-hour workweek. Because excessive exposure to mercury can cause it to build up in the body faster than it is eliminated, it is essential to practice good mercury hygiene. Most dental offices comply with mercury hygiene standards, as demonstrated by studies that have shown mercury levels in most dental offices to be far below OSHA's recommended minimum.

Several measures can be taken by the office staff to minimize mercury exposure. See Methods of Mercury Vapor Reduction in the highlighted text.

Safety for the Environment

In 2003 dental offices were estimated to be responsible for 50% of the mercury contamination from wastewater entering publicly owned treatment works (POTWs). In 2008 the Environmental Protection Agency estimated that the approximately 162,000 dentists who use or remove amalgam discharged 3.7 tons of mercury annually into POTWs. The POTWs typically remove about 90% of the amalgam, so the remaining 10% goes into streams, rivers, lakes, and oceans. Therefore it is vitally important to our environment that the dental profession do all it can to manage amalgam waste.

Special collection devices called **amalgam separators** can collect up to 95% of amalgam particles and mercury that might escape into the wastewater. The Environmental Protection Agency mandated under the Clean Water Act that in July 2017 dental practices must control amalgam waste through the use of amalgam separators.

Practices that place and remove amalgam should follow best practices for handling amalgam scrap and cleaning waterline traps (see Table 11.8).

RESTRICTIONS ON AMALGAM USE

The stance taken in the USA on amalgam safety has been largely retrospective, meaning that no studies so far have shown a harmful effect from the use of amalgam in the general population or in specific groups such as pregnant females or children. So, amalgam can be used until studies show a harmful effect. However, in Europe and some other countries a more precautionary approach is used. They conclude that because mercury is a known toxin, it is prudent to restrict the use in pregnant females and young children unless it is proven safe.

In 1956 in Japan thousands in the city of Minamata died from mercury poisoning caused by seafood contaminated from industrial waste. In the 1980s primarily to reduce mercury in the environment, Japan became one of the first nations to restrict dental amalgam use. Since then, several countries have taken steps to reduce the use of amalgam both for environmental reasons and patient safety, especially in pregnant females and children under 6 years of age. Norway, Sweden, and Denmark have banned amalgam use. In 2013 an international meeting was held to address health and environmental concerns involving mercury pollution. Ninety-three countries signed a treaty to reduce the risks to human health and to the environment from the use and release of mercury. Dental amalgam was exempted from an outright ban. Instead, countries still using it were encouraged to find

TABLE 11.8 Best Practices for Amalgam Waste

DO THESE	DO *NOT* DO THESE
Use factory encapsulated alloy	Do not use bulk mercury
Store in air-tight containers and recycle amalgam scrap, capsules, and extracted teeth with amalgam	Do not dispose of amalgam scrap, capsules, or extracted teeth with amalgam in biohazard bags, infectious waste bags, or regular trash
Use chairside amalgam traps, vacuum pump filters, and amalgam separators. Recycle scrap	Do not clean traps, filters, or separators over the sink
Use line cleaners that do not dissolve amalgam	Avoid cleaners that contain bleach or chlorine
Train all staff in safe handling procedures and review state regulations	Avoid direct contact with amalgam and its scrap

alternatives to amalgam, phase out amalgam over time, and promote best environmental practices.

Sources of Office Staff Exposure to Mercury

1. Placing or removing amalgam
2. Leaking amalgam capsules (less frequent with factory-sealed capsules)
3. Mercury droplets collecting on triturator surfaces
4. Sterilizing instruments contaminated with amalgam
5. Improper disposal of amalgam capsules and waste
6. Improper storage of amalgam scrap
7. Amalgam particles in traps within high-volume evacuation system
8. Carpeted operatories or floors with tile or linoleum seams that can collect spilled mercury

Methods for Mercury Vapor Reduction

- Work in a well-ventilated space.
- Avoid direct skin contact with mixed amalgam or free mercury.
- Use factory-sealed amalgam capsules, not bulk alloy and mercury that could spill. Stock a variety of capsules with various portions of amalgam to avoid excess waste.
- Use an amalgamator with a completely enclosed mixing arm to prevent spread of mercury during mixing.
- Store amalgam scrap and mercury in sealed containers away from heat. Do not use x-ray fixer for amalgam scrap storage because the fixer is another environmental hazard.
- Recap used amalgam capsules and dispose of them in a sealed container. (Used capsules are highly contaminated with mercury and are a source of mercury vapor.)
- Use copious water and high-volume evacuation when removing old amalgam to prevent release of mercury vapor into the air.
- Use a rubber dam whenever possible to prevent patients from swallowing scrap or breathing mercury vapors.
- Use facemask and shield to avoid splatter and vapors.
- Use traps or filters (or both) in evacuation systems. Check and clean regularly.
- Avoid the use of mechanical or ultrasonic condensers. They increase mercury vapor release.
- Clean up spilled mercury promptly with a commercial spill kit. Dispose of it in a sealed container (one comes with the kit).
- Clean instruments of any adherent amalgam before sterilization.
- Avoid carpeted operatories. Use floor coverings that are nonabsorbent, seamless, and easy to clean.
- Remove professional protective clothing before leaving the workplace.
- Amalgam scrap retrieved from dental unit traps should first be disinfected with a diluted bleach solution, then stored with the other amalgam scrap in a sealed container.
- Place contaminated disposable materials into polyethylene bags, seal them and dispose of them following state/province and local regulations.

Handling of Mercury Spills

1. Do not use a vacuum cleaner to removed spilled mercury (dangerous mercury vapor can be released into the air)
2. Do not use cleaning products, especially those that contain bleach, chlorine, or ammonia
3. Do not use a broom or brush to collect the mercury
4. Do not dispose of the mercury in the drain
5. If clothing or shoes have been contaminated with mercury, remove them and leave them at the spill site
6. Use a commercially available cleanup kit to safely contain and remove mercury

> **KEY POINTS**
>
> Amalgam Use
> 1. Cost-effective and safe restorative material.
> 2. Silver in color, which limits esthetics and use to posterior areas of the dentition.
> 3. Frequently used in public health settings for large restorations when crowns may not be an option.
> 4. Manufacturer's instructions should be followed for storage, mixing, and handling.
> 5. Final set of material does not occur until 24 hours after placement.

SUMMARY

Dental amalgam is a widely used restorative material. It is an economical, durable, and useful restorative material, although composite resins have surpassed amalgam in popularity. Dental auxiliaries play an important role in the delivery of amalgam restorations to patients by assisting the dentist or, in some states when properly licensed, the placement, carving, and finishing and polishing of the amalgams. Knowledge of the physical properties, mixing and placement techniques, and finishing and polishing methods is important for the proper handling of amalgam and ultimately the longevity of restorations. Safe mercury hygiene practices in the workplace are essential to the health and well-being of patients, office staff, and to the environment in general.

Patient education is an essential role of the dental auxiliary in the dental practice. The ability to describe the pros and cons of the various materials used in practice to the patient and the ability to aid in the treatment process depends on your knowledge of these materials. As new materials are introduced into dental practice, it is important to stay current about their indications, contraindications, and application techniques. Manufacturers' instructions for their care and use should also be followed. Many manufacturers have websites on which they post information relative to their materials.

INSTRUCTIONAL VIDEOS

See the Evolve Resources site for a variety of educational videos that reinforce the material covered in this chapter.

Procedure 11.1 Placing and Carving Class II Amalgam

See Evolve site for Competency Sheet.

EQUIPMENT/SUPPLIES (FIG. 11.19)
a. Local anesthesia setup
b. Operative dentistry setup: Assorted burs, excavators, hand-cutting instruments
c. Amalgam placement setup: Amalgam carrier and well; large and small condensers; ball burnisher; coronal and interproximal carvers; matrix retainer; pre-burnished bands; wedges; articulating paper and holder and dental floss
d. Encapsulated amalgam alloy and mercury
e. Dental dam setup
f. Disposables: Gauze, cotton pellets, high-volume evacuation tip, air-water syringe tip

PROCEDURE STEPS
1. After the administration of local anesthetic, application of the dental dam, and preparation of the cavity, place the preassembled Tofflemire matrix band and retainer on the tooth and firmly insert the wedge in the interproximal space from the lingual side (Fig. 11.20).
   NOTE: After placement, the band should be burnished against the adjacent tooth with an interproximal burnisher or the blade of a plastic instrument to create the proper contour of the contact area.

The band should:
1. Be sealed against the tooth at the gingival margin by the wedge
2. Extend approximately 1 mm coronal to the level of the marginal ridge
3. Be in contact with the proximal surface of the adjacent tooth

The wedge should:
1. Press the band against the tooth to seal the gingival margin
2. Create a separation of the teeth to make up for the thickness of the matrix band so an open contact is not formed when the band is removed

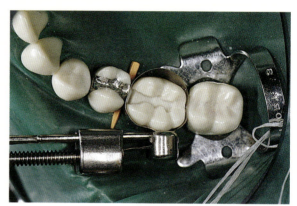

FIG. 11.20

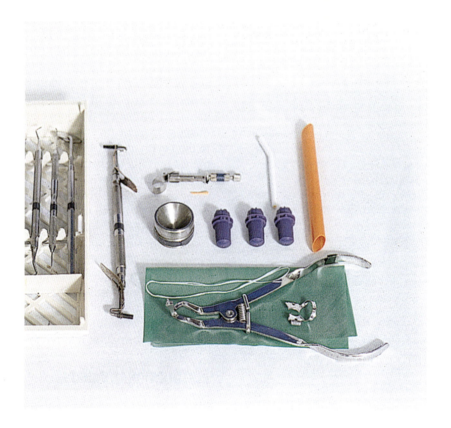

FIG. 11.19

Procedure 11.1 Placing and Carving Class II Amalgam—cont'd

2. Place a base, liner, or cavity varnish, as needed.

   NOTE: Copal resin is seldom used as a cavity varnish, because it quickly washes out of the preparation. Some offices have replaced it with dentin sealers or bonding agents that occlude the dentinal tubules. At present, bases and liners are used less frequently and are applied mostly in deeper cavity preparations. Deeper preparations may need a base or liner for thermal insulation.

3. After the base or liner has set, activate the amalgam capsule (unless it is self-activating), place it into the arms of the triturator, and set for the recommended time and speed (Fig. 11.21).

   NOTE: Do not activate the capsule and let it sit in the triturator before you are ready to mix it. Mercury will start reacting with the alloy powder. Also, do not mix the amalgam and let it set for a couple minutes, because it will start setting and result in a crumbly mix. Do not use it. Make a fresh mix. Careful coordination and timing of mixing and placement between the auxiliary and the clinician are crucial to a successful restoration.

4. Mix the amalgam, open the capsule, and place the mixed amalgam in the amalgam well (Fig. 11.22).

5. Fill both ends of the amalgam carrier and place the amalgam in the proximal box from the small end first (Fig. 11.23).

6. Use a small condenser with vertical and lateral **condensation** to work the amalgam into the corners of the proximal box. The objective is to reduce porosity in the amalgam and adapt it to the walls of the cavity preparation.

   NOTE: Some clinicians who use spherical alloy prefer to place the amalgam in large increments and quickly condense it into the cavity preparation. Spherical amalgam requires much less condensation pressure and displaces easily into the preparation as compared with an admixed amalgam. **Caution:** Ultrasonic condensation devices tend to create mercury aerosols that can be inhaled.

7. Continue to fill the preparation with amalgam. Mix additional amalgam as needed to complete the restoration.

   NOTE: If the amalgam in the preparation starts to stiffen, a new mix placed on top may not join with the

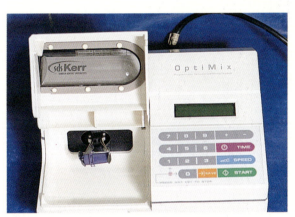

FIG. 11.21

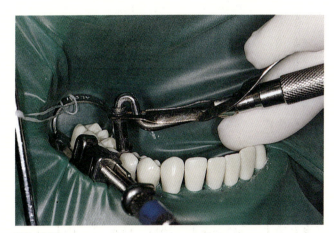

FIG. 11.23

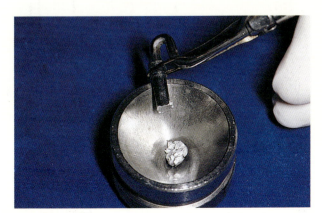

FIG. 11.22

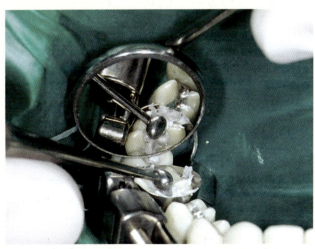

FIG. 11.24

Procedure 11.1 Placing and Carving Class II Amalgam—cont'd

firm material. This will result in a weaker restoration that may fail.

NOTE: Usually, the smaller end of the condenser is used first to condense amalgam onto the gingival floor of the box and against the facial and lingual walls. Both vertical and lateral condensation forces should be used to adapt the amalgam to the preparation. Use larger condensers as the amalgam begins to fill the preparation. Condensers should be used in overlapping steps to prevent voids in the material.

8. After the preparation has been slightly overfilled, the amalgam is burnished with the ball burnisher over its surface and margins (Fig. 11.24). Some clinicians use an anatomic burnisher (e.g., acorn burnisher) to begin the initial contour of the occlusal morphology.

NOTE: The preparation is slightly overfilled to allow adequate material to allow contouring and carving of the amalgam. **Burnishing** creates a denser surface, adapts the amalgam closely to the margins, and brings excess mercury to the surface that is then carved away. Not all clinicians burnish their amalgams.

9. An explorer tip is used to carve excess amalgam away from the band and to begin shaping the marginal ridge (Fig. 11.25). A discoid carver is used to remove large excesses of amalgam from the occlusal surface.

NOTE: Removing excess amalgam adjacent to the band helps prevent fracture of the amalgam during removal of the band.

10. Remove the matrix retainer. While holding the marginal ridge of the amalgam restoration down

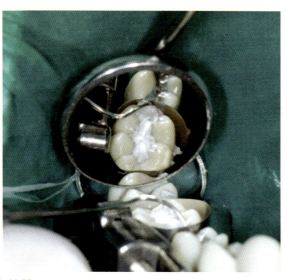

FIG. 11.25

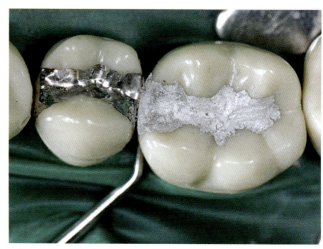

FIG. 11.27

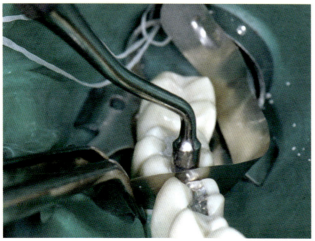

FIG. 11.26

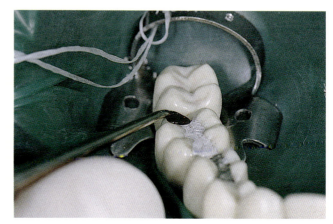

FIG. 11.28

Procedure 11.1 Placing and Carving Class II Amalgam—cont'd

with a large condenser, remove the matrix band in an occlusal direction with a gentle rocking motion (Fig. 11.26).

NOTE: Some clinicians prefer to leave the wedge in place while removing the band to maintain some separation of the teeth. This helps to minimize risk of fracture of the marginal ridge. If the marginal ridge is not held down during removal of the band, the unset amalgam is at risk of fracture, requiring its removal and placement of fresh amalgam.

11. An interproximal carver (e.g., 1/2 Hollenbeck) is used to carve first the gingival margin, then facial and lingual margins to remove any excess material (Fig. 11.27). Next, a discoid/cleoid or similar carver is used to carve the occlusal surface (Fig. 11.28). The blade of the carver is held partially on the adjacent enamel to act as a guide so that the amalgam margins are not overcarved.

12. After the amalgam is firm, pass dental floss through the contact to clear the embrasure of excess carving debris and to test the adequacy of the contact relationship (Fig. 11.29).

NOTE: A weak, open, or poorly contoured contact relationship with the adjacent tooth can lead to food impaction into the gingival tissues and periodontal pocket formation.

13. Remove the dental dam and mark the occlusal contacts with articulating paper (Fig. 11.30). High spots as indicated by heavy marks from the articulating paper are carefully carved away. Repeat the process until contact is no longer heavy and the patient indicates that the restoration does not feel high. As a last step, some clinicians smooth the surface of the amalgam with a wet cotton pellet.

NOTE: Before checking the occlusal contacts, make sure the marginal ridges of the amalgam are at the same level as the ridges of the adjacent teeth. The patient should be instructed to close very lightly and then open again. If the patient closes too firmly and the amalgam is high, especially at the marginal ridge, it might fracture. When patients are still numb from the local anesthetic, they often cannot judge how hard they are biting. Some clinicians prefer to wait a couple of minutes after completing the carving before checking the occlusal contacts to allow the amalgam to gain some firmness, especially for very large amalgams.

In some states, dental hygienists and assistants licensed in expanded functions can place, condense, and carve the amalgam.

14. Instruct the patient to avoid chewing on the new amalgam restoration until the next day. Advise the patient to take care while they are still numb from the anesthetic when chewing or consuming hot foods or beverages due to the risk of biting the lip or tongue or burning the oral tissues or throat.

NOTE: High-copper amalgams, especially spherical ones, have a high strength early and gain about 80% of their compressive strength in the first 8 hours. The set of the material is usually complete within 24 hours.

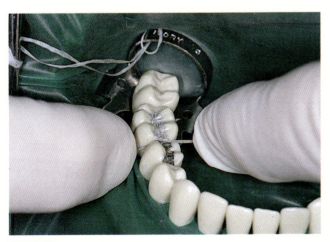

FIG. 11.29

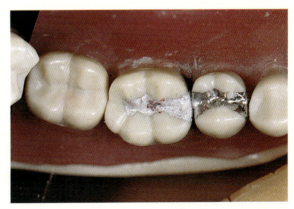

FIG. 11.30

CHAPTER 11 Dental Amalgam

Review and Discussion

Review Questions

Select the one correct response for each of the following multiple-choice questions.

1. In an amalgam restoration, which of the following elements has the greatest effect on reduction of corrosion?
    a. Silver (Ag)
    b. Mercury (Hg)
    c. Copper (Cu)
    d. Indium
2. What are the two main components of the amalgam restoration?
    a. Silver and copper
    b. Copper and tin
    c. Silver and mercury
    d. Mercury and zinc
3. Why should all remnants of amalgam be removed from the placement instruments before they are autoclaved?
    a. The steam causes the amalgam to fuse to the stainless steel.
    b. Amalgam corrosion products produced by the steam are toxic.
    c. The heat causes mercury vapor to be released from the amalgam.
    d. The heat melts the silver component, and it will clog the drain of the autoclave.
4. What factors can affect the strength of the amalgam restoration?
    a. Over-trituration
    b. Under-trituration
    c. Corrosion
    d. All of the above
5. How should a properly mixed amalgam appear?
    a. Dry and crumbly
    b. Soupy and shiny
    c. As a homogeneous mass with a slight shine
    d. Liquid-like and should pour easily out of the capsule
6. Scrap amalgam should be:
    a. Autoclaved before it is sent to the recycler
    b. Thrown into the incinerator
    c. Stored in a sealed container
    d. Put into the general nonmedical waste
7. With high-copper alloys, which metal reacts with copper to reduce gamma-2 phase corrosion?
    a. Tin
    b. Zinc
    c. Silver
    d. Palladium
8. The fact that mercury makes up almost half of amalgam has caused concerns about:
    a. Its safety for patient use
    b. Risks to the office staff
    c. Environmental effects of improper disposal of amalgam waste
    d. All of the above
9. Why has amalgam been popular for the restoration of carious teeth?
    a. It is economical.
    b. It has excellent physical properties.
    c. It is easy to manipulate.
    d. All of the above.
10. For best mercury hygiene practices, which type of flooring is preferred for the dental operatory?
    a. Hardwood plank flooring
    b. Ceramic tile
    c. Seamless vinyl
    d. Tight-knit carpet
11. How does tarnish differ from corrosion?
    a. Tarnish occurs only on the surface.
    b. Tarnish is more harmful to the restoration than is corrosion.
    c. Tarnish contributes to the destructive effects seen in the gamma-2 phase.
    d. Tarnish cannot be removed by polishing, whereas corrosion can.
12. Which one of the following amalgam mixes has the least resistance to condensation pressure?
    a. Lathe-cut low-copper
    b. Spherical high-copper
    c. Admix high-copper
    d. Lathe-cut high-copper
13. Delayed expansion of amalgam is caused by contact of water with which component of amalgam?
    a. Mercury
    b. Copper
    c. Tin
    d. Zinc
14. How should polishing of amalgam be done?
    a. With light pressure, using water as a coolant
    b. With rubber abrasive points without water
    c. Immediately after carving
    d. With heavy pressure, using pumice in a rubber cup
15. Amalgam is strongest in which one of the following?
    a. Tension
    b. Shear
    c. Compression
    d. Torsion
16. All of the following features meet the criteria for a well-placed matrix assembly *except* one. Which one?
    a. The narrow portion of the band is oriented toward the gingival margin.
    b. The matrix band extends apical to the gingival margin of the proximal box by at least 1 mm.
    c. No gap is present between the band and the gingival margin of the proximal box.
    d. The top edge of the band extends 3 mm above the adjacent marginal ridge.
17. Which one of the following statements does *NOT* fit the criteria of a well-placed wedge for a class II cavity preparation matrix assembly?
    a. The wedge is located just coronal to the gingival margin of the proximal box.
    b. The wedge does not deform the contours of the matrix band.
    c. The wedge is seated firmly to produce separation of the teeth.
    d. The wedge holds the band against the gingival margin of the proximal box.

Review and Discussion—cont'd

18. The dental staff is most at risk for mercury overexposure from which one of the following sources?
    a. Inhaling mercury vapor
    b. Handling amalgam with gloved hands
    c. Triturating commerically prepared capsules of amalgam
    d. Polishing amalgam under water spray

For answers to Review Questions, see the Appendix.

Case-Based Discussion Topics

1. A healthy 23-year-old college student reports to the dental office for a routine examination. It is discovered that the patient has several class II carious lesions in molars that require restoration. The patient does not have a lot of money and wants a durable restoration. Esthetics and the restorations showing are not of concern to the patient.

Discuss the advantages and disadvantages of amalgam and composite resin for the patient's situation. Which restoration would you choose for yourself? Why?

2. A 43-year-old patient comes to the dental office and reports that another dentist recommended the removal of all the old amalgam restorations in their mouth due to the mercury content. The patient inquires about the safety of amalgam fillings.

Discuss the safety issues related to amalgam, its mercury content, and the risks involved in removing the restorations.

3. You have just triturated a double mix capsule of amalgam, and mercury has leaked while the capsule was being shaken and can be seen in small puddles on the outer surface of the triturator.

Discuss appropriate ways to capture the spilled mercury and dispose of it. What risks does the spill present to the office staff?

4. While removing the matrix band from a newly placed MOD amalgam on tooth #19, the mesial marginal ridge of the amalgam fractured off.

Can this fracture be fixed by replacing the matrix band and adding more amalgam from a fresh mix? Why or why not? What steps can be taken to avoid the marginal ridge fracture when removing the band?

5. A 36-year-old nurse had an MO amalgam placed on a moderately deep cavity preparation in tooth #3. When the patient drinks hot coffee or eats ice cream, there is a sudden sharp pain in the tooth that lasts two to three seconds.

What is the likely cause of the pain? How could this problem have been prevented?

BIBLIOGRAPHY

ADA Council on Scientific Affairs: Dental mercury hygiene recommendations, *J Am Dent Assoc* 134:1498–1499, 2003.

American Dental Association (ADA) Best Management Practices for Amalgam Waste. Available at https://www.ada.org/resources/research/science-and-research-institute/oral-health-topics/amalgam-separators

Bird DL, Robinson DS: *Modern Dental Assisting,* ed 13, St. Louis, 2021, Elsevier.

DermNet New Zealand: Lichenoid Amalgam Reaction. Available at: http://dermnetnz.org/reactions/amalgam-lichenoid.html, 2010.

Life Sciences Research Office: Executive Summary: Review and Analysis of the Literature on the Health Effects of Dental Amalgam. Available at: http://www.lsro.org/presentation_files/amalgam/amalgam_execsum.pdf.

Mackey TM, Contreras JT, Liang BA: The Minamata Convention on Mercury: attempting to address the global controversy of dental amalgam use and mercury waste disposal, *Sci Total Environ* 472:125–129, 2014.

Marshall GW, Marshall SJ, Bayne SC: Restorative dental materials: Scanning electron microscopy and x-ray microanalysis, *Scanning Microsc* 2:2007–2028, 1988.

Office of Environmental Health Hazard Assessment: Mercury in Dental Amalgam Fillings. State of California, 2022.

Powers JM, Wataha JC: *Dental amalgam.* In *Dental Materials: Foundations and Applications,* ed 11, St. Louis, 2017, Elsevier.

Ritter AV, Boushell LW, Walter R: *Clinical techniques for amalgam restorations in Sturdevant's Art and Science of Operative Dentistry,* ed 7, St. Louis, 2019, Elsevier.

Sakaguchi RL, Ferracane J, Powers JM: *Restorative materials – metals.* In *Craig's Restorative Dental Materials,* ed 13, St. Louis, 2019, Elsevier.

Shen C, Rawls HR, Esquivel-Upshaw JF: *Dental Amalgams.* In *Phillips' Science of Dental Materials,* 13 ed, St. Louis, 2022, Elsevier.

Stafford G.: *The Environmentally Responsible Dentist—Dental Amalgam Recycling: Principles, Pathways and Practice,* July 2011. Available at: https://www.researchgate.net/publication/263370547_The_Environmentally_Responsible_Dentist_-_Dental_Amalgam_Recycling_Principles_Pathways_and_Practice.

U.S. Department of Labor, Occupational Safety and Health Administration. *Permissible Exposure Limits. Annotated OSHA Z-2 Table,* December 19, 2016. https://www.osha.gov/dsg/annotated-pels/tablez-2.html

U.S. Environmental Protection Agency. Mercury in Dental Amalgam. https://www.epa.gov/mercury/mercury-dental-amalgam

U.S. Food and Drug Administration. About Dental Amalgam Fillings, Updated 2/18/2021. https://www.fda.gov/medical-devices/dental-devices/dental-amalgam-fillings

Xu HH, Eichmiller FC, Giuseppetti AA, et al: Three-body wear of a hand-consolidated silver alternative to amalgam, *J Dent Res* 78:1560–1567, 1999.

12 Metals and Alloys

http://evolve.elsevier.com/Eakle/materials/

Chapter Objectives

On completion of this chapter, the student should be able to:

1. Describe the differences among the types of gold alloy used for dental restorations.
2. Differentiate between high-noble, noble, and base-metal alloys.
3. Describe the properties of casting alloys.
4. Describe the properties of metals used for casting partial denture frameworks.
5. Describe the properties needed for porcelain bonding alloys.
6. Explain the biocompatibility issues associated with some alloys.
7. Explain how solders are used.
8. List metals used for solders.
9. Identify how wrought metal alloys differ from casting alloys.
10. Describe the uses of wrought wire.
11. Explain the use of the different types of metal for orthodontic archwire.
12. Explain the differences between cast and preformed endodontic posts.
13. Describe the types of materials used for preformed endodontic posts.

KEY TERMS

Alloy a solid compound made up of two or more elements of which at least one is a metal

High-Noble Alloy alloy containing at least 60% noble metals, 40% of which must be gold

Base-Metal Alloy alloy composed of non-noble metals which corrode more readily

Noble Alloy alloy composed of metals that do not corrode readily; at least 25% must be noble metals

Precious Metal classification of metal based on its high cost

Elastic Modulus a measure of the stiffness of a material. A high modulus indicates a stiff material and a low modulus a more flexible one

Yield Strength amount of stress at which a substance deforms

Annealing controlled heating of a cast metal to modify physical properties

Porcelain Bonding Alloys special casting alloys manufactured for their compatibility with porcelain that is bonded to them at high temperature

Coping a thin covering that serves as a substructure for a porcelain-bonded-to-metal crown (in this case, the coping is metal)

Solder an alloy used to join two metals together or to repair cast metal restorations

Wrought Metal Alloy an alloy that has been mechanically changed into another form to improve its properties (including ductility and malleability)

Wire a wrought metal alloy that can be soft and easily bent or can be heat treated to be hard and resist bending. It has numerous applications in dentistry

Archwire a curved, flexible wire that approximates the general shape of the dental arches and when slightly bent and attached to orthodontic brackets or bands tries to regain its original form, creating forces that move the teeth

Gauge a measure of the thickness of a wire; the lower the gauge, the thicker the wire (e.g., 8 gauge is thicker than 16 gauge)

Endodontic Post a metal or nonmetal dowel placed within the root canal to retain a core buildup for a crown

---

Historically, the most widely used material in restorative and corrective dentistry has been metal. Because a pure metal may not possess the physical and mechanical properties desired for a restoration, it may be combined with one or more other elements to form an alloy with the properties desired. Metal alloys generally have high strength and consequently make durable dental restorations. They melt at high temperatures, conduct temperature and electricity, can be polished to a high shine (luster), and have varying degrees of ductility (ability to be pulled or drawn into a wire). The thin margins of gold restorations can be mechanically pulled or pushed for better adaptation to the tooth preparation margins. Other metals may be more brittle and tend to break rather than bend or stretch. As esthetic nonmetal materials improve in their physical properties, they are gradually replacing metals in many applications.

The dental healthcare worker (clinical or laboratory) is in contact with and involved in the manipulation of metal dental materials in various ways every day. Grinding dust from certain metal alloys can present the dental healthcare worker with health hazards, so personal protective equipment must be used. It is essential that the dental auxiliary have an understanding of the properties of various metal materials to correctly manipulate and care for them and to be able to answer questions by patients relative to a particular material that will be used for their treatment.

STRUCTURE OF METALS AND THEIR ALLOYS

PURE METALS

Pure metals are composed of multiple small interlocking crystals (also called grains). Each crystal is composed of multiple, closely packed metal ions surrounded by a sea of free, circulating electrons that have left the outer shell of the metal atoms. These electrons are shared among all of the atoms. The force of attraction between the metal ions and the electrons circulating among them forms the metallic bond. The metallic bond is very strong and helps the metal to maintain a regular shape.

LATTICE STRUCTURE

The metal ions are arranged in a highly ordered, three-dimensional structure called a lattice (Fig. 12.1). The lattice has layers of metallic ions in a pattern that repeat throughout the metal. There are three types of lattice patterns that are most common but as many as 14 patterns exist. The lattice pattern is responsible for the physical properties of the metal. Because the metallic bonds are strong it takes more energy to break them, resulting in high melting points. Strong metallic bonds also contribute to high strength. The tighter the metal ions are bound together, the harder the metal (more resistant to scratching).

The pattern of the lattice affects physical properties such as malleability and ductility (see Chapter 3). Gold for example is a metal that is highly malleable and ductile because of the arrangement of its lattice. The layers of metal ions in the lattice can slide across each other, allowing the metal to be hammered into thin sections or drawn into a wire.

KEY POINTS

STRUCTURE OF METALS
- Metal atoms are tightly arranged in lattice structures that have layers of repeating patterns.
- Metal atoms each share an electron from their outer shell that is freely moving throughout the lattice.
- The strong metallic bonds, the type of lattice, and the repeating patterns are responsible for the physical properties.

ALLOYS

Since most pure metals lack the properties desired for dental uses, they are combined with other metals or nonmetal elements to form an **alloy**. Alloys are formed by melting the metal and added elements, mixing them together, and then cooling them back into a solid. Alloys typically have higher strength and hardness than pure metals.

Both pure metals and their alloys are crystalline solids. The properties that are desired for dental uses can be controlled by the changes to the crystalline structure that occur when they are processed or heated; for example, the manner in which steel is heated and cooled can increase its hardness but can also make it more brittle.

Do You Recall?

Why are alloys of metals used in dentistry instead of the pure metals?

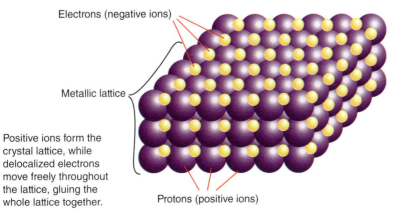

FIG. 12.1 Representation of a crystal lattice structure of a metal. A sea of free electrons in the outer shell are shared among all of atoms. (Modified from HSC Physics, Dux College.)

Metal Casting Alloys

In the early 1900s, W.H. Taggart developed a technique for making dental restorations from metal that was melted and cast into a mold, using the lost wax technique (see Chapter 6). A variation of this technique with improved equipment is still used today for casting metal dental restorations.

Alloys used with the lost wax technique are called *dental casting alloys*. Unlike amalgam, restorations made from these alloys are not placed directly into the preparation but are made outside the mouth, and then are cemented in place (see Chapter 16). The International Organization for Standardization sets specifications for casting alloys; these can be found on its website (www.iso.org).

Classification of Cast Metal Restorations

Cast metal restorations can be classified by the portions of the tooth they restore. They can be intracoronal (restoration is placed within the crown of the tooth) or extracoronal (restoration covers primarily the outside of the crown of the tooth). An inlay is an intracoronal restoration, whereas an onlay has both intracoronal and extracoronal components in that it has an inlay preparation and also covers the outer surface of one or more cusps (Fig. 12.2). Other extracoronal cast restorations include partial-coverage (¾ and ⅞ crowns) and full-coverage crowns (Fig. 12.3). Cast metal alloys can also be used to make fixed partial dentures (bridges) and removable partial dentures for the replacement of missing teeth.

Classification of Casting Alloys

Dental casting alloys can be classified by their use:
- All-metal alloys for crown and bridge
- Ceramo-metal alloys (porcelain fused to metal) for crown and bridge
- All-metal alloys for removable partial dentures

Dental casting alloys can also be classified by the type of metal used:
- Noble metals
- Base metals

Noble Metal Casting Alloys

A noble alloy is one that does not tarnish or corrode very readily in the oral environment. Gold (chemical symbol, Au) is the most corrosion-resistant noble metal and has been used in dentistry for centuries. However, its use in dentistry is declining because of its high cost, and it is not considered esthetic in Western cultures. Gold alloy is classified as karats, percentage, or fineness (obtained by multiplying percentage of gold by 10) according to its gold content. As an example, pure gold is 24 karat, 100%, or 1000 fine, and half gold is 12 karat, 50%, or 500 fine. The term *karat* is used more to signify the gold content of jewelry than dental alloys. Pure gold has limited use in dentistry today but is used in the form of gold foil by a small number of dentists for direct-placement restorations. Pure gold is too soft to use for dental castings; however, gold alloys have excellent properties and handling characteristics.

The American Dental Association classifies dental casting alloys according to their noble metal content and divides them into the following three categories:
- High noble: To be considered a **high-noble alloy**, they must contain at least 60% noble elements (gold, palladium, and platinum), of which 40% must be gold.

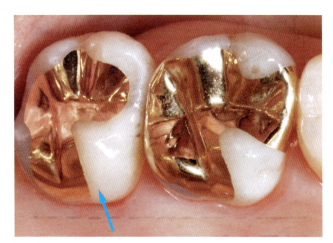

FIG. 12.2 Inlay (*blue arrow*) and onlay using high-noble metal (*gold alloy*). (Courtesy Richard V. Tucker, Department of Restorative Dentistry, University of Washington, Seattle, Washington.)

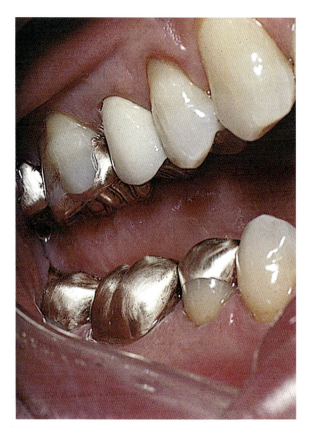

FIG. 12.3 Partial- and full-coverage cast gold restorations. (Courtesy David Graham, University of California, San Francisco, San Francisco, California.)

Base metals (usually copper, silver, or gallium) make up the remaining 40%.
- Noble: **Noble alloys** contain at least 25% noble elements, with no requirement for gold, and the remaining 75% consists of base metals.
- Base metal: **Base-metal alloys** have no requirement for gold and require less than 25% by weight of noble metals.

PROPERTIES OF CASTING ALLOYS

Color of Casting Alloys
Most dental casting alloys are either yellow or silver ("white") in color. Often an assumption is made that yellow casting alloys have a higher gold content than silver-colored alloys. However, this may not be true. It is possible for a yellow casting alloy to have absolutely no gold at all! On the other hand, a silver casting alloy may have a high gold content. Because beauty is in the eye of the beholder, some patients may prefer the yellow color, whereas others prefer the silver color, and others still prefer no metal showing at all.

Melting Range
A dental casting alloy, being composed of more than one metal, will have a temperature range at which it melts rather than a single melting point. The temperature at the start of the range is when the alloy shows an initial shift toward melting and the temperature at the end of the range represents the point at which the entire alloy is liquid. So, an alloy with a range of 1100°C to 1300°C has the first signs of melting at 1100°C and will be totally melted (called *liquidus*) at 1300°C. When cooling a melted metal, the temperature at which it becomes a solid is called *solidus*.

Elastic Modulus
The **elastic modulus** is a measure of stiffness of the alloy. The higher the elastic modulus of the alloy, the stiffer the alloy will be. Alloys used for fixed bridge restorations need to be stiff to avoid bending or distorting. If the crown or bridge has porcelain fused to it, bending would cause the brittle porcelain to fracture. Likewise, alloys used for removable partial dentures need to be stiff so that the framework does not flex too much and stress the abutment teeth when the patient chews. **Wires** used for orthodontic purposes must have a low elastic modulus to allow them to be bent without breaking.

Thermal Expansion
When a metal is heated, atoms within the metal increase in vibration. The result is a small increase in its length, width, and volume known as thermal expansion. How much expansion occurs depends on the particular metal.

Thermal and Electrical Conductivity
Metals are good conductors of heat and electricity. Thermal and electrical conductivity is determined mainly by the movement of free electrons throughout the lattice structure of the metal. Heat excites the tightly packed particles in the metal so that their vibrations quickly pass from one to the next. Electricity causes electrically charged particles—the free electrons—to flow through the lattice structure of the metal.

Density
Gold and platinum are among the densest (and heaviest) of the metals used in dental casting alloys. On the other hand, titanium is less dense and is lighter in weight. Gold alloys are easier to cast than chrome-cobalt alloys because their weight drives the molten metal into the investment better under casting forces than the lighter alloys.

Strength
Dental casting alloys must be strong enough to resist fracture or distortion. Typically, they are strong in both compression and tension. When the strength of alloys is compared, it is their yield strength that is considered. The **yield strength** is the maximum stress the alloy can withstand before it is permanently distorted. Typically, base-metal alloys have greater yield strength than gold alloys.

Hardness
Alloys that have low yield strength (like gold alloys) will be softer than those with higher yield strength (like base-metal alloys). A hard alloy will be more resistant to denting or scratching and will be more difficult to polish. Gold restorations, being softer, will also be kinder to the opposing enamel when chewing.

Crystal Formation (Grains)
After casting alloys have been melted and cast into the mold, they cool and form crystals (also called *grains*). Small crystals produce more desirable properties (especially improved yield strength) in the metal alloy than large crystals. Some elements, such as iridium or ruthenium, are added to gold-based alloys to keep the crystals from growing too large.

A process called **annealing,** or controlled reheating of gold-based alloys, can improve some of the properties. After heating, slow cooling produces a harder metal and rapid cooling keeps the metal soft. However, with base-metal alloys, reheating will degrade the physical properties.

Resistance to Tarnish and Corrosion
It is important that dental casting alloys be composed of materials that resist tarnish and corrosion in the oral environment. The noble metal alloys naturally resist tarnish and corrosion. Base-metal alloys are more likely to corrode in the mouth, so they are blended with other metals such as chromium that make them more corrosion resistant.

Dental gold casting alloys can be classified (Table 12.1) by their:

Table 12.1 Classification of Gold Alloys

CHARACTERISTIC	CLASS I	CLASS II	CLASS III	CLASS IV
Hardness	Soft	Medium	Hard	Extra hard
Use	Inlays (not in heavy function)	Inlays, crowns	Inlays, crowns, bridges	Partial denture framework, bridges
Yield strength (amount of stress at which alloy deforms)	Low	Medium	High	High
Wear resistance	Low	Medium	High	High

- Hardness (resistance to penetration)
- Malleability (ability to be shaped, as by tapping or pounding)
- Ductility (ability to be elongated, as by stretching or pulling)

The more ductile the alloy, the more margins of restorations can be burnished (pushing or pulling the metal at the margins) to close small gaps between the restoration and the tooth.

Dental casting alloys should possess the following properties:
- Strength
- Resistance to corrosion and tarnish
- Melting temperature compatible with investment materials (see Chapter 6)
- Thermal expansion compatible with porcelains (for porcelain-fused-to-metal [PFM] restorations)
- Biocompatibility

Nongold Noble Metals for Casting Alloys
Other noble metals include platinum (Pt) and palladium (Pd):
- Platinum is not used much because of its expense, high melting point, and difficulty mixing with gold.
- Palladium is used widely because it has good corrosion resistance, increases hardness of the alloy, and is less expensive than gold.
- These noble metals are sometimes referred to as **precious metals** because of their high monetary value. Although silver (Ag) is considered to be a precious metal, it is not considered noble because of its tarnish and corrosion in the oral cavity.

Of the seven noble metals, gold, palladium, and platinum are the most widely used in dentistry. The remaining four noble metals (rhodium, iridium, ruthenium, and osmium) are used in very small amounts to enhance the physical properties of a dental alloy.

Other metals that may be added to noble metals to enhance their properties and handling characteristics include copper, silver, zinc, tin, indium, gallium, and nickel (Table 12.2).

Table 12.2 Function of Metals Added to Gold Alloys

METAL (SYMBOL)	FUNCTION	MELTING POINT (°C)	COLOR
Palladium (Pd)	Reduces corrosion and tarnish Improves mechanical properties	1554	White
Platinum (Pt)	Raises melting temperature Improves hardness and elasticity	1772	Blue-white
Copper (Cu)	Hardens and strengthens the alloy Allows heat-treatment properties	1083.4	Reddish
Silver (Ag)	Hardens gold alloy Counters copper's redness	961.9	Silver
Zinc (Zn)	Acts as oxygen scavenger during casting process	419.6	Blue-white
Indium (In)	Used as a replacement for zinc	156.6	Gray-white
Nickel (Ni)	Seldom used. Increases hardness and strength	1453	White
Tin (Sn)	Acts with palladium and platinum to harden the alloy	232	White
Gallium (Ga)	Forms oxides for bonding ceramic to metal	29.8	Gray-white
Iridium (Ir)	Improves yield strength by creating smaller grains	2410	Silver-white
Ruthenium (Ru)	Improves yield strength by creating smaller grains	2310	White

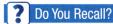 Do You Recall?

Why are some metals used in dentistry called noble metals?

Base-Metal Dental Casting Alloys
The most common base-metal alloys are chrome-cobalt and nickel-chrome. It is the chromium content that gives these metals their corrosion resistance.

Other base metals used in casting alloys are:
- Copper (Cu)
- Nickel (Ni)
- Silver (Ag)
- Zinc (Zn)
- Tin (Sn)
- Titanium (Ti)

Copper and silver are often added to gold alloys to increase their hardness. Zinc is added to reduce oxidation when the alloy is cast.

Because of their low cost, base metals have also been called nonprecious metals. They are inexpensive alternatives to noble metals for all-metal crowns and PFM crowns. Base-metal alloys have about half the density of gold alloys, making them much lighter. Although they are not considered to be as good as the noble metals, the base metals are essential for many applications in dentistry.

Base Metals for Removable Partial Dentures
The metals used today for partial denture frameworks are mostly base-metal alloys with or without minor amounts of noble elements (Fig. 12.4). Because the base metals are less dense than gold, they are lighter in weight. These base metals include:
- nickel
- titanium
- chromium
- aluminum
- cobalt
- vanadium
- iron
- beryllium
- molybdenum
- gallium
- carbon

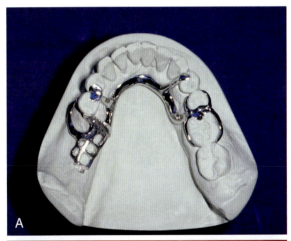
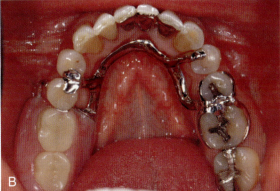

FIG. 12.4 Chrome-cobalt metal framework for a removable partial denture: **(A)** Framework on the cast. **(B)** The completed partial denture in the mouth after processing of acrylic and teeth over the retentive area. (Courtesy Mark Dellinges, University of California School of Dentistry [San Francisco, CA].)

In addition to corrosion resistance, hardness and resistance to deformation under function (**yield strength**) are important properties for these metals. Hardness indicates their resistance to scratching and denting resulting in an increased effort needed to polish them. Their resistance to deformation is especially important for use in partial denture frameworks, where flexing of the framework under chewing forces would put undue stress on abutment teeth. The stiffness (modulus of elasticity) of base alloys is twice as great as that of gold-based alloys.

Base-metal alloys used for partial denture frameworks should also be resistant to fatigue, so that repeated flexing of the clasp arms as the partial denture is seated and removed does not cause them to break off. Cobalt-chromium alloys are the most resistant to this type of fatigue and most commonly used for partial denture frameworks.

Because these metals are among the hardest of the alloys and are quite difficult to cast, they require special casting machines and are cast by commercial dental laboratories.

Uses for Titanium and Its Alloys
Titanium and its alloys can be used for implant fixtures, partial denture frameworks, and all-metal and metal-ceramic crowns and bridges. Titanium and its alloys have very high melting temperatures (approximately 1670°C) and require special equipment to melt and cast them. They have low density and, therefore, are very lightweight and harder to cast into the investment mold. Because of the difficulties in casting titanium, some crowns and partial denture frameworks are fabricated from metal blocks using CAD/CAM techniques (see Chapter 10).

Titanium and its alloys have a low coefficient of thermal expansion. When used for metal-ceramic restorations, they need special low-expansion porcelains so expansion of the metal does not crack the overlying procelain. The most widely used titanium alloy is Ti-6Al-4V (6% aluminum and 4% vanadium). It has high hardness, high strength, and more fatigue resistance than other titanium alloys. Pure titanium is more biocompatible than aluminum and vanadium.

While titanium alloys have good physical and mechanical properties to serve as partial denture frameworks, their high melting temperature and difficulty in casting them make them harder to work with than chrome-cobalt alloys. Surface oxides resulting from casting are more tedious to remove.

 Do You Recall?

What are some uses in dentistry for base metals?

Biocompatibility
Noble metals are more biocompatible with the oral tissues because they tend to corrode less than base metals.

As metals corrode, they release metal corrosion products into the oral cavity and adjacent soft tissues. Some of these products are responsible for allergic responses (Fig. 12.5).

Nickel. Of the base metals, nickel has the highest incidence of allergic response. The overall allergy rate to nickel for the general population is about 9% to 12%. The allergic response is sometimes seen around the free gingival tissues, especially at the margins of base-metal crowns. This is less common for removable partial dentures because the metal often is not in direct contact with the tissues, and they are not worn constantly like fixed bridges or single crowns. Some responses to nickel cause a skin reaction rather than a response in the mouth, even though the oral cavity is the source of the nickel.

Beryllium. Beryllium is a base metal added to nickel-chrome alloys to reduce the fusion temperature for easier casting and to improve physical properties. Laboratory technicians are at risk for nickel and beryllium exposure when casting (metal vapors), grinding, and polishing these metals. Beryllium is toxic and can cause chronic lung scarring and difficulty breathing. It can also cause allergic reactions with skin rashes. Once exposed, the individual is at risk for disease for a lifetime even if exposure is stopped.

Protective Measures. In the laboratory, an exhaust hood should be used for grinding procedures and the room should have good ventilation. When grinding in the mouth, high-volume evacuation should be used as well as isolation with a rubber dam where applicable. In addition, dental personnel should wear personal protective equipment (PPE) when working with these materials.

> **! Caution**
>
> Inhalation of beryllium is known to contribute to a lung disease called *berylliosis*. All dental personnel should wear PPE when grinding these alloys to prevent inhalation of small particles and to prevent fine particles from getting into the eyes. They should follow Occupational Safety and Health Administration guidelines for occupational hazards.

> **? Do You Recall?**
>
> What are some important properties for dental casting alloys?

PORCELAIN BONDING ALLOYS

Porcelain bonding alloys were developed in the late 1950s. They are similar to the other casting alloys with similar physical properties. They are also classified as high-noble, noble, and base-metal alloys (Fig. 12.6). However, they have minor changes in their composition that make them compatible with dental ceramic materials. The most common ceramic materials used with these metals are conventional feldspar-based porcelains (see Chapter 10).

The metals in porcelain bonding alloys are selected and blended so that they have the ability to withstand the high temperatures at which porcelain is fired without melting or distorting. They also have a lower thermal expansion than gold alloys used for all-metal crowns, so they will not expand too greatly and crack the brittle porcelain that lies over top. In addition, small amounts of metals, such as indium, iron, tin, or gallium, are added to form oxides on the metal surface to which porcelain will bond (or fuse) at a high temperature. Most of the alloys are silver ("white") in color. Alloys that are gold colored (yellow) contain mostly gold with platinum and palladium added to increase the melting temperature.

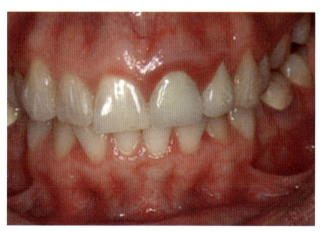

FIG. 12.5 Chronic gingival inflammation due to allergic reaction to a metal substructure of the porcelain-fused-to-metal crown. (Courtesy Dr. Nicole Vane, Encinitas, California.)

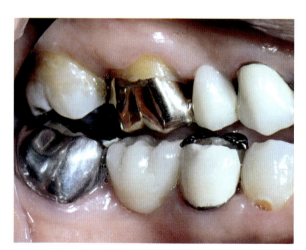

FIG. 12.6 Variety of metal alloys used to restore the teeth. Shown are gold and base-metal alloys and alloys used for porcelain-fused-to-metal crowns. (Courtesy Steve Eakle, University of California, San Francisco, San Francisco, California.)

> **? Do You Recall?**
>
> Why is it important that the dental alloy used in porcelain-fused-to-metal restorations have low thermal expansion?

PORCELAIN-BONDED-TO-METAL RESTORATIONS

Preparing the Metal

Porcelain-bonded-to-metal (also called *porcelain-fused-to-metal* or *PFM*) crowns have a metal substructure (typically 0.3–0.5 mm thick) that is covered with layers of porcelain. The metal substructure (also called a **coping**) must be at least 0.3 mm thick to prevent distortion at high temperatures and must be convex in shape with no sharp angles that would cause stress points in the porcelain leading to fracture. After the metal coping is cast, it is heated at high temperature to form oxides on the surface to which the porcelain bonds.

Porcelain Application to Metal Coping

See Chapter 10, Porcelain-Fused-To-Metal Restorations, for a detailed discussion of porcelain application.

Failure Modes

The metal and porcelain must have compatible rates of thermal expansion or the porcelain will crack as it and the metal cool. Failure can occur within the porcelain or may result from debonding from the metal. Debonding is often a result of contamination of the oxide layer on the metal or an oxide layer that is inadequate or too thick. The American National Standards Institute/American Dental Association (ADA) Specification 38 sets the standard for testing the porcelain-metal bond.

Crown Design

Porcelain-fused-to-metal crowns can have several different designs based on the esthetic demands of the patient and the need for maximal strength.

Occlusal Surface Configuration:
- All-porcelain occlusal surface for esthetic zones where patients do not want metal showing.
  Metal occlusal surface where esthetics is secondary to the need for maximal strength, as with patients who grind their teeth. The buccal surface is covered with porcelain to look like a tooth when the patient smiles.

Margin Configuration:
The margins of the crowns can also have different configurations.
- Porcelain facial margin. It is the most esthetic margin. To create this margin, the metal coping is not extended all the way to the edge of the crown margin so porcelain can be placed to complete the margin (see Fig. 12.7A).
- Disappearing metal margin. The metal at this margin has been ground to a thin, knife edge, where it extends to the edge of the crown margin. Porcelain is applied over the coping (most of the metal disappears from view), except for a thin, dark, metal

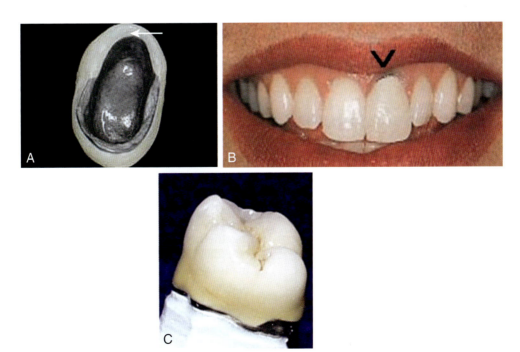

FIG. 12.7 Margin configurations for porcelain-fused-to-metal crowns: **(A)** Porcelain facial margin. **(B)** Disappearing metal margin seen as a dark line at the margin after gingival recession exposes it. **(C)** All-metal margin (metal collar). (A, Courtesy Dr. George Freedman; B, Courtesy Infodentis; C, Courtesy Marotta Dental Studio.)

line (see Fig. 12.7B). Clinicians often place the preparation below the crest of the gingiva to hide this metal line. Over time, the gingiva may recede and expose the dark line of metal. Patients do not like the appearance of this dark line. The dental auxiliary may be asked by the patient what is causing that dark line, so it is important to be able to provide an accurate explanation.
- All-metal margin. The all-metal margin (sometimes called a metal collar) is used only in a nonesthetic zone (Fig. 12.7C).

 Caution

Patients should be advised not to soak their appliances with metal components in household bleach. It will attack and corrode the metal.

IDENTALLOY PROGRAM

Manufacturers of dental alloys have developed a program that certifies the content of the alloys they produce. A certificate (IdentAlloy) is provided for each alloy (Fig. 12.8). It lists the manufacturer, name of the alloy, composition, and the ADA classification and is color coded based on the noble metal content. The certificate is provided with a duplicate, so that both the laboratory and the dentist can have a copy.

Benefits of this program include the following:
1. Assurance the alloy meets the ADA classification criteria
2. Provision of a record for the laboratory in case the US Food and Drug Administration has a recall, the dentist has questions, or future repairs are needed
3. Insurance claims documentation
4. Documentation in the patient's record concerning what was used in case the patient has an allergic reaction to the alloy

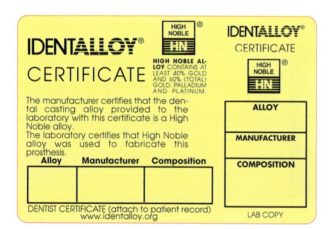

Fig. 12.8 IdentAlloy certificate that indicates the components of the metals used. (Courtesy the IdentAlloy/IdentCeram Council.)

 KEY POINTS

CASTING ALLOYS

Uses
- Partial-coverage and full metal crowns
- All metal bridges or porcelain-fused-to-metal bridges and crowns
- Partial denture frameworks

Types of Metals
- High noble—60% noble metals of which 40% is gold
- Noble metals—at least 25% noble metals (gold, platinum, and palladium), no gold required
- Base metals—no gold, less than 25% noble. Chrome-cobalt and nickel-chrome are the most common
- Small amounts of other elements added to enhance properties and handling

Properties of Casting Alloys
- Melting range rather than point because they are a combination of metals
- Elastic modulus—stiffness needed for partial dentures and bridges
- Thermal expansion—for porcelain-fused-to metal crowns, metal must not expand much when heated or porcelain will crack
- Strength—must resist fracture
- Hardness—resists scratching and denting but is more difficult to polish
- Biocompatible—most alloys are biocompatible, but those containing nickel cause the most allergic response. Beryllium grinding dust is toxic
  IdentAlloy sticker lists name, composition, manufacturer, and ADA classification of alloy for the dental record.

SOLDERS

Metals are joined by three processes:
1. Soldering
2. Brazing
3. Welding

Soldering and brazing are similar and use a molten filler metal to join two other metals together. The difference between soldering and brazing is the temperature at which the procedure is completed. Soldering is performed at temperatures below 450°C and brazing is done at temperatures above 450°C. Because the term *soldering* is the one most commonly used, we use it here to discuss both soldering and brazing. Welding, on the other hand, is a process that uses high heat to fuse two metals together where they contact each other without the use of a filler metal. At one time, custom matrix bands were made by spot welding two ends of a strip of matrix band material together by a device using an electric current.

GOLD SOLDERS

Solders used for crown and bridgework are generally gold-based alloys because they are used with gold alloys that make up the crowns. They generally contain gold, silver, and copper with small portions of zinc and tin. Gold-based solders are used to join together units of a bridge, add proximal contacts, or close holes (before the crown is cemented) accidentally ground in the occlusal surface by adjusting the bite.

Gold-based solder is often categorized according to its fineness. The higher the fineness number, the higher the gold content and the lower the melting point of the solder. Gold solders are available with different melting ranges (690°C to 870°C), depending on their composition, to accommodate the melting ranges of the gold alloys to which they will be soldered. This is important when two gold castings are soldered together or when a proximal contact is added to a gold crown because the solder must melt before the casting. Tin is often added to the solders to lower the melting range and improve the flow of the molten metal.

FLUX

Flux is a chemical compound in paste or powder form applied to the alloy surfaces to be soldered. Flux for gold alloys usually contains borax. Flux removes surface oxides so that the solder will flow freely and will wet the alloy surfaces as it melts. The alloys are heated with a torch until they turn red. The solder is added and heated until it melts and flows over the desired surfaces of the bridge units.

Soldering of units of PFM is much more challenging because the ceramic and the metal alloy have different melting temperatures, and uneven heating of the unit can cause the porcelain to crack. Often soldering of PFM units is done in a special furnace where the temperature can be better controlled than with a torch.

SILVER SOLDERS

Silver-based solders are used more often in orthodontics and pediatric dentistry to solder fixed-space maintainer components (e.g., wire loop soldered to an orthodontic band) and to solder wire components to removable and fixed orthodontic appliances (Fig. 12.9). These solders contain varying amounts of silver, copper, and zinc and small amounts of tin. Silver solder is selected because it melts at a lower temperature (620°C–700°C) than gold solder. The higher heat required to melt gold solder sometimes will degrade the wire adjacent to the solder joint and weaken it.

WROUGHT METAL ALLOYS

Wrought metal alloys are different from casting alloys in that they are formed after the metal is cast. Usually the metal is drawn or extruded through a die or formed in a press to the desired shape, such as a flat plate or a wire or other instrument shape (Fig. 12.10). The mechanical forming of the wrought metal changes the crystalline patterns of the cast metal into a fibrous form. The result is an alloy that is harder and has greater yield strength (the point at which a force can create permanent deformation of the metal). Wrought

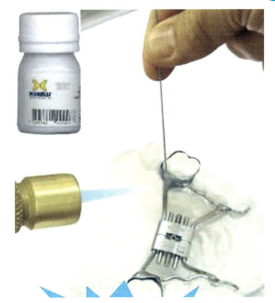

Fig. 12.9 An arch expander unit is attached to a metal orthodontic band with silver solder. (Courtesy Royal Dent.)

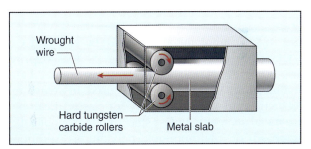

FIG. 12.10 Wrought wire is formed from a slab or thick rod of metal: **(A)** by pulling it through a hard metal die or **(B)** forcing it through rollers.

metal has the characteristic of being able to be heat modified, or annealed, to create differing resistance to deformity. However, overheating can degrade the properties of the metal and make it easier to break.

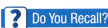 **Do You Recall?**

How do wrought metal alloys difffer from casting alloys?

STAINLESS-STEEL ALLOYS

Steel is made from iron to which a small amount of carbon has been added. Stainless steel is steel to which chromium (12% or more) has been added to reduce tarnish and corrosion. Other metals, such as molybdenum and nickel, may also be added to stainless steel to improve its physical and mechanical properties.

Stainless-steel alloys have the following features that make them popular:
- Low cost
- Good mechanical properties
- Corrosion resistance
They have several applications in dentistry:
- Preformed stainless-steel crowns

- Orthodontic wires, brackets, and bands
- Fixed-space maintainers
- Endodontic files

PREFORMED PROVISIONAL CROWNS

Wrought alloys of stainless steel are used for the fabrication of preformed provisional crowns. They are the most durable of the preformed crowns and can last for months or even years. They come in a variety of sizes that fit most molars and premolars (see Chapter 15). Because more esthetic alternatives are available, they are no longer used much for anterior teeth. These provisional crowns are thin and flexible to fit over minimally prepared teeth.

They are used in pediatric dentistry when trying to protect a primary tooth until it exfoliates. These durable, stainless-steel crowns protect primary teeth following pulpotomy or pulpectomy, caries involving multiple surfaces or fractured teeth. They are occasionally used for adults to protect a tooth when the patient cannot afford a cast metal crown.

Wires

Wire is a wrought metal that may be soft and easily shaped or it may resist bending, as does a spring. Various degrees of resistance to bending can be created by annealing. Wrought metal is used in removable prosthetic appliances, primarily for clasps. It can be a base metal such as stainless steel or a high-noble alloy composed of platinum-gold-palladium. Additional examples of wrought wire used in dentistry include arch bars and ligature wires used in oral surgery for stabilization of a jaw fracture or applications in orthodontics (discussed below).

METALS USED IN ORTHODONTICS

In the early days of orthodontics, wires were made from alloys of noble metals such as gold, platinum, and iridium. Alloys of silver (although not a noble metal) were also used. The development of stainless steel rapidly led to a decline in the use of noble metals. Currently, orthodontic wires are composed mostly of base metals. They may be in single strands of material in a variety of diameters or may be composed of several fine strands twisted or braided together. The wire can be purchased in long strands to be bent by the orthodontist or may be in preformed shapes.

ARCHWIRES

An **archwire** is a curved wire that approximates the general shape of the dental arches.

Special characteristics are manufactured into these archwires to create the desired amount of resistance to being deformed. Resistance to deformity creates "memory" in the wire so that it tries to reassume its original shape. When the archwire is bent slightly, then tied into orthodontic brackets attached to the teeth, it is the "memory" in the wire that exerts the forces that move the teeth.

Archwire Materials

Archwires are composed of three types of base-metal alloys:
- Stainless Steel
  - Readily formed or shaped into the configuration needed
  - Stiff and not very springy
  - Strongest of the archwire materials
- Nickel-Titanium (Ni-Ti)
  - Very resilient and have the most springback or memory to return to their original shape compared with the other alloy wires
  - Readily facilitate tooth movement with lower, more constant force
    - Usually used as preformed archwires because they are difficult to bend at chairside
    - Prone to fracture if bent sharply
- Beta-Titanium
  - Beta-titanium archwire has better springback and ability to be shaped than stainless steel
  - Formulated to produce low force and slow movement of teeth through bone to prevent root damage seen when movement is too fast

See Table 12.3 for the composition of these alloys.

Arch Forms for Archwires

Archwires can be bought preformed to conform to average arch shapes. There are three basic arch forms (Fig. 12.11A):
- Round
- Oval
- Square

Table 12.3 Archwires

ALLOY TYPE	COMPOSITION	FEATURES
Stainless steel	Iron (72%–74%) Chromium (18%) Nickel (8%) Carbon (0.1%)	Inexpensive high strength Corrosion resistant Low springiness Readily shaped
Nickel-titanium (Ni-Ti)	Nickel (55%) Titanium (45%)	Low stiffness Superelastic (rubber like) High springback Shape memory (returns to original shape readily)
Beta-titanium	Titanium (79%) Molybdenum (11%) Zirconium (6%) Tin (4%)	Produces lower forces and better springback than stainless steel Elasticity and strength fall between stainless steel and Ni-Ti

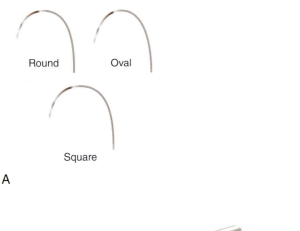

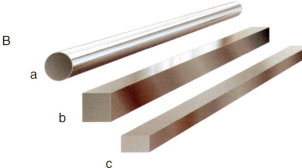

FIG. 12.11 Arch forms for archwires: **(A)** Archwires can be preformed to the three basic arch forms: round, oval, square as seen in the curved part of the wire. **(B)** Orthodontic wire shapes in cross-section: (a) round, (b) square, and (c) rectangular.

The orthodontist must custom shape archwires when the arch shape varies significantly from these basic forms.

Archwire Shapes in Cross-Section
Archwires come in three shapes, as seen in cross-section (Fig.12.11B):
- Round
- Square
- Rectangular

Each shape has a use in different phases of orthodontic treatment. Often the round wire is used in the initial stages to get the teeth moving. In the latter stages, the rectangular wire more closely fits the shape of the bracket and provides more control in finalizing the position of the teeth. However, orthodontists have their own preferences as to which wires to use and when to use them.

Archwire Size
The size refers to the diameter or thickness of the wire. The diameter of wire is sometimes referred to as its gauge. The thicker the wire, the smaller its gauge; thus 8-gauge wire is thicker than 16-gauge wire. The diameter of wire is more commonly described in hundredths of an inch (e.g., 0.36 inches). Smaller diameter wires are more flexible and elastic. Thicker wires are much stiffer.

Archwire Ligation
Two basic methods have been used to tie (ligate) the archwire to the brackets:
- Ligature wire
- Elastics

For years, fine stainless-steel wires were used. A ligature wire was wrapped around the bracket and over the archwire and the ends twisted to hold the archwire in place. Lips and cheeks could rub against the ligature wire and cause soreness.

For the most part, elastics resembling tiny rubber bands have replaced ligature wires. They are stretched over the arms of the bracket and hold the archwire in place. They are soft and less likely to cause mouth irritation and easy to apply.

BRACKETS AND BANDS

Orthodontic brackets and bands are bonded or cemented on the teeth, and they retain the archwire that the orthodontist has shaped. When the wire is tied to the brackets of the teeth, the wire tries to assume its ideal form, and as a result, exerts a force on the teeth that gradually moves them in the desired direction.

Metal orthodontic brackets are cut and shaped from stainless-steel alloy and are attached to a stainless mesh backing (Fig. 7.32). They are bonded to the tooth with bonding resin or other appropriate luting cement that locks into the mesh backing. The edgewise bracket, which is the most common, has a horizontal slot between four wings. The slot is where the archwire is placed, and the wings are used to hold the elastics or ligature wire that secures the archwire (Fig. 12.12). Orthodontic bands are formed from a stainless-steel alloy and are preformed. Stainless-steel brackets, tubes, and hooks are welded onto the bands or brackets for the purpose of attaching intraoral wires, elastics, or extraoral headgear (see Fig. 12.12).

 Do You Recall?

What is an archwire and what does it do?

RETAINERS AND REMOVABLE ORTHODONTIC APPLIANCES

A retainer is often placed to help maintain the position of the teeth after orthodontic treatment. Retainers are of two general types:
- Fixed
- Removable

A fixed lingual retainer is simply a wire adapted to the lingual surfaces of the lower or upper anterior

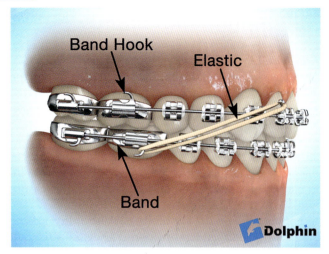

FIG. 12.12 Orthodontic bands with tubes and hooks, edgewise brackets, archwires, and elastics used for tooth movement. (Courtesy North Coast Orthodontics.)

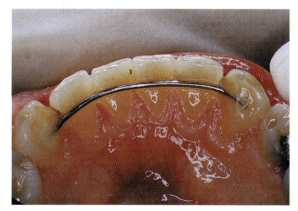

FIG. 12.13 Orthodontic bonded wire lingual retainer. (Courtesy Steve Eakle, University of California, San Francisco, San Francisco, California.)

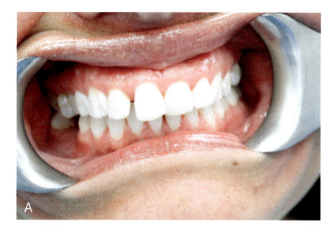

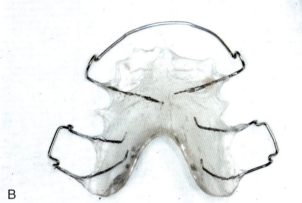

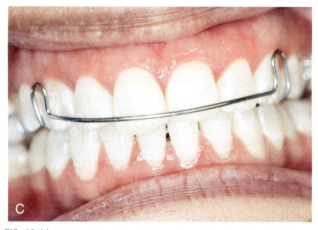

FIG. 12.14 Removable orthodontic appliance to retract tooth 8. It can serve as a retainer after tooth movement has been accomplished: **(A)** Protruding maxillary central incisor. **(B)** Hawley appliance with adjustable labial wire bow to move tooth lingually. **(C)** Tooth has been repositioned. (Courtesy Dr. Scott Rooker, Bend, Oregon.)

teeth and bonded in place with composite resin (Fig. 12.13).

A removable retainer often uses a wire embedded in acrylic to engage the facial surfaces of the teeth and holds them in position. Some removable appliances can be used for minor tooth movement. In this case, the wire is activated to put pressure on the teeth to be moved (Fig. 12.14). After the teeth have moved into their desired position, the appliance can be used as a retainer by keeping the wire resting passively against the facial surfaces of the teeth.

SPACE MAINTAINERS

When teeth are lost prematurely, it is desirable to prevent adjacent teeth from drifting into the space. If the space of a primary tooth is lost, the permanent tooth may not have room to erupt into its proper position.

If a drifting neighbor takes up the space of a lost permanent tooth, there may not be adequate room for a bridge or implant and the drifting tooth may tip into the space. Fixed and removable space maintainers are often used temporarily to hold the space. Common fixed-space maintainers consist of a wire loop that is attached to a stainless-steel crown or an orthodontic band. The loop rests against the adjacent tooth and holds it in position (Fig. 12.15).

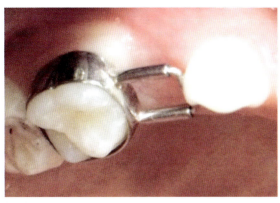

FIG. 12.15 Fixed band and loop space maintainer. (Courtesy Brent Lin, Pediatric Dentistry, University of California, San Francisco, California.)

METALS USED IN ENDODONTICS

ENDODONTIC FILES AND REAMERS

Endodontic files and reamers are other examples of wrought metal used in endodontics. They are made of wrought wire that has been twisted to produce multiple cutting edges (Fig. 12.16).

Files

Files are made of stainless steel or nickel-titanium and are used within the root canal to clean and shape it for final filling. Stainless-steel files become stiffer as the diameter of the file increases. This stiffness is not desirable when curved canals are instrumented because the files tend to remove more dentin at the point of the curvature. Nickel-titanium (nitinol) files are far more flexible than stainless-steel files. They have an enhanced elastic characteristic that allows them to return to their original shape after they have had a load or force put on them. When used for instrumenting curved canals, they will regain their shape, unlike stainless-steel files.

Rotary Instruments

Some files are used to instrument root canals by hand, and some are used in slow-speed dental handpieces at low speeds and are called *rotary instruments*. Rotary instruments are usually composed of nickel and titanium alloys. Rotary instruments are very popular and allow root canal therapy to proceed much faster and more efficiently. Their flexibility is highly desirable in a curved canal because they can follow the curvature of the canal more easily and remove less dentin than stainless-steel files.

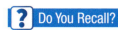

Do You Recall?

Why is nickel-titanium alloy popular for rotary endodontic files?

File Breakage

Both hand files and rotary files are subject to metal fatigue that can cause fracture of the file after repeated use. If the file fractures within the root canal, it might not be able to be removed. This could result in failure of the root canal treatment. The dentist and the assistant should determine how many times a file can be used, and then should discard the file when it has reached that limit. A tracking system must be developed to document how many times each file has been used.

Reamers

Reamers are similar to files except that they have fewer twists in the metal and cut faster. Reamers are made by twisting a tapered triangular or square rod so that its cutting edge is parallel to its long axis. It is used for cutting canal walls to enlarge and shape them. A reamer will remove debris from the canal more efficiently than a file.

ENDODONTIC POSTS

Teeth in which the pulpal tissues are infected or die often receive root canal therapy (endodontic treatment). Conventional root canal therapy generally entails making an access preparation through the crown of the tooth to the pulp chamber, removing the diseased pulpal tissue from within the root canal with a series of fine files, and sealing the root canal space with a special sealing material (gutta percha) and a sealing cement so that bacteria cannot grow in the space.

PURPOSE OF THE POST

Endodontic posts are metal or nonmetal dowels or rods placed within the root canal space after a root canal treatment. The purpose of a post is to retain the core buildup over which the final restoration (crown) is placed. If there is adequate tooth structure remaining to hold the core buildup without a post, a post should not be used. While the choice of using posts or other retaining designs is up to the dentist, it is important for all clinicians to be familiar with the various types of posts that might be used. Dental auxiliaries are often asked questions by patients about the materials they see in their teeth on the radiographs mounted on the view box or seen on the monitor. Some patients may confuse the post with an implant and need to be educated as to the differences.

CLASSIFICATION OF POSTS

Post can be classified in several ways:
- Active or passive posts: Active posts engage the root canal surface with threads like a screw. Passive posts are simply cemented into the canal space without actively engaging the canal walls.

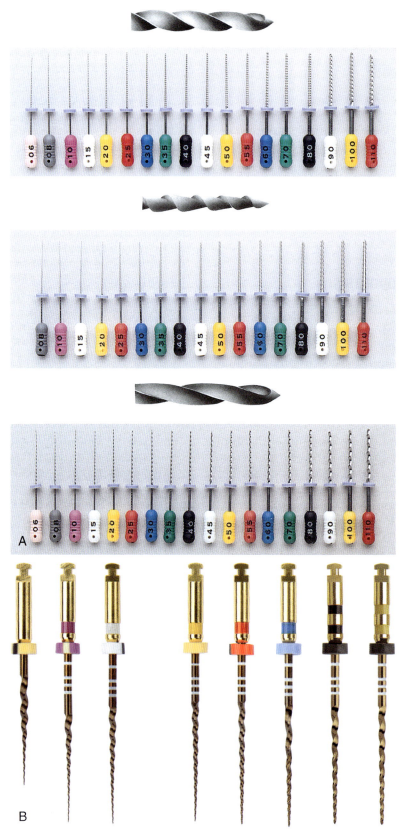

FIG. 12.16 A variety of endodontic files: **(A)** Types of hand files. **(B)** Rotary files. ((A) From Robinson DS, Bird DL: Endodontics. In *Essentials of dental assisting*, ed 6. St. Louis, 2017, Elsevier. **(B)** Courtesy Dentsply Sirona.)

- Parallel or tapered posts: Classified by the shape of their sides: parallel or tapered. Parallel posts have been shown by in vitro studies (meaning they were done in a laboratory) to transmit less stress to the root than tapered posts. Tapered posts, when loaded, place a wedging force on the root, with a higher risk of root fracture.
- Metal or nonmetal posts: Made of metal or can be nonmetal such as ceramic (Table 12.4).
- Custom-made or preformed posts can be custom made in the laboratory (cast posts) or can be purchased preformed in various sizes and materials.

Custom posts are made from a wax or resin pattern made directly on the tooth or in the laboratory on a replica of the preparation (a die) poured from an impression of the tooth and canal space. They are cast into metal or ceramic using the lost wax technique, or can be milled using CAD/CAM techniques (see Chapter 10). Noble or base-metal alloys or ceramic-fired materials are used. Cast and CAD/CAM posts generally are made as one unit with the core already attached.

Preformed posts are available from many commercial sources and are by far the most commonly used posts (Fig. 12.17). They can be used in most clinical situations, are inexpensive, and can be placed in one appointment (Fig. 12.18). Preformed posts are much more time efficient than cast posts, which take two appointments. The designs of these preformed posts are active or passive, parallel or tapered, and metal or nonmetal. They rely on retention by their length, diameter, and shape and by the use of a cementing or bonding medium (see Chapter 7 and 16). Preformed posts come in kits with drills specific to the size and style of the post. Preformed metal posts are made of stainless steel, titanium, or titanium alloy. Preformed nonmetal posts are made of fiber-reinforced resin or ceramic materials. Preformed posts generally do not have a core attached by the manufacturer, so one must be added (Fig. 12.19). The core can be made of amalgam, composite resin, or resin-modified glass ionomer cement.

Table 12.4	Composition of Posts
CUSTOM CAST POSTS	
Nickel-chromium alloy (Ni-Cr)	
Cobalt-chromium alloy (Co-Cr)	
Gold alloy (ADA type IV)	
Palladium-silver alloy	
PREFORMED POSTS	
A. Metal	
Titanium (99% pure)	
Stainless steel (Fe-Ni-Cr)	
Titanium-aluminum-vanadium alloy (Ti-Al-V)	
B. Nonmetal	
Ceramic (zirconia)	
Fiber-reinforced resin	

ADA, American Dental Association.

KEY POINTS

WROUGHT METAL ALLOYS
Uses
1. Wire—orthodontic archwire or retainers (fixed or removable)
2. Preformed crowns
3. Endodontic files

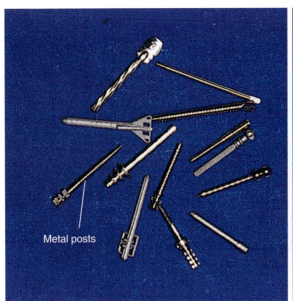
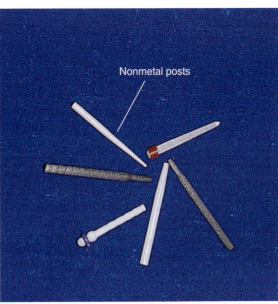

FIG. 12.17 A variety of preformed metal and nonmetal posts.

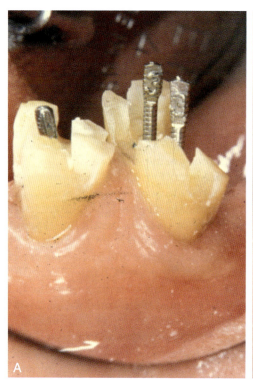
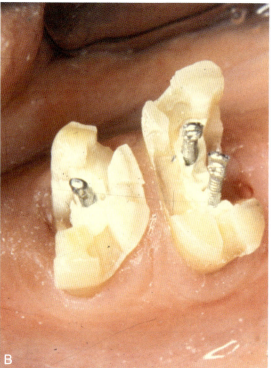

FIG. 12.18 Clinical photographs of preformed metal posts: (**A** and **B**) show two views of preformed metal posts that will be used to retain a composite resin core. Supplemental retention boxes have been cut to lock in the core material. (Courtesy Dr. Dennis J. Weir, Novato, California.)

> ### KEY POINTS—cont'd
> **Materials**
> 1. Stainless steel—strong but stiff; when used for orthodontic wire, has low springback to original shape
> 2. Nickel-titanium—for archwire has greatest springback; for endodontic files, has good flexibility and useful for rotary files. Very popular material for these uses
> 3. Beta-titanium—good springback for archwire and generates low force for moving teeth
>   **Other alloy uses**
> Endodontic posts—to support a core buildup for crown or bridge
>   Types—preformed or cast
>   Materials used—metal or nonmetal
>   1. Metals—stainless steel, titanium and its alloys, cast gold
>   2. Nonmetals—ceramic and resin

SUMMARY

Metals play a major role in restorative and corrective dentistry. Gold and alloys of gold are some of the most biologically compatible materials and have many uses, even with the shift toward cosmetic dentistry. Noble and non-noble cast metals have a significant role in modern prosthetic dentistry. They are the main support for removable partial dentures, fixed bridges, and prostheses used in combination with implants. Orthodontic treatment relies heavily on the use of metal. Brackets are predominantly metal, although some are ceramic. Wrought wire, with its "memory,"

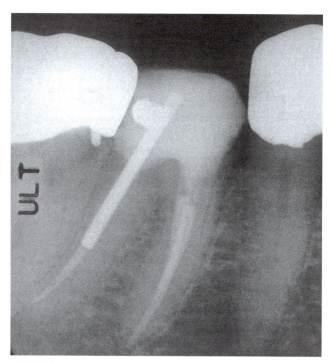

FIG. 12.19 Radiograph of lower first molar with endodontic gutta percha filling and metal preformed post in the distal canal. A composite core has been added. The post retains the core. (Courtesy Dr. Steve Eakle.)

exerts predictable forces and has made the job of the orthodontic clinician easier, improved comfort for the patient, and reduced the time needed for treatment. Titanium is a lightweight metal and has good characteristics of strength and elasticity. Titanium alloy is the main alloy used for dental implant fixtures (see Chapter 13). It is used as an alloy with nickel for archwires in orthodontics and for endodontic hand files and rotary instruments. Endodontic treatment has moved into the modern era with the use of rotary files and the controlled speed of the electrical handpiece. Likewise, the restoration of endodontically treated teeth and the use of post and core materials have changed dramatically. Now, both metal and nonmetal posts are available for the dentist to select for the process of restoring endodontically treated teeth. The indications for each are important for the clinician to understand.

Patient education is an important aspect of the role of the dental auxiliary in dental practice. The auxiliary's ability to describe to the patient the pros and cons of the various materials used in practice and to aid in the treatment process depends on their knowledge of these materials. As new metal-based materials are introduced into dental practice, it is important to stay current on their properties, indications, contraindications, and application techniques. Manufacturers' instructions for the care and use of materials should be followed. Many manufacturers have websites on which they post information relative to their materials.

INSTRUCTIONAL VIDEOS

See the Evolve Resources site for a variety of educational videos that reinforce the material covered in this chapter.

Review and Discussion

Review Questions

Select the one correct response for each of the following multiple-choice questions.

1. The ADA recognizes which three major categories of alloys?
   a. High noble, noble, and low noble
   b. High noble, noble, and base metal
   c. Precious, semiprecious, and nonprecious
   d. Class I, II, and III
2. High-noble metal classification must contain what percent by weight of gold?
   a. 40%
   b. 60%
   c. 75%
   d. 90%
3. Noble metal elements include all of the following except:
   a. Palladium
   b. Gold
   c. Silver
   d. Platinum
4. How does porcelain bond to metal alloys?
   a. By fusing to oxides formed on the surface of the metal
   b. By sandblasting the metal surface to roughen it
   c. By the use of metal bonding adhesive systems
   d. By melting the surface of the metal and embedding the porcelain in it
5. When bonding porcelain to metal for a crown, the metal must have which one of the following properties to prevent cracking of the porcelain?
   a. High hardness
   b. High density
   c. Low melting range
   d. Low thermal expansion
6. Metal that is formed by casting into an ingot or bar and then is altered in its form by extruding or pressing it is known as:
   a. Stainless steel
   b. Wrought metal
   c. Milled metal
   d. Brazed metal
7. High-noble alloys usually have which metals added to increase their hardness?
   a. Silver or copper
   b. Nickel or beryllium
   c. Iron or aluminum
   d. Chromium or cobalt
8. Which type of orthodontic wire has the most springiness and tendency to maintain its original shape?
   a. Stainless steel
   b. Cobalt-chrome nickel
   c. Gold
   d. Nickel-titanium
9. Which one of the following statements about an archwire is true?
   a. It comes as a long, straight wire that must be bent by the dentist to the shape of the arch.
   b. It breaks easily when bent.
   c. The thicker the wire, the more springback it has.
   d. Its resistance to being shaped creates memory in the wire that helps to move teeth.
10. Allergy to nickel:
    a. Occurs in less than 3% of the population
    b. Is seen only in the oral cavity
    c. Occurs 10 times more often in females than in males
    d. Is associated more often with orthodontic wire than with crowns

Review and Discussion—cont'd

11. Solder has all of the following uses *except* one. Which one?
    a. Adding a proximal contact to a crown
    b. Joining a pontic to a bridge retainer
    c. Repairing a hole in the occlusal surface of a crown cemented in a patient's mouth
    d. Joining a wire loop to a band to make a space retainer
12. The purpose of flux used during soldering is to:
    a. Lower the melting point of the solder
    b. Make the solder harden quickly
    c. Prevent the solder from flowing to areas where the solder is not needed
    d. Remove oxides from the surfaces of the metals so the solder can flow and wet the surfaces better
13. Preformed metal posts are available in all of the following materials *except* one. Which one?
    a. Pure gold
    b. Stainless steel
    c. Titanium
    d. Titanium alloy
14. The purpose of a post is to:
    a. Retain the core buildup material
    b. Put a permanent seal over the root canal filling material
    c. Strengthen the core material
    d. Strengthen the root
15. An all-metal crown that is yellow in color has which one of the following?
    a. A high gold content
    b. A high copper content
    c. A high palladium content
    d. Cannot tell the composition from the color
16. All of the following statements about cast posts are true *except* one. Which one?
    a. They may be formed from a wax or acrylic resin pattern.
    b. They can be cast using high-noble, noble, or base-metal alloys.
    c. They usually have the core already attached to the post.
    d. They are used in practice far more often than preformed posts.
17. The alloy most used for partial denture frameworks and most resistant to fatigue failure of the clasps is which one of the following?
    a. Cobalt-chromium alloy
    b. Stainless steel
    c. Gold alloy
    d. Titanium alloy

For answers to Review Questions, see the Appendix.

Case-Based Discussion Topics

1. A 33-year-old schoolteacher comes to the dental office to have a crown placed on tooth 18. The dentist has told the patient that they should have a gold crown. After the dentist has left the room, the patient asks you if there are any cheaper metals that could be used. The patient says that they have no insurance and is short of money at this time. *What can you tell the patient about the general types of metals used for cast crowns and what the pros and cons are for each?*
2. A 65-year-old retired accountant comes to the dental office with a gold crown for tooth 19 in their hand. It came off last night while eating sticky candy. The patient complains that since the crown was placed last year, food has been packing between the crown and tooth 20, which has a disto-occlusal amalgam. Floss passes without resistance in that interproximal space. The crown has an acceptable fit to the tooth and no dental caries are present. The amalgam is also acceptable. *While the crown is off, what procedures can you suggest to solve the food impaction problem without making a new crown or replacing the amalgam? What materials should be used? Describe the correct sequence for the procedure(s).*
3. A 46-year-old business professional complains that the gum has receded on tooth 12 and now a dark line can be seen at the margin of a porcelain-bonded-to-metal crown that was placed 5 years ago. The patient is unhappy with the appearance and is concerned that it might be "decay." When you check, there is no decay present. *What is the likely cause of the dark line the patient is referring to? How might the dentist have prevented this from occurring?*
4. A 34-year-old schoolteacher presents to your dental office complaining that a cusp has broken off the lower-left first molar. Visual inspection reveals that tooth 19 is missing the distolingual cusp down to the gingival crest, and a large MOD amalgam is present. The patient is a heavy bruxer and admits to nighttime teeth grinding. The dentist recommends a crown to restore the tooth. *From a strictly functional perspective, what type of crown would be the most trouble free and durable? If the patient selects a PFM crown with porcelain on the occlusal surface, what should the patient be told regarding the risks and benefits of this type of crown?*
5. As you are preparing for a cementation appointment for a porcelain-bonded-to-metal crown for tooth 5, you notice several small cracks in the porcelain. The crown has just come from the lab and has not been in the patient's mouth. *If the crown was not dropped or otherwise mishandled, what is one explanation for how these occurred? Discuss compatibility problems as they relate to the physical properties of the porcelain and the porcelain-bonded alloy. Should the dentist proceed with the cementation of the crown?*
6. A 58-year-old mail carrier presents for an annual periodic examination. The patient has noticed some inflammation in the gum around tooth 14 that started 2 weeks after a base-metal crown was placed last year. The patient has been brushing and flossing carefully but the inflammation does not go away. *What are some possible causes for the inflammation? If a prophylaxis and application of antibiotics to the sulcus have no effect, what now becomes a greater suspect for the cause? If the dental laboratory uses IdentAlloy labels, what information can you obtain that might help in determining the likely cause?*

BIBLIOGRAPHY

American Dental Association (ADA): *Council on scientific affairs: products of excellence: ADA seal program,* Chicago, 1999, ADA.

Bird DL, Robinson DS: *Endodontics.* In *Modern Dental Assisting,* ed 13, St. Louis, 2021, Elsevier.

Department of Health and Human Services, Agency for Toxic Substances and Disease Registry: *Beryllium toxicity: patient education care instruction sheet.* 2008. Accessible at https://www.atsdr.cdc.gov/csem/beryllium/patient_education.html.

Leinfelder KF: An evaluation of casting alloys used for restorative procedures, *J Am Dent Assoc* 128:37–45, 1997.

Powers JM, Wataha JC: Casting alloys, wrought alloys and solders. In *Dental Materials: Foundations and Applications,* St. Louis, 2017, Elsevier.

Roach M: Base metal alloys used for dental restorations and implants, *Dent Clin N Am* 51(3):603–627, 2007.

Robinson DS, Bird DL: Endodontics. In *Essentials of Dental Assisting,* St. Louis, 2017, Elsevier.

Rosenstiel SF, Land MF, Walter RD: *Laboratory procedures. Contemporary Fixed Prosthodontics,* ed 6, St. Louis, 2023, Elsevier.

Sakaguchi RL, Ferracane J, Powers JM: Restorative materials—metals. In *Craig's Restorative Dental Materials,* ed 14, St. Louis, 2019, Elsevier.

Sansone V, Pagani D, Melato M: The effects on bone cells of metal ions released from orthopaedic implants. A review, *Clin Cases Miner Bone Metab* 10(1):34–40, 2013.

Shen C, Rawls HR, Equivel-Upshaw JF: Metals. In *Phillips' Science of Dental Materials,* ed 13, St. Louis, 2022, Elsevier.

Van Noort R: Structure of metals and alloys. In *Introduction to Dental Materials,* ed 4, St. Louis, 2013, Elsevier.

13 Dental Implants

http://evolve.elsevier.com/Eakle/materials/

Chapter Objectives

On completion of this chapter, the student should be able to:
1. Describe the components of an implant used for a crown.
2. List the most common materials used for dental implants.
3. Explain osseointegration of an implant.
4. Discuss the indications and contraindications for dental implants.
5. Identify risks to the patient for implant surgery.
6. Compare the one-stage, two-stage, and immediate surgical procedures.
7. Make an impression for an implant using the open- or closed-tray procedure (as permitted by state law).
8. Identify the uses for mini-implants.
9. Describe the assessments that should be done for dental implants at the hygiene visit.
10. Demonstrate to a patient the use of home care aids for dental implants.
11. Explain the rationale for the selection of instruments for cleaning titanium implants.
12. List the different types of sutures.
13. Demonstrate the removal of sutures.

KEY TERMS

Endosseous Implant implant placed into the bone
Implant Fixture metal or ceramic component placed into bone to support a crown or prosthesis
Implant Abutment metal or ceramic component that connects the implant crown to the implant fixture
Healing Abutment a component placed temporarily on the implant fixture during the healing phase to allow the gingiva to adapt to it and form a cuff that will function around the implant
Cover Screw component placed in the top of the implant fixture to prevent tissue from growing into the screw hole when the fixture is covered with the flap in a two-stage surgical procedure
Osseointegration bone growing into intimate contact with an implant fixture after placement (a microscopic space exists between the bone and the implant surface)
Biointegration a total integration of the implant fixture with the bone (without a microscopic space) that occurs with ceramic implant materials
Mini-Implant a very small-diameter implant that can be placed with minimal surgery involved
Cone Beam Computed Tomography (CBCT) type of digital tomographic radiography used to produce three-dimensional images of the jaws; useful for analyzing the structures before surgery
Impression Abutment component used in the implant impression to align the implant analog in the same way as the implant fixture was in the mouth
Implant Analog a substitute for the implant fixture used during the laboratory fabrication of the implant crown

Open-Tray Impression impression for implants that uses a tray with a hole over the impression abutments to be able to remove the abutments with the impression
Closed-Tray Impression impression for implant that removes the impression with the impression abutment still attached to the implant fixture; the abutment is later removed and placed in the impression
Temporary Anchor Devices (TADs) small, tack-like mini-implants used on a temporary basis as anchors for orthodontic tooth movement
Autograft graft tissue harvested from the patient's own body
Allograft tissue taken from a donor (usually deceased) for grafting in another human
Xenograft graft tissue taken from an animal (usually bovine) for use in a human
Alloplast synthetic graft material
Sinus Lift a surgical procedure that lifts up the floor of the maxillary sinus to allow placement of a bone graft. It is used to provide adequate bone for an implant when there was not enough available over the maxillary sinus
Peri-implantitis an infection around an implant that can cause gingival inflammation and loss of bone around the implant
Sutures natural or synthetic material with the appearance of thread used to hold tissues together or to reposition tissues after trauma or surgical procedures
Absorbable Sutures sutures broken down naturally by the body's enzymes and absorbed
Nonabsorbable Sutures sutures made of materials that are not broken down by the body and require removal by a dental professional

For centuries people have attempted to replace missing teeth with some form of implant. Over the years, many materials and implant designs have been used with limited success. A major breakthrough came in 1969 when P.-I. Brånemark and coworkers, using medical implants, reported their finding of integration of bone with an implant surface. The Brånemark dental implant system was introduced into the United States in 1982. The development of endosseous root-form implant treatment has rapidly progressed over the last 40+ years with high success rates. Advances in technology with cone beam computed tomography (CBCT) and computer-aided design software have helped dentists more accurately plan for and place dental implants. Bone grafting and guided tissue regeneration have helped to improve bone in sites for implant placement where previously the patient would have not been considered a candidate for implants. The use of implants in modern dentistry has accelerated rapidly, with sales of implant components exceeding $3.5 billion worldwide.

This chapter emphasizes endosseous implants because they are the most widely used. The materials used for implants and the indications, contraindications, placement, restoration, integration with bone, components, and maintenance are discussed. It is essential that the dental hygienist have an understanding of the characteristics of the various implant materials to correctly manipulate and care for them. The dental auxiliary must be able to answer questions by patients relative to the material and techniques that will be used for their treatment. In addition, they must have an understanding of the process of restoring implant fixtures so they can skillfully assist the dentist. Where allowed by state law, dental auxiliary trained in expanded functions can make impressions for implant restorations and play an important role in implant maintenance.

DENTAL IMPLANTS

Dental implants are of three main types (Fig. 13.1):
- Subperiosteal
- Transosteal
- Endosseous

SUBPERIOSTEAL IMPLANTS

With subperiosteal implants a surgical excision exposes the bony ridge and an impression is made. A metal framework is fabricated and placed over the bony ridge (and beneath the periosteum) with metal struts protruding through the soft tissues to support a prosthesis.

TRANSOSTEAL IMPLANT

The transosteal implant (also called a *mandibular staple*) is placed from under the chin and has a flat plate from which two to four threaded posts projected through

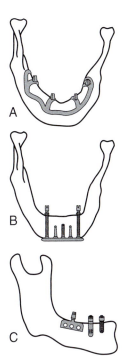

FIG. 13.1 Older implant types: **(A)** Subperiosteal. **(B)** Transosteal. **(C)** Older variety of endosseous implants. (From Phillips RW, Moore BK: *Elements of Dental Materials for Dental Hygienists and Dental Assistants*. WB Saunders; 1994.)

the anterior mandible into the oral cavity. The posts are used to support a complete denture.

Subperiosteal and transosteal implants are rarely done because of the high success rate of endosseous implants. **Endosseous implants** are the most commonly used implants in dentistry today and are the focus of this chapter.

ENDOSSEOUS IMPLANTS

Endosseous implants are surgically placed into the bone and act like a root substitute for missing teeth to support a crown or prosthesis (Fig. 13.2). Implants can be used to replace one or more single units as individual crowns or as fixed bridges, or they can support a partial or full denture. Their use is expanding as implant materials and techniques continue to improve, and their success rate remains high with careful case selection. Clinical studies have shown these implants to be very successful, with long-term survival (greater than 10 years) of approximately 90% in the maxilla and 95% in the mandible. The difference in success rates between the two jaws is related to the quality of the bone in each jaw. The bone in the mandible is generally much denser.

INDICATIONS FOR IMPLANTS

Implants are indicated for a variety of clinical situations. Because of the excellent survival rate of implants, they are often the treatment of choice in place of a partial denture or a fixed bridge when a single tooth has been

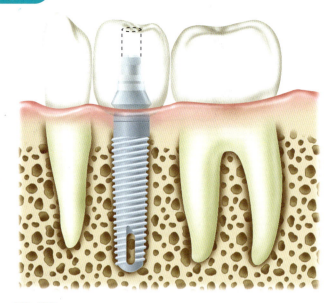

FIG. 13.2 Contemporary endosseous dental implant. (From Rosenstiel SF, Land MF, Fujimoto J. *Contemporary Fixed Prosthodontics*. 4th ed. Mosby; 2006.)

lost, particularly when the potential abutment teeth are unrestored. When a patient has a problem stabilizing a denture because of extreme ridge resorption, implants can be used to anchor the denture. Implants may also be indicated to improve function and esthetics.

CONTRAINDICATIONS FOR IMPLANTS

Implants are contraindicated in patients who have medical conditions (such as advanced cardiovascular or respiratory disease) that make them poor candidates for surgery. Patients with conditions that can affect their ability to fight infections or heal properly (such as diabetes) are not good candidates for implants. Patients who have recently taken bisphosphonates (such as Boniva and Zometa) to prevent osteoporosis or that have had radiation therapy affecting the implant site are not candidates for implants because of the risk of delayed bone healing and bone infection (osteonecrosis). Patients with compromised immune systems are also not candidates for implants. Smokers are not good candidates because their healing may be compromised. In addition, patients who are mentally or physically not able to maintain good oral hygiene or those with unrealistic expectations are not candidates for implants.

BENEFITS OF IMPLANTS

Dental implants have several benefits that make them a desirable means for restoring the dentition. When implants are used in place of a fixed bridge, the tooth structure is preserved because abutments do not have to be prepared. The individual implant units are easier to keep clean than a fixed bridge, so the gingiva stays healthier and the caries incidence of adjacent teeth is lowered. When teeth are extracted, the bone at the site begins to resorb (shrink from bone loss) fairly rapidly soon afterward and then continues more slowly over time. When an implant is placed it helps to preserve the bone both in ridge height and width.

Patients with complete dentures can bite and chew with only a small fraction of the force they could with their natural teeth. The muscles of mastication weaken and show signs of atrophy and the ridges resorb. With an implant-supported denture, biting, chewing, and speaking are improved. Muscle tone is regained and the implants help preserve bone. The patient is more comfortable, especially when chewing hard foods, and does not have the discomfort associated with shifting of the denture and pressure on the soft tissues. The esthetic result is often improved because the teeth can be set where they are most attractive rather than being limited to placement over the center of a ridge.

IMPLANT COMPONENTS

Numerous components are used for restoration with an implant. Some components are permanent parts of the implant, and others are used temporarily for healing phases, impression making, or crown construction. Different terms may be used to describe them, depending on the manufacturer. Conventional dental implants used to support crowns and bridges have three basic components: the implant fixture, abutment, and crown (or bridge) (Fig. 13.3).

Implant Fixture
The *implant fixture* is that portion of the implant that is placed in the bone and remains there to support the crown (or other prosthesis).

Implant Abutment
The *implant abutment* is attached to the implant fixture that protrudes through the gingiva and acts like a tooth preparation on which the crown attaches or the prosthesis rests. The abutment is usually attached to the fixture with a screw.

Healing Abutment
Another type of abutment is the healing abutment. It is attached to the fixture and is placed temporarily to allow the gingiva to heal around it and form a gingival cuff and sulcus.

Preformed or Custom Made Abutment. Both the abutment for a crown and the healing abutment may be prefabricated or custom made. Prefabricated abutments are generally round, so the gingiva conforms to the round shape. However, teeth are rarely round in shape. Custom abutments are shaped more like the root form of the teeth they are replacing. The custom abutment may be made by a laboratory technician or milled by a CAD/CAM (computer-aided design/computer-aided machining) unit.

Implant Crown or Prosthesis
When a single tooth is being replaced, a crown is made to fit to the abutment much like a crown is made to

fit to a prepared tooth. When multiple teeth are being replaced, an implant supported fixed bridge, removable complete denture, or partial denture is used.

Other Components

Additional components are needed in the implant procedure. Titanium alloy screws are used to attach the abutment to the implant fixture and in some cases will attach the crown to the abutment. Of course, a screwdriver is also needed. The **cover screw** is the component that is placed in the top of the implant fixture to prevent bone and tissue growth into the top of the implant while it is covered with the surgical flap during the healing phase. The healing abutment replaces the cover screw after the top of the implant is uncovered (see Fig. 13.3A). A torque wrench is used to tighten various components of the implant to very specific amounts of force. Impression and laboratory components are discussed in the section "Implant Impression and Laboratory Components."

IMPLANT MATERIALS

Various materials have been used for implant fixtures over the years, but metal and ceramics are the materials currently used. The metals of choice are titanium and titanium alloy.

Titanium

Titanium (Ti) and titanium alloys are the metals most commonly used because of their favorable biocompatibility with the oral tissues. Their elastic modulus is the closest to bone of the materials used for implants. As a result, forces placed on the implant will be more evenly distributed between the implant and the bone. Those implant materials with an elastic modulus much greater than bone will concentrate stress within the implant.

Titanium is a lightweight, corrosion-resistant, biocompatible material that is 99% titanium with oxygen and trace elements. Bone will grow around and closely adapt to titanium and titanium alloy implants (a process called **osseointegration**) when they are placed intimately in contact with the bone (Fig. 13.4). There should be no fibrous connective tissue formed at the interface, but there will be a microscopic space present between the fixture surface and the bone. There will be no mobility of the implant.

Titanium is not as rigid or strong as titanium alloy, and this property can occasionally lead to fracture of an implant if it is placed under heavy loading forces (such as with patients who grind their teeth frequently). Titanium quickly forms a thin surface layer of oxides that will integrate with the bone. Titanium alloys

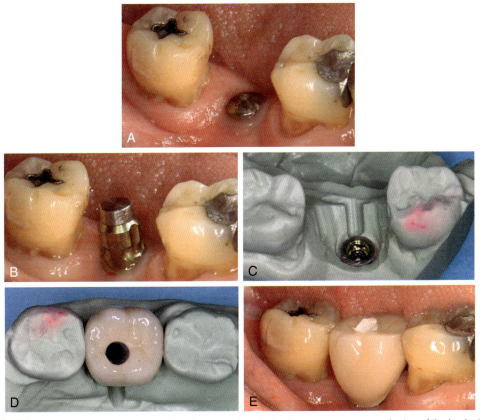

FIG. 13.3 Implant components: **(A)** Healing abutment placed after the surgeon uncovers the top of the implant fixture to allow the soft tissue to adapt. **(B)** Impression abutment facilitates orientation of an implant analog to the cast in the same way the implant fixture was oriented in the mouth. **(C)** Implant analog is used in the laboratory as a substitute for the implant fixture, so the implant crown can be made. **(D)** Screw-retained implant crown with occlusal screw-access hole. **(E)** Implant crown in the mouth with the access hole filled. (Courtesy Fritz Finzen, University of California School of Dentistry, San Francisco, California.)

Table 13.1 Mechanical Properties of Dental Implant Materials

MATERIAL	YIELD STRENGTH (MPA)*	ELASTIC MODULUS (GPA)*	TENSILE STRENGTH (MPA)*
Titanium	170	102	240
Titanium alloy (Ti-6Al-4V)	860	113	930
Zirconia	1200	200	350

*1 MPa = 145 psi (pounds per square inch); 1 GPa = 1000 MPa
Adapted from Shen C, Rawls HR, Esquivel-Upshaw JF. *Phillips' Science of Dental Materials.* 13th ed. Elsevier; 2022.

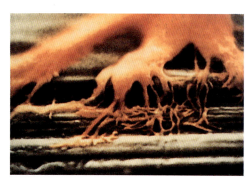

FIG. 13.4 Osseointegration: bone cells growing in contact with a titanium implant. Courtesy Professor Per-Ingvar Branemark, Institute for Applied Biotechnology, Gothenburg, Sweden.

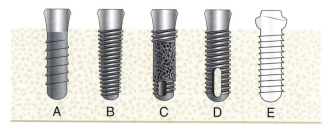

FIG. 13.5 Implant designs. From left to right: **(A)** Cylinder. **(B)** Tapered. **(C)** Textured. **(D)** Vented. **(E)** Ceramic cylinder.

contain small amounts of vanadium (decreases corrosion) and aluminum (increases strength, decreases density) to improve their mechanical properties, particularly their tensile strength. Ti-6Al-4V is a commonly used titanium alloy containing 6% aluminum and 4% vanadium. Because of the favorable mechanical properties of titanium alloys, they are also used for the screws that hold the implant components together.

Ceramics and Other Implant Materials

Other materials that have been used for dental implant fixtures are:
- ceramics
- composites
- vitreous carbon
- polymers
- other various metals including gold.

These materials have been used with limited success. Composite, vitreous carbon, and polymer implant fixtures did not integrate with the bone. Negative aspects of the early ceramic materials were their brittleness and lack of flexibility, causing them to transmit greater stress to the implant site. These implant fixtures were at greater risk of fracture from functional forces.

Newer ceramics such as zirconia (see Chapter 10) are much stronger and hold up better than older ceramics (see Table 13.1 for properties of implant materials). Ceramic implants will integrate with the bone more intimately than titanium implants. It is thought that they integrate chemically with the bone so that that there is no interruption between the ceramic surface and the bone (no microscopic space as seen with osseointegration); this is called **biointegration**.

Ceramics are also used for implant abutments in the esthetic zone, particularly where all-ceramic crowns are used to restore the implants. Metal abutments tend to show through and cause a gray coloration in the cervical area of the crowns due to the partial translucency of the ceramic crowns. Zirconia and titanium are equally biocompatible implant fixtures.

 Do You Recall?

How does osseointegration differ from biointegration?

IMPLANT FIXTURE DESIGNS

Over the years, various endosseous implant designs have been used. Today, the most commonly used implant fixtures are the threaded type with a cylindrical or tapered shape. The threads vary in their spacing and angulation. Some designs include the use of very small threads at the coronal aspect of the implant to aid in directing forces away from the implant top. This helps to prevent loss of bone at the crest.

Some threads are sharp and will cut into the bone. An initial pilot hole is made slightly smaller than the implant, which is screwed into place, making for a very close adaptation to the bone.

Some designs have a hollow core with or without holes in the apical portion. The holes were placed to allow bone to grow into them and mechanically lock the implant in place. The expectation is that these surface designs will help the integration of bone with the implant (Fig. 13.5).

Early implant fixtures were flat on top, allowing bacterial contamination of the internal portion of the implant with an ensuing inflammatory response from the tissue. Current implants use a conical connection that provides a seal against bacteria and as a result a healthier periodontium.

Implant Dimensions

The dimensions of implant fixtures can vary in diameter and length to fit the implant site and amount of available bone. The size of the tooth being replaced is a factor in determining the diameter and length of the implant fixture used. A wider-diameter implant fixture provides more surface area for support of the crown or prosthesis. When an implant is placed between two adjacent teeth, approximately 1.5 mm of bone should remain between the implant and the adjacent tooth root to prevent compromising the bone. Likewise, there should be 1.5 mm of bone on the facial and lingual surfaces to prevent bone remodeling and gingival recession. When the patient is partially or totally edentulous, implant size in the mandibular anterior may be 3 mm or smaller, 4 mm in the premolar area, and 6 mm in the molar area. Wide-bodied implants have diameters ranging from 8 to 10 mm. They are often used when a shorter length of implant is needed; their larger diameter provides additional surface area for support to make up for the lack of length. Very small-diameter implants (*mini-implants*) are growing in popularity for mandibular complete denture support (they are discussed in the section "Retention of the Removable Prosthesis").

Surface Treatment

Oxides. Titanium and its alloys are very reactive and will readily form oxides on their surfaces. Manufacturers will create these oxides in a controlled environment to prevent contamination of the oxide layer. To further protect from contaminants, after manufacturing, the implant fixtures are sealed in containers to protect them until they are ready to be placed in bone. The oxide layer is very thin but is essential to integration with bone. Special care must be used when cleaning implants in the mouth to prevent scratching the implant surface. Scratching will disrupt the oxide layer and allow contaminants to form on the damaged surface.

Roughening. Manufacturers may roughen the surfaces of the implant fixtures to increase the surface area available for integration with bone. Roughening has been accomplished by sandblasting, etching with acid, or coating with titanium plasma spray. Some studies show faster healing and greater integration with the bone with rough-surface implants. Bone apposition of 80% or more occurs when surface roughening is used as opposed to only 40% bone-to-implant contact with implants that were not roughened.

Coating. Ceramic coatings have been used on titanium alloys to promote more rapid integration with the bone. The ceramic materials are applied in thin layers by a plasma spraying process. The bond of the ceramic coating may break down with time, and therefore use of this process is controversial.

Epithelial Seal

Epithelial cells will adapt to and adhere to the surface of the implant to provide a seal to prevent the ingress of bacteria along the implant interface with the bone. This seal is important to the longevity of the implant.

American Dental Association Seal of Acceptance

Of the many companies that manufacture implants, only a few (including Nobel Biocare, Astra, and Straumann) have obtained the American Dental Association (ADA) Seal of Acceptance. The ADA requires companies to submit information about the materials used, research, and 5 years of clinical testing. The US Food and Drug Administration does not require clinical testing. Although the ADA seal is not required to sell implants, it demonstrates a commitment by the companies to produce a reliable product.

 Do You Recall?

What is the benefit of roughening the implant fixture surface?

IMAGE-GUIDED IMPLANT PLANNING

Before the introduction of **cone beam computed tomography (CBCT)**, most surgeons relied on their clinical examination and two-dimensional radiographs. The use of CBCT provides the dentist with very accurate three-dimensional images of the dental structures. With CBCT, the density of the bone, the thickness and height of the ridge at the planned implant site, the location of nerves and major blood vessels, and the size and configuration of the maxillary sinuses can all be assessed. Therefore the surgeon can have an image of the anatomy of the patient's jaw with all of its concavities and irregularities prior to the surgery.

IMPLANT PLANNING SOFTWARE

Treatment planning software can import CBCT images, allowing the surgeon and restorative dentist to plan for the implant placement surgery by:
- Virtually extracting teeth
- Determine precisely where the implant should be placed
- Plan for the type of implant
  - Proper diameter and length of the implant
  - Proper position in the buccolingual, mesiodistal, and apicocoronal dimensions.

Once the proper placement is determined, then CAD/CAM technology can be used to create accurate acrylic models of the patient's jaws, if needed, and make precision surgical guides for placement of the implants (Fig. 13.6).

ADVANTAGES OF GUIDED IMPLANT SURGERY

Implant surgery that is precision guided by this technology affords several distinct advantages. Among these advantages are the following:
- The option to place the implant without laying a flap; this leads to less postoperative discomfort and faster healing
- Fewer perforations of bone by a misaligned drill

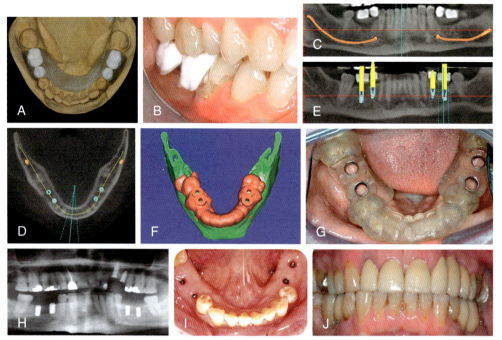

FIG. 13.6 Image-guided implant planning and surgery combines cone beam computed tomography (CBCT) and implant planning computer software: **(A)** Plastic guide with barium-filled teeth marks positions in the CBCT scan. **(B)** Scan guide in the mouth. **(C)** Barium-filled teeth show up in the scan (white opaque). **(D)** Scan lines (orange) orient position of transverse cross-section of the mandible. **(E)** Software allows simulation of implant placement. **(F)** Software-designed surgical guide for correct position of implants. **(G)** Surgical guide positioned in the mouth. **(H)** Implant fixtures seen in panoramic radiograph. **(I)** Implant fixture heads seen in the mouth. **(J)** Restored implants in the mouth. (From Rosenstiel SF, Land MF, Fujimoto J. *Contemporary Fixed Prosthodontics*. 4th ed. Elsevier; 2006.)

- Improved prosthetic outcomes of treatment and enhanced esthetics because of better implant placement
- Increased survival rates for the implants

Minimally invasive surgical techniques are greatly facilitated by image-guided surgery.

COMPUTER-AIDED DESIGN/COMPUTER-AIDED MACHINING TECHNOLOGY

In Chapter 10 on ceramics, CAD/CAM technology was discussed regarding fabrication of ceramic restorations. The same technology can be applied to fabrication of custom implant abutments and crowns. Additionally when implants are placed in the socket immediately after extraction of the tooth, a provisional restoration can be fabricated to support the gingival tissues and help maintain their contours during healing.

Milling or 3D printing can be used to fabricate the provisional restoration to fit the implant. After the soft tissues and bone have healed, a custom abutment and crown can be made from a new digital scan.

IMPLANT PLACEMENT

Variations are seen in the surgical approaches to implant placement and in healing times before the crown or other prosthesis is placed. Decisions underlying these variations depend on whether there is already a healed edentulous space with adequate bone or whether a tooth needs to be extracted first. The surgery for implant placement is often done by an oral surgeon or a periodontist. However, many well-trained general dentists are now placing implants in the more straightforward cases—those patients who are healthy and have adequate bone. Implants are restored by general practitioners and prosthodontists.

INFORMED CONSENT

Before the surgical procedure, the patient must be fully informed of the risks, benefits, and alternatives to implants. The patient must be given the opportunity to ask questions and have things explained in terms they can understand. Many times the patient will ask the dental auxiliary questions about implants or the surgery, so it is important to be knowledgeable about the entire implant process.

SURGICAL RISKS

Risks from the implant surgery include the usual surgical risks of excessive bleeding and swelling, infection, and necrosis of the gingival flap. In addition, there are risks of perforation of the bone or the maxillary sinus, puncture of major blood vessels, and damage to nerves. Also, bone grafting material may not develop a blood supply and new bone, and the implant fixture may not integrate with the bone.

PREPARATION OF THE PATIENT FOR SURGERY

Several steps can be taken to enhance the success of the surgery. An oral hygiene appointment should be scheduled a week or so before the surgery to improve gingival health and remove any calculus that could break off and fall into a surgical site. Prior to the surgery, postoperative instructions should be reviewed with the patient while they are still capable of listening to and understanding the instructions. The patient should also be given written instructions as many patients will forget or misunderstand portions of the instructions given verbally.

Just before the surgery, all removable prostheses should be removed and the mouth rinsed with an antibacterial rinse such as chlorhexidine (e.g., Peridex or PerioGard) to reduce bacterial levels in the mouth. Some clinicians like to administer an antibiotic and an antiinflammatory medication (e.g., ibuprofen) to minimize the risk of infection and reduce swelling. The surgery can be done under a local anesthetic, but some patients prefer oral or intravenous sedation. Sedated patients may be kept in recovery for an hour or more and should have someone drive them home after the surgery.

POSTSURGICAL INSTRUCTIONS

First, provide the patient with a cold pack to place on the face in the area of the surgery to help minimize swelling. The patient can apply an ice pack at home—10 minutes on, 10 minutes off—for a couple of hours. Postsurgical instructions should be reviewed again or reviewed with a companion who will be with the patient at home. A pack of sterile gauze should be provided to use with pressure for an hour or two on the surgical site to control bleeding. The patient should rest and limit physical activity, eat soft foods, drink plenty of fluids but not through a straw (to avoid disrupting any clots), avoid smoking, and avoid vigorous rinsing. All medications should be taken as prescribed. Warm saltwater rinses three or four times a day can be started the day after the surgery and continued for about 4 days (unless the patient has high or uncontrolled blood pressure which would limit sodium intake). The surgical site should not be brushed but can be cleaned gently with a cotton swab or gently wiped with a piece of gauze during the first week. Heavy or prolonged bleeding, abnormal swelling, intense pain, and allergic reactions should be reported to the surgeon at once. For any adverse reactions perceived to be life threatening, the patient or companion should call 911.

IMPLANT PLACEMENT SURGERIES

Presently there are three modes of implant placement surgery:
- Two stage
- One stage
- Immediate placement

TWO-STAGE SURGICAL PROCEDURE

The surgical procedures are done in two stages.

First Stage

Drilling the Hole. The first stage involves exposing the bone at the chosen placement site with a surgical flap. Next, a hole (called an *osteotomy*) is drilled in the bone at low speed and with sterile saline irrigation to prevent overheating the bone. A series of burs will be used, starting with a small-diameter bur and increasing to the size of the implant fixture being used. The hole is the shape and length of the implant fixture and a size that is just slightly smaller than the fixture. Depending on the implant fixture design, the implant is either lightly tapped into place to have a frictional fit with the bone, or it is screwed into place.

Surgical Guide. Often an acrylic resin surgical guide (called a *stent*) is made ahead of time with holes drilled through it at the same angulation at which the implant should be positioned. The surgeon places the guide over the ridge at the time of surgery and inserts a bone-cutting bur through the predetermined holes to cut the hole for the implant at the correct angulation. The stent is particularly helpful when the surgeon must place several implants that need to be parallel to each other for purposes of the restoration that will be placed on the implants.

Precaution. It is important that excessive heat not be generated during drilling of the bone. The bone can be damaged easily and then will not integrate with the implant fixture.

Cover Screw. After the implant fixture is placed in the bone, a cover screw is placed into the opening at the top of the fixture (Fig. 13.7). The cover screw prevents tissue from growing into the screw hole to which the future abutment will be attached. The surgical flap is repositioned and sutured closed over the implant.

Second Stage

Healing Abutment. Approximately 3 months later, the surgeon uncovers the top of the implant fixture, removes the cover screw, and places a smooth, prefabricated or custom healing abutment (see Fig. 13.3A) that screws onto the top of the fixture.

Forming the Gingival Cuff. Next, the soft tissue (gingiva) is positioned around the healing abutment, leaving it exposed to the oral cavity while the gingiva heals around it. This process allows the gingiva to form a cuff around the implant, which will adapt to the crown when it is placed. After a few weeks, the crown impression procedure can begin.

ONE-STAGE SURGICAL PROCEDURE

With the one-stage procedure, surgery for placement of the implant fixture is performed just as with the

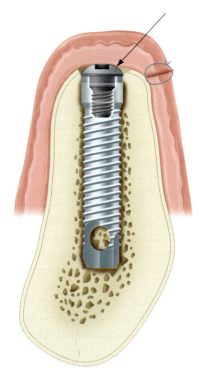

FIG. 13.7 Cover screw (also called a healing screw) used in a two-stage surgical procedure. It prevents tissue from growing into the screw hole after the implant fixture is covered with the surgical flap. (From Rosenstiel SF, Land MF, Fujimoto J. *Contemporary Fixed Prosthodontics*. 4th ed. Mosby; 2006.)

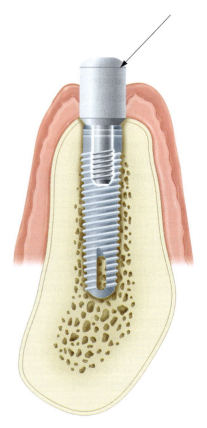

FIG. 13.8 Healing abutment used immediately in a one-stage surgical procedure or in a two-stage procedure after initial healing of 2–3 months. The healing abutment is placed to allow the gingiva to form a cuff around it. (From Rosenstiel SF, Land MF, Fujimoto J. *Contemporary Fixed Prosthodontics*. 4th ed. Mosby; 2006.)

two-stage procedure. The difference is that with the one-stage procedure, a cover screw is not placed at the top of the fixture and it is not covered with the gingival flap. Instead, the healing abutment is placed and the gingiva is positioned around the healing abutment and sutured (Fig. 13.8).

The one-stage procedure is increasing in popularity because it saves the patient from having to go through a second surgery. Occasionally, a provisional crown is placed that is out of occlusion while healing takes place.

Research has shown that there is no difference in survival of the implant between the one-stage and the two-stage surgery.

IMMEDIATE-PLACEMENT SURGICAL PROCEDURE

When the implant procedure involves the extraction of a tooth, some clinicians place the implant fixture at the time of extraction directly into the new socket. This is called an *immediate-placement implant*. A soft tissue flap is used to cover the extraction site until bone fills in and integrates with the fixture. Often an artificial bone material is also placed in the socket to aid the growth of new bone into the socket and to help stabilize the fixture. There is a slightly higher rate of failure of the implant after initial placement with this procedure compared with the one- or two-stage surgical approaches.

IMMEDIATE LOADING

Initially it was thought that 3 to 6 months of healing was needed so that osseointegration could occur before the implant could be loaded. Loading, it was thought, would cause movement of the fixture that would result in failure to integrate with the bone and loss of the implant. However, more recent findings suggest that it is the stability of the implant in bone that is important for loading rather than osseointegration. Therefore, many clinicians are placing the abutment and a provisional crown at the same visit as the placement of the implant fixture. Usually, this is done when the implant is long and wide enough to engage sufficient bone in the socket and beyond to have a stable fixture. If needed, bone grafting material is packed around the fixture to provide additional stability. Loading of the implant under chewing forces, then, occurs before integration of the fixture with the surrounding bone. However, forces still need to be controlled, distributed, and directed along the long axis of the implant.

If the surgical procedure is performed in accordance with a careful protocol and the fixture is very stable, then the success rate for implants with immediate loading is equivalent to that of implants with conventional loading (after healing), according to a meta-analysis (i.e., a review of many similar but independently conducted experiments).

Do You Recall?
When is a healing abutment used and what is its purpose?

RESTORATIVE PHASE

Restoration of a single-tooth implant is usually achieved with a prosthetic crown. With one- or two-stage procedures, once the soft tissue has healed around the top of the implant, the impression for the crown can begin. Dental auxiliary may need to become familiar with the implant impression techniques and the impression and laboratory components because they may be called on to assist the dentist with the impressions and pour the impressions, or, if allowed by state dental practice acts, may be asked to make the impressions.

IMPLANT IMPRESSION AND LABORATORY COMPONENTS

Impression Abutment
Some laboratory components are used during the impression-making process to facilitate the correct alignment of the implant to the cast. An **impression abutment** (also referred to as the *impression post*, *transfer post*, or *impression coping*) is attached to the implant fixture (see Fig. 13.3B), and an imprint of it is captured in the impression. The abutment is transferred from the mouth to the impression, and when the impression is poured, it becomes part of the cast.

Implant Analog
The **implant analog** is the component used during laboratory construction of the implant crown. It attaches to the impression abutment and is used to replicate the implant fixture for the laboratory cast (see Fig. 13.3C); the impression abutment orients the analog in the cast in the same way that the implant fixture is oriented in the mouth.

IMPRESSION PROCEDURES
There are two conventional impression techniques used for dental implants:
- Open-tray impression
- Closed-tray impression

Open-Tray Impression
The **open-tray impression** (also called a *pick-up impression* because it picks up the abutments in the impression) is the easiest for the inexperienced clinician. The legend in Fig. 13.9 briefly describes the steps. The open-tray procedure cannot be used if there is a lack of interarch space to allow access to unscrew the abutments.

Clinical Tip
When making an open-tray impression, be sure to wipe away impression material from the ends of the abutments after the tray is fully seated. Otherwise you will be frantically searching for the abutments in set material! Do not forget to fully loosen the abutments fully before removing the tray!

Closed-Tray Impression. With the **closed-tray impression** (also called a *transfer impression*), there is no hole cut in the impression tray. The impression abutments are screwed to the fixtures and the impression is made using the same types of materials as with the open-tray procedure (Fig. 13.10). When the set impression is removed from the mouth, the abutments remain in the mouth, attached to the fixtures. The abutments are removed from the fixtures, and then the implant analogs are attached to them. The abutments are reinserted into the impression in their proper orientation. The impression is poured in stone and the cast will look the same as with the open-tray procedure.

The biggest drawback of the closed-tray procedure is the potential source of error if the abutments are not placed back into the impression fully or in their proper orientation.

Digital Impressions. Digital impression techniques are discussed in detail in Chapter 5. Intraoral scanners take digital images of the implant components so that custom implant abutments and crowns can be made. The precise location of the implant can be captured.

For the digital impression, a scannable impression coping is placed into the implant fixture and its seating verified with a radiograph. The scan is made and checked to see that all necessary components have been captured, including:
- Opposing teeth
- The bite
- Contact areas of adjacent teeth
- Gingival contours (Fig. 13.11)

The laboratory prescription is completed containing the tooth shade and abutment and crown materials.

RETENTION OF THE IMPLANT CROWN
Implant crowns can be retained by screws or by cementing.

Screw-Retained Implant Crowns
The implant crown can be attached to the implant fixture core by a small screw often made of titanium alloy or gold alloy (Fig. 13.12). Screw-retained crowns are retrievable so that the implant fixture or abutment can be evaluated or the crown replaced or repaired. Special wrenches called *torque wrenches* are set to deliver the recommended amount of force to tighten the screws.

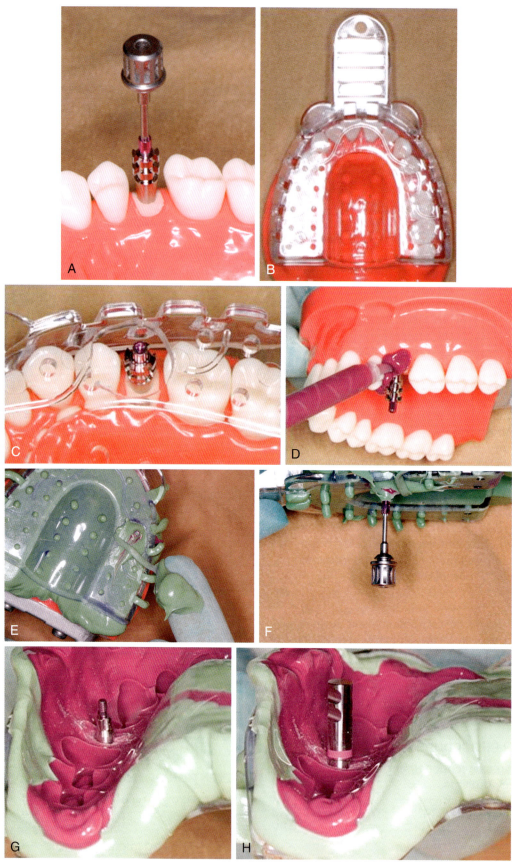

FIG. 13.9 Open-tray impression procedure: **(A)** Screw impression abutment into the implant fixture. **(B)** Select a plastic impression tray to fit the arch. **(C)** Cut a hole in the tray over the top of the impression abutment to allow access to it after the impression material is placed. **(D)** Monophase or light-bodied impression is syringed around the abutment and heavy-bodied impression material is placed in the tray, and then the tray is seated. **(E)** Impression material is wiped away from the abutment through the hole in the tray. **(F)** After the impression material has set, unscrew the impression abutment before removing the impression. **(G)** Impression with impression abutment in place. **(H)** Carefully attach the implant analog to the end of the impression abutment, making sure it does not shift position within the impression. When poured in stone, the analog will represent the implant fixture (see Fig. 13.3C). (Courtesy Arun Sharma, University of California San Francisco School of Dentistry.)

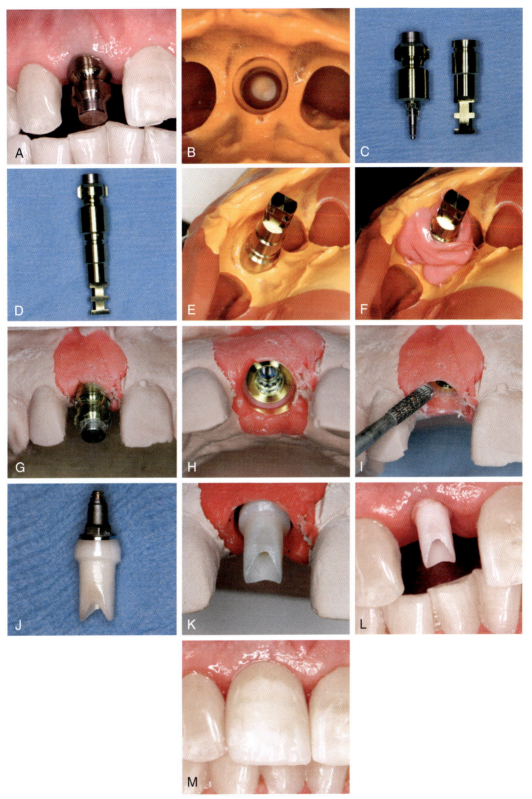

FIG. 13.10 Closed-tray impression technique for a single implant crown: **(A)** Impression abutment in place in the implant fixture. **(B)** Closed-tray impression showing imprint of the impression abutment. **(C)** Impression abutment (on *left*) has been removed from the mouth and is next to the implant analog. **(D)** Impression abutment is attached to the implant analog. **(E)** Impression abutment is seated into its imprint in the impression. **(F)** Soft tissue simulation material is placed around the top of the implant analog before casting in dental stone. **(G)** Poured cast with the impression abutment showing. **(H)** Implant analog can be seen after the impression abutment has been removed. Impression abutment positions the analog the same way the implant fixture is in the mouth. **(I)** Soft tissue material can be shaped to develop the emergence profile of the crown. **(J)** Ceramic abutment selected. **(K)** Zirconia abutment seated on the cast for crown fabrication. **(L)** Zirconia abutment seated in the mouth. **(M)** Ceramic crown cemented on the abutment. (From Rosenstiel SF, Land MF. *Contemporary Fixed Prosthodontics.* 5th ed. Elsevier; 2016.)

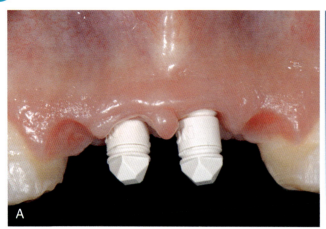
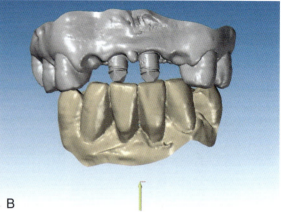

FIG. 13.11 Digital impression for fabrication of implant abutments and cantilevered bridge 7–10: **(A)** Impression abutments on implant fixtures 8 and 9. **(B)** Digital impression scan captured the impression abutments, gingival contours, opposing teeth, bite relationship, and proximal contact areas of adjacent teeth. (Courtesy Sang J. Lee, DMD, MMSc.)

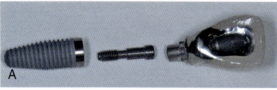
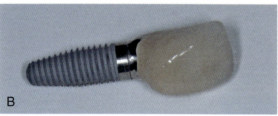

FIG. 13.12 Assembly of implant components: **(A)** Screw-retained implant crown with implant fixture and retaining screw. The screw-access hole can be seen on the lingual surface of the crown, and the implant abutment can be seen at the apical end of the crown. **(B)** Crown retained on implant fixture by the screw. (Courtesy Fritz Finzen, University of California School of Dentistry, San Francisco, California.)

> **⚠ Caution**
> After cementing an implant crown, it is critically important to ensure that all cement has been removed from the gingival sulcus. Cement retained under the gingiva can lead to infection and loss of the implant!

RETENTION OF THE REMOVABLE PROSTHESIS

Implants can be used to support a partial or full denture. In the mandible, atrophy (loss of bone through resorption) of the alveolar ridge is common in patients who have lost teeth at a relatively young age. A complete denture often has very little retention in this circumstance. Implants are a viable option for support and stability of the prosthesis (Fig. 13.15). They can also be used to anchor a prosthesis used to replace missing facial parts, such as a nose, eye, or ear lost to trauma or cancer surgery.

MINI-IMPLANTS

Mini-implants (also called *narrow-body implants*) are smaller in diameter than conventional implants and typically range in diameter from 1.8 to 2.9 mm. They can be placed in sites where the available bone would be inadequate for conventional implants. They are minimally invasive in that a soft tissue flap is usually not needed and the hole made by the implant is much smaller than conventional implants. Healing is faster with less discomfort. The survival rates for mini-implants are similar to conventional implants, ranging from 91% to 96%. They are less costly than conventional implants because they require less of a surgical procedure and can be placed in one visit. Two to four mini-implants can be placed by an experienced operator in under 2 hours, using local anesthesia. Most commonly they are loaded immediately after placement.

Screw-retained crowns require an access hole in the crown (see Fig. 13.3D and Fig. 13.12A) for placement or removal of the screw. After the screw is tightened, a soft material such as cotton, gutta percha, or Teflon tape is placed over the screw head (to make retrieval easier), and then a restorative material, usually composite, is placed into the hole (see Fig. 13.3E).

Cement-Retained Implant Crowns

Cementing the implant crown (Fig. 13.13) is a much more popular technique, particularly for anterior crowns. If the crown is cemented with permanent cement, it will not likely be retrievable. But if it is cemented with provisional cement, then retrievability is possible.

The downside is that the crowns may come off unexpectedly. It is very important to ensure that no cement remains under the tissue. Cement remnants could cause peri-implantitis and loss of the implant (Fig. 13.14).

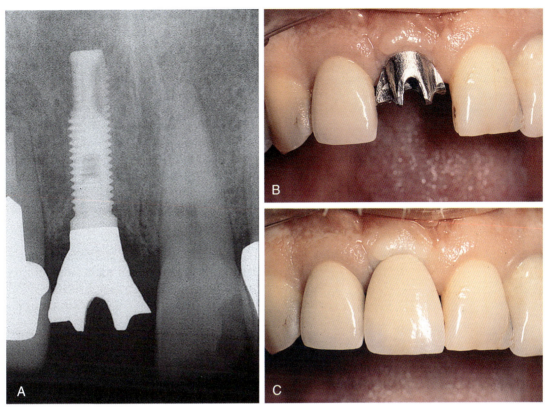

FIG. 13.13 Single-tooth implant with a cemented crown: **(A)** Radiograph of fixture in bone and the attached implant abutment. **(B)** Abutment is attached to the fixture by a screw. **(C)** Crown is cemented onto the abutment. (Courtesy Mark Dellinges, University of California School of Dentistry, San Francisco, California.)

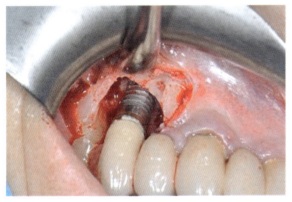

FIG. 13.14 Peri-implantitis resulting in bone loss around the dental implant. (Courtesy Toronto Implant Institute.)

USES FOR MINI-IMPLANTS

Stabilize Denture

One of the main uses for mini-implants is to stabilize a denture. The denture rests gently on the ridge and gains support and retention from the mini-implants (Fig. 13.16).

Narrow Spaces

Mini-implants are also used in sites with minimal bone that could not accommodate a conventional implant unless grafting was done. They are used to replace teeth with narrow roots, such as lower incisors or upper lateral incisors, and then restored with a crown. Conventional implants are often too wide for these sites.

Temporary Anchor Devices

A growing use for mini-implants is as **temporary anchor devices (TADs)** in orthodontic treatment when adequate anchorage is not naturally present (Fig. 13.17). They are even smaller than the typical mini-implant, with diameters ranging from 1.2 to 2.0 mm. They can be useful as anchors to move molars distally, intrude them, or to help close open bites. The TADs are used short term (about 6–12 months), and then are easily removed.

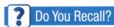

Do You Recall?

When are mini-implants used?

BONE GRAFTING

PURPOSE OF BONE GRAFTING

In order for a dental implant to be successful, it must be anchored in an adequate amount of bone to withstand the forces placed on it. Bone grafting is needed when the proposed implant site lacks an adequate amount and quality of bone. Common bone graft procedures are done to increase the width or height of bone at the implant site.

TYPES OF BONE GRAFTS

The basic types of bone grafts can be put into four general categories:

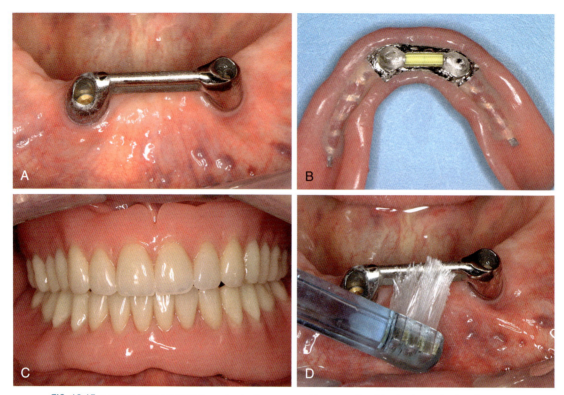

FIG. 13.15 Implant-supported denture. Implants were used because the ridge had resorbed and was inadequate to retain the denture: **(A)** Implants supporting a connector bar onto which a lower denture will attach. **(B)** A metal clip inside the denture slides over the bar **(A)** to retain the denture. **(C)** Lower denture supported by the implants. **(D)** The implants and the bar are cleaned with a brush. (Courtesy Fritz Finzen, University of California School of Dentistry, San Francisco, California.)

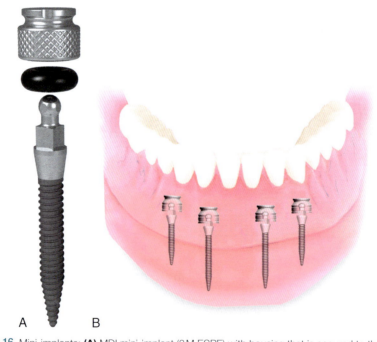

FIG. 13.16 Mini-implants: **(A)** MDI mini-implant (3M ESPE) with housing that is secured to the inside of the denture. The rubber O-ring resides in the housing and snaps over the ball on the head of the implant for retention. **(B)** Complete denture is retained by the mini-implants. (Courtesy 3M ESPE MDI Mini Dental Implants, 2010. All rights reserved.)

- Autografts
- Allografts
- Xenografts
- Alloplasts

Autografts

Autografts are those harvested from the patient's own body. Typical sites for harvesting this bone are the back of the lower jaw (ramus), chin, hip (iliac crest), or shin (tibia). This grafting material is very effective because it

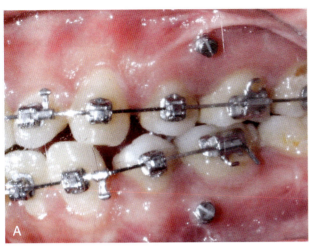
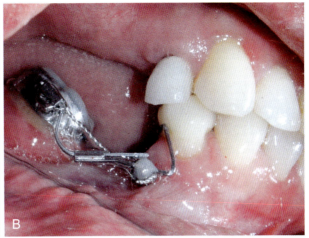

FIG. 13.17 Temporary anchor devices (TADs) are used when there is not enough anchorage in the natural dentition to orthodontically move teeth. They are removed after tooth movement is complete. **(A)** TADs for additional anchorage for retraction of teeth. **(B)** TAD anchor for molar uprighting. (Courtesy Jesse Patino, University of California, San Francisco, California.)

contains the patient's own bone marrow with cells that can promote bone growth and healing. The negative aspect is that it requires another surgery with a certain amount of discomfort, healing time, and expense.

Allografts

Allografts are human bone taken from donors who have donated body parts at the time of their death (cadaver bone). The bone is rigorously washed and sterilized. It is freeze-dried and stored in a tissue bank. The rigorous processing protocol eliminates concerns of transmitting disease from the donor to the recipient. Allograft materials are commercially available (Fig. 13.18).

Xenografts

Xenograft material is obtained from animals, usually cows (bovine bone), but occasionally pigs (porcine bone). The bovine bone is very similar in structure to human bone, so it works well for grafting. The bovine graft material is processed to make it sterile and biocompatible. Only the mineral components are used, and it acts as a matrix or filler around which new bone grows (Fig. 13.19).

Alloplasts

Alloplasts are inert, synthetic materials that stimulate new bone growth. They are commonly composed of calcium phosphate or hydroxyapatite, components found in human bone (Fig. 13.20). Often the material is mixed with the patient's bone marrow or with growth factors to stimulate bone activity. It also acts as a matrix or scaffold on which new bone is laid.

Sinus Lift

A sinus lift is a surgical procedure that adds bone in the molar and premolar region when the maxillary sinus has extended into that area, bone has resorbed from the alveolar ridge after teeth were lost, or both (Fig. 13.21).

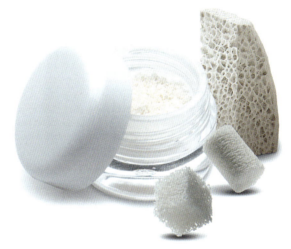

FIG. 13.18 Allograft cadaver bone in granules and large and small pieces. (Puros, Zimmer Dental.)

IMPLANT LONGEVITY

LONG-TERM SUCCESS

Long-term success is found with implants that have integrated with the bone, and when the implant components are kept clean, the surrounding gingiva is maintained in a healthy state, and forces on the implant are not excessive and are aligned with the implant. Forces on the implant must be properly managed. Because the implant has no periodontal ligament, patients cannot sense how much pressure they are applying to the implants. Therefore, forces must be distributed across the arch to other teeth or prostheses. Excessive force can result in loss of bone around the implant as well as fracture of ceramic crowns, denture bases, denture teeth, and implant components. Bruxers can stress the implant components to the point of fracture, resulting in implant failure. Occlusal guards are often indicated for bruxers.

When the negative factors are well controlled, implants have success rates of 95% or more and the implant crowns may last 10 to 20 years or more.

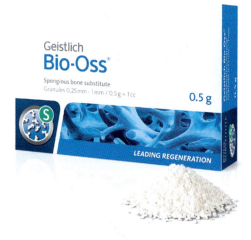
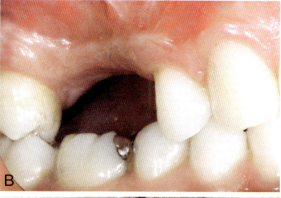
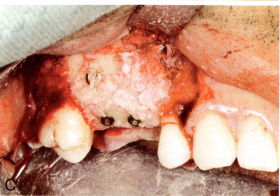

FIG. 13.19 Xenograft mineral granules used for bone graft: **(A)** Granular xenograft bone substitute material (also available in blocks). **(B)** Edentulous site with inadequate bone for implant. **(C)** Xenograft granular bone substitute material packed around newly placed implant fixtures. (**(A)** Courtesy Geistlich Pharma AG, Wolhusen, Switzerland; (**B** and **C**) Courtesy Prof. Dr. M. Chiapasco, Milan, Italy, and Geistlich Pharma AG, Wolhusen, Switzerland.)

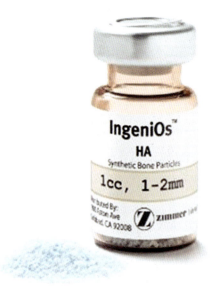

FIG. 13.20 Alloplast synthetic bone made from hydroxyapatite (HA). (Courtesy Zimmer Dental.)

IMPLANT FAILURE

Early Failure

Early failure of an implant is usually due to failure of the bone to integrate with the implant. Lack of integration can be due to poor surgical technique, lack of proper infection control, excessive generation of heat when the implant hole is drilled in the bone, infection of the implant site, poor quality of bone, or placement of loading forces too soon on the implant.

Later Failure

Failure of the implant that occurs after the initial integration is often caused by bacterial infection extending from the peri-implant tissues into the bone, or overloading of the implant during function, leading to loss of the supporting bone.

Potential Adverse Outcomes From Implant Placement

- Failure of implant to integrate with bone
- Loss of integration
- Infection around the implant
- Systemic infection
- Perforation of maxillary sinus, nasal cavity, inferior alveolar canal, buccal or lingual cortical plate of bone
- Inadequate sterility of implant fixture, leading to infection and implant loss
- Heat damage to bone during drilling for implant site
- Improper angulation of implant that compromises esthetics or function
- Damage to adjacent teeth during implant placement
- Nerve damage
- Lingering numbness or pain

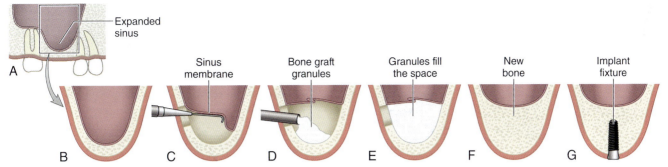

FIG. 13.21 Sinus lift procedure and implant placement: **(A)** Maxillary sinus expanded into edentulous space reducing the amount of bone at the ridge. **(B)** Frontal section through the sinus and ridge. **(C)** Entry is made through the lateral sinus wall and an instrument is used to lift the sinus membrane off the sinus floor. **(D)** Bone grafting granules are placed on the sinus floor. **(E)** Graft material fills the space that was created. **(F)** New bone formed around the graft material. **(G)** Adequate bone is present and an implant fixture is placed.

KEY POINTS

IMPLANT COMPONENTS: PLACEMENT AND RESTORATION

Endosseous Implants
- Surgically placed in the bony ridge
- Used for single tooth crown, fixed bridge, or denture stabilization
- Three main components:
  1. Implant fixture—the portion placed in bone
  2. Implant abutment—attaches to the fixture and acts as the support for the crown
  3. Implant crown—the final restoration
- Temporary components:
  1. Healing abutment—attaches to the fixture and extends through the tissue to allow gingiva to form around it
  2. Cover screw—placed on top of the fixture in two-stage surgery to prevent bone and soft tissue from growing into the fixture hole where the abutment attaches.

Implant Fixture Materials
- Metals—bone grows in close contact with the metal (osseointegrates)
  1. Titanium
  2. Titanium alloy—Ti-6Al-4V; stronger than pure titanium
- Ceramics—bone integrates into the ceramic surface (biointegrates)
  1. Zirconium oxide—ceramic; the strongest material

IMPLANT PLACEMENT SURGICAL APPROACHES

- Two-stage
  - Fixture is placed in bone, covered with soft tissue flap and allowed to heal
  - Second stage fixture is uncovered and healing abutment is placed until ready to restore
- One-stage—fixture is placed, healing abutment is attached and flap positioned around the abutment
- Immediate placement—fixture is placed in the socket when a tooth is extracted

RESTORATIVE PHASE

Impression for crown: open- or closed- tray technique or digital impression
Implant crown retention—titanium alloy screw or cemented in place
Mini-implants—small-diameter implants placed directly through the soft tissue without a surgical flap; used to stabilized a denture

IMPLANT MAINTENANCE

BIOLOGICAL SEAL

In addition to its interface with the bone, the implant has an interface with the soft tissue where it protrudes through the gingiva or mucosa. Although no connective tissue fibers (i.e., periodontal ligament or junctional epithelium) are connected to the implant surface, as they are to the cementum on the root surface of a natural tooth, close adaptation and attachment of the sulcular epithelium to the implant surface are noted (Fig. 13.22). This close adaptation helps to develop a biological seal that prevents microorganisms from invading the tissues.

PERI-IMPLANTITIS

The implant surface can accumulate bacterial plaque and calculus, just as teeth do. If this occurs, the tissues surrounding the implant (peri-implant tissues) will become inflamed, much like the gingiva around the teeth. If it is not controlled, this inflammation and bacterial invasion can progress into the bone (**peri-implantitis**) surrounding the implant and can contribute to its loss.

TISSUE MANAGEMENT

It is critically important to the success of the implant that the patient employ meticulous oral hygiene techniques and work with the dentist and dental hygienist to implement an effective tissue management program. The dental hygienist plays an integral role in helping the patient maintain the health of the implants and in reinforcing home care techniques. Likewise, the dental assistant can reinforce oral hygiene techniques when the patient comes in for periodic examinations or treatment.

HOME CARE

Patients should thoroughly clean the implant surfaces no less than once a day. If the patient has an implant-supported complete or partial denture, the prosthesis should be removed to facilitate cleaning of the implant and the prosthesis. The number and type of implants and the prostheses used for restoration will

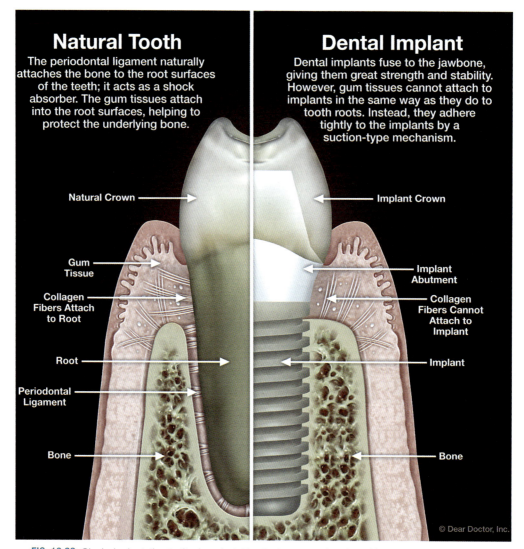

FIG. 13.22 Gingival adaptation to titanium dental implant compared to that with a natural tooth. (Courtesy Dear Doctor, Inc., Hopewell Junction, New York.)

vary from patient to patient. Therefore it is important to customize the home care regimen for each patient. Home care aids that are beneficial to patients with implants include a variety of the following:
- Disclosing agents
- Brushes
- Flosses
- Wooden plaque removers
- Antibacterial agents
- Oral irrigators

Disclosing Agents

Plaque-disclosing agents can help patients visualize the location of plaque in difficult-to-reach areas. These agents should be used daily for the first few weeks until the patient becomes more proficient in keeping the implants clean, and then periodically to check on the effectiveness of hygiene techniques. The patient should be given a disposable mouth mirror to help visualize all areas of the mouth. Adequate lighting is important to visualize all the areas of the mouth.

Brushes

Conventional. Gentle sulcular brushing is recommended to help maintain peri-implant tissue health. Brushes also need to be positioned at a variety of angles to clean around and under the prosthesis. In many cases conventional toothbrushes can be used, but selection of brushes will depend in part on the number and spacing of the implants.

Interproximal. For single-tooth implants, as well as for implant-supported fixed bridges, interproximal (also called interdental) brushes are helpful for reaching between the implant and the adjacent tooth or pontic (artificial replacement tooth that is part of a fixed bridge). Interproximal brushes that have a plastic coating on the wire holding the bristles together are recommended to avoid scratching the implant (Fig. 13.23).

End-tuft. End-tuft brushes can be helpful when the space between implants is greater than is practical for interproximal brushes (Fig. 13.24). For most brushes with plastic handles, the angulation of the brush head can be altered by heating the handle in hot water and bending it to the desired angle.

Power. Patients who have problems with manual dexterity because of arthritis, stroke, or other medical problems can use power brushes. Rotary brushes with bristles forming a point are useful for reaching between implants that are spaced far apart. If a dentifrice is used, one should be selected that is not abrasive.

Foam tip. A foam tip (Oral B, Procter & Gamble) is also useful for interproximal cleaning (Fig. 13.25). It can be soaked in chemotherapeutic agents to deliver them to specific sites.

Floss

Dental floss is often used to remove dental plaque from dental implant surfaces. However, it can be a contributor to the development of peri-implantitis. After implants are placed it is common for some of the bone at the crest to gradually resorb, and this may leave some of the top implant threads exposed to the oral cavity. These threads are relatively rough and can snag and retain bits of the floss. These floss bits harbor bacteria and lead to inflammation and infection of the bony and soft tissues surrounding the implant. If left untreated, the implant can be lost. If the crestal bone is intact and floss would be used against the smooth implant abutment (see Fig. 13.22), the risk of floss shredding is minimized. The dentist or hygienist can advise the patient whether or not floss can be safely used for implant cleaning.

Several types of flosses are available. Regular-thickness floss, dental tape, flossing cord, and fuzzy-type floss with threader (Oral-B Superfloss; Procter & Gamble) all have applications for plaque removal, depending on the nature of the implants and the overlying prosthesis (Fig. 13.26). Floss threaders are helpful for carrying floss under prostheses such as implant-supported complete dentures or fixed bridges, particularly where access is difficult.

Wooden Plaque Removers

Balsa wood triangular sticks (e.g., Stim-U-Dents [Revive Personal Products]) and toothpicks can be used with care to aid in plaque removal. These items will not scratch implants.

Antibacterial Agents

Chlorhexidine gluconate solution (0.12%) is an effective antibacterial agent. It may be used as a rinse for about a week after implant placement or during the second surgical stage when the implant is uncovered. It is also useful when inflammation is found in peri-implant tissues after placement of the prosthesis. It is often used as a 30-second daily rinse for 1 to 2 weeks. It can also be applied directly to the problem site on an interproximal brush, end-tuft brush, foam tip, or cotton swab. Frequent use of chlorhexidine will cause brown staining of the prosthesis and natural teeth.

An alternative antibacterial agent that is beneficial in controlling gingivitis but is not as effective as chlorhexidine is a phenolic compound (e.g., Listerine; Johnson & Johnson).

When a patient has inflammation around the implant that is not responding to good oral hygiene measures and hygiene visits, then prescription antibacterial

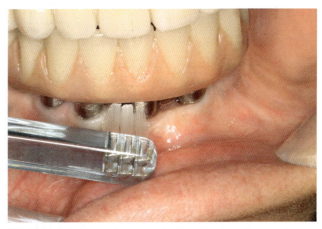

FIG. 13.24 End-tuft brush to clean implant. (Reprinted by permission from McKinney RV. *Endosteal Dental Implants.* Mosby; 1991:404.)

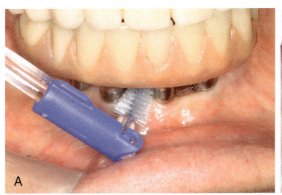
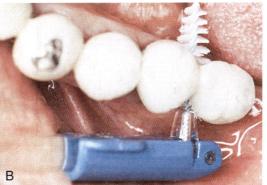

FIG. 13.23 **(A)** Interproximal brush used to clean implant. **(B)** Nylon-coated proxy brush to clean between individual implants. (A, Reprinted by permission from McKinney RV. *Endosteal Dental Implants.* Mosby; 1991:404; B, From Darby ML, Walsh MM. *Dental Hygiene: Theory and Practice.* 4th ed. Elsevier; 2015.)

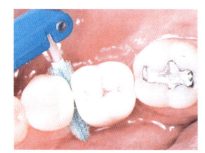

FIG. 13.25 Use of foam tip for cleaning interproximal surfaces of an implant. (Courtesy Procter & Gamble.)

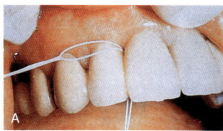

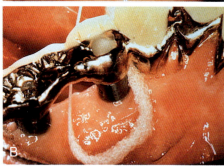

FIG. 13.26 Floss threader used to pass floss under a bridge: **(A)** Use of floss threader to go under a bridge pontic. **(B)** Superfloss used to clean under implant-supported bridge. **(A)** Floss passed under the connector between the implant and the pontic. **(B)** Superfloss used to clean the proximal surfaces of the implant and pontic. (A, From Babbush CA. *Dental Implants: The Art and Science*. Saunders; 2001; B, Courtesy Procter & Gamble.)

agents may be needed. Arestin (OraPharma) is a powder of slow-releasing minocycline that can be placed in the sulcus around the implant to help manage bacteria. Orally administered doxycycline hyclate (Periostat, 20-mg tablets; Galderma Laboratories) taken twice a day may help to manage the inflammation.

Oral Irrigators

Oral irrigators (e.g. Waterpik by Water Pik Inc) use a narrow tip to deliver a pulsing jet of water to the gingiva and implant surface. They can help flush out food particles and can aid in plaque removal from the implant surface. They can also be used to deliver antibacterial solutions at low pressure so as not to damage the biological seal between the epithelium and the implant.

Home Care Aids for Implant Patients

BRUSHES
Regular soft-bristled toothbrush
Interproximal brush with plastic-coated wire
End-tuft brush
Power brushes: standard or rotary with pointed brush tip

FLOSSES
Regular floss or tape
Superfloss
Cord

WOODEN STICKS
Balsa wood sticks (Stim-U-Dents)
Toothpicks

ANTIBACTERIAL AGENTS
Chlorhexidine solution
Phenolic compound rinse (Listerine)

ORAL IRRIGATORS

HYGIENE VISIT

The patient should return to the dental office 3 to 4 months after implant placement for assessment and maintenance. The interval between subsequent visits should be based on how well the patient is doing with oral hygiene measures, the health of the peri-implant tissues, and how rapidly calculus accumulates. At the maintenance visit, review of the health history and vital signs and examination of extraoral and intraoral structures are conducted in the same manner as for patients without implants. However, questions specific to implants should be asked, such as those involving the presence of implant mobility, soreness, bleeding of peri-implant tissues, pain with chewing, and looseness of the prosthesis.

Radiographic Assessment

The dentist may request periodic radiographs to check the bone level surrounding the implants. It is common in the first year for about 1 mm of crestal alveolar bone to be lost around the top of the implant. Conventional bitewings may not extend far enough apically to capture the bone around the crest of the implant, and therefore vertical bitewings should be used. Periapical radiographs alone usually are angled, so the true level of the bone around the top of the implant cannot be determined.

Visual Assessment

The hygienist should perform a visual inspection of the peri-implant soft tissues to evaluate for swelling, redness, bleeding with gentle probing, recession, and other indications of a developing problem. Exudate (pus) may be discovered on probing or palpation of the area with a cotton tip applicator. Usually, when these signs are limited to the tissue around the top of the implant, it is caused by bacterial plaque on the implant. Problem areas can be pointed out to the patient, and a review of oral hygiene techniques should be done. If the patient has a particular problem area, alternative cleaning aids and techniques can be recommended.

Probing
Perform gentle probing at maintenance visits. When probing the peri-implant sulcus, use a light touch so as not to disturb the biological seal (Fig. 13.27). A plastic probe is thought to allow for proper adaptation to the surface of the implant as it is flexible to adapt to the contour of the implant. Sites with increased probing depths, exudate, and bleeding should be recorded.

Mobility
Implants should be checked for mobility. An implant that has integrated with the bone should not be mobile. Mobility can be tested by using the handles of two dental instruments to try to push the implant back and forth buccolingually. Do not use your fingers because the soft pads of tissue on the fingertips will compress when trying to move the implant. This can be mistaken for mobility of the implant. On occasion, the patient may complain that the implant is loose, but careful examination may determine that a component of the implant, such as a retention screw, has loosened or been broken. If the implant is loose, there should be some radiographic finding of bone loss.

> **Do You Recall?**
> What assessments should be done at the hygiene visit?

Cleaning the Implant Surface
The clinically accessible surfaces of the implant should be thoroughly cleaned of plaque and calculus at each maintenance visit. Stainles- steel scalers and curettes should not be used on titanium implants because they will scratch them. When titanium is exposed, special scaling instruments should be used to avoid damage to the surface of the implant. Titanium scalers are preferred because they will not scratch the titanium implant components and the blades are narrower, allowing greater access to tight spots (Fig. 13.28). Titanium-coated, gold-coated, or Teflon-coated instruments may lose their coating with time and the underlying metal could scratch the implant. Plastic curettes and scalers (Fig. 13.29) or ultrasonic implant tips with plastic or rubber coating or sleeve (Fig. 13.30) should not be used. Research has shown that tiny bits of the plastic or rubber can become lodged on these rough surfaces, remain subgingival, and act as soft tissue irritants and plaque traps.

Prophylaxis pastes with coarse or medium grit should not be used on titanium. Even very fine paste can produce some surface scratches on the implant. If polishing is deemed necessary, tin oxide or other nonabrasive polishing paste in a rubber cup applied with light pressure can be used.

> **Do You Recall?**
> Instruments made from which materials are best suited for cleaning implants? Which materials should be avoided?

Air Polishing. Air-polishing devices (also called air-powder polishing devices) spray a stream of compressed air and water containing an abrasive powder through a nozzle onto the implant surface to remove plaque and stain.

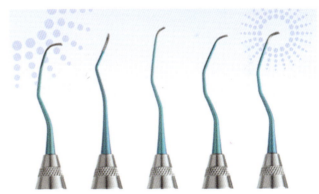

FIG. 13.28 Titanium scalers for titanium implants. (Courtesy Hu-Friedy Manufacturing Company, Inc., Chicago, Illinois.)

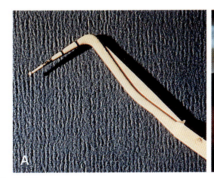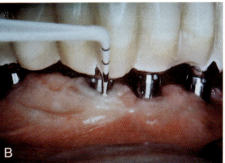

FIG. 13.27 Use of plastic probe around implant: **(A)** Plastic probe for measuring sulcus around implant. **(B)** Probe measuring sulcus without scratching implant (Sensor Probe, Pro-Dentec, Courtesy J. Kleinman). (From Darby ML, Walsh MM. *Dental Hygiene: Theory and Practice.* 4th ed. Elsevier; 2015.)

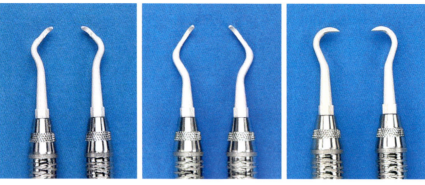

FIG. 13.29 Scaling instruments for implants with replaceable high-grade resin tips. (From Implacare Maintenance Instruments, Courtesy Hu-Friedy Manufacturing Company, Inc., Chicago, Illinois.)

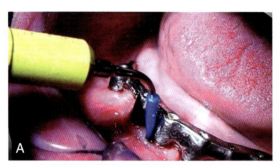

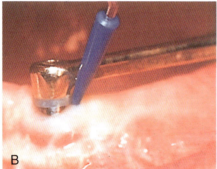

FIG. 13.30 Plastic tips for ultrasonic scalers: **(A)** Disposable polysulfone plastic tip (Cavitron SofTip, Courtesy Dentsply International, York, PA.). **(B)** Plastic ultrasonic scaler insert for titanium implants. (Courtesy Tom Riso Company, North Miami Beach, Florida.)

They are not meant to remove calculus. High-volume evacuation should be used with air polishing to capture as much of the aerosol as possible to minimize the amount the patient inhales and swallows.

Air-powder polishers are generally considered safe to use on implants, according to in vitro studies. However, these systems must be used with caution. The use of incorrect powders can scratch titanium implant surfaces and can injure surrounding soft tissues. Incorrect use or too much air pressure can result in air being forced into tissue spaces (called tissue emphysema). The risk is greatest if the stream is aimed directly into the gingival sulcus rather than angled toward the implant.

Abrasive Particles. Sodium bicarbonate to which flavoring agents have been added is the most common powder used with supragingival air polishing. The size of the powder particles is kept small, 60 to 80 μm. Sodium bicarbonate is less than half as abrasive as pumice, which is used in prophylaxis paste. Glycine (an amino acid) with a particle size of 20 to 30 μm and erythritol (a sugar alcohol) with a particle size of 14 μm are mildly abrasive powders used as alternatives to sodium bicarbonate to remove biofilm. One air polisher (Air-Flow Perio, Hu-Friedy EMS) uses glycine or erythritol and, with its nozzles designed for subgingival use, has been found to be highly effective at removing subgingival biofilm (Fig. 13.31). In one study comparing glycine to sodium bicarbonate, glycine was found to be 80% less abrasive.

Contraindications for Air Polishing. Contraindications for air polishing include patients with respiratory problems, such as chronic asthma or pulmonary disease, that may be aggravated by inhaling the powder spray. Patients with transmissible diseases that could be spread by the aerosol created and those with compromised immune systems are also not good candidates for air polishing.

Do You Recall?

What is peri-implantitis?

KEY POINTS

IMPLANT MAINTENANCE
Home Care Aids
- Disclosing agents
- Variety of brushes
- Interdental cleaners
- Wooden plaque removers
- Antibacterial agents
- Oral irrigators

Hygiene Visit Assessment—check the health of the implant site
- Radiographs—vertical bitewings are preferred
- Visual inspection—check for redness, swelling, bleeding, pus, and recession
- Probing—check sulcus around implant using light touch
- Mobility check—a well-integrated implant should not be mobile

Implant Cleaning
- Hand instruments and ultrasonic tips chosen that will not scratch the implant
- Air polisher with mild abrasive particles

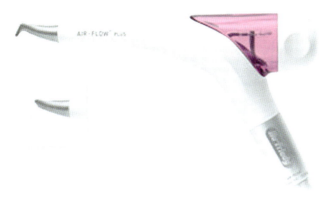

FIG. 13.31 Air polisher with subgingival nozzle (Air-Flow 3.0 Premium, Hu-Friedy EMS). Inset: Enlarged view of nozzle. (Courtesy Hu-Friedy Manufacturing Company, Inc., Chicago, Illinois.)

SUTURES

Extraction of teeth, placement of implant fixtures, bone grafting, and sinus lift procedures often require sutures. Sutures, also known as stitches, are used to hold tissues together so they can grow together or to reposition tissues after trauma or surgical procedures. Initial healing is considered the point at which sutures are no longer needed, typically 7 to 10 days. Until initial healing has occurred, sutures aid in bleeding control and prevent blood clots from being dislodged after tooth extraction. They also hold tissues together to keep debris and bacteria out.

The dental assistant or hygienist frequently will assist in placement of sutures and may be asked to remove them (as permitted by state dental practice acts) after initial healing has occurred. It is important for these dental auxiliaries to know why sutures were needed, which suture materials were used, how long they should remain in place, what to do if sutures come out prematurely, and which suture materials need to be removed or will absorb on their own.

TYPES OF SUTURES

Sutures can be made from a variety of materials consisting of those that are naturally occurring and those manufactured from human-made materials. Two general categories of sutures are absorbable and nonabsorbable.

Absorbable Sutures

Absorbable sutures do as the name indicates; they are broken down by the body's proteolytic enzymes and absorbed, thereby eliminating the need for a second removal appointment. Absorbable sutures include synthetic polyglycolic acid and surgical gut in plain or chromic. Surgical gut sutures are composed of purified collagen taken from the intestines of cattle, sheep, or goats. With chromic gut sutures, the collagen has been treated with chromic acid that almost doubles the length of time over plain gut before they absorb (Fig. 13.32).

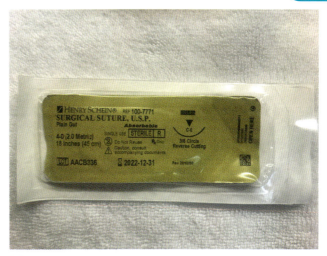

FIG. 13.32 Chromic gut sutures, size 5-0 derived from animal collagen.

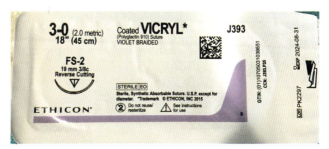

FIG. 13.33 Synthetic polyglycolic acid sutures, size 2-0 (Vicryl, Ethicon Inc.), are made from a biodegradable thermoplastic polymer. (Courtesy Matt Crimaldi.)

Synthetic polyglycolic acid (Vicryl) (Fig. 13.33) sutures are made from a biodegradable thermoplastic polymer.

Nonabsorbable Sutures

Nonabsorbable sutures are not dissolved by the body's enzymes and must be removed at a later appointment. If not removed, the body will see the sutures as a foreign body and initiate the inflammatory process. Nonabsorbable sutures include surgical silk (Fig. 13.34), polyester fiber, and nylon.

Characteristics of Sutures

Sizes. Sutures may be a single filament or multifilament in a braid or twist. The diameter (size) of sutures is identified by a number of zeros. The sizes range from 0 (or ought) to 8-0 (eight ought). The size of the suture declines as the number increases such that 8-0 is smaller than 2-0.

Needles. To place sutures, the filament is pulled through the tissue with a needle (Fig. 13.35).

Needles come in a variety of shapes and sizes. The majority of needles used in dentistry are curved in an arc. Needles are tapered with a round cross-section or cutting with a triangular cross-section. Cutting needles have a sharp triangular apex. Needles are predominately composed of stainless steel.

Needles can have an opening (eye) that the suture material passes through and a knot is tied to hold the suture to the needle. The second needle option does not have an eye and is called a swaged needle. The end opposite the sharp tip is a tube into which the suture material is inserted, and the tube crushed (swaged) onto the suture binding it to the needle. Due to the absence of a knot, swaged needles pass through the tissue more easily and cause less tissue damage.

SUTURING TECHNIQUES

Interrupted sutures are those placed where each stitch is tied and knotted separately. Examples include a single interrupted suture and a mattress interrupted suture. The continuous suture is a series of sutures made with one thread that is tied at the beginning and end of the series. Examples include the continuous blanket suture and the simple continuous suture (Fig. 13.36).

Suture Removal
See Procedure 13.1 for suture removal technique.

Do You Recall?

What types of sutures are nonabsorbable and must be removed?

SUMMARY

Dental implants are increasing in use, with more than 2 million placed annually. Screw-type titanium alloy implants are the most commonly used and have a success rate of approximately 95% with proper case selection and careful surgical technique. Image-guided implant planning and surgical procedures have minimized surgical complications. Two-stage surgical procedures were once the norm but are being replaced by the more popular one-stage and immediate-placement procedures. Dental assistants and hygienists can play an integral role in making the impressions for the implant restorations.

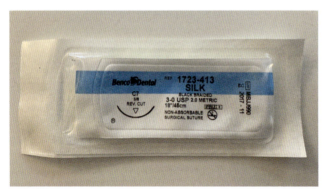

FIG. 13.34 Nonabsorbable suture made of braided silk, size 3-0.

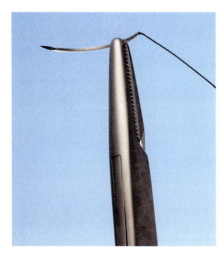

FIG. 13.35 Suture needle attached to suture. (From Hupp JR, Ellis E III, Tucker M. *Contemporary Oral and Maxillofacial Surgery*. 6th ed. Mosby; 2014.)

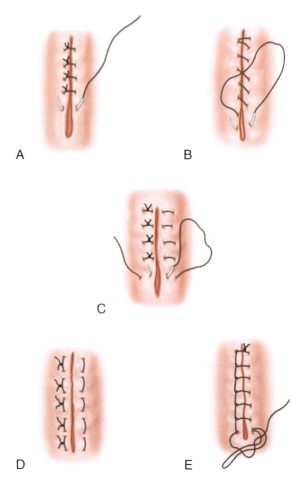

FIG. 13.36 Types of suturing techniques: **(A)** Interrupted sutures. **(B)** Continuous suture. **(C)** Vertical mattress suture. **(D)** Horizontal mattress suture. **(E)** Continuous box suture. (From Singh PP, Cranin AN. *Atlas of Oral Implantology*. 3rd ed. Mosby; 2010; Bird DL, Robinson DS. *Modern Dental Assisting*. 11th ed. Elsevier; 2015.)

Mini-implants have been introduced that are minimally invasive and can be used in sites where conventional implants could not. They are very useful for supporting dentures where there is little remaining alveolar ridge, and variants of them, called TADs, are used as temporary anchorage for orthodontic tooth movement. Bone grafting can improve sites for implants by building bone both in width and height.

It is not enough to just place and restore implants; they must be routinely maintained to ensure the success of the implants. Patients must be shown how to use the various aids for cleaning implants. In addition, a detailed assessment of the implants should be done at each hygiene visit. Care must be taken when providing periodontal preventive care around titanium fixtures to prevent scratching their surfaces. Hygienists must know which hand instruments and ultrasonic tips can be used with implants to avoid damaging them.

Patient education is an important aspect of the role of the dental assistant and the dental hygienist in dental practice. The ability to describe to the patient the pros and cons of the various materials used in practice and to aid in the treatment process depends on your knowledge of these materials. As new materials are introduced into dental practice, it is important to stay current on their indications, contraindications, and application techniques. Manufacturers' instructions for their care and use should be followed. Many manufacturers have websites on which they post information relative to their materials.

Sutures are often placed with implant surgeries. The dental auxiliary may be called upon to help with their placement and removal.

INSTRUCTIONAL VIDEOS

See the Evolve Resources site for a variety of educational videos that reinforce the material covered in this chapter.

Procedure 13.1 Suture Removal

See Evolve site for Competency Sheet.

EQUIPMENT/SUPPLIES (FIG. 13.37)
- Mouth mirror
- Explorer
- Hydrogen peroxide or diluted mouthwash
- Cotton tip applicator
- Suture scissors
- Cotton pliers
- Gauze squares

PROCEDURE STEPS

1. Using a cotton tip applicator, swab the teeth and tissues with antiseptic agent (hydrogen peroxide or diluted disinfectant mouthwash) to remove bacteria and debris (Fig. 13.38).

   NOTE: Inspect surgical site for closure of the wound, absence of drainage, and inflammation.
2. With cotton pliers, grasp the suture knot.
   NOTE: Be sure not to pinch tissues.
3. Lift knot gently away from the tissues, creating a space to insert the scissor blade (Fig. 13.39).

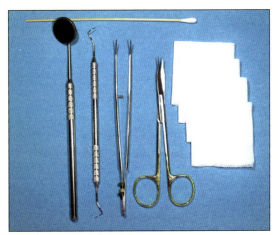

FIG. 13.37 (From Bird DL, Robinson DS. *Modern Dental Assisting.* 12th ed. Elsevier; 2018.)

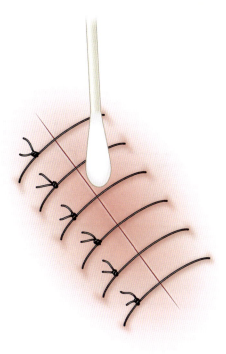

FIG. 13.38

Continued

Procedure 13.1 Suture Removal—cont'd

NOTE: This will expose a portion of the suture that has been under the tissue and thought to be free of bacteria.

4. Insert one cutting tip of the suture scissors into the space between the suture and tissue (Fig. 13.40).

NOTE: If the suture scissors have a half moon cut out in one of the blades, this blade should be inserted under the suture.

5. Snip one thread close to the tissue, taking care not to cut the tissue (Fig. 13.41).

NOTE: Cutting suture material close to the knot will allow the suture previously exposed in the oral cavity to pass through the tissue. This will contaminate sub-epithelial tissues with bacteria.

NOTE: Cutting both ends of the suture may result in the suture material being left in the tissue.

NOTE: If cutting scissors are used, the blade is inserted in the space with the tip curved away from the tissue to prevent laceration/cutting of the tissue.

6. Using a smooth, continuous action to pull the suture out of the tissue in one piece.

NOTE: Do not pass the knot through the tissue, as this would cause the patient discomfort.

7. Place the suture on the gauze square.
8. Remove all visible sutures and place them on the gauze square.

NOTE: To control bleeding, apply pressure to the area with a gauze square.

9. When all sutures have been removed, count the number of sutures on the gauze square to confirm the number is equal to the number recorded in the patient chart during the surgical appointment.
10. Record the number of sutures removed in the patient chart and any significant observations about the wound healing.

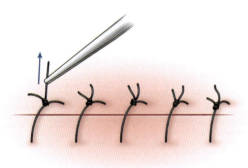

FIG. 13.39

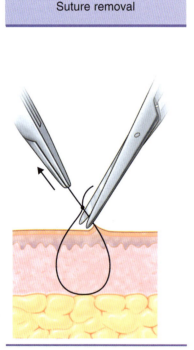

FIG. 13.40 (From Robinson JK, et al. *Surgery of the Skin*. 1st ed. Mosby; 2005.)

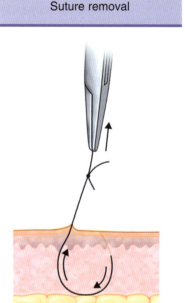

FIG. 13.41 (From Robinson JK, et al. *Surgery of the Skin*. 1st ed. Mosby; 2005.)

Review and Discussion

Review Questions

Select the one correct response for each of the following multiple-choice questions.

1. Which metal is most commonly used for dental implants?
    a. Gold
    b. Silver
    c. Stainless steel
    d. Titanium
2. An implant inserted into a hole drilled into bone is which of the following types?
    a. Subperiosteal
    b. Endosseous
    c. Transosteal
    d. Exosteal
3. Why is the surface of a titanium implant fixture roughened?
    a. To remove oxides
    b. To provide a larger surface area for osseointegration
    c. To remove adherent bacteria
    d. To prevent the implant from rotating under function
4. With a two-stage implant, after the fixture is placed, which one of the following occurs?
    a. The implant crown is placed.
    b. The fixture is covered with bone.
    c. A cover screw is placed and the fixture is covered by the soft tissue flap.
    d. The healing abutment is placed and the soft tissue is allowed to heal around it.
5. Potential adverse outcomes when an implant fixture is surgically placed include:
    a. Infection around the implant
    b. Perforation of one of the cortical plates of bone
    c. Improper angulation of the implant
    d. Damage to a nerve or a large blood vessel
    e. All of the above
6. Immediate-placement implants are done:
    a. About 3 weeks after the extraction of a tooth
    b. At the time of extraction of the tooth that will be replaced
    c. Only when a bone graft is needed
    d. To plug the hole made when the maxillary sinus is accidentally perforated
7. Implants can be used to support which of the following prostheses?
    a. Single crowns
    b. Fixed bridges
    c. Partial or complete dentures
    d. All of the above
8. Implant crowns are fixed to the implant abutment by which method?
    a. Cemented only
    b. Cemented or held by screws
    c. Held in place by screws only
    d. Welded on
9. Which instrument(s) should be used to remove calculus from implants where titanium is exposed?
    a. Carbon steel curettes
    b. Air polishers
    c. Metal ultrasonic tips
    d. Titanium curettes and scalers
10. The closed-tray impression procedure requires that one of the following components be repositioned in its proper alignment into the set impression after it is removed from the mouth. Which one is it?
    a. Impression abutment
    b. Implant analog
    c. Fixture
    d. Healing abutment
11. What is the purpose of the cover screw?
    a. Cover the screw hole on top of the fixture to prevent tissue from growing into it
    b. Allow a cuff of gingiva to heal around it after the surgical flap has been repositioned
    c. Hold the abutment to the fixture
    d. Cover the screw hole in the implant crown used to place the retention screw
12. Mini-implants can be used for which of the following purposes?
    a. To support complete dentures
    b. To support crowns for narrow-rooted teeth such as mandibular incisors
    c. To serve as anchors for orthodontic tooth movement
    d. All of the above
13. Which type of bone graft is derived from animal tissue?
    a. Allograft
    b. Autograft
    c. Xenograft
    d. Alloplast
14. Which one of the following statements regarding the gingiva around an implant is *false*?
    a. The gingiva has connective tissue fibers that connect or integrate with the surface of the implant.
    b. When healthy, the gingiva produces a biological seal against the implant that prevents microorganisms from invading the deeper tissues.
    c. The gingiva is closely adapted to the implant but is not attached to the surface.
    d. Chronic inflammation of the gingiva around the implant could lead to peri-implantitis.
15. The consequences of not maintaining good oral hygiene around an implant include all of the following *except* one. Which one?
    a. Inflammation and swelling of the gingiva
    b. Loss of the biological seal
    c. Bacterial invasion and potential loosening of the implant
    d. Increased bone growth due to chronic irritation
16. Biointegration, where the bone totally integrates with the implant, is seen with which implant material?
    a. Ceramics
    b. Stainless steel
    c. Gold
    d. Titanium
17. Which part of the implant is placed in bone?
    a. Healing abutment
    b. Fixture
    c. Analog
    d. Impression coping

Continued

Review and Discussion—cont'd

18. Which type of suture will be absorbed naturally by the body's enzymes?
    a. Silk
    b. Nylon
    c. Gut
    d. Polyester fiber
19. When removing sutures, the suture material should be cut close to the knot to prevent contamination of the subepithelial tissues with_____ as the suture is pulled through the tissue.
    a. Viruses
    b. Bacteria
    c. Mucus

For answers to Review Questions, see the Appendix.

Case-Based Discussion Topics

- The dentist has discussed a treatment plan with a patient who is a candidate for implants to support a mandibular complete denture. The dentist has described to the patient both conventional endosseous implants and mini-implants. After the dentist leaves the operatory, the patient is somewhat confused and asks you to explain the difference.

In layperson's terms, describe the difference to the patient. If the patient asks you specific details about why the dentist is recommending one type of implant over another, what should you do?

- A 74-year-old retired plumber comes to the dental office for a maintenance visit. The patient has several implants supporting two fixed bridges in the posterior part of the maxilla.

When the patient has the implants cleaned, describe the types of instruments the hygienist will likely use and the instruments that should be avoided if titanium will be scaled. Explain the selection of these instruments.

- The patient described in the preceding discussion topic is found to have inflammation in the peri-implant tissues around three implants and moderate amounts of calculus and plaque on the proximal surfaces of the implants. The patient explains that two previously scheduled maintenance appointments were missed and home care consists of using a regular toothbrush with hard bristles to clean the teeth, including the implants.

What can you do to reinforce the need for regular maintenance visits? What home care aids can you recommend to help the patient keep the implants clean? Should an antibacterial agent be suggested? If yes, which one?

- You are in the room when the dentist reviews the informed consent for implants with a patient. The patient is 78 years old and seems to be confused about upcoming procedures that were just explained. You question whether the patient has the mental capacity to give informed consent.

What should you do? What topics should be covered in an informed consent discussion?

BIBLIOGRAPHY

American Dental Association (ADA): *Council on scientific affairs. Products of excellence: ADA seal program*, Chicago, 1999, ADA.

Bird DL, Robinson DS: Dental implants. In *Modern Dental Assisting*, ed 13, St. Louis, 2021, Elsevier.

Bird DL, Robinson DS: Oral and maxillofacial surgery. In *Modern Dental Assisting*, ed 13, St. Louis, 2021, Elsevier.

Darby ML, Walsh MM: Dental implant maintenance. In *Dental Hygiene Theory and practice*, ed 4, St. Louis, 2015, Elsevier.

Edel A: *Air polishing for implant maintenance*, CDE World, 2017. Available at https://cdeworld.com/courses/20704-Air_Polishing_for_Implant_Maintenance.

Grisdale J: The clinical applications of synthetic bone alloplast, *J Can Dent Assoc* 65:559–562, 1999.

Kotick PG, Blumenkopf B: Abutment selection for implant restorations, *Inside Dent* 7:7, 2011.

McKinney RV: Oral hygiene protocol for implant patients. In *Endosteal Dental Implants*, St. Louis, 1991, Mosby.

Perry DA, Beemsterboer PL, Taggart EJ: Dental implants. In *Clinical Periodontics for the Dental Hygienist*, Philadelphia, 2001, Saunders.

Powers JM, Wataha JC: Dental implants. In *Dental Materials: Foundations and Applications*, ed 11, St. Louis, 2017, Elsevier.

Rethman M.P.: *Introduction and historical perspectives on dental implants*. White paper commissioned by Hu-Friedy. Available at http://www.friendsofhu-friedy.com/userfiles/file/Implant.Maintenance White Paper/Implant Maintenance White Paper Final.pdf.

Robinson DS: Oral and maxillofacial surgery. In *Essentials of Dental Assisting*, ed 7, St. Louis, 2023, Elsevier.

Sakaguchi RL, Ferracane J, Powers JM: Dental and orofacial implants. In *Craig's Restorative Dental Materials*, ed 14, St. Louis, 2019, Elsevier.

Shen C, Rawls HR, Esquivel-Upshaw JF: Dental Implants. In *Phillip's Science of Dental Materials*, ed 13., St. Louis, 2022, Elsevier.

Wilk BL: Intraoral digital impressioning for dental implant restorations versus traditional implant impression techniques, *Compend Contin Educ Dent* 36(7):529–533, 2015.

Wilkins E: Sutures and dressings. In *Clinical Practice of the Dental Hygienist*, Philadephia, 2017, Wolters Kluwer.

Polymers for Prosthetic Dentistry

14

http://evolve.elsevier.com/Eakle/materials/

Chapter Objectives

On completion of this chapter, the student should be able to:
1. Describe the formation of long-chain polymers from monomers.
2. Explain the effect that cross-linking has on the physical and mechanical properties of polymers.
3. Describe the stages of addition polymerization.
4. List the important properties of acrylic resins.
5. Compare the properties of hard and soft lining materials.
6. List the indications for long- and short-term soft liners.
7. Compare the advantages and disadvantages of chairside and laboratory-processed hard liners.
8. List the indications for the use of acrylic denture teeth versus porcelain teeth.
9. Demonstrate proper adjustment of a denture to relieve a sore spot as permitted by state law.
10. Demonstrate accurate use of the ultrasonic cleaner for cleaning complete and partial dentures in the office.
11. Describe how patients should be educated regarding the home care regimen for complete and partial dentures and necessary precautions to be taken when cleaning these appliances.
12. Demonstrate proper fabrication of custom impression trays for upper and lower arches.

KEY TERMS

Polymers long-chain, high-molecular-weight molecules produced by chemically linking many low-molecular-weight monomer molecules

Monomers low-molecular-weight molecules that are joined to form polymers; as used in dentistry, monomers are usually liquids

Polymerization the act of forming polymers by chemically linking monomers into long chains; the process can be activated by chemicals, heat, or light

Cross-Linked Polymers adjacent long-chain polymers joined by the bonding of short chains along their sides to enhance the properties of the polymer

Addition Polymerization common form of polymerization for dental materials; a chain reaction that links monomer units to form a long chain called a polymer.

Free Radical an atom with one unpaired electron in its outer shell making it highly reactive. It initiates the joining of adjacent monomer molecules to form a polymer.

Poly(Methyl Methacrylate) (PMMA) a polymer composed of numerous methyl methacrylate monomers linked together into a long chain. Methyl methacrylate is commonly used in denture fabrication

Plasticizer liquid added to acrylic resin to soften it and make it more pliable

Porosity numerous microscopic holes or voids within a material; often caused during polymerization of resins when monomer vaporizes and is lost; can also be caused by entrapping of air during mixing of powder and liquid

Prosthesis a device used for the replacement of missing teeth and/or soft tissues. It can serve both cosmetic and functional roles

Long-Term Soft Liner a soft liner that is used in patients who have problems with hard acrylic denture bases; it is expected to last for 1 to 3 years

Short-Term Soft Liner a soft provisional (temporary) liner used to improve tissue health; also called a *tissue conditioner*; typically, it lasts from a few days to a few weeks

Hard Liner a rigid reline material used inside a denture to improve the fit and stability

---

Acrylic resins are **polymers** used in the fabrication of complete and partial dentures, as well as maxillofacial prostheses (used to replace missing oral or facial structures). They can be used to simulate the oral mucosa, gingiva, and teeth. They are also used to reline these prostheses to improve their fit and to repair them when they break. With CAD/CAM technology prostheses can be fabricated by milling or three-dimensional (3D) printing.

Even though a commercial dental laboratory fabricates most of the removable prostheses, dental auxiliaries need to be familiar with the materials and their uses, care, and repair. They must understand the materials used in prosthetic dentistry to better care for the patient and to assist the dentist. Patients who wear removable prostheses will often ask dental auxiliary questions that relate to the fit or home care of their prosthesis.

REVIEW OF POLYMER FORMATION

Polymers are large, long-chain molecules formed by chemically joining together smaller molecules, called *monomers*. The polymer chains will vary in length as the monomer is being consumed and may contain from 10,000 to 100,000 monomer units. The chains will lengthen until no more monomer is available. Most of the polymers shrink as they form, and this creates undesirable features in the final product.

COPOLYMERS

When two or more different types of monomers join together, the polymer formed from them is called a *copolymer*. Copolymers are produced to enhance the physical and mechanical properties of the material. They are used in dentures to make them more resistant to fracture, in soft reline materials to make them soft and pliable, and in mouth guards to improve their shock-absorbing capacity.

POLYMERIZATION

The act of forming polymers is called polymerization. In general, less than 100% of the monomer is used up. The remaining unused monomer is called the *residual monomer*. The best clinical results occur when there is little residual monomer.

Polymerization (Curing) Methods

There are three types of curing methods:
- Chemical curing (self-curing or autopolymerizing)
- Heat curing
- Light curing (photo-curing)

Whether initiated by chemical means, light, or heat, the polymerization process releases heat (i.e., it is an exothermic reaction). The heat must be controlled during the process. If the temperature becomes too great, the monomer will vaporize and produce porosity in the material.

CROSS-LINKED POLYMERS

Polymer chains often have short chains of atoms attached to their sides. When the side chains of adjacent polymers bond together, the polymers are termed cross-linked polymers. When side chains of adjacent polymers are joined by weak bonds, the polymers are easily manipulated, bent, or stretched. When adjacent polymers are joined by highly charged side chains, the bond is stronger, and the cross-linked polymers are stronger and stiffer. They also are more wear resistant and, consequently, can be used in denture teeth. They polish more easily and are less affected by solvents such as alcohol.

POLYMERIZATION REACTIONS

There are two types of polymerization:
- Addition polymerization
- Condensation polymerization

Addition Polymerization

Addition polymerization is the most common form of polymerization for dental materials. It occurs in three stages:
Stage 1: Initiation (or induction)
Stage 2: Propagation
Stage 3: Termination

See video on Evolve Resources entitled "Free Radical Polymerization (addition polymerization)."

Unlike condensation polymerization, the reaction does not produce any by-products.

Initiation. A free radical initiates the reaction by opening the bond between the two carbon atoms of the monomer. The broken carbon bond causes the monomer molecule to bond to another monomer. Each linkage leaves a free radical available for further reaction.

Propagation. The process of linking monomer units is termed *propagation*, and it continues until the monomer units are used up, or until a substance reacts with the free radical to tie it up.

Termination. When the free radicals are tied up or destroyed, the process is terminated.

Condensation Polymerization

Materials formed by a condensation reaction do not have many uses in dentistry. The reaction itself produces by-products such as water, hydrogen gas, or alcohol that may compromise the physical properties or handling characteristics.

ACRYLIC RESINS (PLASTICS)

Synthetic polymers used in prosthetic dentistry are called acrylic resins because they are derived from acrylic acid. Acrylic resin forms when a liquid monomer (commonly methyl methacrylate) is mixed with a powder of small polymer beads, and the mixture undergoes polymerization. The polymerized resin is **poly(methyl methacrylate) (PMMA)**.

USES OF ACRYLICS

Acrylic resins are especially useful because they can be shaped to any contour and custom colored to match the shade of the teeth, gingiva, or skin. The resins are used for denture bases, denture teeth, relining and repair of prostheses, provisional acrylic partial dentures (flippers or stayplates), tissue conditioners, and custom impression trays. They also have uses as orthodontic retainers and removable tooth movement devices (Fig. 14.1), bruxism mouth guards, and provisional restorations. Specialized acrylic resins are used in esthetic tissue replacement for severe gingival recession and for facial reconstruction due to trauma, surgery, or birth defects.

MODIFIERS

Acrylic resins used in dentistry are often modified by the addition of plasticizers, rubbers, and fillers to change their physical and mechanical properties.

- **Plasticizers** are oily liquids added to soften the acrylic plastics and make them more pliable.
- Rubbers may be added to increase the impact fracture resistance of the acrylic resin.
- Fillers are added to strengthen the resin or change its optical properties.
- Chemical coupling agents may be used to bond the filler to the acrylic resin to make the resin more wear resistant (similar to the use of silane to couple fillers in composite resins). These bonded fillers can be found in light-cured denture repair or impression tray materials.

PROPERTIES

Polymerization Shrinkage

Polymers undergo shrinkage as a result of the polymerization process. Heat-cured acrylic resins shrink about 6% by volume and about 0.2% to 0.5% linearly (from one point on the denture to another).

Dimensional Change

Sources of dimensional change in addition to polymerization shrinkage include water sorption and thermal expansion. A denture base will increase slightly in its overall size when it absorbs water. This expansion may help offset some of the shrinkage that occurs during polymerization. Heat can cause the resin to expand. The coefficient of thermal expansion is more than twice that of composite resins.

Strength

The strength of the acrylic resins is fairly low, with a compressive strength of approximately 11,000 pounds per square inch (psi) and a tensile strength of 8000 psi. By comparison, amalgam has a compressive strength of about 60,000 psi. Acrylics are not very hard materials and as a consequence are not very wear resistant. While they have fairly good resistance to fatigue failure (can be flexed repeatedly before they break), they have low-impact failure and will break if dropped on the floor or in an empty sink during cleaning. To combat the brittleness and breakage problem, some manufacturers add butadiene-styrene rubber to the MMA to create a high-impact acrylic resin.

Thermal Conductivity

Denture bases do not conduct temperature well. Patients wearing dentures will notice a marked difference when they eat foods such as ice cream or drink hot beverages. Because the denture partially insulates against the temperature of the food or beverage, patients may burn themselves when they attempt to swallow foods that are too hot.

 Do You Recall?

Why is rubber added to acrylic resin for dentures?

CURING

Chemical-Cured Versus Heat-Cured Acrylics

The type of processing has some effect on the properties. Polymerization is never 100% complete, and varying amounts of free monomer may be present in the polymerized material. In general, chemical-cured acrylic resins are weaker, softer, more porous, and less color stable than heat-cured acrylic resins.

After polymerization, there is more residual monomer in chemical-cured acrylic (up to 5%), and it initially adversely affects many of the physical and mechanical properties until the monomer leaches out in minute amounts over several days or weeks. Some dimensional change can occur during the first 24 hours in chemical-cured acrylic. For this reason, custom acrylic trays should not be used immediately, but should sit for 12 to 24 hours to allow most of the dimensional change to occur, so the impression will not be distorted.

Heat-cured acrylics are harder, stronger, and less porous and have less than 1% residual monomer that leaches out of the surface relatively quickly. Properties of heat-cured acrylic resins are summarized in Table 14.1.

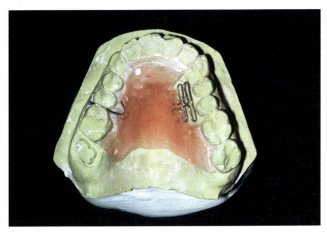

FIG. 14.1 Removable acrylic orthodontic tooth movement device.

Table 14.1	Properties of Heat-Cured Acrylic Resins (PMMA)	
PROPERTY	VALUE
Polymerization shrinkage (by volume)	6%
Polymerization shrinkage (linear)	0.2%–0.5%
Coefficient of thermal expansion	More than twice that of composite
Compressive strength	75.8 MPa (11,000 psi)
Tensile strength	55.2 MPa (8000 psi)
Hardness (Knoop)	15–18 kg/mm^2
Biocompatibility	Good
Thermal conductivity	Poor
Wear resistance	Fair
Fatigue resistance (to flexing)	Good
Impact resistance (to breakage when dropped)	Poor

PMMA, Poly(methyl methacrylate). 1 MPa (megapascal) = 145.038 psi (pounds per square inch)

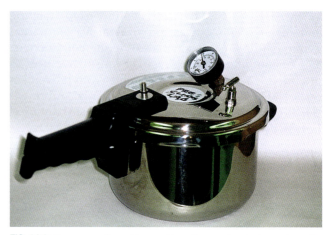

FIG. 14.2 Pressure pot used to provide a denser chemical-cured acrylic.

Porosity

Porosity in polymerized acrylic resin is characterized by the presence of many small or microscopic voids or pores. Porosity in the acrylic weakens it and makes it prone to collect debris and microorganisms. Denture odor and stains develop more readily.

Porosity is a result of loss of monomer or inadequate pressure during processing. The monomer is highly volatile and can evaporate rapidly at room temperature during handling of the mixed powder and liquid. Monomers can vaporize during heat curing of the resin if the temperature rises too much. Porosity can also occur by the entrapment of air during mixing of the powder and liquid acrylic resin components.

Curing under pressure helps keep the monomer from evaporating during polymerization and creates a denser acrylic. When chemical-cured acrylic is cured in room temperature water and 15 to 20 pounds of air pressure in a pressure pot (Fig. 14.2), the resulting acrylic is stronger and has less porosity and shrinkage. A pressure pot is a laboratory device that resembles a pressure cooker and can be pressurized by the addition of air through a one-way valve in its lid.

❗ Caution

When using a pressure pot, it is not necessary to pressurize it with air to more than 20 psi. Although the pressure pot is constructed of heavy materials and has a pressure release valve, it can usually withstand high pressure, but excessive pressure—more than 30 psi—increases the risk of a mishap should the release valve malfunction.

ALLERGIC REACTION

Sensitive patients can react to the components of the denture materials. If excessive free monomer is present in the denture base, some people's tissues may be irritated and inflamed by the methacrylate monomer. Other components such as hydroquinone, benzoyl peroxide, and pigments can also cause irritation. Dental personnel who work with the materials can develop contact dermatitis (an itchy rash) through repeated exposure of unprotected skin. Personal protective equipment (PPE) should be used when handling these materials. Dental resins are not known to cause systemic toxic reactions.

❗ Caution

To prevent contact dermatitis, avoid contact with methyl methacrylate even with gloved hands. Most resin monomers easily pass through gloves. Remove gloves and wash hands thoroughly if contact occurs.

❓ Do You Recall?

Why do chemical-cured acrylic resins have poorer physical properties than heat-cured acrylic resins?

ACRYLIC RESINS FOR DENTURE BASES

The functions of the acrylic resin denture base are to:
- Retain the artificial teeth in the **prosthesis**
- Adapt to the supporting oral structures for stability
- Distribute forces of mastication over a wide area to reduce pressure on the ridges that might contribute to resorption of the underlying bone
- Replace missing tissues or rebuild the contours of tissues lost when the underlying bone resorbs
- Establish a seal along the periphery of a complete denture that aids in retention (Fig. 14.3)

POLYMERIZATION REACTION

Acrylic resins polymerize by an addition reaction. Acrylic resins are supplied as a powder and a liquid.

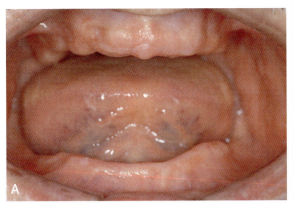
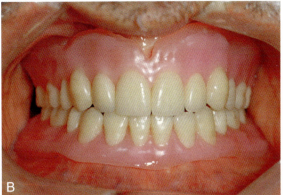
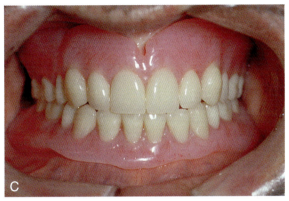

FIG. 14.3 Complete dentures: **(A)** Edentulous ridges. **(B)** Denture teeth set in wax for try-in. **(C)** Dentures processed in acrylic, polished, and delivered to patient.

Powder

The powder is composed mostly of small beads of PMMA and benzoyl peroxide (the initiator). Inorganic pigments are added to give the acrylic resin colors resembling those of the oral mucosa, and titanium dioxide is added to keep the acrylic from being too transparent. Small, colored fibers may be added to simulate small blood vessels. Several shades of acrylic are available so that the clinician can attempt to match the variations of racial pigmentation that can occur in the gingiva and mucosa of patients (Fig. 14.4).

Liquid

The liquid contains MMA, hydroquinone as an inhibitor or preservative to prevent polymerization of the MMA during storage, and glycol dimethacrylate as a cross-linking agent. Cross-linking of the acrylic polymer chains helps prevent surface cracks, and it improves resistance to structural fatigue that can lead to fracture. The liquid is supplied in dark brown bottles to prevent ultraviolet light from initiating polymerization during storage.

When the powder and the liquid are mixed, chemical- and heat-cured materials go through a similar reaction, except that chemical-cured materials have a tertiary amine in the liquid as an activator, whereas heat-cured materials do not (Table 14.2).

Steps in Complete Denture Fabrication

1. Make preliminary alginate impressions of edentulous ridges (by dental auxiliay).
2. Pour impressions into stone for preliminary casts (by dental auxiliary).
3. Fabricate custom impression trays from preliminary casts (by dental auxiliary or laboratory technician).
4. Border mold trays with compound (or other thermoplastic material) and make final impressions with elastomer (by dentist or extended-function dental auxiliary).
5. Box impressions with utility wax and pour into die stone for master cast (by dental auxiliary or sent to lab).
6. Fabricate record bases (used to capture relations between upper and lower jaws; also called *wax rims*) (by dental auxiliary or laboratory technician).
7. With record bases, record jaw relations, midline, and lip line. Make facebow transfer—not used by all dentists (by dentist or expanded functions dental auxiliary).
8. Select shade and mold of teeth (by dentist with help from the dental auxiliary and patient).
9. Mount casts on articulator and set teeth in wax on record bases (by dentist or laboratory technician).
10. Try teeth in wax in the patient's mouth to check appearance and occlusion (by dentist).
11. Return wax try-in to laboratory for final processing in acrylic resin.

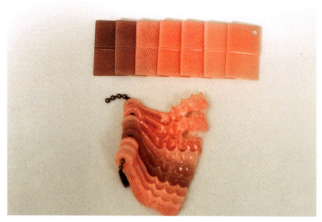

FIG. 14.4 Acrylic shade guides for matching the color of the gingiva. (Courtesy Mark Dellinges, School of Dentistry, University of California, San Francisco, San Francisco, California.)

Table 14.2 Ingredients of Acrylic Resin and Their Function

COMPONENT	FUNCTION
Liquid Components	
Methyl methacrylate	Monomer
Hydroquinone	Inhibitor to prevent polymerization of monomer during storage
Glycol dimethacrylate	Cross-linking agent
Tertiary amine	Activator for chemical-cured resin
Powder Components	
Poly(methyl methacrylate)	Polymer beads
Benzoyl peroxide	Initiator
Titanium dioxide	Reduces translucency
Pigments	Simulate tissue colors
Colored fibers	Simulate small blood vessels

> **! Caution**
> Liquid monomer should be considered a hazardous material. It is flammable and vaporizes easily when the lid is off of the container. Use in a well-ventilated area, ideally under a vapor hood. Avoid prolonged direct breathing of the vapor. Because all of its potential hazards have not been defined, it is advisable for pregnant workers and patients to avoid breathing the fumes. It can irritate eyes, nose, skin, and lungs and may affect the nervous system.

Physical Stages of Polymerization

Sandy Stage. The first stage seen when the powder (polymer) and the liquid (monomer) are mixed is called the *sandy stage* because the mixture looks grainy, similar to sand and water, and has a runny consistency.

Stringy Stage. The second stage occurs when the powder particles absorb the liquid into their surface. It is called the *stringy stage* because the mixture is stringy when handled and is thicker in consistency.

Dough Stage. In the next stage, called the *dough stage*, more of the powder goes into the solution and the mixture changes from stringy to doughy and is more easily manipulated.

Rubber Stage. In the final stage, called the *rubber stage*, the mixture has a rubbery consistency that can no longer be manipulated for forming the denture base. At the end of this stage, the acrylic is hard.

PROCESSING METHODS FOR COMPLETE DENTURES

Compression Molding

The most common method for processing denture bases uses heat and pressure during the polymerization of the acrylic resin.

Processing the Complete Denture by Compression Molding

After the dentist has tried in the denture teeth set in wax and the patient approves the appearance, the denture is returned to the laboratory, where the technician places the cast of the edentulous arch, along with the denture setup in a specially designed processing flask. The flask separates in the middle into two sections. The denture setup mounted on the cast is invested in a plaster investing material in the flask in such a manner that the flask can be opened in the middle to allow removal of the wax and record base after heating in a water bath. The teeth are held in place by the plaster. All remnants of the wax are removed. A liquid, called a *separating medium*, is placed and air-dried on the plaster and the cast to prevent the acrylic resin from sticking to or absorbing moisture from the gypsum materials (Fig. 14.5).

Mixed acrylic resin in the dough stage is placed in the space created by the removal of the wax and record base. This space is where the denture base will be formed. A sheet of polyethylene material is placed over the resin and the flask is reassembled and closed under pressure. The flask is reopened to remove excess material that exudes out of the sides of the flask. This process is repeated until no excess material appears and the polyethylene sheet is removed. The flask is put into a device called a *pneumatic press* that maintains pressure on it, and it is placed into a temperature-controlled water bath for at least 8 hours (Fig. 14.6).

Heat activates the benzoyl peroxide, causing the formation of free radicals and allowing polymerization to occur. Applying pressure and controlling the heat minimize porosity by preventing the monomer from vaporizing. More of the monomer is consumed during the polymerization, so less free monomer is present in the cured denture base with heat-processed dentures.

Polymers for Prosthetic Dentistry **CHAPTER 14** 281

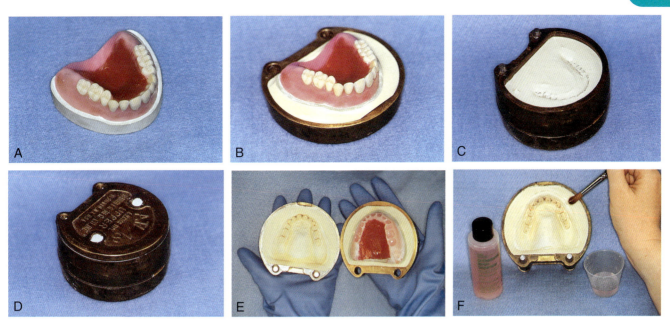

FIG. 14.5 Steps in preparing the mold for the compression mold technique: **(A)** Completed tooth arrangement prepared for flasking process. **(B)** Master cast embedded in properly contoured dental gypsum. **(C)** Occlusal and incisal surfaces of the denture teeth are exposed to facilitate subsequent denture recovery. **(D)** Fully flasked maxillary denture. **(E)** Separation of the flask segments during the wax elimination process. **(F)** Placement of separating medium.

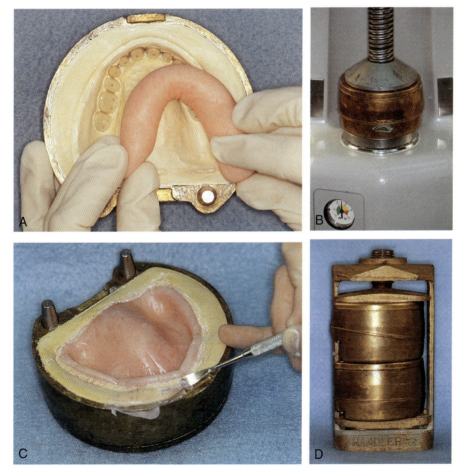

FIG. 14.6 Steps in packing the resin for the compression mold technique: **(A)** Resin at the dough stage is bent into a horseshoe shape and placed into the mold cavity. **(B)** The flask is reassembled and placed into a press under pressure. **(C)** Excess resin material is removed from the flask. **(D)** The flask is put into a carrier that maints pressure on the flask during processing.

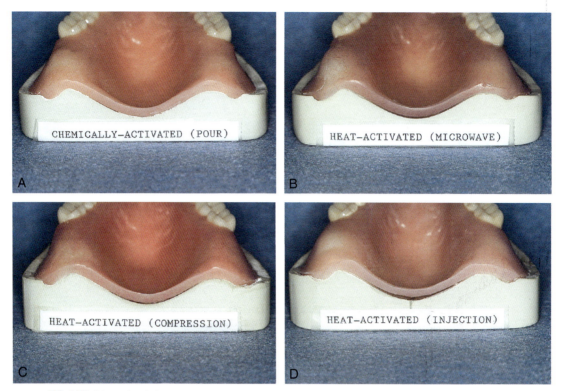

FIG. 14.7 Dimensional changes from polymerization shrinkage with four processing techniques seen mostly in the mild-palatal area: **(A)** Chemically activated resin using pour technique. **(B)** Microwave resin using compression molding. **(C)** Heat-activated resin using compression molding. **(D)** Heat-activated resin using injection molding.

Similar to the chemical-cured resins, the material is hard and stiff when the polymerization is complete. It also shrinks when it is polymerized. Shrinkage is seen most readily in the palatal area and can cause the acrylic to lift from the cast as much as 0.25 mm. Fig. 14.7 shows the dimensional changes in the palatal area from polymerization shrinkage using four different processing techniques.

Components of a Complete Denture

- Denture Base—acrylic resin component that rests on the edentulous ridge and adjacent oral mucosa and contains the denture teeth. In the maxillary denture it also covers and rests on the hard palate.
- Flange—that portion of the denture that extends vertically from the base of the denture into the facial or lingual vestibule. In Fig. 14.3, panel B, it is the pink acrylic that extends on the facial from the base of the denture teeth to the depth of the vestibule.
- Peripheral Seal—a seal created around the outer edge of the denture by its intimate contact with the oral soft tissues. It is needed to provide retention of the denture.
- Posterior Palatal Seal (also called Postdam)—a seal formed in the posterior extent of the maxillary denture base at the junction of the hard and soft palates. It is the part of the peripheral seal of the denture that resists tipping of the denture when biting with the anterior teeth.
- Denture Teeth—acrylic, composite resin or porcelain teeth used to replace missing natural teeth.

Injection Molding

Some vinyl acrylic resins can be processed by injecting the material into a mold when it is in a doughy form. With some materials, shrinkage and porosity are reduced by injection molding. Some laboratories use this technique because it is faster than traditional heat/compression molding.

Microwave Processing

The same denture resins used for the heat/compression processing technique can be used for processing in a microwave oven. If a special monomer liquid is used in place of regular monomer, less porosity is found. Processing time is greatly speeded up, and processing is completed in about 5 minutes instead of several hours as needed for heat processing.

Chemical-Cured Resins

Polymerization of chemical-cured acrylic resins is an addition reaction facilitated by free radicals. An inhibitor increases the working time so that the materials can be manipulated for a reasonable period of time. The reaction releases heat, and when the reaction is complete, the material is hard and stiff.

Pour Technique

Some chemical-cured materials can be mixed to a thin, fluid consistency and poured into a mold and cured under pressure.

Light-Cured Resins

Light-polymerized resins have photoinitiators such as camphorquinone and amine activators. These react to form free radicals when exposed to blue light and initiate the polymerization reaction. Silica fillers may be added for thickening the material and reinforcing it. The materials come in flat sheets or ropes depending on the application. Sheets are individually packaged in thick black plastic bags to prevent room light from reaching them and causing premature polymerization. Light-cured materials are fast and easy to use but require the purchase of a light-curing unit. The material is available in limited acrylic colors. It is used for denture bases, record bases, custom trays, and denture repairs. It also has applications for removable orthodontic appliances.

PROCESSING OF A REMOVABLE PARTIAL DENTURE

A similar process is performed for applying a denture base to a removable partial denture, except that the partial denture will have a metal framework (see Fig. 14.8 for framework components) invested in the mold, as well as the teeth set in wax. Because the acrylic resin does not adhere well to the metal, a retentive mesh or lattice is made as part of the partial denture framework to lock the acrylic in place (Fig. 14.9).

Components of a Removable Partial Denture (RPD) Framework

The framework is the structure that supports the denture base and the teeth and provides stability and retention of the prosthesis. Its components include:

- Major Connector—joins the components of the framework on one side of the arch to the other side. In Fig. 14.8 it is the lingual bar. A maxillary RPD would have a palatal connector (as seen in Fig. 14.9). The major connector provides cross-arch stability and aids in resisting displacement of the RPD by functional forces.
- Minor Connectors—join the major connector to the other components of the framework such as the retentive clasp assembly, occlusal or cingulum rests, and indirect retainers.
- Direct Retainer—the clasp assembly that has a retentive clasp arm (that engage undercuts on the crown of the support tooth), a reciprocal arm opposite the retentive arm (that braces against lateral stresses) and rests (metal stops on the occlusal of posterior teeth or cingulum of anterior teeth that prevent the partial denture from seating too far).
- Indirect Retainer—when an RPD has no support teeth at the distal extent of the arch on one or both sides, the indirect retainer aids the direct retainer in preventing displacement of the distal extension denture base. In Fig. 14.9 the upper-right quadrant has a distal extension denture base replacing teeth 2 to 5.
- Retentive Meshwork—a metal grid overlying the edentulous ridge into which the denture acrylic will be forced during processing for retention of the denture base.
- Denture Base—acrylic resin component that rests on the edentulous ridge and adjacent oral mucosa and contains the denture teeth.
- Denture Teeth—acrylic, composite resin or porcelain teeth used to replace missing natural teeth.

KEY POINTS

POLYMER FORMATION AND ACRYLIC RESINS

1. Addition polymerization—long chain polymers form by linking small monomer molecules activated by free radicals
2. Cross-linking of adjacent polymer chains make the polymer:
    - Stronger
    - Stiffer
    - More wear resistant
    - Easier to polish
3. Acrylic resins—synthetic polymers
    - Used for denture bases, teeth, reline and repair
    - Custom colored to match teeth, gingiva and skin
4. Physical properties manipulated by adding
    - Plasticizers
    - Rubbers
    - Fillers
    - Affects flexibility, impact resistance and strength
5. Acrylic resins
    - Shrink when polymerized
    - Slightly increase in size when they absorb water
    - Are brittle unless rubber is added
    - Do not conduct temperature well
    - Have better properties when heat processed rather than chemical cured
    - If porous, have increased staining and odor and reduced strength
6. Types of processing
    - Chemical curing
    - Heat and pressure
    - Microwave processing
    - Injection molding
    - Light curing

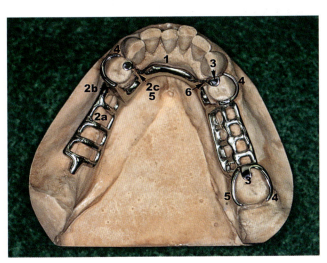

FIG. 14.8 Components of a removable partial denture framework. (From Carr AB, Brown DT. *McCracken's Removable Partial Prosthodontics*. 13th ed. Mosby; 2016.)

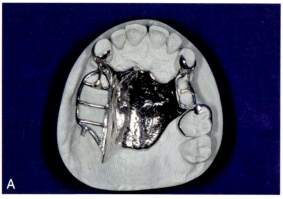
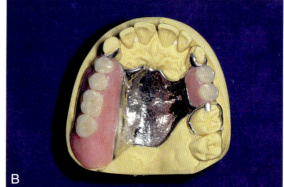
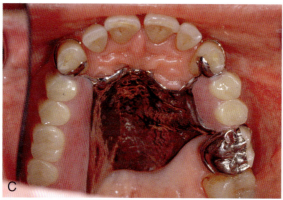

FIG. 14.9 **(A)** Metal frameworks for upper removable partial denture with retentive areas to hold acrylic. **(B)** Acrylic processed over retentive structure with denture teeth added. **(C)** Maxillary partial denture in the mouth.

DIGITAL DENTURES

The use of computer-assisted design/computer-assisted machining (CAD/CAM) technology in dentistry has expanded beyond crown and bridge applications to many other clinical aspects of dentistry including removable partial and complete dentures. Digital scanners can scan the edentulous ridges for complete denture construction. However, the scanners are not able to determine with accuracy where the flange of the denture should end in the vestibule. Therefore they cannot be used for complete denture final impressions since the peripheral seal needed for retention cannot be established from the scan. A mix of traditional denture construction techniques and CAD/CAM techniques are needed.

The clinician that wants to provide digital dentures has two options. First, the clinician can use traditional denture methods up to the point of processing the denture and then can have the records entered into a CAD/CAM system for design and fabrication by milling or 3D printing. The second option is to use methods and devices developed by companies for their digital denture systems. These systems allow final impressions and records of the bite and other jaw relations, occlusal plane orientation, tooth shade and mold and maxillary anterior tooth position all to be gathered in the first appointment and sent to the company to be scanned and entered into their CAD/CAM software. Then, the denture can be designed and processed.

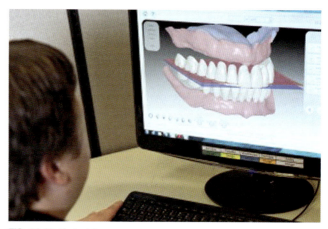

FIG. 14.10 Technician scans the clinical records and designs the denture. (Courtesy AvaDent.)

The two main systems currently in use differ in the way they fabricate the dentures: one system uses CAD/CAM milling and the other uses 3D printing. There are also some differences in their records collections methods and design software. The two systems use trays that can be customized to take final impressions at the first visit and use their own devices for capturing jaw records and the other features (mentioned above) needed to design the denture.

The impression and other records are sent to the company. A technician scans the records into the software and designs the denture based on the records (Fig. 14.10). The dentist can receive this image and

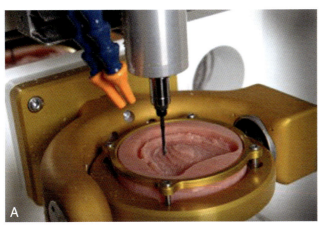 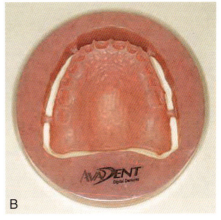

FIG. 14.11 Denture base is being milled from a preformed, thick acrylic disk: **(A)** Milling of the denture base. **(B)** Completed denture base with spaces created for the denture teeth. (A, Courtesy Loma Linda University Dentistry Summer/Autumn 2012, CAD/CAM technology: application to complete dentures by Mathew Kattadiyil, DDS, MSD and Charles J. Goodacre, DDS, MSD; B, Courtesy AvaDent.)

view it with the patient in the dental office and make adjustments on the arrangement, size, and shade of the teeth before the denture is processed. If desired, a try-in denture can be made and sent to the dentist for the patient to evaluate.

One system mills the denture base from large, thick, preformed disks of acrylic that have been polymerized under heat and much more pressure than conventionally processed denture bases (Fig. 14.11). As a consequence, when the denture base is milled there will be no polymerization shrinkage because it occurred when the disk was made and porosity will be greatly reduced. The acrylic disk is highly cross-linked, producing a stronger acrylic. Denture teeth are bonded to the denture base (Fig. 14.12).

The other system also designs the denture and allows the clinician to review it with the patient. Processing of the denture is by 3D printing. The denture base and teeth are printed as one unit. It produces a denture with similar improvements in physical properties as with the first technique.

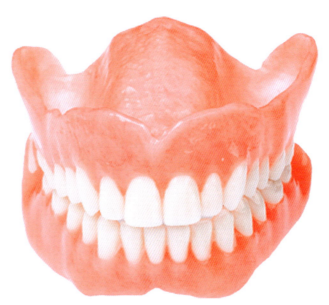

FIG. 14.12 Completed dentures after teeth have been bonded to the denture base. (Courtesy AvaDent.)

Advantages of Digital Dentures

- Reduced number of appointments—usually two instead of five for conventional denture techniques
- Time savings for dentist and patient
- Dentures can be ready in a matter of days rather than weeks with conventional dentures
- Better fit of the denture because polymerization shrinkage is eliminated
- Porosity is reduced or eliminated reducing staining and development of odor
- Records can be stored for futures needs
- Duplicate or replacement dentures can be made without additional appointments

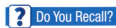 Do You Recall?

Why do digital dentures fit better than heat-processed dentures?

KEY POINTS

DIGITAL DENTURES
- Produced by CAD/CAM technology or 3D printing
- Reduced steps to make
- No polymerization shrinkage

DENTURE RELINE MATERIALS (LINERS)

Relining a denture is done for several reasons:
- To fix looseness that occurs as the bony ridges resorb and the gums shrink
- To prolong the life of a denture
- To fix minor cracks that may have developed under a loose denture
- To allow sore tissues to heal by using a soft, temporary liner

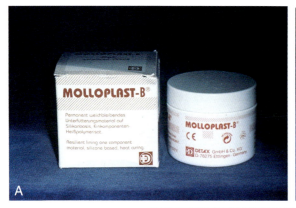
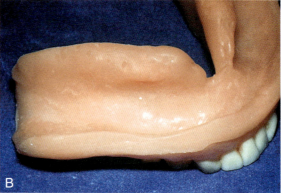
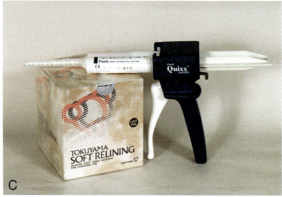

FIG. 14.13 Long-term soft liners: **(A)** Heat-cured, silicone-based soft lining material. **(B)** Soft liner processed in lower denture. **(C)** Chairside, chemical-cured, silicone-based soft liner in cartridges dispensed with a mixing gun and tip. (Courtesy Mark Dellinges, School of Dentistry, University of California, San Francisco, San Francisco, California.)

Long-term denture relines can be made with either a hard-setting material or a soft, flexible one.

SOFT RELINING MATERIALS

Complete and partial dentures sometimes have a soft lining material placed on the tissue-bearing surface of the denture base. Materials applied can be for long-term or short-term use.

Long-Term Soft Liners

Uses for **long-term soft liners** include:
- Treatment for patients with bony tissue undercuts that cannot be surgically corrected. A hard denture base rubs the mucosa in the area of the undercut, whereas a soft liner cushions the tissues and will flex in and out of the undercut when the denture is placed and removed.
- Treatment for patients who have chronic soreness with hard denture bases because of sharp, bony spicules or thin mucosa over narrow ridges. Patients feel more comfortable with a lining that has a cushioning effect.
- Management of palatal defects such as cleft palate or tissue loss from cancer surgery or trauma.

Long-term soft liners:
- Are made from silicone rubber or acrylics that have been made pliable by the addition of plasticizers (Fig. 14.13).
- May be processed at room temperature or with the application of heat.
- Can be placed at chairside or placed at the commercial laboratory.

Heat-cured silicone liners are processed in the laboratory because they release acetic acid that can cause tissue burns. They are more stable over the long term (1–3 years) because they do not have softeners to leach out. However, they can be difficult to adjust. Special burs and stones are needed to make these adjustments.

Chairside soft relines are more porous and stain more easily. Long-term liners composed of acrylic will harden over time as the plasticizers leach out and will need replacement. Long-term soft liners often do not form a good bond to old acrylic. Therefore they may separate from the denture base at the edges and leak between the liner and the denture base.

Short-Term Soft Liners (Tissue Conditioners)

Short-term soft liners are referred to as *tissue conditioners* or *treatment liners* and are usually placed at chairside. They are supplied as a powder composed of poly(ethyl methacrylate) and softeners or plasticizers (Fig. 14.14).

Application of Short-Term Liner. The powder and liquid are mixed thoroughly according to the manufacturer's directions and are flowed onto the tissue-bearing surface of the denture, which was previously cleaned with soap and water. The denture is reseated in the patient's mouth, and the patient is instructed to gently close into normal occlusion until the material cures (see sequence in Fig. 14.15).

These liners are capable of readapting to the patient's tissues as they heal because they have a high degree of flow. Because this flow property is greatest the first day, hard foods should be avoided to prevent distortion of the material. As the plasticizers leach out, the resin becomes stiffer. The plasticizers leach out more quickly in the short-term liners than in the long-term liners and therefore need frequent replacement. Some short-term liners last for only 1 week; others last for 2 to 4 weeks.

HOME CARE FOR SOFT LINERS

Soft liners cannot be cleaned effectively, and consequently patients complain about a bad taste and odor. Accumulation of food debris in pores of the silicone liners supports the growth of yeasts such as *Candida albicans* and may cause tissue irritation that requires antifungal therapy. Cleaning soft liners on a daily basis in benzalkonium chloride will reduce the growth of yeasts.

Use of appropriate denture soaks (those with enzymes are preferred) can prolong the useful life of soft liners, and therefore the manufacturer's recommendations are important. Soaks containing dilute bleach-like substances can degrade soft liners. Scrubbing soft liners can be damaging. If brushing is needed to remove debris, a soft brush and a nonabrasive toothpaste or mild soap solution can be used carefully.

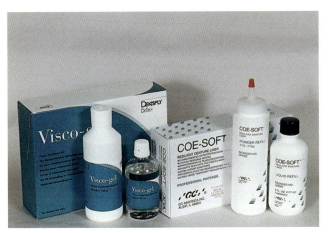

FIG. 14.14 Two tissue conditioners (short-term soft liners). They come with two components—powder and liquid. (Visco-gel, Courtesy Dentsply International, York, Pennsylvania; Coe-Soft, Courtesy GC America, Alsip, Illinois).

The dental auxiliary must be familiar with materials and procedures for the placement of liners at chairside and for the home care of both chairside and laboratory-processed liners.

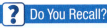

What problems do long-term soft liners alleviate?

HARD RELINING MATERIALS

Immediate dentures are those placed immediately after extraction of the teeth. They become loose rapidly (usually within 6–12 months) as the extraction sites heal and the bone resorbs. These loose dentures can often be made to fit well again by placement of a **hard liner** to fill in the spaces. Conventionally placed dentures will loosen as well but over a longer period of time. The most common material used for relining is an acrylic resin similar to the original denture base material. This hard liner is placed directly into the patient's mouth at chairside or indirectly in the dental laboratory using an impression of the arch.

When to Use a Hard Reline Material
- Inadequate seal of denture borders
- Lack of retention of the denture
- Looseness and poor denture stability
- Overclosed bite (loss of vertical dimension of occlusion)

Chairside Reline

Chairside reline material is composed of chemical-cured acrylic resin [poly(methyl methacrylate)]. It is supplied as polymer powder and liquid (methyl methacrylate) monomer.

Application Technique. First, an acrylic bur is used to remove a thin layer of the tissue-bearing surface of the denture base, so that a fresh, clean surface is available for chemical bonding of the lining material. A lubricant such as petroleum jelly is applied to the denture teeth and to non–tissue-bearing surfaces to which the liner should not adhere. The freshened surface is primed with some of the liquid to make it ready for the liner. The monomer is a good solvent and will slightly soften the surface, allowing the liner to bond better.

The powder and the liquid are mixed thoroughly and applied to the primed denture base. The patient should be advised that the material has a strong smell and bad taste. The denture is reseated in the patient's mouth. The lips, cheeks, and tongue are moved through appropriate motions to reestablish the peripheral borders (a process called *border molding*). In essence, the reline material makes an impression of the tissues. The patient is asked to close into the normal occlusion. This

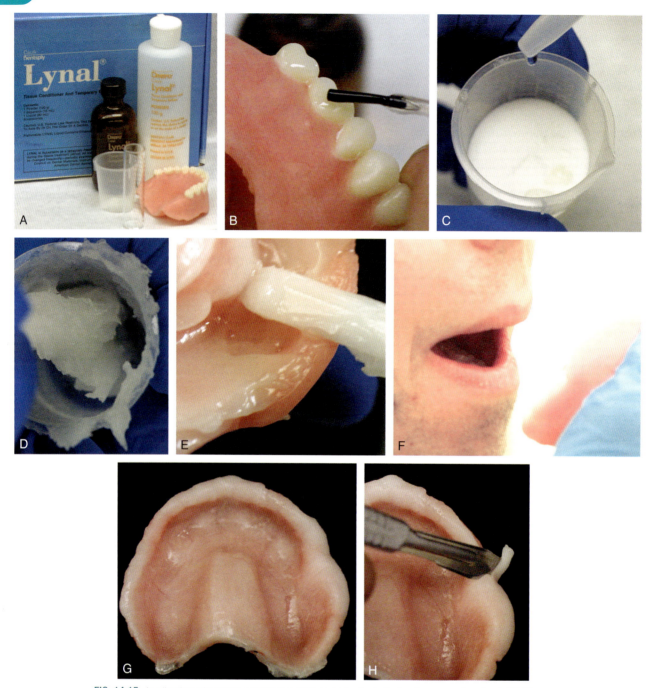

FIG. 14.15 Application of a tissue conditioner. It flows and adapts to the tissues as they heal: **(A)** Tissue conditioner. **(B)** Separating material to keep conditioner from sticking to outer surfaces of denture. **(C)** Liquid added to powder. **(D)** Mixed conditioner material. **(E)** Conditioner added to tissue-bearing surfaces. **(F)** Denture inserted into patient's mouth, seated evenly, and left until it gels. **(G)** Excess material around denture border. **(H)** Scalpel blade used to trim excess from border. (From Powers JM, Wataha JC. *Dental Materials: Properties and Manipulation*. 10th ed. Elsevier; 2013; Courtesy Richard Lee, Sr., and Bradley Jones, Department of Restorative Dentistry, University of Washington, Seattle, Washington.)

position is held until the material just begins to harden. It should be removed from the mouth before polymerization is complete because the chemical reaction is exothermic and the heat generated could burn the tissues. Also, the hardened material could lock into tissue undercuts, making it difficult and painful to remove.

Gross excess material extending over the borders is removed with sharp iris scissors or a scalpel blade before it hardens completely. The denture is placed into a plastic bag and sprayed with an appropriate disinfectant before taking it to the laboratory. The denture is placed into warm water (not hot) in a pressure pot in the office laboratory at 20 psi of pressure for about 15 to 20 minutes while the final set occurs. Once completely hardened, excess material is trimmed away and the denture borders are carefully polished.

The denture is disinfected before returning it to chairside. Pressure indicating paste (PIP) is used to detect pressure spots (see "Denture Sore Detection" below). After all of the pressure spots have been removed, the occlusion is checked with articulating paper and adjustments made as needed.

The patient is advised that the interior of the denture is now entirely new and may cause sore spots, much like a new denture. One or more visits may be necessary to complete the adjustments.

An alternative hard reline material (Ufi Gel hard; VOCO) is free of methyl methacrylate. It uses polymer beads and dimethacrylate as the monomer. It is hand-mixed or is available in a cartridge for direct application to the denture. The self-mixing cartridge makes it easy to use and provides a homogeneous, bubble-free mix. The liner does not generate heat as it polymerizes, so it can be left in the patient's mouth until it fully cures, improving the accuracy of the fit. It is more pleasant for the patient because it is odorless and tasteless.

Problems Associated with Chairside Reline with Poly(Methyl Methacrylate)

- Porosity from mixing or applying, causing staining and odor
- Bad taste and smell
- Potential soft tissue irritation from free monomer
- Poor bonding with the denture base
- Heat generation with potential tissue burn if not removed soon enough

Caution

When doing a chairside hard reline with poly(methyl methacrylate), be sure to remove the denture before the reline material completely hardens. The heat released can burn the tissues and the material could lock into undercuts, making it difficult and painful to remove.

LABORATORY RELINE

The laboratory reline uses an indirect technique in which an impression of the tissues is made inside the existing denture and a cast is made from this impression. Because daily use of the denture will compress the underlying tissues, prior to taking the impression the denture should be left out 12-24 hours to allow the tissues to return to a normal, uncompressed state. This will produce a more accurate impression for placing the denture reline.

The technician uses an indexing instrument called a *reline jig* or device to establish the relationship between the cast and the denture. The impression material is removed, along with a thin layer of the tissue-bearing denture base surface, as with the chairside technique. The lining material is placed inside the denture, and the denture is returned to the reline jig, and then the lining material is heat- and pressure-processed to the denture base.

This process produces a denser, longer-lasting reline that is less prone to staining than a chairside reline. However, the negative aspect of the laboratory reline is that the patient will be without the denture for a period of time.

OVER-THE-COUNTER LINERS

Some patients are "do-it-yourselfers" who purchase reline materials over-the-counter in the drugstore and apply them at home. They do not receive professional advice on the use and care of these liners and often use the liners far beyond their useful life. These materials can stiffen with time and can cause damage to the tissues, particularly if the occlusion is not properly reestablished with the new lining in place. They are usually porous and promote the growth of fungi, and patients can end up with fungal infection of the oral tissues. These over-the-counter products are not recommended.

DETECTION AND MANAGEMENT OF DENTURE SORES

Denture sores are common with new dentures as the tissues adapt to the new prosthesis. Older dentures may also produce sore spots as the bony ridges slowly resorb and the denture becomes loose. Sore spots can also occur after a denture reline since a whole new tissue-bearing surface has been created.

SIGNS AND SYMPTOMS

Typically the patient first senses some mild soreness under the denture when eating or placing and removing the denture. After a few days, mild soreness may become outright pain. Initially the affected area may be slightly red as inflammation begins, and then can become a larger, bright-red area in a couple days (Fig. 14.16). If not treated right away, the tissue can ulcerate, leaving a painful raw area that will take longer to heal.

CAUSES OF DENTURE SORES

Common Causes of Denture Sores

- Bony or soft tissue undercuts
- Sharp, bony edges to sockets of extracted teeth
- Overextended denture borders
- Loose dentures
- Uneven occlusion on the denture, causing pressure areas

TREATMENT OF DENTURE SORES

The denture requires some adjustment to eliminate the source of the irritation. The source needs to be detected. Sometimes there is an obvious projection on the inside of the denture that can readily be removed with rotary instruments such as an acrylic bur (a metal bur made

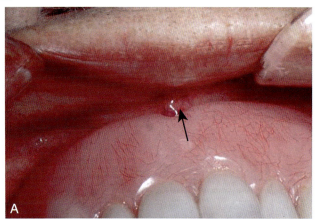
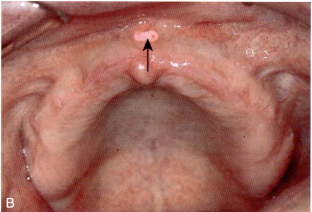

FIG. 14.16 Denture sore: **(A)** Denture flange impinged on maxillary frenum. **(B)** Denture sore resulted. (Courtesy Dr. Mark Dellinges.)

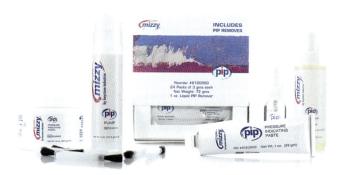

FIG. 14.17 Pressure indicating paste (PIP; Keystone Industries) Available in bulk jar, pump, tube, or single-use packets with brush. Spray bottles of PIP removal agent and wetting agent (to keep PIP from sticking to the tissues).

for grinding acrylic) or abrasive stone. Other times it is necessary to discover precisely where the offending acrylic is located.

There are two common methods for finding the high spots in the acrylic and acrylic that rubs the tissues:
- Use of a paste painted inside the denture that shows the area of pressure
- Colored dye that is applied to the denture sore and transferred to the inside of the denture

Use of Pressure Indicating Paste

Paste used to show pressure areas inside the denture (pressure indicating paste [PIP]) is an opaque, white silicone paste (Fig. 14.17) that is painted inside the denture with a brush. A thin layer of the paste should be evenly distributed across the entire tissue-bearing surface of the denture if there are multiple sore areas or limited to one area if there is only one sore. See Fig. 14.18 for the technique for using PIP.

Use of Dye Transfer Method

A small wooden applicator with dry purple dye on one end (Dr. Thompson's Sanitary Color Transfer Applicators) is used to mark the denture sore (Fig. 14.19). Excess moisture is wiped away from the denture sore with gauze. Next, the tip of the applicator with dye is wet with a drop of water and touched to the sore depositing the dye (Fig. 14.20). The inside of the denture should be dry. The denture is seated over the ridge and gently held in place for 10 to 20 seconds. The denture is removed and the purple dye will have been picked up by the denture in the area of the sore. This marks the spot to be adjusted (Fig. 14.21).

HOME CARE FOR DENTURE SORES

Warm salt-water rinses can be useful to reduce inflammation and speed healing when used three to four times a day. Warm salt-water rinses should not be recommended for patients with hypertension or a salt restricted diet. Going to a soft diet will also reduce the pressure on the tissues produced with eating. When possible, leaving the dentures out for a few hours a day will also help with healing. Good oral hygiene is necessary to reduce oral debris and bacteria. Over-the-counter numbing pastes, gels, and rinses can be helpful in reducing symptoms and help to reduce pain while eating. Acidic and spicy foods may irritate the ulcerated tissue, so they should be avoided.

Do You Recall?

What are two methods used to find the part of a denture causing a denture sore?

DENTURE TEETH

Acrylic resin (plastic), composite resin, and porcelain teeth are used for complete and partial dentures. Each has certain advantages and disadvantages.

ACRYLIC RESIN TEETH

The vast majority of denture teeth used for removable dental prostheses are made from acrylic resin.

Advantages and Disadvantages

Acrylic teeth are tough and chemically bond to the acrylic base of the denture. They are easy to grind to

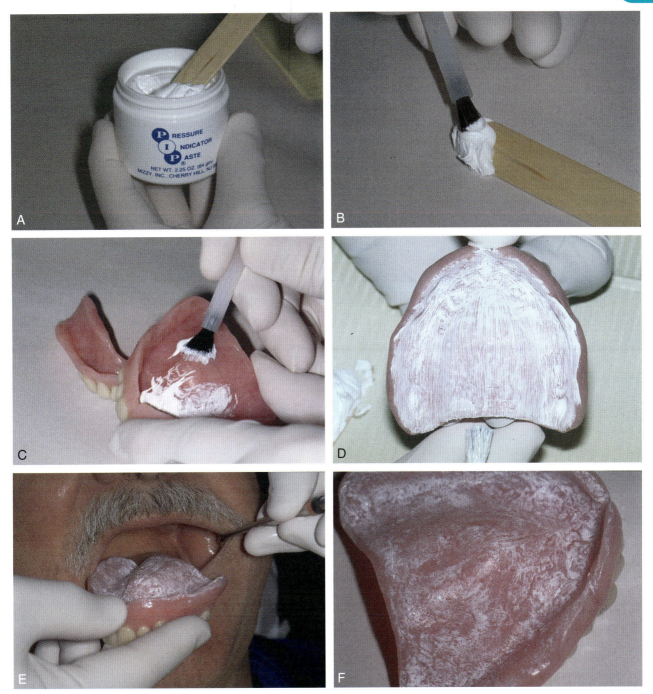

FIG. 14.18 Use of pressure indicating paste (PIP) at delivery of a new denture or after a hard reline: **(A)** A tongue blade is used to remove enough PIP to coat the denture a couple times. **(B)** PIP is picked up on a disposable brush. **(C)** PIP is spread on the tissue-bearing portion of the denture. **(D)** PIP is spread in a even coating leaving brush marks that all course in the same direction. This pattern helps in reading tissue contact with the denture. **(E)** Denture with PIP is seated in the mouth with light pressure for about 20 s. **(F)** When the denture is removed, the brush marks are gone and an even distribution of PIP has occurred. No pressure spots are evident. Pressure spots would show as areas where PIP was displaced and the denture base exposed. Areas where the denture did not have contact with the tissues would show as PIP with remaining brush marks. (Courtesy Dr. Mark Dellinges, University of California, San Francisco, California.)

adjust the occlusion or to reshape a tooth to fit the available space and easy to repolish. They do not wear down the opposing natural or artificial teeth or restorations. Acrylic resin teeth are used more often than porcelain teeth because they are somewhat resilient and are thought not to stress the underlying ridges as much as porcelain teeth. Their main disadvantage is that they are softer and wear more readily than porcelain teeth.

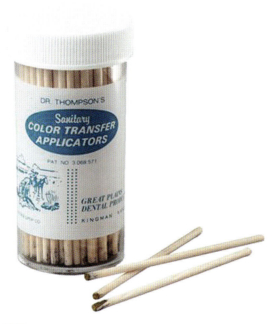

FIG. 14.19 Color transfer applicators. (Dr. Thompson's Sanitary Color Transfer Applicators, Great Plains Dental Products).

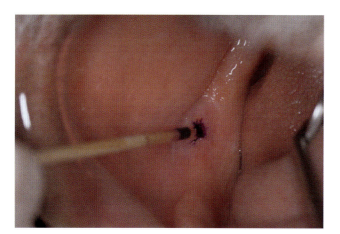

FIG. 14.20 Color transfer applicator used to mark denture sore and transfer the location to the denture. (Courtesy Dr. Mark Dellinges, University of California, San Francisco, California.)

Cross-Linking

Acrylic resin teeth are made in layers to simulate the colors and translucencies of natural teeth. The gingival portion of the teeth is manufactured so that the acrylic has minimal cross-linking. The bond of the acrylic tooth to the denture base is better without cross-linking. Cross-linking in the other portions of denture teeth makes them tougher and better able to hold up under function.

COMPOSITE RESIN TEETH

Nanohybrid composite material is used to make denture teeth that have improved properties compared with the simple acrylic resin teeth. Composite resin teeth have a more natural appearance and translucency.

Filler Particles

Various filler particles have been used often in combination. Highly cross-linked macrofillers increase strength and color stability. High-density microfillers improve wear resistance, and silane-treated silica-based nanofillers improve optical properties, such as light reflection.

PORCELAIN TEETH

Porcelain teeth are brittle, hard, and very resistant to wear. Because of their brittleness, they are prone to fracture if the denture is dropped or is overstressed by hard foods or accidental biting on a fork. They do not bond to the acrylic of the denture base and must have mechanical retention, such as metal pins or retention holes to keep them in the acrylic denture base (Fig. 14.22). They have a good esthetic appearance, until the surface glaze is lost through wear or abrasive polishing. Porcelain teeth cannot be easily repolished, as can acrylic resin teeth. They are highly stain resistant, whereas some acrylic resin teeth will stain over time.

Porcelain teeth are not indicated for use against the natural dentition or most restorative materials because they are very abrasive (Fig. 14.23). They also transmit heavier occlusal forces to the ridge and therefore may be a factor in patient discomfort, denture sores, and accelerated ridge resorption. Some patients prefer porcelain teeth because they sense a better ability to chew harder or more fibrous foods.

> **? Do You Recall?**
>
> How are porcelain teeth retained in a denture?

CHARACTERIZATION OF DENTURES

Dentures can be given individual characteristics to make them seem more lifelike. Denture teeth can be arranged in the standard "ideal" arch alignment, or teeth can be arranged to re-create spaces (diastemas) (Fig. 14.24) or overlapping or crooked teeth that the patient had with the natural teeth. The denture teeth can be all one shade or can be selected to simulate the lighter and darker teeth that most people have in their mouths (e.g., canines are usually darker than incisors). Some patients request that restorations be placed in the denture teeth to simulate restorations they had in their natural teeth.

The denture base acrylic itself is made in several shades, and these can be selected to replicate the color of the patient's mucosa and gingiva (see Fig. 14.4). The dental technician can do custom shading with pigmented resins to simulate racial pigmentation in the denture base, because racial pigmentation is not always uniformly distributed in the tissues.

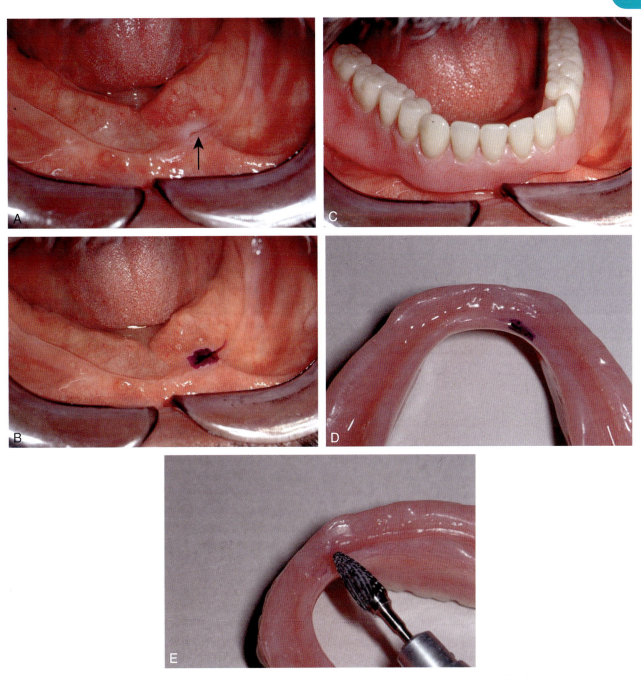

FIG. 14.21 Denture sore: **(A)** Ulcer in soft tissue lingual to mandibular edentulous ridge caused by the lower denture. **(B)** Denture sore marked with dye from color transfer applicator. **(C)** Denture dried and reseated. **(D)** The dye is transferred to the denture indicating the location of the offending pressure area. **(E)** An acrylic bur in a low speed handpiece is used to relieve the pressure area. **(F)** Now that the location of the irritating denture part has been located, pressure indicating paste (PIP) is used to detect any remaining pressure spots. **(G)** The denture is reseated and the interior inspected. Areas where pressure from the denture is evenly distributed will show a thin layer of PIP. PIP will be wiped away in areas of heavy pressure. **(H)** Readjust areas of heavy pressure. **(I)** Final check with PIP shows no pressure spots. (Courtesy Dr. Mark Dellinges, University of California, San Francisco, California.)

PLASTICS FOR MAXILLOFACIAL PROSTHETICS

A specialized aspect of a prosthodontic practice may include the fabrication of maxillofacial prostheses to replace facial tissues lost as the result of trauma, disease, surgery, or birth defect. These prostheses must have specialized characteristics so that they can be colored to match the surrounding skin, tear resistant in thin layers, resistant to staining, very flexible, and able to be attached to the surrounding skin with adhesives (Fig. 14.25). Materials that have been used are synthetic latex, plasticized vinyl resins, and silicone rubbers. Of these materials, the best for maxillofacial prostheses is silicone rubber.

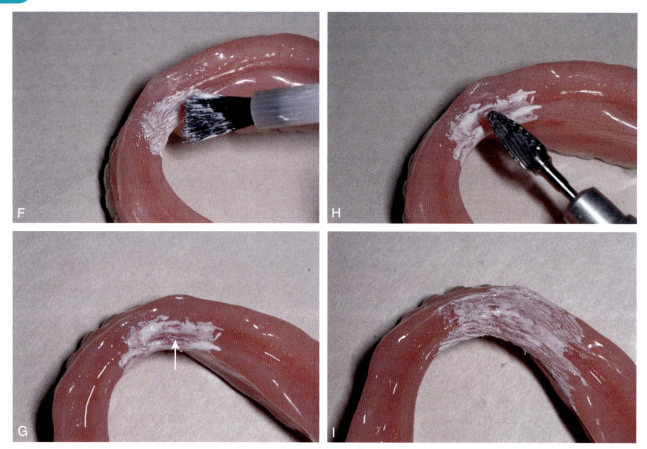

FIG. 14.21, cont'd

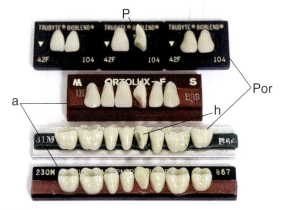

FIG. 14.22 Plastic and porcelain denture teeth. Porcelain teeth (*Por*) do not chemically bond to the denture base, as do plastic teeth (*a*); therefore they have metal pins (*P*) or retention holes (*h*) to lock into the acrylic.

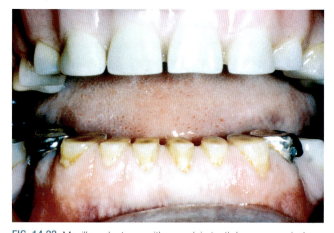

FIG. 14.23 Maxillary dentures with porcelain teeth have excessively worn opposing natural teeth. (Courtesy Steve Eakle, University of California School of Dentistry, San Francisco, California.)

DENTURE REPAIR

Acrylic complete and partial dentures usually can be repaired when they are broken. The repair of a partial denture with a metal framework is more complex, depending on the location of the break. Broken denture bases can be repaired if the fragments can be reassembled. Lost or broken teeth can be chemically bonded in place with repair acrylic. If the break occurs through the framework or the clasp, it can sometimes be repaired by welding in the dental laboratory. However, many times such a break means that a new partial denture must be made.

CHEMICAL-CURED ACRYLIC REPAIR MATERIAL

Repair Technique

The broken prosthesis should be disinfected at chairside before it is transported to the laboratory. For repair of an all-acrylic denture or partial denture, the broken

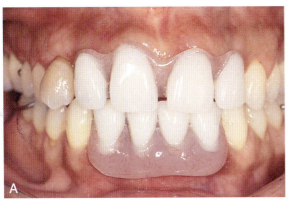 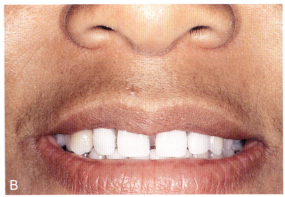

FIG. 14.24 Characterized temporary partial denture (stayplate) to create a lifelike appearance. Patient had naturally occurring diastemas between her maxillary incisors and wanted to have diastemas in the prosthesis: **(A)** Stayplate with diastemas between the incisors. **(B)** Natural-looking smile. (Courtesy Arun Sharma, School of Dentistry, University of California, San Francisco, San Francisco, California.)

parts are pieced together and are held with sticky wax. Plaster or stone is poured into the prosthesis to create a cast on which the parts can be stabilized while they are being repaired.

After the plaster has set, the fracture line is cut with an acrylic bur to create room for a sufficient bulk of repair material, and the adjacent surfaces several millimeters around the fracture line are ground to expose fresh surfaces for bonding. Often mechanical locks or dovetails are cut into the acrylic fragments to ensure a good, strong union between fragments. A coating of the liquid monomer is placed on the roughened surfaces to wet and prime them.

Often the repair material is the same as the chairside reline material. The repair material is applied to the fracture in bulk or by the "salt and pepper" technique. With the salt and pepper technique, a small quantity of powder is sprinkled onto the monomer-wet fracture site and is wet with more liquid. This process of alternately adding powder and liquid continues until the fracture site is slightly overfilled. The prosthesis on the cast is then placed into a pressure pot with warm (not hot) water and about 20 pounds of pressure until cured (at least 20 minutes). Once the repair acrylic has cured, the prosthesis is removed, and excess material is cut back and polished. The prosthesis is disinfected and returned to chairside to try in the patient's mouth to confirm the fit and comfort.

 Caution

Liquid monomer repair material is highly flammable; do not use it around an open flame, such as a Bunsen burner.

LIGHT-CURED REPAIR MATERIAL

Light-cured dimethacrylates have a number of useful applications, including repair of broken acrylic prostheses and fabrication of custom trays and record bases. Dimethacrylate is an acrylic resin that contains a chemical activated by light in the blue wavelength range, as well as an accelerator, inorganic fillers, and pigments to simulate tissue colors. These materials are cross-linked to improve their stiffness and strength.

Repair Technique

When used for denture repair, the prosthesis is prepared in the same manner as for chemical-cured material, except that a different liquid is painted on the fractured pieces before the repair material is applied. The repair material is removed from its lightproof package and is pressed onto the prepared fracture site. The repair material is coated with a liquid to prevent the development of an oxygen-inhibited layer of uncured material on the surface. Uncured material at the surface makes it more difficult to polish.

The prosthesis on the cast is placed into a curing unit with intense blue light for about 10 minutes. These curing units are more commonly found in a dental laboratory than a dental office. A high-intensity, hand-held curing light can be used, but the process will take much longer.

After curing, it is finished and polished, The repaired denture is disinfected before it is delivered to the patient. This technique is somewhat faster than the chemical-cured method.

CUSTOM IMPRESSION TRAYS AND RECORD BASES

Chemical-cured and light-cured acrylic resins can be used to construct custom impression trays and the record bases on which wax rims are placed during the process of making dentures. These acrylics contain a high proportion of filler particles to impart strength to the material.

CHEMICAL-CURED TRAY MATERIAL

Custom Tray Fabrication

Similar to other chemical-cured acrylics, tray materials are supplied as polymer powder and monomer liquid. See Procedure 14.1 for details.

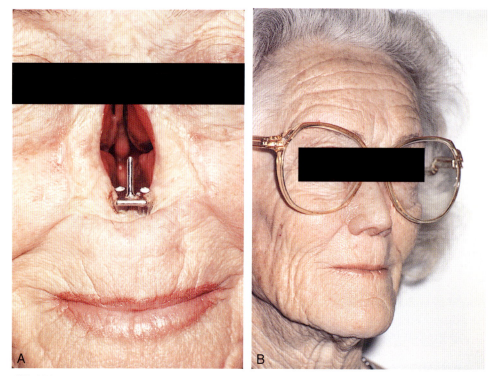

FIG. 14.25 Flexible acrylic prosthesis for nose lost to cancer: **(A)** Metal implant at site of lost nose will hold the prosthesis in place. **(B)** Lifelike prosthesis made of silicone rubber replaces the nose. (Courtesy Arun Sharma, School of Dentistry, University of California, San Francisco, San Francisco, California.)

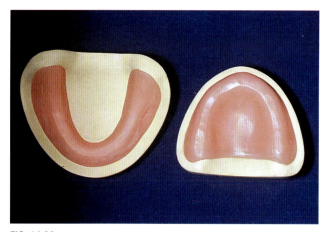

FIG. 14.26 Mandibular and maxillary record bases on casts. (Courtesy Mark Dellinges, School of Dentistry, University of California, San Francisco, San Francisco, California.)

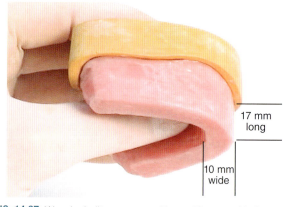

FIG. 14.27 Wax rim built up on record base. (Courtesy Mark Dellinges, School of Dentistry, University of California, San Francisco, San Francisco, California.)

Record Bases

Record bases are rigid bases that correspond roughly to the denture base (Fig. 14.26). They are used in the construction stage of the denture and have wax rims added to them over the ridge areas (Fig. 14.27). They are used initially to establish the proper dimension between upper and lower arches, as well as the position of centric occlusion (Fig. 14.28). Marks can be made in the wax to denote the location of the border of the upper lip, the "smile" line, and the midline of the face as guides for placement of the denture teeth. Later, the denture teeth are set in the wax rims, and the record bases serve to stabilize the wax rims during the try-in appointment. The record bases are discarded during denture processing to make room for the denture base material.

Record Base Fabrication

Record bases are also constructed from the same materials as the trays. The difference in their construction is that wax spacers, tissue stops, and handles are not used. If significant tissue undercuts are present on the cast, they are blocked out with wax before the record bases are constructed.

LIGHT-CURED TRAY AND RECORD BASE MATERIAL

Light-cured dimethacrylates can be used for construction of custom trays and record bases. They are similar to light-cured repair materials but come in one color and do not have fibers to simulate blood vessels.

The technique for making custom trays and record bases is the same as for the chemical-cured materials, except that instead of mixing powder and liquid, a sheet of the preformed material is removed from its light-proof package and adapted over the cast or wax spacer (Fig. 14.29). After excess material is trimmed (and a handle is formed if a tray), the tray or record base on the cast is placed in a light-curing unit as described previously for light-cured repair materials. The light-cured material generates very little heat during polymerization and is much easier to use because no mixing is required. It eliminates the concerns about inhaling and handling the monomer associated with the chemical-cured material.

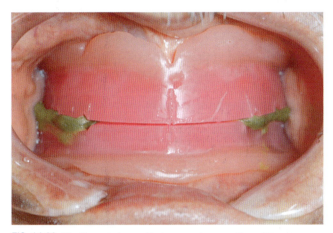

FIG. 14.28 Maxillary and mandibular wax rims positioned in centric occlusion and locked together using soft, green wax. A vertical groove in the wax marks the patient's midline. (Courtesy Mark Dellinges, School of Dentistry, University of California, San Francisco, San Francisco, California.)

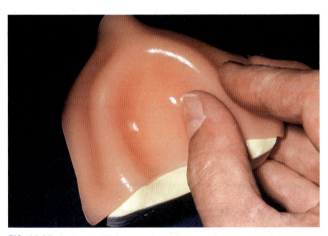

FIG. 14.29 A sheet of light-cured acrylic material is adapted over the cast. It can be used for making a record base or a custom tray. (Courtesy Mark Dellinges, School of Dentistry, University of California, San Francisco, San Francisco, California.)

Do You Recall?
What are record bases used for?

KEY POINTS

DENTURE RELINE AND REPAIR MATERIALS

1. Long-Term Soft Liners
   - Last 1–3 years
   - Made with silicone rubber or acrylics made pliable with plasticizers
   - Used for patients that cannot wear hard denture bases
   - Applied chairside or in laboratory (better results)
2. Short-Term Soft Liners
   - Last days to weeks
   - Tissue conditioners placed chairside
   - Used to treat sore tissues
3. Denture sore markers identify offending areas in the denture
   - Pressure indicating paste
   - Color transfer applicators
4. Hard reline material used to correct:
   - Loose dentures
   - Dentures lacking retention and border seal
   - Applied chairside or lab (better results)
5. Denture repair materials
   - Similar to hard reline materials
   - Also used for custom trays and record bases
   - Chemical-cured and light-cured materials

INFECTION CONTROL PROCEDURES

Contaminated dentures, custom trays, record bases, laboratory relines and other materials that are transported back and forth between the dental office and the dental laboratory should be treated following proper infection control procedures. The dental office is responsible for disinfecting these items that have been in the patient's mouth before they are sent to the laboratory. Likewise, the laboratory should disinfect the items before delivering them to the dental office. However, the dental office is ultimately responsible for assuring that items have been disinfected (or sterilized when possible) before placing them in the patient's mouth (see the box "Disinfecting Prostheses").

Instruments and materials used for finishing and polishing the dentures whether they are used chairside or in the laboratory need to be sterilized or disinfected. Rag wheels and pumice are commonly used in the laboratory for polishing the denture. The rag wheel should be rinsed to remove residual pumice and autoclaved. Pumice should be used in single-use quantities. The hooded polishing pan that contains wet pumice should be lined with plastic that can be disposed of after each use. Cross-contamination can easily occur in the laboratory if careful precautions are not taken.

> **Disinfecting Prostheses**
>
> - Properly disinfect all prostheses before trying in the patient's mouth.
> - Disinfect at chairside all prostheses going from the patient to the commercial or office laboratory, and package properly for transport.
> - Iodophors and synthetic phenols are suitable disinfectants for most prostheses.
> - Immerse prostheses for 15 minutes in one of these disinfectants in a denture cup or a plastic bag.

INSTRUCTIONS FOR NEW DENTURE WEARERS

Approximately 44 million people in the United States wear dentures. Losing one's teeth can have a physical and psychological effect on some people. Trying to adjust to acrylic prostheses can become a frustrating experience if patients do not know what to expect from their new dentures. It is vitally important to the patient's acceptance of the dentures that dental auxiliaries as part of the dental team be able to instruct patients on what to expect, how to manage use of their new dentures, and how to care for them. The following is information you can provide to the new denture wearer.

WHAT TO EXPECT WITH YOUR NEW DENTURES

Speaking

Dentures may create a feeling of fullness to the mouth as you adapt to the additional thickness of the dentures. Some people may feel a gagging sensation as they swallow. The tissues and muscles will adapt with time.

Most people will have some difficulty pronouncing some words, especially those with "f" and "s" sounds. Try reading out loud and practice words that are difficult to pronounce. The lower denture will move when you talk or eat because the tongue and cheeks move. Avoid the tendency to thrust your tongue forward because it will dislodge your dentures.

Eating

The biting force with your dentures is about 20% of that with your natural teeth. The dentures sit on top of tissues that are compressible, so there will be some movement of the dentures while eating. Start with soft foods that are easy to chew. Biting into food with the front teeth will tend to dislodge the dentures. People with dentures tend not to chew the food long enough to grind it into small pieces, because it takes longer than with natural teeth. This can put you at risk for choking. Cut the food into smaller pieces than you usually do. Chew the food well before swallowing. To help balance the dentures, chew with food on both sides of your mouth at the same time.

Your dentures cover many of your oral tissues, so you may not be aware of foods or beverages that are very hot. Take care not to burn yourself.

Excess Saliva

Saliva is important to help you swallow your food, lubricate your mouth tissues, and help form a seal with your dentures. However, your mouth will react to the presence of the new dentures by producing more saliva than usual. Your mouth will usually adapt and return to its normal salivary flow in a week or 2.

Fit

Your upper denture rests on the bony ridges and the hard palate. The borders of the denture help create a seal with the tissues and saliva fills in the gaps between the denture and the tissues, so suction is created to hold the denture in place. Your lower denture will feel looser because it does not have the large surface area of the palate for support and the tongue is continually moving and lifting the lower denture. You will need to learn how to position your tongue to help keep the lower denture seated. Avoid using denture adhesive if possible while you learn to adapt to the new dentures.

Soreness

Like a new pair of shoes, your dentures may rub the tissues and create sore spots. Biting your cheeks is not unusual in the first few weeks. Do not attempt to adjust the dentures yourself. Call the office and we will get you in quickly to relieve the soreness. It might take several visits to eliminate all of the pressure spots.

Looseness

If you had teeth extracted just before placement of the dentures, some looseness will occur as the extraction sites heal and the gum shrinks. Your dentist will discuss with you when it is time to put a lining material inside the dentures to adapt them to the new position of the gums.

Regular Dental Checkups

Even though you no longer have your natural teeth, you will need to visit the dentist periodically to have your mouth checked for cancer or other mouth disorders. In addition, your dentist will check the fit of your dentures and professionally clean them. The dentist will advise you as to how often you should come in.

You should come in sooner than your regular checkups if you notice soreness, exceptional looseness, chipped teeth or acrylic, or if you have dropped and broken your dentures. Do not attempt to repair them yourself, as you could cause damage that may make a repair more difficult or impossible.

CARE OF ACRYLIC RESIN DENTURES

Cleaning the dentures is important in maintaining the health of the oral tissues. Improper or inadequate home care can lead to fungal infections of the tissues or damage to the dentures. The most commonly used home cleaning aids for dentures are denture brushes and denture soaks or cleaners. Denture brushes, when used with water or mild soaps, are not abrasive to the acrylic surface. Household cleaners can be very abrasive to the acrylic and should not be used.

Denture cleaners can be found as tablets (Efferdent and Polident) or powders. They may contain detergents, sodium perborate, alkaline compounds, and flavoring agents. When sodium perborate is placed in water it releases oxygen and effervesces, loosening debris.

Diluted household bleach (sodium hypochlorite) will remove some stains and will have an antimicrobial effect. However it will remove the tissue color from the denture base over time. Bleach should not be used with prostheses containing metal such as partial denture frameworks or removable orthodontic appliances because it will attack the metal and corrode it.

HOME CARE

The patient needs to be instructed on how to care for new dentures. The following are home care instructions you can provide.

Clean the dentures every day, twice if possible, to remove plaque and debris. Hold them over a towel or put water in the sink, so if you drop them they will not break. Clean the tissue surfaces and the teeth and outer surfaces of the denture with a denture brush. Many denture brushes have medium or hard bristles. The stiffness of the bristles is not as critical to the abrasion of the acrylic as the cleaner used on the brush. Use liquid soap, mild hand soap, or a nonabrasive denture cleaning paste to remove surface debris.

Expect some food to get under the denture when you eat. Remove and rinse the dentures after each meal if you cannot brush them, but do not use hot water as it may warp the dentures. Rinse your mouth as well to remove food particles.

At bedtime, clean the tissues that the dentures sit on and those surrounding the dentures. Use a soft toothbrush and water to gently clean your gums, palate, tongue, and lining of your cheeks.

Remove the dentures overnight or at least for 4 hours during the day to give the gums a rest. You can prepare a denture soak with commercial denture cleaning tablets (such as Efferdent or Polident). Calculus that accumulates on the denture can be softened and more easily removed by soaking the denture in a solution of white vinegar diluted 1:1 with water for 30 minutes or more. Dentures are soaked overnight in commercial or homemade soaks. Be sure to rinse them thoroughly before putting them back into your mouth because the soaks may contain chemicals that can irritate the tissues.

Bleach is an effective organic solvent and eliminates yeasts. It should be diluted: 1 part bleach to 10 parts water. Undiluted household bleach should not be used as an overnight soak for complete or partial dentures. It will fade the color from the acrylic and attack the metal framework and clasps of a partial denture, causing them to darken and corrode. Partial dentures with metal components should be soaked in commercial products that do not contain bleach.

Store your denture in water when you are not wearing it to keep it from drying and distorting.

Clasps on partial dentures can be cleaned with the pointed brush on the end of the denture brush if the two-headed variety is used. Use care to keep from damaging or distorting the clasps. Gently clean the tissue-bearing surfaces of dentures with soft liners, using a soft toothbrush. Liquid soap can also be used (Fig. 14.30).

Long- and short-term soft liners may be adversely affected by some of the effervescent commercial soaks (Efferdent or Polident). Do not soak them in mouthwash containing alcohol because it dries out the material. Use only cleaners recommended by the manufacturer. Clean soft temporary liners with damp cotton balls or cotton-tipped applicators for a few days. After about a week it will harden enough to clean with a soft-bristle toothbrush and light pressure.

Wearing a partial denture increases your risk of getting tooth decay. Be sure to brush your remaining teeth at least twice a day with a fluoride toothpaste, and floss at least once a day. Avoid starchy or sugary snacks.

IN-OFFICE CARE

Patients will accumulate calculus on the denture around the surfaces of the maxillary molars and the mandibular anterior teeth, just as they did with their natural dentition. The dental hygienist can provide a service by removing the calculus before returning the denture to the patient. Calculus can be removed by placing the prosthesis in a denture cleaning solution inside a zippered bag placed into an ultrasonic cleaner. It can also be carefully scaled off with hand instruments and the area polished with flour of pumice, then tin oxide or acrylic polishing compounds (Fig. 14.31). Care must be taken not to wear down the teeth and

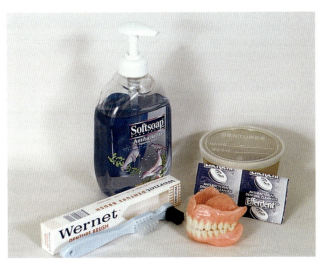

FIG. 14.30 Home care products for cleaning dentures: brush, liquid soap, denture cleaner tablets, denture cup.

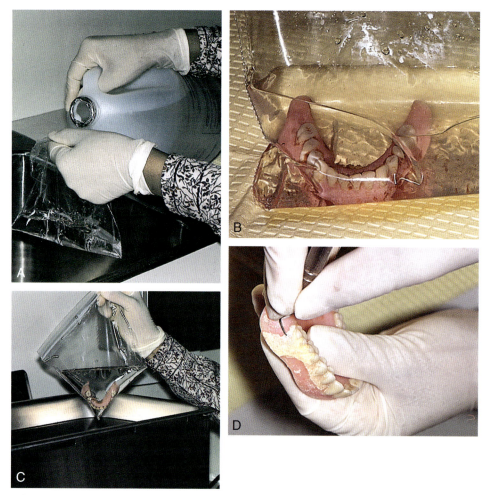

FIG. 14.31 Cleaning a denture in an ultrasonic cleaner: **(A)** Cleaning solution (to remove stain and calculus) placed in plastic zippered bag. **(B)** Denture placed in bag and sealed. **(C)** Bag placed in ultrasonic cleaner for 10–14 min. **(D)** Dentures with large calculus deposits need initial scaling with hand instruments before placing in ultrasonic cleaner. (From Darby ML, Walsh MM. *Dental Hygiene: Theory and Practice.* 4th ed. Elsevier; 2015; Courtesy Bertha Chan.)

acrylic base during the polishing process. In addition, tissue-bearing surfaces of the complete denture or partial denture should not be polished.

 Do You Recall?

What measures can patients take to clean their dentures?

STORAGE OF DENTURES

Acrylic resin prostheses absorb water and also are sensitive to water loss. The patient should be instructed to keep the prosthesis wet during periods of storage. This will prevent dimensional changes and distortion that can affect the fit. The prosthesis should be kept wet during the dental appointment. It can be stored in a denture cup to which water and a little mouthwash have been added to freshen it. Prostheses with soft liners should not be placed in mouthwash containing alcohol because the alcohol may adversely affect the properties of the soft liner. Instructions for care of complete and partial dentures should be given to nursing home staff and to caregivers for homebound or incapacitated individuals.

Precautions for Patients With Partial or Complete Dentures

- Store dentures in water to prevent warping from loss of moisture.
- Do not clean dentures in hot water because they may warp.
- Avoid soaking dentures in undiluted chlorine bleach because it will remove color from the resin and will attack metal components of partial dentures.
- Clean dentures over a sink partially filled with water or a towel to avoid breaking the denture if dropped.
- Avoid abrasive toothpastes or household cleaners because they will scratch or wear the plastic.

SUMMARY

Acrylic resins are vitally important to the success of prosthetic dentistry. They are versatile materials that can be used to replace missing oral structures. The ability of these resins to chemically bond to one another is important when plastic teeth are linked to the denture base or when dentures are relined or repaired. When properly handled, they are strong and durable. They can readily be relined to improve the fit as the alveolar bone resorbs over time. Lining materials can be similar to the denture base material or can be modified with plasticizers to create soft liners for tissue conditioning or long-term cushioning for patients who cannot tolerate hard liners. Many relining procedures can be accomplished in the office at chairside, so that the patient does not have to be without the prosthesis for any length of time. Simple fractures of the resin also can be repaired readily in the dental office. The acrylic resins can be colored with pigments to simulate racial pigmentation, so the denture can be customized to match the tissue coloration of the patient.

Other resins chemically similar to the methyl methacrylate resins are also used in prosthetic dentistry. The addition of photoinitiators and amine activators produces light-cured materials that are easy to use, require no mixing, and eliminate the volatile monomer that is potentially hazardous. Light-cured resins have application for fabrication of custom trays and record bases and for denture repair. Acrylic and vinyl resins to which plasticizers have been added to soften them are often used in maxillofacial prosthodontics for replacement of facial tissues after trauma or cancer surgery. Noses, cheeks, ears, and other structures can be made from these materials and colored to match the surrounding skin.

Dental auxiliaries play an important role in delivering care to individuals who require prostheses. They may be called on to mix, place, remove, or repair any number of these materials. Therefore an intimate knowledge of the properties and handling characteristics of these materials is very important. In addition, patients need instructions in proper home care of the prostheses to maintain them and to prevent injury to the oral tissues. Knowledge of proper cleaning agents and methods is also necessary.

INSTRUCTIONAL VIDEOS

See the Evolve Resources site for a variety of educational videos that reinforce the material covered in this chapter.

Procedure 14.1 Fabrication of Custom Acrylic Impression Trays

See Evolve site for Competency Sheet.

Consider the following with this procedure: safety glasses are recommended for the patient, PPE is required for the operator, and ensure appropriate safety protocols are followed.

NOTE: Figs. 14.32–14.39 (Courtesy Mark Dellinges, School of Dentistry, University of California, San Francisco, San Francisco, California).

EQUIPMENT/SUPPLIES (FIG. 14.32)

- Maxillary or mandibular edentulous cast
- Sheet of baseplate wax, Bunsen burner, laboratory knife
- Tray powder and liquid, tongue blade or cement spatula, waxed paper cup
- Laboratory handpiece and acrylic bur, sandpaper drum (arbor band), and dental lathe
- Cast-separating medium, disposable brush, petroleum jelly

PROCEDURE STEPS

1. Using the disposable brush, coat the cast with separating medium and allow it to dry.

   NOTE: The separating medium keeps the tray material and the wax from sticking to the cast.

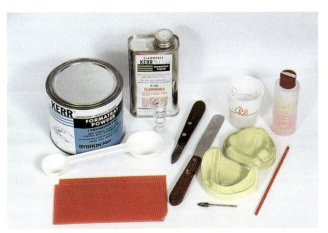

FIG. 14.32

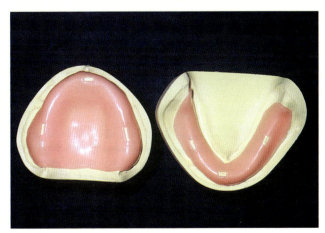

FIG. 14.33

Procedure 14.1   Fabrication of Custom Acrylic Impression Trays—cont'd

2. Warm a sheet of baseplate wax over the Bunsen burner and place it on the cast. Adapt it to the cast over the edentulous ridges and into the vestibular folds. Use the laboratory knife to trim excess wax away until it is about 2 mm from the depth of the folds.

   NOTE: The wax will be removed after the tray is fabricated and will create an even space within the tray for the impression material.

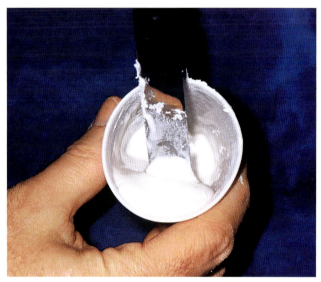

FIG. 14.34

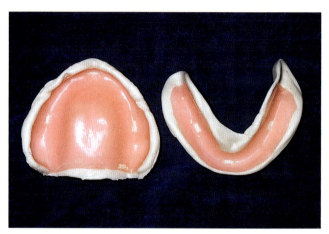

FIG. 14.37

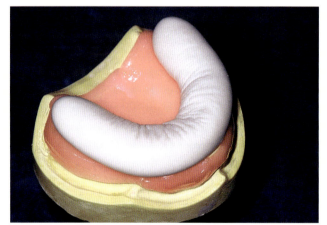

FIG. 14.35

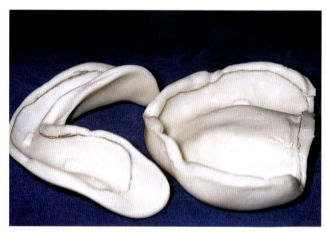

FIG. 14.38

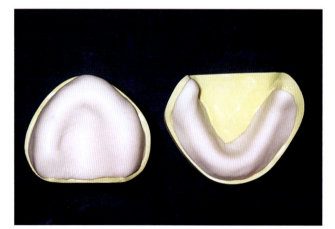

FIG. 14.36

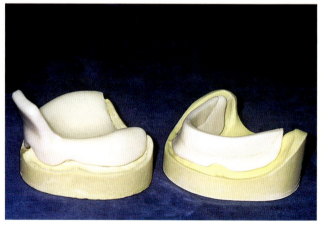

FIG. 14.39

Procedure 14.1 Fabrication of Custom Acrylic Impression Trays—cont'd

3. Cut three 2- × 2-mm square holes in the wax over the ridges for the maxillary and mandibular casts: two in the molar area, and one in the incisor area.

   NOTE: As tray material is adapted into these holes, resin squares will appear inside the tray. When the impression is taken, these squares will contact the tissues over the ridges and act as stops. The stops will create an even thickness of impression material within the tray (except for the very small area of the square) and will prevent an uneven seating of the tray (Fig. 14.33). Some clinicians do not use these stops.

4. Mix the powder and liquid components of the tray material in the wax cup, in proportions recommended by the manufacturer. Stir with a tongue blade or cement spatula until thoroughly mixed (Fig. 14.34).

   NOTE: The mix will be too wet to handle at this stage. Use only in a well-ventilated area.

5. Apply petroleum jelly to the gloved hands. When the mixture is doughy, form it into a thick, wide rope that is long enough to fit around the entire ridge (Fig. 14.35).

   NOTE: Petroleum jelly keeps the tray material from sticking to the gloves.

6. Adapt the resin over the wax, into the holes in the wax, and into the depth of the vestibular folds. The tray should be 1 to 2 mm thick (Fig. 14.36).

   NOTE: If the tray is too thin, it might be too flexible to keep the impression from distorting.

7. Cut away excess tray material with the laboratory knife and quickly adapt it into the shape of a handle. Wet the tray end of the handle with monomer and place it on the tray. Smooth it into place with the fingers. The handle should be positioned so that it will not be in the way of the lips when seated in the patient's mouth.

   NOTE: Wetting the end of the tray with monomer (liquid) dissolves some material at the surface and allows it to stick to the polymerizing tray material.

8. Readapt the tray material to the cast continually as polymerization takes place.

   NOTE: The tray material shrinks as it polymerizes and tends to pull away from the cast.

9. Remove the tray from the cast once the heat of the reaction has cooled. Remove wax from inside the tray. If difficult to remove, heat the wax in warm (not hot) water (Fig. 14.37).

   NOTE: Residual wax must be removed, or it might prevent the impression material from adhering to the tray.

10. Trim the tray with an acrylic bur or arbor band to remove excess material (Fig. 14.38), and smooth the rough edges. The completed tray should extend 2 mm short of the vestibular folds. Confirm the fit of the tray on the cast (Fig. 14.39).

    NOTE: The tray must be smooth to the touch, or it will be uncomfortable in the patient's mouth. The tray is left short of the depth of the folds to allow room for stick compound to be added for border molding. Border molding uses softened compound to shape the location for the borders of the denture as the patient's cheeks and tongue are manipulated through simulated functional movements.

    NOTE: Some dentists use addition silicone putty or special thermoplastic materials for border molding.

11. Disinfect the tray by immersion in appropriate disinfectant and store in a sealed bag labeled with the patient's name until ready for use.

Review and Discussion

Review Questions

Select the one correct response for each of the following multiple-choice questions.

1. A polymer is formed by:
   a. Breaking down chains of complex, high-molecular-weight molecules by heating them
   b. Mixing polysulfide and polyether
   c. Joining monomer molecules together in a long chain through carbon bonds
   d. Fusing acrylic powder beads together at high temperature

2. Cross-linking of polymers:
   a. Is used to improve the physical and mechanical properties of the final resin product
   b. Occurs when long-chain polymers are mixed together and the chains physically wrap around each other
   c. Usually results in a weaker material as the degree of cross-linking increases
   d. Occurs when long chains link end to end

3. Addition polymerization:
   a. Always results in increased porosity in the final material
   b. Is the least common method of polymerization used in dentistry
   c. Produces numerous by-products such as alcohol and acetone
   d. Is initiated by a free radical

Continued

Review and Discussion—cont'd

4. What are the physical stages of the addition polymerization reaction?
   a. Sandy, stringy, dough, and rubber
   b. Wet, flexible, and stiff
   c. Sol, gel, and solid
   d. Initial, thermal, and terminal
5. A heat-processed denture differs from a chemical-cured denture. Which one of the following is NOT true for the heat-processed denture?
   a. It is stronger.
   b. It is more porous.
   c. It is harder.
   d. It has less dimensional change during the first 24 hours after curing.
6. High-impact resins are created by:
   a. Removal of free monomer
   b. Use of additional liquid monomer in the mix
   c. Heat treating the resin after it has polymerized
   d. Addition of rubber particles to the acrylic
7. Which stage of polymerization of acrylic resins is longer for heat-cured resins during denture processing to allow adequate time to pack the acrylic resin into the denture flask?
   a. Sandy
   b. Stringy
   c. Dough
   d. Exothermic
8. What is the effect on a denture if it is left on the nightstand overnight?
   a. It will lose water and shrink.
   b. It will expand.
   c. It will crack.
   d. It will oxidize and lose color.
9. What is the effect on a partial denture framework if it is soaked in a chlorine-containing cleaner?
   a. Nothing will happen.
   b. The metal will clean rapidly and become shiny.
   c. The metal will dissolve and fracture.
   d. The metal will darken and corrode.
10. The effect that porosity has on an acrylic denture can be seen as all of the following EXCEPT one. Which one?
    a. It contributes to staining.
    b. It contributes to growth of microorganisms.
    c. It weakens the acrylic.
    d. It decreases the thermal conductivity of the acrylic.
11. The purpose of the use of a pressure pot during polymerization of a chemical-cured acrylic resin is:
    a. To increase the strength of the acrylic
    b. To decrease the porosity
    c. To decrease the shrinkage
    d. All of the above
12. Which type of hard liner has the best physical properties?
    a. Chairside chemical-cured liner
    b. Laboratory chemical-cured liner
    c. Laboratory heat-cured liner
    d. None (they are all the same)
13. Methyl methacrylate is which one of the following?
    a. An inhibitor
    b. An accelerator
    c. Powder polymer
    d. Liquid monomer
14. Long-term soft liners are indicated for all of the following reasons EXCEPT one. Which one?
    a. Chronic soreness with hard acrylic denture bases
    b. Severe soft tissue undercuts
    c. Sharp, knife-edge ridges
    d. Soft tissues with chronic fungal infection
15. Acrylic resins can be made soft and pliable by the:
    a. Use of less monomer in the mix
    b. Use of less powder in the mix
    c. Addition of plasticizers
    d. Addition of filler particles
16. All of the following statements about short-term soft liners are true EXCEPT one. Which one?
    a. They are also called *tissue conditioners*.
    b. They can readapt to the tissues as healing takes place because they have a high degree of flow.
    c. They do not need frequent replacement because they absorb water and get softer over time.
    d. They are adversely affected by some commercial denture soaks.
17. Over-the-counter denture liners have which of the following shortcomings?
    a. May not reestablish proper occlusion
    b. Are generally porous
    c. Promote growth of yeasts
    d. All of the above
18. All of the following are advantages of acrylic denture teeth over porcelain teeth EXCEPT one. Which one?
    a. They are more wear resistant.
    b. They chemically bond to the denture base.
    c. They are kind to the opposing teeth or ridges.
    d. They can easily be ground and shaped to fit the available space.
19. When a denture is repaired with a chemical-cured acrylic resin, all of the following procedures are performed EXCEPT one. Which one?
    a. The pieces are reassembled and held with sticky wax while a cast is poured inside the denture.
    b. A layer of the old resin surrounding the fracture site is removed.
    c. The resin surrounding the fracture site is wet with monomer to enhance the chemical bond with the repair acrylic.
    d. The repair acrylic is mixed, applied to the fracture site, and allowed to cure at room temperature on the laboratory bench for the best results.
20. Which one of the following statements regarding construction of custom impression trays is FALSE?
    a. Tray material may be chemical-cured or light-cured.
    b. Tray material is adapted directly to the cast.
    c. During polymerization, the chemical-cured material gets very hot.
    d. Baseplate wax is adapted over the cast to develop space for the impression material.
21. Which one of the following statements is FALSE regarding the care of dentures by the patient?
    a. Dentures should be stored in water to prevent warping.
    b. Dentures should be cleaned over a sink filled with water or over a towel to prevent fracture if dropped.

Review and Discussion—cont'd

    c. Abrasive pastes or cleaners should not be used, or they will scratch the acrylic.
    d. The denture should be cleaned in hot water periodically to kill microorganisms.
22. Which one of the following statements about liquid monomer is FALSE?
    a. Gives a pleasant taste to a hard reline done at chairside
    b. Is potentially harmful to breathe
    c. Can cause allergic reactions or skin irritation
    d. May be present in small quantities in a new denture
    e. Evaporates readily so do not leave the cap to the bottle off
23. All of the following can have an adverse effect on soft denture liners EXCEPT one. Which one?
    a. Some effervescent commercial denture soaks
    b. Liquid hand soap
    c. Mouthwash containing alcohol
    d. Hot water

For answers to Review Questions, see the Appendix.

Case-Based Discussion Topics

1. A thin, frail 76-year-old widow had complete dentures made about 3 years ago. The chief complaint is "my lower denture hurts me when I eat." In the 3 years since the dentures were made, the lower denture has been relined twice with hard acrylic. This has not improved the comfort level. The lower ridge is sharp and thin.
Can you suggest a process that might improve the comfort level? Is the procedure best done in the office or in a commercial dental laboratory? What kinds of materials are often used?

2. A 62-year-old retired janitor comes to the dental office for a dental cleaning. The patient wears an upper complete denture and a lower partial denture with a metal framework that replaces teeth 22 to 26. In addition to calculus on the teeth, there are light amounts of calculus on the denture and partial denture.
Describe a method of removing the calculus without scratching the acrylic. What home care measures can you recommend for care of the prostheses? What type of cleaner should be avoided on the partial denture? What types of brushes should be used to clean the prostheses?

3. A 57-year-old truck driver comes to the dental office with a broken maxillary denture. It is broken in two pieces through the midline of the palatal portion of the denture base. The pieces fit together easily. The patient said the denture was dropped it in the sink while cleaning it.
What steps should be taken to prepare the denture for repair in the office? What materials could be used for the repair? What is the function of the pressure pot? What advice can be given to the patient to avoid a similar mishap in the future?

4. A 71-year-old retired teacher had an upper denture made 6 months ago. At the next dental visit, the patient complains that the denture has stained heavily in the palatal portion of the denture base and has developed a foul odor.
When you inspect the denture, you confirm a dark stain in the mid-palate but also notice numerous small porosities in the acrylic. Cite causes of porosity during processing of the denture. Why has the denture stained and developed a foul odor? What effect does porosity have on the physical and mechanical properties of the acrylic?

5. A 43-year-old beautician lost all of the upper teeth last year due to rapidly progressing periodontal disease associated with uncontrolled diabetes. A maxillary denture replaced the missing teeth. At a periodontal maintenance visit the patient complains of soreness in the palate beneath the denture. It has been getting progressively worse over the past 3 weeks. The denture is worn all night so.
What is the likely cause of the soreness? What should the dentist prescribe to help? What can you advise the patient to do regarding home care? If the denture had been new, had only been worn for a few days and was taken out at night, what else could cause irritation of the palatal tissues?

BIBLIOGRAPHY

Bird DL, Robinson DS: *Removable prosthodontics*. In *Modern Dental Assisting*, ed 13, St. Louis, 2021, Elsevier.

Darby ML, Walsh MM: Persons with fixed and removable prostheses. In *Dental Hygiene Theory and Practice*, ed 9, St. Louis, 2015, Elsevier/Saunders.

Ferracane JL: *Polymers for prosthetics*. In *Materials in Dentistry*, Philadelphia, 2001, Lippincott Williams & Wilkins.

Leinfelder KF, Terry DA, Connelly ME: The art of denture relining, *Inside Dentistry* 3(5), 2007.

Powers JM, Wataha JC: *Polymers in prosthodontics*. In *Dental Materials: Foundations and Applications*, ed 11, St. Louis, 2017, Elsevier.

Robinson DS: *Removable prosthodontics*. In *Essentials of Dental Assisting*, ed 7, St. Louis, 2023, Elsevier.

Sakaguchi R, Ferracane J, Powers J: *Prosthetic applications of polymers*. In *Craig's Restorative Dental Materials*, ed 14, St. Louis, 2019, Elsevier.

Shen C, Rawls HR, Esquivel-Upshaw JF: *Prosthetic polymers and resins*. In *Phillips' Science of Dental Materials*, ed 13, St. Louis, 2022, Elsevier.

Vaidyanathan J, Vaidyanathan TK: Dynamic mechanical analysis of heat, microwave and visible light cure denture base resins, *J Mater Sci Mater Med* 6:670–674, 1995.

15 Provisional Restorations

http://evolve.elsevier.com/Eakle/materials/

Chapter Objectives

On completion of this chapter, the student should be able to:

1. Explain the purpose of provisional coverage.
2. Describe circumstances that may require provisional coverage.
3. Identify the criteria necessary for a high-quality provisional restoration.
4. Describe the properties of provisional materials.
5. Distinguish among properties that are important for coverage in both the posterior and anterior areas.
6. Differentiate between intracoronal and extracoronal restorations.
7. Summarize the advantages and disadvantages of preformed and custom crowns.
8. Differentiate among direct and indirect fabrication techniques.
9. Summarize the advantages and disadvantages of acrylic and composite resin provisional materials.
10. Describe the technique for fabrication of preformed metal and polycarbonate crowns, custom crowns, and intracoronal cement provisional restorations.
11. Summarize patient education and home care instructions.
12. Fabricate and cement metal, polycarbonate, and custom provisional crowns.
13. Place an intracoronal cement provisional restoration.

KEY TERMS

Provisional Coverage a restoration that temporarily holds the place of a permanent restoration, typically for up to 2 to 4 weeks. In the case of an implant or complex prosthodontic and periodontal treatments, provisional restorations may be required to last for extended periods of time and are called interim restorations

Finish Line the continuous edge that borders the preparation to which the restoration is fit or finished; it is also called the *margin*

Extracoronal Restoration a restoration that covers all or part of the external surface of the clinical crown of the tooth and may extend over the cusp tips on facial or lingual surfaces or may include the removal of cusps, such as onlays, three-quarter crowns, full crowns, and veneers

Indirect Fabrication provisional restorations made on a cast or milled by computer-assisted design/computer-assisted machining outside the patient's mouth before delivery

Intracoronal Restoration a restoration within the crown of the tooth, such as an inlay

Direct Fabrication provisional restorations made directly on the prepared tooth/teeth inside the patient's mouth

---

The increased retention of natural teeth and advances in technology to restore and replace tooth structure have increased the need for high-quality fixed prosthodontic, pedodontic, and endodontic treatments. Fabricating provisional restorations, also referred to as temporary or interim restorations, is an important component of fixed prosthodontic treatment. While the final restorations are being fabricated, provisional restorations are critical for both the biological and biomechanical health of the tooth and periodontium as well as the comfort of the patient. Once the tooth has been prepared, the exposed dentin must be protected from thermal, chemical, mechanical, and bacterial effects from the oral environment. Adjacent soft tissues must be protected, and the position of the tooth must be maintained. All of this is accomplished with provisional restorations, with additional considerations of esthetics, function, and patient comfort.

The dental auxiliary may be called on to provide a variety of functions such as fabricate, repair, remove, or maintain the provisional restoration as well as give home care instructions. Good provisional coverage not only helps to ensure the success of the final restoration, it is also an important component in patient satisfaction. Patients who need to return to the dental office to have their provisional crowns recemented or replaced or do not like the esthetics of the restoration may lose confidence in the doctor's ability.

DENTAL PROCEDURES THAT MAY REQUIRE PROVISIONAL COVERAGE

Provisional coverage may be required in:
- General cases
- Pediatric dental cases
- Endodontic cases
- Prosthodontic cases

Whenever a situation arises wherein a permanent restorative material cannot be placed at the time of preparation, a provisional (temporary) material will be chosen (Table 15.1).

The patient wears this provisional restoration to protect the tooth for a short period of time, generally 2 weeks to a month while the final restoration is being fabricated. In cases involving complex treatments, such as implants and complex prosthodontic procedures, a longer time of 6 to 15 months may be required.

This short-term or interim period of time may be used to:
- Make a final diagnosis
- Develop a treatment plan
- Allow hard or soft tissue healing
- Communicate with the laboratory for the optimal success of the final restoration

In some cases, the patient may be asked to evaluate the provisional restoration to make cosmetic decisions regarding the final restoration. For instance, the patient wishing to close a large diastema (space) between teeth #8 and #9 may find that the resultant size of the restorations necessary to close this space is less esthetically pleasing than the space they wished to close.

Table 15.1 Dental Procedures Requiring Provisional Coverage

PROCEDURE	FUNCTION OF PROVISIONAL COVERAGE
Endodontic access preparation	Closes endodontic access preparations between appointments
Vitality of the tooth is in question	Allows the pulp to respond to therapeutic agents or to recover from the trauma of preparation
Emergency care	Prevents additional damage and improves esthetics and function while awaiting a permanent solution
Awaiting permanent restoration	Allows time for laboratory fabrication of cast and ceramic restorations
Restoration of implants	For long-term provisional coverage while the implant site is allowed to heal
Restoration of primary teeth	Placed on primary teeth because of extensive caries, pulpotomies, or pulpectomies until permanent teeth erupt

CRITERIA FOR PROVISIONAL COVERAGE

Criteria for a properly fabricated and cemented provisional restoration include the following:
- Maintenance of tooth function and position in the arch
- Protection of hard and soft oral structures including the pulp
- Establishment of esthetics and retention
- Provide patient comfort

If the criteria for provisional coverag are not met, the following is very likely to occur:
- Pulpal and periodontal irritation
- Tooth migration
- Patient dissatisfaction

Keeping these criteria in mind, the clinician can choose the most appropriate material, technique, provisional cement, and postoperative instructions for the patient.

MAINTAIN PREPARED TOOTH POSITION RELATIVE TO ADJACENT AND OPPOSING TEETH

When a tooth has been prepared to receive a crown, sufficient tooth structure has been removed to create a space between the adjacent teeth and the opposing teeth. The provisional restoration must contact the adjacent teeth on the mesial and distal sides as well as be in occlusion with the opposing teeth. If these criteria are not met, the tooth's position can shift within a couple days. When shifting of the prepared tooth occurs, the restoration, which was designed to fit the tooth in its original position, may now be too high because of occlusal/incisal migration or may not seat properly as a result of lateral migration of the prepared tooth. This shifting will likely require the patient to have additional chair time for adjustments to the final restoration before cementation or possibly result in the need to retake the impression to fabricate a new restoration. Provisional restorations should share the load from forces during normal masticatory function or bruxing. If the provisional restoration itself is too high, the results may be those associated with trauma from occlusion, which may cause the tooth to become sore and mobile.

PROTECT THE EXPOSED TOOTH SURFACES AND MARGINS

When the tooth is prepared, the dentinal tubules become exposed to potentially harmful insults such as:
- Thermal
- Chemical
- Mechanical
- Bacterial

Provisional materials placed near the pulp must have no adverse chemical effect and be sufficiently insulating to protect the pulp from thermal assaults.

Some provisional materials generate heat as they set and must be handled properly to avoid pulpal damage. Maintaining the comfort of the patient is essential.

The **finish line (or margin)** of the tooth preparation is particularly susceptible to fracture if not adequately protected. Well-adapted provisional restorations protect the finish line from fracture and from exposure to oral fluids and bacteria. If the finish line is damaged, the permanent restoration will no longer fit precisely, leaving space for future leakage of oral fluids and bacteria. The process of caries may even begin during the time the provisional restoration is in place.

> **Caution**
>
> Because provisional luting agents (cements) are highly soluble and may wash out from under a provisional restoration, they cannot be expected to make up for marginal deficiencies in the restoration.

PROTECT THE GINGIVAL TISSUES

Many crown preparations extend 0.5 to 1 mm subgingivally, making the margins and the overall contour of the provisional restoration critical to periodontal health. Periodontal tissues are susceptible to irritation from:
- Overcontoured
- Overextended or overhanging margins
- Trauma from food impaction
- Buildup of plaque

Margins of the provisional must be flush with the preparation. If a margin is overextended, the resultant tissue irritation may lead to bleeding, inflammation, and gingival recession, adversely affecting the cosmetic effect of the permanent restoration. If the margin is short of the finish line, the tooth may experience sensitivity.

All surfaces of the provisional restoration must be:
- Properly contoured
- Properly polished
- Maintain contact with adjacent teeth

If surfaces are undercontoured the process of chewing will excessively force food directly onto the gingiva rather than deflecting it facially and lingually. An overcontoured restoration may trap plaque by not allowing for any self-cleansing or gingival stimulation from the chewing process (Fig. 15.1). Inadequate or open contacts likewise can lead to food impaction. Rough surfaces will act as plaque traps and may abrade the tongue or oral mucosa. These scenarios may also lead to irritation, inflammation, and recession.

> **Clinical Tip**
>
> A properly contoured, polished, and well-fitting provisional restoration is critical to maintaining periodontal health around the prepared tooth. Inflamed gingival tissue will bleed profusely at the delivery of the final restoration and potentially interfere with bonding or cementation.

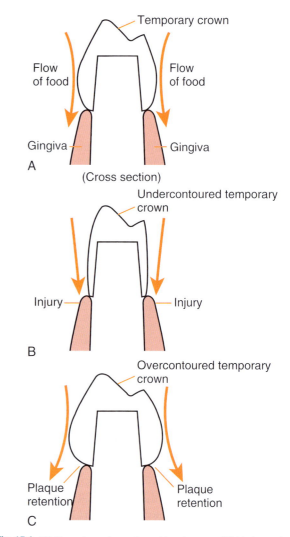

Fig. 15.1 **(A)** Properly contoured provisional crown. **(B)** Undercontoured provisional crown. **(C)** Overcontoured provisional crown.

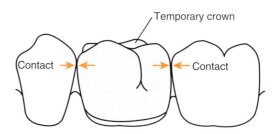

Fig. 15.2 Provisional crown duplicates natural tooth contour, contact, and occlusion.

PROVIDE FUNCTION

The provisional restoration should restore ideal occlusal/incisal contact with the opposing teeth and have functional contours and proximal contacts (Fig. 15.2). Patients must be able to chew normally and clean the provisional restoration as they would a permanent restoration. However, the provisional restoration is not intended to function exactly like the permanent restoration due to it being worn for a brief period of time. Modifications in diet, including the avoidance of sticky and hard foods, may be necessary to prevent dislodging or fracturing of the provisional restoration.

ESTHETICS AND SPEECH

In addition to function, it is important to consider esthetics of the provisional. Provisional restorations must have the appearance of natural tooth structure whenever esthetics is important. For anterior esthetic restorations, provisional restorations may be used as a guide for the final restoration as it relates to:
- Color
- Contour
- Length
- Positioning

This is an important component for patient satisfaction, as the patient now has an opportunity to give input concerning the esthetics of the final restoration.

Speech is also influenced by the position of the teeth and the provisional restoration must not interfere with normal speech patterns. Anterior provisionals that are too bulky, thin, long, short, or do not occlude properly can change the patient's speech patterns causing lisps or whistling sounds when they speak.

Do You Recall?

Why is provisional coverage important while a patient is awaiting the placement of a permanent restoration?

Clinical Tip

Matching shades and customizing provisional materials to duplicate the natural teeth will greatly enhance patient acceptance and thus the success of the provisional restoration.

RETENTION

The cementation of the provisional restoration is accomplished with temporary cement, which is not designed to be retentive for extended periods of time. Like a permanent restoration, the fit of the provisional crown contributes to its retention. The design, height, and taper of the crown preparation are also responsible for the retention of the provisional restoration. For many patients, a well-fabricated provisional restoration is a direct reflection on how the final restoration will turn out. The provisional restoration must be retentive enough to ensure patient confidence during the period in which the final restoration is being constructed.

Criteria for Provisional Coverage

Provisional coverage must:
- Reproduce proper proximal contacts and occlusal alignment
- Fit the tooth at the finish line (margins)
- Reproduce natural tooth contours
- Promote gingival health
- Provide pulpal protection
- Provide function, esthetics, and phonetics (speech)
- Remain stable and retentive
- Provide smooth surfaces

KEY POINTS

GOAL OF PROVISIONAL COVERAGE
1. Maintain tooth function and position
2. Protect the hard and soft oral tissues
3. Establish esthetics and retention
4. Provide comfort

PROPERTIES OF PROVISIONAL MATERIALS

Materials used to fabricate provisional restorations must have properties that meet the specific requirement of the clinical treatment and the part of the mouth in which they are placed. Strength and hardness are important for single and multi-unit **extracoronal restorations**. Biocompatibility with hard and soft tissues is also important. Provisional restorations located in the smile zone must be esthetic. In areas of the mouth with difficult access, the ability to manipulate the materials is also an important consideration.

STRENGTH

Materials must have sufficient compressive and tensile strength to resist the forces of mastication. Materials that are used for provisional bridges must also have sufficient flexural strength to resist deformation from flexing during mastication. Acrylics have more fracture toughness than brittle materials such as composite resins that do not hold up well when used for long-span bridges or with patients who are bruxers. The material chosen must be able to resist the forces of chewing without breaking or coming off the tooth. In addition, the restoration should remain intact when removed so that it can be reused when necessary.

HARDNESS

Acrylic materials wear more readily than composite resin materials. Surface hardness must be sufficient to resist abrasion and wear for the period the provisional restoration is to be worn. The material should also be able to be polished to a smooth finish and retain that smooth surface throughout its use. Smooth, polished surfaces will not irritate the tongue or oral mucosa, attract less plaque and make home care easier resulting in healthier gingival tissues.

TISSUE COMPATIBILITY

Ideally, the material should not produce any additional irritation to pulpal or gingival tissues during or after setting reactions. Materials that generate heat when setting must be carefully selected depending on the clinical situation (i.e., deep preparation) and may be more appropriate for the **indirect fabrication** technique. In addition, for patient comfort, materials should not absorb or give off odors or poor taste.

ESTHETICS

Materials used in areas of esthetic concern must match adjacent teeth and must have good color stability and stain resistance. Shade selection is important in the management of patient expectations; many materials are not accurate in this area. Color stability is influenced by the surface quality and porosity of the material chosen as well as by the patient's oral hygiene and consumption of foods and beverages that tend to stain (e.g., berries, red wine, coffee, tea).

> **KEY POINTS**
>
> Properties needed in a provisional restoration
> - Strength
> - Hardness
> - Tissue compatibility
> - Esthetics

> **Clinical Tip**
>
> It is advisable to pick a shade before a tooth is prepared; enamel dehydration from isolation during preparation procedures leaves the teeth lighter in color.

PROVISIONAL CROWN MATERIALS

The selection of provisional materials is typically based on:
- Cost
- Ease of handling
- Esthetics
- Strength
- Accuracy of margins

Provisional materials include:
- Metals
- Polycarbonate
- Acrylics
- Composites
- Cements

These materials may be used alone or in combination, such as an aluminum shell crown lined with acrylic. Provisional restorations may be preformed (e.g., stainless steel, tin-silver, aluminum, or polycarbonate crowns) or made specifically for individual procedures (e.g., custom acrylic or composite crowns and intracoronal restorations).

Provisional materials, whether they are cement, acrylic, or bis-acrylic composite, are mixed and placed in a plastic state and allowed to harden directly in/on the preparation or on a stone model. Cements are limited to intracoronal placement; provisional acrylic and composite resin can be used for extracoronal coverage as well.

Preformed crowns have the advantage of convenience, in that they are already premade in a variety of sizes and anatomic forms. This saves time because it eliminates the need for a crown template and is particularly useful in emergency situations and for badly broken-down teeth. Even though they come in different sizes, time must be spent in establishing contact, contour, occlusion, and marginal integrity.

Customized crowns are more versatile and more consistently meet the criteria for successful provisional restorations. They do, however, require the additional step of making a template or matrix for the final product. This template captures the external shape of the tooth structures as they exist before the preparation. This additional step can be further complicated if the original tooth is badly broken down or fractured.

PREFORMED CROWNS

The process of temporization using preformed crowns includes the use of various metals (including stainless steel, aluminum or tin-silver), polycarbonate, and celluloid crown forms lined with acrylic, bis-acrylic composite, or zinc oxide eugenol materials (Fig. 15.3). The preformed crown will become the outer surface of the provisional crown, and an acrylic or bis-acrylic composite material or thick, hard cement will occupy the inner portion of the crown.

Preformed crowns come in kits containing anterior and posterior crown forms in many sizes. Because the prepared tooth is much smaller than this preformed shell, a reline of acrylic or bis-acrylic composite material is generally required to fill the shell to allow for a close fit. Metal crowns are typically used only in posterior cases, while polycarbonate and celluloid forms are used on anterior teeth or premolars. Preformed crowns may only be used for single crowns and are not appropriate for temporary bridges.

> **Clinical Tip**
>
> If the kit of provisional crowns does not come with a measuring gauge, use a millimeter ruler to select the most appropriate crown size, measuring the width from mesial-to-distal contacts. All crowns that are tried in and not used must be sterilized before they are returned to the crown kit.

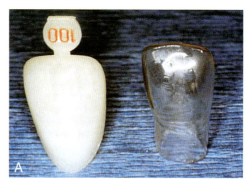
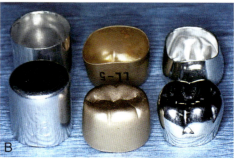

Fig. 15.3 **(A)** Polycarbonate and celluloid crown forms. **(B)** Aluminum shell, anodized aluminum, and silver-tin crowns. (From Rosenstiel SF, Land MF, Fujimoto J. *Contemporary Fixed Prosthodontics.* ed 5th ed. Elsevier, 2016.)

STAINLESS-STEEL CROWNS

The stainless-steel crown (SSC) does not tarnish or corrode and is the most durable and abrasion-resistant of the preformed crowns, The SSC can provide provisional coverage lasting months and even years, if necessary (Fig. 15.4). Traditionally the SSC has been used to restore primary teeth (Fig. 15.5). These durable and economical restorations are also used for adults, in cases where financial or health concerns would otherwise prohibit restoration of the tooth and result in the recommendation to extract. The primary advantage of SSC crowns is their malleability, which allows them to be bent and burnished to provide for good contacts, occlusion, and marginal integrity. The margin of the crown is cut with crown and bridge scissors and is crimped (curved inward to fit to the preparation margins) and contoured at the contact and margins with crimping and contouring pliers. Some manufacturers make their crowns precrimped at the cervical.

If the SSC is an alternate to a cast restoration for prolonged periods of time, minimal reduction of the tooth is ideal to preserve natural tooth strength and provide protection for the pulp. With the marginal seal and occlusion intact, these crowns may be a solution to long-term provisional coverage of posterior teeth even though the adaptations of margins, the occlusion, and overall contours are never as precise as those of cast restorations.

An alternative to SSCs is nickel-chromium crowns, which have similar durability, handling characteristics, and appearance.

ALUMINUM SHELL AND TIN-SILVER ALLOY CROWNS

Aluminum, anodized aluminum shell crowns and tin-silver alloy crowns are used for provisional coverage of posterior teeth (see Fig. 15.3B). They are lined with acrylics, bis-acrylic composites, or a thick mix of reinforced ZOE cement to support the soft metal. Without adequate support, the crown will distort and come off under functional forces. For patients who brux their teeth, a hard liner is preferred over ZOE. A well-fitted aluminum shell or tin-silver crown can last a few weeks.

Tin-silver crowns are the softest and most ductile of the preformed metal crowns and as a consequence, are easily burnished. They may be precrimped (constricted) at the cervical margins. For crown preparations with a thin finish line, these precrimped crowns when seated on the prepared tooth will stretch over the margins and be closely adapted to the tooth. For crowns with wider finish lines such as a shoulder margin, the crown may need to be expanded to allow it to fit over the margins. A plastic stretch block with a series of tapered stumps is supplied with the Iso-Form kit to expand the crown. The crown is pressed down on the tapered stumps that come in a variety of diameters (Fig. 15.6).

FITTING THE CROWN

The mesial-distal width is measured for the most appropriate fit, and some crown kits provide a gauge for measuring the mesial-distal width (Fig. 15.7). To confirm the correct width of the selected provisional crown without trying it on the tooth, simply turn it upside down and see if the coronal portion fits the space. The softness of the metal allows for easy manipulation of the contact, occlusion, and margins because the metal can be stretched and burnished without wrinkling.

Generally, the crowns are too tall for most preparations and require trimming at the cervical margins to attain the correct height. To accomplish this:
- Hold the crown on the prepared tooth with a dental mirror and use an explorer to scribe a line on the crown at the level estimated to be the correct crown length that follows the contour of the finish line of the preparation.
- Using crown and bridge scissors begin trimming away a little material at a time to avoid overtrimming.
- If ragged edges are present after trimming, the margins should be smoothed with a finishing bur, sandpaper disk, a fine stone, a rubber wheel, or polishing points.

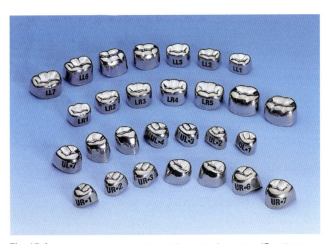

Fig. 15.4 A selection of pedatric stainless-steel crowns. (Courtesy Denovo Stainless Steel Crowns.)

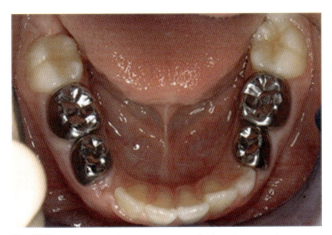

Fig. 15.5 Stainless-steel crowns on mandibular primary molars. (Courtesy DentalGama.)

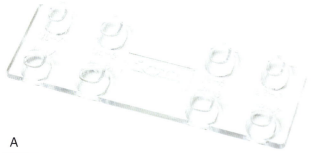

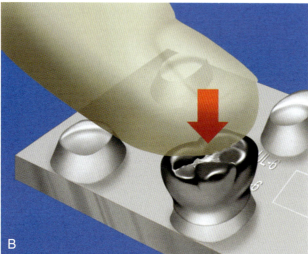

Fig. 15.6 Plastic stretch block for tin-silver alloy provisional crowns: **(A)** Series of tapered stumps of various sizes for different size crowns. **(B)** Preformed crown is precrimped at the cervical and needs to be stretched by pressing it down on the tapered stump. This will allow it to pass over the margins of the prepared tooth. (Courtesy 3M ESPE.)

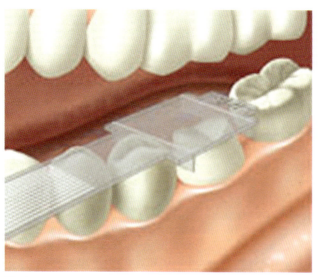

Fig. 15.7 Plastic measuring gauge used to determine the mesiodistal width for selecting a posterior provisional crown. (Courtesy 3M ESPE.)

- Contouring pliers are used to form the cervical contours and crimp the margins so they will closely adapt to the tooth.
- Prior to placing the supporting liner, the patient can bite on the crown a few times to begin forming the occlusal contacts.

Because of their softness, these crowns wear easily, especially in patients who brux and must be checked for occlusal integrity if they will be worn for more than a few weeks (Procedure 15.1).

> **Clinical Tip**
>
> When selecting a preformed provisional crown, it is better to choose one that is slightly larger than the space rather than one that is smaller, because a larger one can be shaped and trimmed to fit the space. The smaller one cannot.

POLYCARBONATE CROWN FORMS

Preformed polycarbonate crown forms are composed of polycarbonate resin, which contains microglass fibers allowing the margins to be crimped with pliers and provide strength and durability. These crowns come in kits with several sizes and shapes for primary and permanent teeth and are available in tooth-colored shades, predominately in the A and B shades (see Fig. 15.3A). Polycarbonate crowns are more rigid than the soft metal provisional crowns and may require adjustment with acrylic burs and disks or may be carefully cut with sharp crown and bridge scissors. The primary advantage of the polycarbonate crown is their esthetics for replacement of anterior and premolar teeth (some manufacturers even have molar forms) and their compatibility with acrylic resins to further customize the fit and margins. As an alternative to polycarbonate, tooth-colored crown forms are also made from polymethyl methacrylate.

Fitting the Crown

An appropriate size crown can be selected by measuring the mesial-to-distal space between the adjacent teeth of the prepared tooth to ensure adequate proximal contacts and confirming that it is long enough to cover the preparation. Most crowns are too long initially and must be trimmed at the cervical margin with scissors or an acrylic bur (Procedure 15.2). After the crown has been adjusted for width and height, it is filled with acrylic resin or bis-acrylic composite, which is matched to tooth shade, and then placed onto the prepared tooth. The acrylic mix should reach the dough stage before seating the crown on the moistened (keeps the acrylic mix from sticking) preparation. Acrylic resins will chemically bond with the polycarbonate crown and composites will bond if the interior of the crown is first primed with methyl methacrylate liquid or by roughening the interior of the crown.

> **Do You Recall?**
>
> Why are provisional crowns intended to be worn for a short period of time?

> **Clinical Tip**
>
> Keep the tab of the polycarbonate crown form in place during fitting; it makes for a convenient handle for trying in and removing the crown.

Celluloid Crown Forms

Celluloid crown forms are thin, transparent shells made of cellulose acetate (Fig. 15.8). They are available in:
- Primary and permanent anterior tooth shapes and sizes
- Primary posterior teeth

Fitting the Crown Form

To select the appropriate form size, a measurement is made of the incisal width of the preparation space between the two adjacent teeth. The size of the celluloid crown form can be enlarged by warming the round end of an instrument such as a ball burnisher and pressing it into the form at the location requiring enlargement. The size can also be reduced by slitting the crown form vertically on the lingual surface, overlapping the cut edges to fit the crown preparation and then fusing the edges with a couple drops of acetone or a hot instrument (use caution). Like other crown forms, preformed celluloid crown forms are filled with acrylic or composite resin provisional material to create the tooth shape presented by the form. Usually, one or two small holes are placed in the incisal corners of the crown form to allow excess resin or composite material to flow out when the crown form is seated on the prepared tooth. This prevents trapping air and the creation of voids in the material. After the fill material cures, the shell is slit with a scalpel and peeled off the tooth and adjustments to margins, contours, or occlusions are done with an acrylic bur. Final smoothing and polishing can be done with standard acrylic or composite polishers.

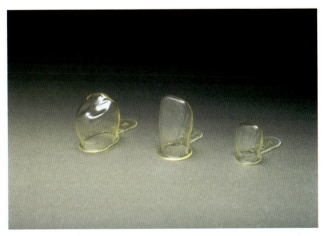

Fig. 15.8 Clear celluloid crown forms for permanent premolar and incisor and primary incisor. (Courtesy 3M ESPE.)

Advantages and Disadvantages

The advantage with the transparent form is that the shade selected to match the teeth is not affected by a predetermined color of the crown form allowing for a superior color match. The disadvantage is that after the crown form is removed, there is often a space left by the thickness of the crown form preventing contact with adjacent teeth and acrylic must be added to reestablish the interproximal contacts.

> **Clinical Tip**
>
> If the margins of the preformed crown are overextended when fitting, the gingival tissue will blanch when the patient bites on the crown or as the auxiliary seats the crown under finger pressure. This can be a useful sign to know where to trim the excess material from the preformed crown, especially in areas where the margins cannot be viewed directly, such as interproximal areas.

CUSTOMIZED PROVISIONAL CROWNS

Custom provisional crowns more consistently meet the criteria for successful provisional restorations than preformed provisional crowns. A customized provisional allows for better function and fit. Superior

Modifying Preformed Crowns to Close Open Contacts

Metal crowns: Place the proximal surface on a paper pad or small stack of 2 × 2 gauze squares and burnish the internal surface at the contact area with a ball burnisher. This stretches the metal outward to extend the contact area.

Polycarbonate crowns: Roughen the contact area and prime it with a drop of methyl methacrylate liquid. Add freshly mixed acrylic to the contact area. When it reaches the doughy stage, reseat the crown on the prepared tooth to establish contact. Remove the crown and place in warm water to accelerate the set of the acrylic. Once set, remove excess acrylic and very lightly polish the contact area.

An alternative material to use is flowable composite resin. The composite is added to the roughened and primed contact area, seat the crown on the prepared tooth, and then light-cure the composite. Remove the crown and shape and polish the composite as with the acrylic material.

Celluloid crown forms: Use a warm ball burnisher to push out the contact area from the interior when extension of the contact area is needed. Try the crown form on the prepared tooth and check the contact.

An alternative method is to make an opening (hole) where the contact area is located and allow the provisional crown material (acrylic or composite resin) to flow into contact with the adjacent tooth when the filled crown form is seated. Remove from the tooth before the acrylic sets fully so it does not get locked on the tooth. Remove excess material and reseat on the preparation a few times as it sets. With composite resin, use a 2- to 3-second tack cure and remove excess material from the margins and interproximal embrasure spaces before the final cure.

esthetics improves patient acceptance and the ability to fabricate multiunit provisional bridges makes these materials extremely popular.

Handling

Customized provisional materials must be:
- Fast and easy to use
- Reliable
- Inexpensive
- Have sufficient working time
- Have a simplified technique
- Economical
- Efficient to use
- Cost-effective

For many customized provisional materials, the working time must also allow for removal from the mouth while still elastic for trimming before reinsertion. For these materials, tear strength is a consideration. The setting time must be fast and must accommodate difficult-to-access areas when light-cured materials are used. Materials should be repairable to account for defects and to modify fit. Adding provisional material directly to the margins for repair will help provide good marginal integrity and relining the provisional crown with a new mix of material will ensure a good fit.

MATERIALS FOR CUSTOM PROVISIONAL RESTORATIONS

Materials used for the fabrication of custom provisional restorations fall into two main categories:
- Methacrylates
- Composite resins (Fig. 15.9)

METHACRYLATE PROVISIONAL MATERIALS (ACRYLICS)

Acrylic materials in the form of methacrylates have been used for many years to fabricate custom provisionals. They have been a good choice due to their:

- Good esthetics
- Ease of manipulation
- Low cost

However, these self-curing materials have high shrinkage and release heat (exothermic reaction) during polymerization. Additionally, patients complain about the acrylic odor and bad taste. They have a low modulus of elasticity (relatively flexible), have adequate strength, but wear easily. For the short time they will be in use, they are stain resistant and dimensionally stable.

The methacrylates can be placed into two subgroups:
- Methyl methacrylate
- Ethyl methacrylate

These acrylics have several features in common:
- Powder—liquid formulation
- Come in a variety of tooth colors
- Self-curing
- Shrink and release heat on setting
- Relatively strong
- Good polishability
- Material can be added to repair them

When the powder and liquid are mixed, the liquid partly dissolves the powder to produce a doughy mass that can be used to make provisional restorations.

Methyl Methacrylate

Methyl methacrylate (also called *polymethyl methacrylate* or *PMMA*) is the provisional material that has been used the longest. It consists of:
- Powder
  - Dibutyl or diethyl phthalate (polymer) powder
- Liquid
  - Methyl methacrylate (monomer)

It is available in a variety of tooth colors (Fig. 15.10). It has good strength for both single units and long-span bridges with good marginal fit.

Of the two categories of methacrylates, PMMA has the most shrinkage and heat generation on setting. The greater

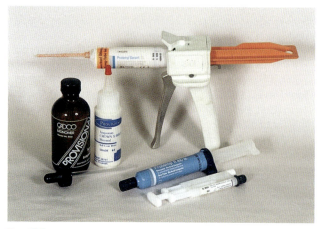

Fig. 15.9 Acrylic (liquid and powder) and composite provisional crown materials mixed by hand and automix.

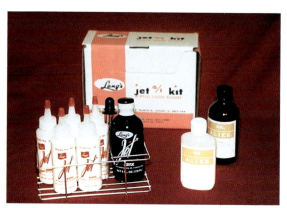

Fig. 15.10 Kit of methyl methacrylate (acrylic) materials: powders in a variety of shades and a bottle of liquid (monomer). (From Rosenstiel SF, Land MF, Fujimoto J. *Contemporary Fixed Prosthodontics.* 4th ed. Elsevier; 2006.)

the volume of material, the more heat will be generated. As an example, the pontic area of bridges has the most volume and care must be taken so the patient does not receive a tissue burn from the heat. The monomer can be toxic to the pulp if in close proximity and any free monomer not reacted with the powder can cause irritation to the oral mucosa in sensitive individuals. Additionally, the taste and odor is unpleasant. The setting time is approximately five to six minutes but fast set formulations are available with a four-minute setting time.

Caution
Methyl methacrylate monomer is flammable, care should be used to keep it away from an open flame. The material should be used in a well-ventilated area as it is not good to inhale the fumes or allow the material to contact the skin.

Ethyl Methacrylate

Ethyl methacrylates (also called *polyethyl methacrylates* or *PEMA*) provide some improvements over methyl methacrylates. It consists of:
- Powder
  - Polymer powder with coloring pigments
- Liquid
  - Benzoyl peroxide
    - Initiates the chemical reaction
  - Ethyl methacrylate

PEMA generates less heat and shrinkage when setting compared to methyl methacrylate and is better tolerated by the pulp and oral mucosa. However, they are not as strong as the methyl methacrylates and have less surface hardness. They are not suitable for long-span provisional bridges or for use in patients who brux their teeth.

Caution
Heat generated during the polymerization of self-cured acrylic can potentially damage the pulp or burn soft tissues, especially when used in a large volume such as a bridge.

Clinical Tip
Do not allow acrylic to set completely on a model or prepared tooth; this will cause the material to lock onto the preparation. Remove gross excess from the interproximal and "pump" the material on and off the tooth preparation until initial polymerization is complete.

COMPOSITE RESIN PROVISIONAL MATERIALS

Composite resin provisional materials were developed to overcome the undesirable features of methacrylates. Composites are biocompatible and kinder to the pulp. They can be grouped into three categories:
- Bis-acryl composite resin
- Bis-GMA composite resin
- Urethane dimethacrylate resin

They are a bit more expensive, but are easier to handle, have less odor and poor taste, and present with better esthetics.

Bis-acrylic Composite Resin

Bis-acrylic composite provisional materials (Fig. 15.11) have a chemical structure between that of acrylic resins and dental composite materials. Low shrinkage and heat release during curing, unnoticeable odor, good shade selection, and biocompatibility are distinct advantages over acrylic resins. The presence of micro- and nanosized glass fillers makes bis-acrylic composite resin provisionals more wear resistant than acrylics, and they have good marginal fit. Early versions were self-curing but a newer variation is dual-cured. A thin layer of unset resin remains on the surface (oxygen inhibited layer) of freshly polymerized bis-acrylic composite resin that should be removed. The material is are more brittle (higher modulus of elasticity) than the acrylics and, therefore, must be limited in use to single units or short-span bridges that are not under significant occlusal loading. They are esthetically more pleasing in the anterior area of the mouth than the acrylics but more prone to stain.

Bis-Glycidyl Methacrylate Composite Resin

Bis-GMA (bisphenol-A-glycidyl methacrylate) composite resins are an improvement over bis-acryl composites. They are stronger and less brittle, making them suitable for both single- and multiple-unit temporaries as well as long-term temporization. They have better esthetics, a wider shade selection, and are less prone to staining. Polymerization shrinkage and exothermic heat are reduced, making them kind to the pulp. They also have good margins and polish well. The newest materials, made with nano-fillers, provide a smooth and lustrous surface with little finishing and polishing required. These smoother surfaces are more comfortable for the patient and are easier to keep clean, thereby promoting better periodontal health.

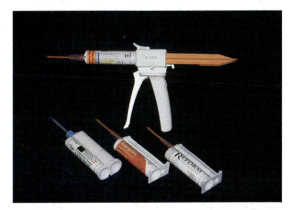

Fig. 15.11 Composite resin provisional materials in two-paste cartridges with automixing delivery tips. (From Rosenstiel SF, Land MF, Fujimoto J. *Contemporary Fixed Prosthodontics.* 4th ed. Elsevier; 2006.)

Manipulation of Material

The two-paste material is typically dispensed from a double-barrel cartridge placed into a dispensing gun and appropriate amounts of catalyst and base are mixed with a specific automix tip as the material is dispensed. Automixing helps to prevent operator error and unnecessary waste as well as ease of cleanup. Additionally, automix syringes allow for direct delivery into a template without the incorporation of air voids.

Light-cured, self-cured, and dual-cured versions of these materials are available.

- Automixed self-cured materials are dispensed from syringes and may be used with any template.
- Light-cured materials require clear plastic templates and are difficult to cure in deep areas or those with limited access.
- Dual-cured materials require additional time to chemical-cure in areas the curing light cannot reach, but they allow for removal from undercut areas while the materials are still flexible. Then they are trimmed and replaced for final curing (Table 15.2). They, too, are used with a template procedure.

KEY POINTS

ADVANTAGES OF COMPOSITE RESIN PROVISIONAL MATERIALS
1. Easy to use
2. Set quickly
3. Flexible so easier to insert and remove
4. Minimal polymerization shrinkage and heat
5. Color stable and stain resistant
6. Minimal bad taste and odor
7. Easy to repair using flowable composite
8. Radiopaque

Clinical Tip

When using automix dispenser guns, ensure the cartridges and dispenser gun are compatible. There are varying sizes of the catalyst and base depending on the manufacturer of the material being used.

Table 15.2 Features of Acrylic and Composite Provisional Materials

ACRYLIC	COMPOSITE
High heat during polymerization	Low heat during curing
High shrinkage during polymerization	Low shrinkage during curing
Possible tissue irritation	Good tissue biocompatibility
Poor taste and smell	No unpleasant smell and mild taste
Difficult to repair	Easily repaired
Variety of color shades	Excellent esthetics
Inexpensive	Expensive

METHODS OF FABRICATION OF CUSTOM PROVISIONALS

Custom provisional crowns can be made by:
- Direct fabrication
  - Made directly on the prepared tooth
- Indirect fabrication
  - Out of the mouth on a stone cast or by a combination of the two

Often a template is used as a carrier for the provisional material.

Types and Uses of Templates

A template (also called a *mold* or *matrix*) shapes the external contours and anatomy of the provisional, and the prepared tooth or stone cast creates the internal dimensions. Template materials include:
- Hard wax
- Impression materials (such as alginate, silicone, or polyvinyl siloxane)
- Vacuum-formed plastic and thermoplastic resins (Fig. 15.12)

A template can be made directly in the mouth prior to the preparation of the tooth or teeth or on a stone cast of the unprepared teeth. If the teeth are broken or require a change in shape for a more natural provisional, some repair or reshaping must be done in the mouth or on the stone cast, so the template will capture the new tooth form.

Alginate and wax are the easiest to use, least expensive, and used extensively for single-unit, direct-technique provisionals. Polyvinyl siloxane (PVS) impression material is very popular and is often used in its putty form or regular body consistency in a tray. PVS, while more expensive, has an advantage over wax or alginate in that it can be reused multiple times, especially days later if the provisional should break and need to be remade.

Vacuum-formed plastic is the most common choice for multiunit and indirect provisional techniques. The vacuum-formed plastic template is made using a technique similar to the process of making a whitening trays. A stone cast of the unprepared teeth is trimmed to remove borders that might entrap air. A thin sheet of the stiff plastic material (0.02 mm) is heated on a vacuum former until it sags 1 to 1.25 inches, and then the machine is activated to adapt the molten plastic to the cast. After the material cools it is removed from the cast and trimmed to include one or two teeth mesial and distal to the tooth/teeth to be prepared and approximately 3 to 4 mm below the gingival margin of the area of interest. The template is, then, ready for use with a direct or indirect fabrication technique.

DIRECT TECHNIQUE

Using the direct technique for provisional coverage, the provisional is fabricated directly on the prepared tooth using one of the provisional materials in a template

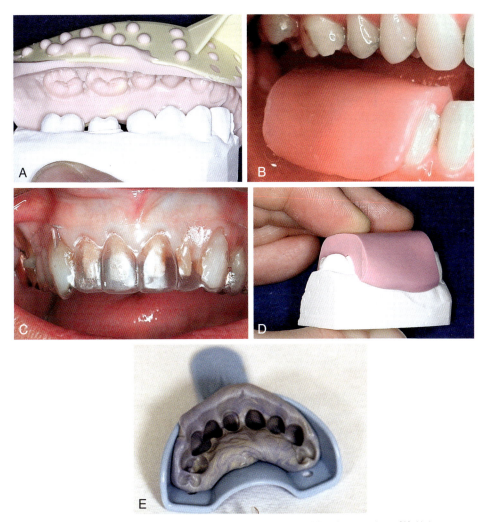

Fig. 15.12 Variety of templates used for fabrication of custom provisional restorations: **(A)** Alginate impression. **(B)** Baseplate wax. **(C)** Clear vacuum-formed plastic. **(D)** Silicon putty. **(E)** Polyvinyl siloxane impression. ((A–D) From Rosenstiel SF, Land MF, Fujimoto J. *Contemporary Fixed Prosthodontics*. 5th ed. Elsevier; 2016.)

(Procedure 15.3). One popular technique uses a disposable triple tray impression with fast-set material or bite registration material as the template. The impression used for the template is taken before the tooth is prepared. After the tooth is prepared, the impression is filled with a provisional material and seated on the prepared tooth.

If using an acrylic material for the provisional, powder and liquid must be mixed together to form a paste (see Fig. 15.30). It must be hand-mixed to the proper consistency, and care must be taken to avoid trapping air during mixing or in delivering the material into the template. After placing the paste in the template, the template is inverted and seated over the moist prepared teeth. If gross voids are found on the occlusal or incisal, it may be necessary to place small holes in the occlusal or incisal corners of the template to alleviate hydrostatic pressure that has prevented the material from flowing into these areas.

Caution must be taken when using this technique so that the provisional crown does not get locked on the prepared tooth. Locking happens when excess provisional material flows out of the template and hardens in the interproximal embrasure spaces under the contact areas of the adjacent teeth (Fig. 15.13). Not only is the crown very difficult to remove (and occasionally excess material must be cut from the undercuts with a bur), but heat generated during setting can

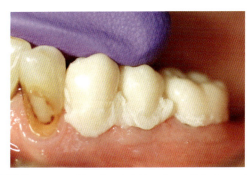

Fig. 15.13 Excess provisional material has flowed into the embrasure spaces and must be removed before it sets or the provisional restoration must be lifted and reseated several times before it sets to keep the restoration from being locked on the teeth. (From Rosenstiel SF, Land MF, Fujimoto J: *Contemporary fixed prosthodontics*, ed 4, St Louis, 2006, Elsevier.)

burn tissues or damage the pulp. To avoid this error, the template with acrylic in place is "pumped" on and off the preparation when the material reaches a rubbery consistency. It can be removed just prior to its final set and the acrylic provisional crown can be removed from the template. Gross excess can be trimmed away with crown and bridge scissors. The provisional should, then, be placed in a cup of room temperature water to finish polymerization. (Hot water will accelerate the set but will cause more shrinkage and distortion.) If these materials are removed from the mouth too early and allowed to polymerize off the preparation, the amount of shrinkage may be sufficient to prevent them from seating back on the prepared tooth or the margins may be short. However, more material can be added to fill voids or correct deficient margins. This is accomplished by adding some liquid (monomer) to a clean surface to wet the surface so a new mix will bond to it. After the material has set completely the rough provisional should be finished and polished for tissue health and patient comfort.

Clinical Tip
Make sure the prepared tooth is slightly moist when seating the template containing acrylic. If the preparation is dry, the acrylic might stick to it and the provisional restoration may distort on removal.

If using a composite resin paste-paste system in an automixing device with a delivery tip, be sure to keep the tip in the material as it is extruded into the impression prevent the introduction of air bubbles. After placing the mixed material in the impression, reinsert it into the mouth. If using the triple tray, the patient is asked to bite into their normal occlusion while the material sets.

The impression is removed from the patient's mouth and the provisional crown is removed from the impression. If the triple tray is used, the occlusion should be very close to perfect. However, if the tray did not seat correctly, the occlusion could be quite high.

This technique is fast and provides a provisional restoration that duplicates the original tooth. Some clinicians use a clear PVS bite registration material so that they can speed the initial set by light-curing the material through the clear impression material.

Clinical Tip
If bits of the provisional composite resin crown margins are going to come off, it is usually when the impression is removed from the prepared tooth. If the margins are thin, some of the material may tear or stick to the prepared tooth. If the marginal defect is minor, seat the provisional crown back on the moistened preparation and add some flowable composite to repair the margin, then light-cure it. Be sure to lap the composite up onto the crown a couple millimeters so it has enough surface area to affect a good bond with the crown.

Caution
Before using the direct technique, make sure there is adequate access to the preparation site, the template does not unduly impinge on the tissues, and tissues in the area are not inflamed and likely to bleed.

Indirect Technique

With the indirect technique the entire provisional is made outside of the mouth, then tried in and adjusted for fit. Any needed corrections to margins, contacts, or voids can be made with the addition of new material either in the mouth or on the cast. Using the indirect technique, a pre-preparation impression of the area is made and poured into stone; the template is then made on this model. If it is necessary to account for missing tooth structure caused by caries or trauma, the defect can be corrected on the model with:
- Wax
- Acrylic
- Light-cured resin
- Other materials

The template can be used indirectly with fabrication of the provisional on the model of the prepared teeth.

The indirect technique has several advantages over the direct technique:
- Superior access to the preparations (stone replicas)
- Saves chair time
- Is more convenient for making multiunit bridges or crowns in difficult-to-access areas
- Is desirable when the patient reports previous tissue irritation from methacrylate monomer
- Has difficulty maintaining an open mouth during the procedure
- Is recommended when there is a concern for the health of the pulp due to deep caries or extensive prepping with the high-speed handpiece

By fabricating the crown indirectly, the tooth is not subjected to exothermic heat and chemical irritants of some provisional materials before they are set. The marginal fit is better when the material is allowed to set completely on the stone cast rather than with the direct technique where it is removed from the mouth before fully set.

Clinical Tip
Although the indirect technique requires additional time to fabricate a stone model or PVS die, this technique can end up saving time in complicated cases and may be required if hard or soft tissue conditions would be further traumatized by direct fabrication. The indirect procedure can be delegated to the laboratory.

INDIRECT-DIRECT TECHNIQUE

With the indirect-direct technique:
- A template is made on a pretreatment cast.
- The template is filled with a provisional material.
- The template is The template is seated on a lubricated stone cast.
  - The teeth on the cast to be restored have been lightly prepared so that they are under-reduced compared to the actual tooth preparation.
  - The result is a thin provisional shell that has the external form of the finished provisional.
  - It is too thin to serve as the functioning provisional restoration.
- At chairside, it is relined with freshly mixed provisional material.
- Then the filled provisional shell is seated directly on the prepared tooth or teeth.

Half of the procedure is completed out of the mouth and half is completed directly on the teeth.

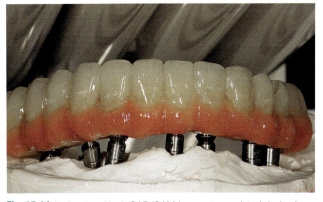

Fig. 15.14 Indirect multiunit CAD/CAM (computer-assisted design/computer-assisted machining) acrylic provisional restorations customized by a skilled laboratory technician (Luke Kahng, CDT) with glaze and gingival colored composite resin. (From Kahng LS. Step-by-step: fabricating temporaries with PMMA material. *Dental Esthetics*, May 2016.)

> **Clinical Tip**
>
> To prevent the provisional material from sticking, coat the gypsum model with a separating medium. (If you use vaseline to lubricate the model, be sure to wash it off the provisional material before advancing to the next step.) If placing the provisional material in the patient's mouth, make sure the tooth is moist with saliva.

If using light-cured material, follow the manufacturer's directions for the required curing time. If using acrylic, remove the template while it is still doughy, trim away the excess with scissors, and then "pump" the provisional up and down on the preparation to prevent it from locking in the embrasures. When final set is achieved, remove the provisional from the template and trim and polish.

> **Clinical Tip**
>
> If the custom provisional restoration is thin in areas, it is likely the result of one of two things:
> 1. The preparation has not been reduced enough to allow for adequate material.
> 2. The template was pressed too hard onto the preparation causing it to compress toward the preparation.

Fabricating and cementing provisional restorations in many states are functions relegated to registered dental assistants and hygienists, while in other states they may be considered expanded functions requiring additional education. Check your state dental practice act for details.

ADVANCED TECHNIQUES

Many experienced dental auxiliary are equally capable of fabricating provisional coverage for complicated cases. At times, the dental laboratory technician may be called on to help in the fabrication of more difficult provisional coverage. Fabrication of provisional coverage over implants, for inlay and onlay preparations, and for long-term coverage will require specialized skills, knowledge of the requirements of the restorative procedure, and specialized alterations to provisional materials.

CAD/CAM Provisional (Temporary) Materials

Acrylate polymer (PMMA) blocks are available for use with computer-assisted design/computer-assisted machining (CAD/CAM) units to fabricate provisional restorations. These products provide many advantages over traditional provisional materials. Because the PMMA blocks are processed with heat and pressure, there is no free monomer to irritate tissues and produce a bad taste. The polymers undergo more complete conversion and the materials have improved physical and mechanical properties, such as:

- Higher flexural strength
- Improved esthetics
- Available in up to six shades
- Longer lasting color stability (due to decreased porosity)
- Elimination of polymerization shrinkage and exothermic heat
- Superior fit and marginal integrity
- Durability
- Extended duration of wear (up to a year)

They are indicated for single crowns, inlays, onlays, and anterior and posterior bridges with up to two pontics. Disks for multi-unit cases can also be used to fabricate provisional restoration in the office or in the laboratory using CAD/CAM technology and custom glazing and gingival effects (Fig. 15.14).

Provisional Materials for Inlays and Onlays

Any of the provisional materials discussed in this chapter could be used to make provisional restorations for inlay or onlay preparations using direct or indirect techniques. However, some of the materials, especially acrylics, are much more difficult to handle in these complex cavity preparations with multiple walls and box forms.

Materials that are easier to use include:
- *Bis-acrylic and Bis-GMA Composite Resins*
  - Less shrinkage, low exothermic reaction
- *Urethane Dimethacrylate Resins*
  - Very strong, light-cured, putty consistency
- *CAD/CAM Materials*
  - Acrylate polymer blocks; eliminate exothermic reaction and polymerization shrinkage because they are already cured; increased strength and better fit
  - Drawback: requires in-office milling machine to deliver at the same appointment as the preparation
- *Cements for Provisionals*
  - Use limited to preparations that are entirely intracoronal; not retentive enough for onlays

 Clinical Tip

If a light coating of a water-soluble lubricant or petroleum jelly is applied to the cervical half of the exterior of the provisional restoration before loading it with cement, cleanup of the restoration after the cement sets will be much easier.

 Do You Recall?

What type of cement should not be used for a provisional restoration prior to cementation of a final restoration with composite resin cement?

 Clinical Tip

Lightly coat the walls of the provisional crown with the cement. Do not fill the entire interior of the crown with cement since the prepared tooth will displace the majority of it and the crown might not seat completely. All excess cement must be thoroughly removed, especially subgingivally, to prevent tissue irritation.

HANDLING THE PROVISIONAL RESTORATION

CEMENTING THE PROVISIONAL RESTORATION

Provisional luting cements are used to cement provisional crowns. The choice of appropriate provisional luting cement is based on several factors:
- Properties of the provisional luting cement
- How long the provisional restoration will be in place
- How naturally retentive the preparation is
- What type of provisional restoration is being used
- What type of permanent restoration is being fabricated
- What type of permanent cement will be used

The cement must be:
- Retentive
- Have limited solubility to protect the tooth margins
- Not detract from the esthetics of the provisional restoration
- Be easily and completely removed
- Not interfere with the bond of the permanent restoration

A wide variety of provisional cements are available for the cementation of provisional restorations. A detailed description of each type of provisional cement is discussed in Chapter 16.

Before cementation of the provisional restoration, the preparation is dried and isolated with cotton rolls and the cement is mixed according to the manufacturer's directions. The walls of the provisional crown are coated with the cement and then seated onto the tooth. Finger pressure is exerted, or the patient is asked to bite down firmly on a cotton roll placed on the occlusal surface of the provisional restoration. Excess cement is removed when appropriately set. Removal of excess cement and the consequences of incomplete cement removal are covered extensively in Chapter 16.

REMOVING THE PROVISIONAL RESTORATION

The provisional restoration must be fabricated in a way that allows for easy removal without damage to the preparation. It is also desirable to preserve the provisional restoration in the event it may need to be reused.

Methods to remove the provisional restoration include the following:
- Using an instrument to engage the crown margin, pry the provisional off the preparation. Use caution not to damage the preparation margins.
- Using a chisel and mallet or crown and bridge removal instrument (also called a *reverse hammer*) to gently tap the restoration off the preparation. Keep the force directed along the long axis of the tooth to prevent damage to it.
- Using a pair of temporary removal forceps to grasp the provisional restoration, gently rock it back and forth and apply mild force in an occlusal direction until the cement loosens and then lift it from the preparation (Fig. 15.15).

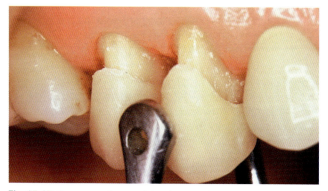

Fig. 15.15 To remove the provisional restoration, grasp it with removal forceps and gently rock it back and forth while applying mild force in an occlusal direction until the cement loosens. (From Rosenstiel SF, Land MF, Fujimoto J. *Contemporary Fixed Prosthodontics*. 4th ed. Elsevier; 2006.)

If the provisional crown had a very snug fit when trying it on, only apply provisional cement to 3 or 4 mm of the crown walls around the margins. There will be less cement internally to hold the provisional crown, making removal easier. Do not use this technique if the patient bruxes. Another technique to make removal easier with a snug-fitting crown is to add a small amount of petroleum jelly to the cement mix.

Caution
All remnants of provisional cement must be completely removed and the tooth surface cleaned completely to prevent interference with bonding of the permanent restoration.

CLEANUP

After the provisional restoration has been removed, there will be remnants of cement stuck to the tooth preparation. If the patient's tooth has been sensitive, a local anesthetic may be required prior to removal of the provisional restoration. Carefully remove as much cement as possible with an instrument such as an explorer, interproximal carver or spoon excavator using light pressure so as not to damage the preparation. Usually very small fragments of cement will still remain. These must be removed to allow complete seating of the final restoration and prevent interference with bonding procedures. Use a slurry of flour of pumice and water on a rubber prophy cup or a soft brush to complete the removal of these fine pieces of cement and rinse thoroughly. Do not discard the provisional restoration until the final restoration has been successfully cemented in case it is needed.

INTRACORONAL PROVISIONAL CEMENT RESTORATIONS

The main uses for intracoronal provisional cement restorations are for emergency treatments, such as for deep caries or painful teeth, for protecting preparations for metal or ceramic inlays, and to close endodontic access preparations. These cements are discussed in Chapter 16.

Clinical Tip
It should be noted that zinc oxide eugenol (Fig. 15.16) provisionals should not be used if a permanent restoration is to be cemented with a resin luting agent because eugenol-containing cements inhibit polymerization of the resin cement.

Cements are placed directly into the cavity preparation with the aid of a matrix band and wedge when appropriate. The cement is carved and contoured, and then allowed to set. The final check of occlusion is done with articulating paper followed by additional carving as necessary (Procedure 15.4).

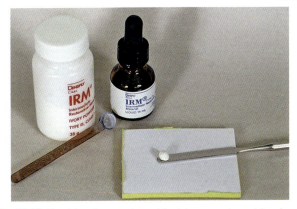

Fig. 15.16 Provisional cement used for intracoronal provisional coverage.

 Do You Recall?

Why it is important to remove all remnants of provisional cement prior to cementation of the permanent restoration?

PATIENT EDUCATION

Scheduled appointment times for fabricating provisional restorations must allow sufficient time to instruct the patient on appropriate home care techniques and permit of these techniques, educate patients as to the limitations and expectations of the provisional restoration, and address patient concerns. Patients should understand that provisional restorations, although functional, are not as durable, well-fitting or esthetic as permanent restorations.

Because of limitations in the strength of provisional materials and the weak cements used to retain them, patients must be instructed that:
- Sticky foods may dislodge the provisional.
- Hard foods may crack it.
- Chewing gum may stick to it.

Patients must be informed that there may be temperature sensitivity and an unpleasant taste associated with the provisional material. To avoid complications with treatment resulting from tooth movement or loss of tooth structure, patients must be told to immediately call the office if the provisional becomes dislodged, fractured, or lost, even if the tooth is not sensitive. Teeth can shift in as little as 24 hours after loss of the provisional restoration. Strict adherence to appointment intervals is extremely important. Patients must return to the office at the appropriate time for placement of the permanent restoration due to the potential wear and breakdown of the provisional material or washing out of the provisional cement. Limitations in esthetics of the provisional restoration may include:
- Imperfections in color matching
- Anatomic contour
- Smoothness
- Staining by certain foods and beverages
  - Such as tobacco, coffee, tea, red wine, berries, and fruit juices

To avoid dissatisfaction, patients must be reminded that provisional restorations are not the same as permanent ones.

> **Clinical Tip**
>
> If a provisional crown comes off during a time that the dental office is closed, the patient can be instructed to replace it after cleaning the interior of the crown and placing a small amount of denture adhesive into the crown. The patient should be instructed never to use any household cements.

HOME CARE INSTRUCTIONS

Home care instructions include brushing the entire dentition, inclusive of the restoration carefully at least twice a day. Flossing should be done at least once a day and the floss should be pulled out to the side under the contact of the provisional rather than back in an occlusal/incisal direction. Removing the floss back through the contact in an occlusal/incisal direction might dislodge the provisional restoration. If the provisional restoration includes a pontic, the additional use of floss threaders, Superfloss (Oral B), or end-tufted brushes must be stressed for cleaning the surface of the pontic contacting the tissue and the proximal embrasures. Maintenance of healthy tissue during provisional coverage is crucial to the success of the permanent restoration. Inflamed gingival tissues can result in bleeding at the time of cementation of the permanent restoration that may compromise the cement seal.

> **KEY POINTS**
>
> **PATIENT EDUCATION AND HOME CARE**
> 1. The patient should be instructed that the provisional is intended to be worn for a limited time.
> 2. Regular brushing and flossing of the provisional is important to maintain the health of the oral tissues.
> 3. Floss should be pulled through the interproximal area to prevent dislodging of the provisional.
> 4. Sticky foods should be avoided to prevent removal of the provisional.
> 5. If the provisional comes off or becomes loose, the patient should contact the office for recementation immediately.

SUMMARY

Provisional restorations protect teeth and periodontal structures in a variety of dental procedures. Regardless of the material and technique selected, a high-quality provisional restoration must be well adapted to the preparation, have proper contact, contour, and occlusion and must be functional and acceptable to the patient. If these criteria are not met, pulpal and periodontal irritation, tooth migration, and patient dissatisfaction will likely occur. There are many choices in the selection of provisional restorations and techniques for the fabrication of provisional restorations. The clinician must select materials and techniques on the basis of each patient's clinical needs and situation.

INSTRUCTIONAL VIDEOS

See the Evolve Resources site for a variety of educational videos that reinforce the material covered in this chapter.

Procedure 15.1 Metal Provisional Crown

See Evolve site for Competency Sheet.

Consider the following with this procedure: safety glasses are recommended for the patient, PPE is required for the clinician, ensure appropriate safety protocols are followed, and check your local state guidelines before performing this procedure.

EQUIPMENT/SUPPLIES (FIG. 15.17)
- Mirror and explorer
- Selection of silver-tin alloy crowns
- Crown and bridge scissors
- Contouring pliers
- Ball burnisher
- Articulating paper
- Dental floss
- Isolation materials
- Cement and armamentarium
- Sandpaper disk and rubber wheel

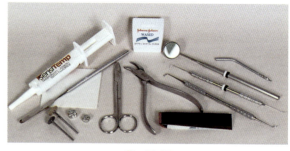

Fig. 15.17

PROCEDURE STEPS
1. Measure the mesiodistal width of the space between adjacent teeth.
2. Choose a crown that has a mesiodistal width equal to that of the original tooth.
   NOTE: If the crown does not fit, it may be sterilized and placed back in the kit.

Continued

Procedure 15.1 Metal Provisional Crown—cont'd

3. Try in the crown, noting the occlusal relationship to adjacent and opposing dentition.
   NOTE: The crown will be considerably higher than the adjacent teeth (Fig. 15.18).
4. Scribe a line on the facial and lingual crown surfaces to match the contour of the gingiva and approximate the amount of crown length that needs to be trimmed.
   NOTE: The crown is longer on the facial and lingual surfaces and shorter on the mesial and distal surfaces, forming a wavy line.
5. Trim to within 1 mm of the scribed line, using curved crown and bridge scissors.
   NOTE: Try to blend your cutting junctions to avoid producing burs of metal that will irritate the tissues (Fig. 15.19).
6. Contour the trimmed areas, using contouring pliers. Advance the pliers around the crown periphery as you continually squeeze the pliers with the ball portion of the pliers inside the crown and the curved beak on the outside of the crown.
   NOTE: This crimps the crown edge, adapting its circumference to the finish line (Fig. 15.20).
7. Retry the crown on the preparation to confirm fit. Adjust as needed.
8. Have patient tap the teeth together to adapt the soft metal to the occlusion
9. Check the bite with articulating paper; make sure the crown is occluding properly when the patient's teeth are fully together.
   NOTE: If the crown is interfering with occlusion, some reduction will be necessary. Only minor adjustments can be made on the occlusal surface before the surface is perforated (Fig. 15.21).
10. Check the contacts, using dental floss, to determine whether contacts are present and in the proper location.
    NOTE: If contact points need to be established, use the ball burnisher or contouring pliers with the ball portion inside and the curved beak outside, and gently squeeze to establish contact at the appropriate location.
11. Trim and polish the crown margins with disks and a rubber wheel to make the crown smooth and to prevent tissue irritation (Fig. 15.22).
12. Isolate the area and mix the cement according to the manufacturer's directions.
    NOTE: Because the metal is soft, the occlusal portion must be supported by a reinforced cement such as IRM. Plain ZOE cement such as TempBond is too weak for this purpose.

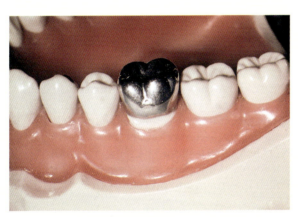

Fig. 15.18

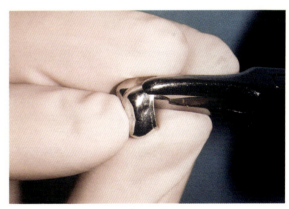

Fig. 15.20

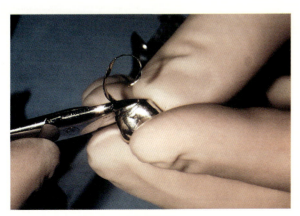

Fig. 15.19

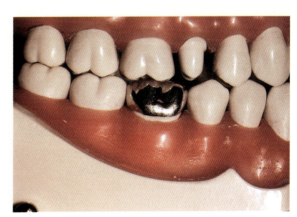

Fig. 15.21

Procedure 15.1 Metal Provisional Crown—cont'd

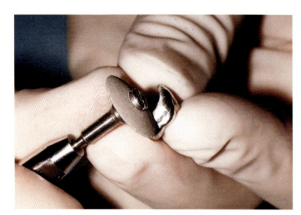

Fig. 15.22

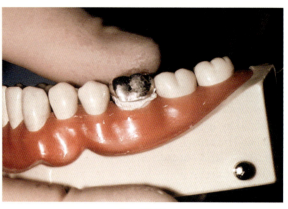

Fig. 15.23

13. Seat the crown onto the preparation and have the patient bite on a cotton roll or a wooden stick in a mesiodistal direction to improve force distribution.
   NOTE: Make sure the patient is not biting only on the crown, but also on the adjacent teeth in the quadrant; biting only on the crown may force the crown too far in a gingival direction (Fig. 15.23).
14. When appropriate, remove excess facial and lingual cement. Remove interproximal cement by drawing a knotted piece of dental floss through the contact (Fig. 15.24) followed by an explorer.

Optional Steps

NOTE: The crown may be lined with an acrylic or bis-acrylic composite provisional material to further customize the internal fit and support the occlusal portion.

1. Mix the acrylic or composite provisional material according to the manufacturer's directions.
2. Place the material into the prepared crown, making sure to line the crown to avoid trapping air.
3. Place the crown back on the preparation, and have the patient bite in occlusion.

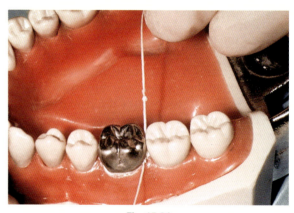

Fig. 15.24

4. After the material has reached the desired consistency, remove the crown and remove the excess.
5. Because the acrylic supports the occlusal portion of the crown, it may be cemented with weaker ZOE cement such as TempBond or a noneugenol version.
   NOTE: Material should be removed while still elastic to avoid trapping the crown in undercuts.
6. Polish the crown and proceed with steps 12 through 14 above.

Procedure 15.2 Polycarbonate Provisional Crown

See Evolve site for Competency Sheet.

Consider the following with this procedure: safety glasses are recommended for the patient, PPE is required for the clinician, ensure appropriate safety protocols are followed, and check your local state guidelines before performing this procedure.

EQUIPMENT/SUPPLIES (FIG. 15.25)
- Mirror and explorer
- Selection of polycarbonate crowns
- Articulating paper
- Dental floss
- Acrylic burs and sandpaper disks
- Pumice and rag wheel
- Isolation materials
- Cement and armamentarium

PROCEDURE STEPS

1. Measure the mesiodistal width of the space between adjacent teeth.
2. Choose a crown that has a mesiodistal width equal to that of the original tooth.
   NOTE: Choose a crown that is slightly larger if an exact size cannot be found.

Continued

Procedure 15.2 Polycarbonate Provisional Crown—cont'd

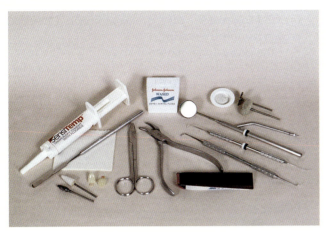

Fig. 15.25

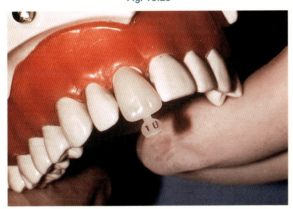

Fig. 15.26

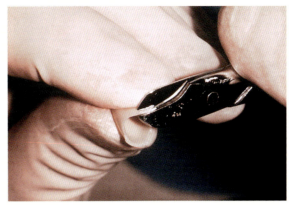

Fig. 15.27

3. Try in the crown, noting the occlusal or incisal relationship to adjacent and opposing dentition.
   NOTE: The crown will be considerably higher than the adjacent teeth. If the crown does not fit, it may be sterilized and placed back in the kit (Fig. 15.26).
   NOTE: Keep the incisal identification tab in place to use as a handle for try in and removal.
4. Scribe a line on the facial and lingual crown surfaces to match the contour of the gingiva and approximate the amount of crown length that needs to be trimmed.
   NOTE: The crown is longer on the facial and lingual surfaces and shorter on the mesial and distal surfaces, forming a wavy line.
5. Trim to within 1 mm of the scribed line with scissors or an acrylic bur on a slow-speed handpiece. Do not trim from the incisal/occlusal surface to adjust the length.
   NOTE: Trim a small amount at a time while continuing to try and retry the crown until the desired amount is removed. If the crown was slightly larger than the space, it may be necessary to trim the proximal surfaces to establish a good seat (Fig. 15.27).
6. Check bite with articulating paper; make sure the crown is occluding properly when the patient's teeth are fully together.

NOTE: If the crown is interfering with occlusion, further reduction will be necessary. Only minor adjustments can be made on the incisal or occlusal surface before the surface is perforated. If the crown is fully seated and adjusting the occlusion has caused a perforation in the crown, it is possible that the preparation is under-reduced.

7. Check the contacts, using dental floss, to determine whether contacts are present and in the proper location.
   NOTE: If contact points are too tight or are not at appropriate locations, it will be necessary to trim the proximal surface of the crown to establish correct location. If contact points are not present, you may have to add to the proximal surface with acrylic.
8. Trim and polish the crown margins with disks and pumice on a rag wheel to make the crown smooth and to prevent tissue irritation.
9. Isolate the area and cement the crown, following the manufacturer's directions for mixing the appropriate cement.
   NOTE: Completely coat the inside surfaces of the crown to avoid trapping air.
10. Seat the crown onto the preparation and have the patient bite on a cotton roll or a wooden stick in a mesiodistal direction to improve force distribution.
    NOTE: Make sure the patient is not biting only on the crown, but also on the adjacent teeth in the quadrant; biting only on the crown may force the crown too far in a gingival direction (Fig. 15.28).
11. When appropriate, remove excess facial and lingual cement. Remove interproximal cement by drawing a knotted piece of dental floss through the contact.

Optional Steps

NOTE: If the crown is loosely fitting, it may be lined with an acrylic or bis-acrylic composite provisional material to further customize the internal fit.

1. It may be necessary to place one or two small vent holes on the incisal corners or occlusal surface to

Procedure 15.2 Polycarbonate Provisional Crown—cont'd

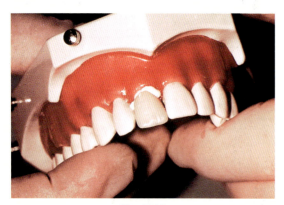

Fig. 15.28

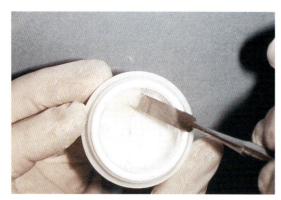

Fig. 15.29

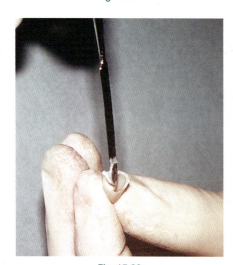

Fig. 15.30

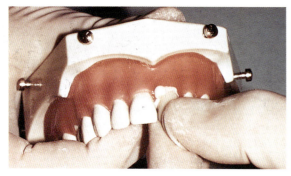

Fig. 15.31

prevent hydrostatic pressure from keeping the crown from fully seating.

2. Mix the provisional material according to the manufacturer's directions (Fig. 15.29).
3. Place the material into the prepared crown, making sure to line the crown to avoid trapping of air (Fig. 15.30).
4. Place the crown back on the preparation, and have the patient bite in occlusion (Fig. 15.31).
5. After the material has reached the desired consistency, remove the crown, place it in room temperature water until set, and then remove the excess.

   NOTE: Crown should be pumped on and off the tooth while the lining material is still elastic to avoid trapping the crown in undercuts (Fig. 15.32).
6. Polish the crown and proceed with steps 8 through 11 above (Figs. 15.33 and 15.34).

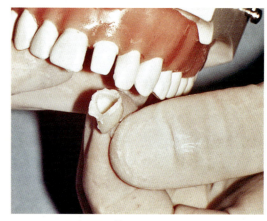

Fig. 15.32

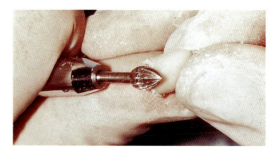

Fig. 15.33

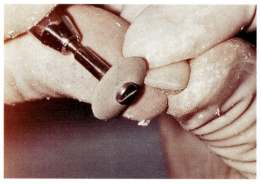

Fig. 15.34

Continued

Provisional Restorations CHAPTER 15 327

Procedure 15.3 Custom Provisional Coverage: Direct Technique

See Evolve site for Competency Sheet.

Consider the following with this procedure: safety glasses are recommended for the patient, PPE is required for the clinician, ensure appropriate safety protocols are followed, and check your local state guidelines before performing this procedure.

EQUIPMENT/SUPPLIES (FIG. 15.35)
- Mirror and explorer
- Template of the tooth before preparation
- Acrylic or composite provisional material
- Separating medium
- Dispensing syringe
- Acrylic stones and sandpaper disks
- Pumice and rag wheel
- Isolation materials
- Cement and armamentarium

PROCEDURE STEPS
Preparing the Template
1. Before preparing the tooth, make a template by taking an alginate or triple tray impression of it or by using a thermoplastic resin button or vacuum-formed plastic sheet on a stone cast of the unprepared tooth.
   NOTE: Alginate impressions should be kept moist until used.
2. Trim the template to remove undercuts or excess material.

Preparing the Provisional Coverage
1. Coat the prepared tooth with a water-soluble lubricant such as K-Y jelly or glycerin.
   NOTE: This will aid in separating the provisional material from the preparation while in a doughy stage (Fig. 15.36).
2. Remove excess moisture from the template.
3. Prepare the acrylic or composite resin provisional material according to the manufacturer's directions.

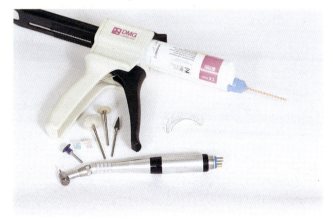

Fig. 15.35

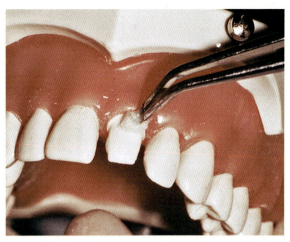

Fig. 15.36

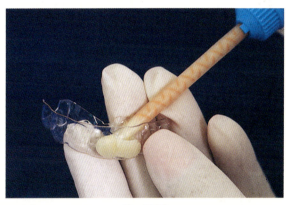

Fig. 15.37

   NOTE: Custom shading must be considered at this time, with matching of adjacent teeth.
4. Dispense the provisional material directly into the template, making sure not to trap air.
   NOTE: An automixing tip on the syringe or cartridge that allows delivery of the mixed provisional material directly into the template is useful. Begin loading the template from the bottom and keep the tip buried in material until loading is complete to avoid introducing air into the mix (Fig. 15.37).
5. Place the template back into the patient's mouth or onto the lubricated model, aligning it precisely on the prepared tooth.
   NOTE: A notch cut in the template at a visually accessible location in the mouth will facilitate replacement of the template to the correct position (Fig. 15.38).
6. Check the initial set of the material in the patient's mouth which occurs within 1 to 3 minutes.
   NOTE: Check material in the patient's mouth, as heat and moisture will accelerate the set; use the material that has extruded from the location notch to test the set.

Procedure 15.3 Custom Provisional Coverage: Direct Technique—cont'd

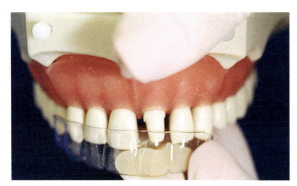

Fig. 15.38

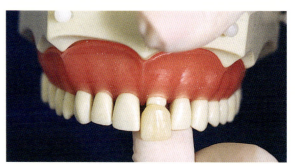

Fig. 15.39

7. Remove the template with provisional material in place when firm but a still elastic consistency is reached.
   NOTE: If the material is too soft, it will tear or stretch; if it is too hard, it may be difficult to remove it from undercut areas.
8. Remove the provisional material from the template and allow it to reach its final set.
   NOTE: If acrylic materials are used, you must "pump" the provisional on and off the preparation when it reaches the doughy stage to avoid locking the material on the tooth or interproximal undercuts. Remove it from the mouth when it starts to get firm and warm.
   If bis-acrylic composite resin materials are used, you should allow the material to reach its final set outside the mouth.
9. Trim excess material with acrylic burs and disks.
   NOTE: If bis-acrylic composite material is used, you will first have to remove the greasy air-inhibited layer of unset resin with alcohol or it will tend to clog your disks and burs.
10. Reinsert the provisional and check margins, occlusions, and contacts, adjusting as needed.

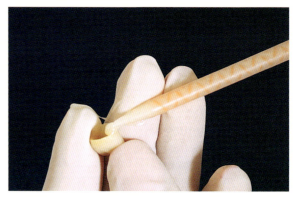

Fig. 15.40

NOTE: For acrylic: If slight air voids are present, they may be repaired with freshly mixed material (Figs. 15.39 and 15.40). For composite resin, fill voids or repair margins or contacts with flowable composite.

11. Finish polishing with flour of pumice or whiting polishing compound on a rag wheel.
12. Cement provisional with an appropriate luting agent and remove excess.
    NOTE: The custom provisional may be completely fabricated on a stone model and then tried into the mouth and adjusted as necessary (indirect technique).

Procedure 15.4 Intracoronal Provisional Cement Restoration

See Evolve site for Competency Sheet.

Consider the following with this procedure: safety glasses are recommended for the patient, PPE is required for the clinician, ensure appropriate safety protocols are followed, and check your local state guidelines before performing this procedure.

EQUIPMENT/SUPPLIES (FIG. 15.41)
- Mouth mirror and explorer
- Isolation materials
- Matrix band and wedges
- Matrix retainer
- Cotton pliers
- Burnisher
- Temporary cement (powder/liquid)
- Paper mixing pad
- Cement spatula
- Plastic instrument
- Condenser
- Occlusal carver
- Interproximal carver
- Articulating paper
- Dental floss

Continued

Procedure 15.4 Intracoronal Provisional Cement Restoration—cont'd

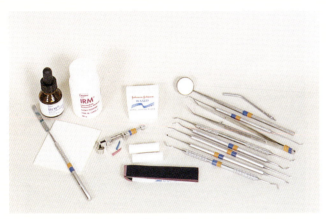

Fig. 15.41

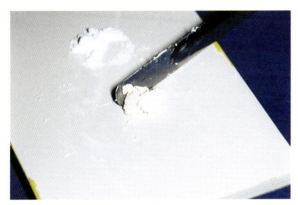

Fig. 15.42

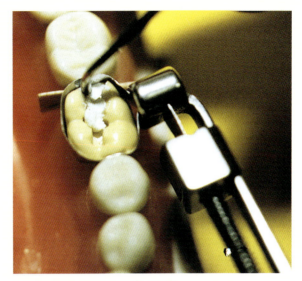

Fig. 15.43

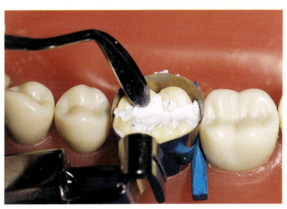

Fig. 15.44

PROCEDURE STEPS

1. Isolate the tooth, and note size and class of the cavity preparation.
   NOTE: This will determine the amount of cement necessary and the size of the matrix for placement.
2. Place the matrix and wedge.
   NOTE: Be sure to obtain contact with adjacent teeth; insert the wedges firmly to create some separation of the teeth and use a burnisher to press the band to the adjacent tooth at the contact area.
3. Prepare a mix of the temporary cement to a putty-like consistency.
   NOTE: The mix should be lightly coated in cement powder and should not stick to your gloved fingers (Fig. 15.42).
4. Roll the mix into a small ball and place a portion into a proximal area.
   NOTE: Begin by filling the proximal areas, and then across the pulpal floor (Fig. 15.43).
5. Use the condenser to condense into the preparation, while packing the cement firmly to avoid trapping of air.
   NOTE: Tap the end of the condenser into the remaining loose cement powder to prevent the instrument from sticking to the cement.
6. Place and pack cement into the rest of the cavity with the condenser.
7. Do not overfill; pack cement only slightly higher than the cavosurface margin of the preparation.
8. Using the blade of the plastic instrument, wipe material toward the margin to ensure a good seal.
   NOTE: Always wipe toward the margins; wiping away from the margins will pull material away from this important area (Fig. 15.44).
9. Remove excess material around the matrix in proximal areas and at occlusal margins.
   NOTE: Remove excess material carefully, as the material has not set. The material must be set enough so it is not pulled from the preparation margins.
10. Remove wedges, retainer, and matrix.
    NOTE: Be careful not to pull material away with the band.
11. Seal any open proximal margins by wiping still pliable cement toward them.
12. Remove proximal and gingival excess with an interproximal carver, and then from the marginal ridge.

Procedure 15.4　Intracoronal Provisional Cement Restoration—cont'd

NOTE: The marginal ridge should be at the same height as that of the adjacent tooth.

13. Create embrasure.
14. Remove excess from the occlusal surface and carve the anatomic form with an occlusal carver.

NOTE: The occlusal anatomy should approximate the original tooth form; it is not necessary to carve detailed anatomy as the restoration is temporary (Fig. 15.45).

15. Carve from tooth to filling material, keeping half the instrument on the tooth and half on the filling.

NOTE: This prevents breaking the material from the margins or ditching the margins of the material.

NOTE: If you wish to accelerate the set of the material, pat a cotton pellet saturated in hot water on the surface of the material.

16. Check the occlusion with articulating paper, and adjust as necessary.
17. Check contacts with dental floss.

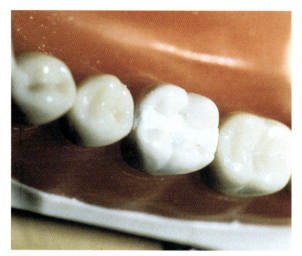

Fig. 15.45

Review And Discussion

Review Questions

Select the one correct response for each of the following multiple-choice questions.

1. Intracoronal provisional Class II restorations must:
   a. Contact adjacent teeth and be crimped with crimping pliers to fit snugly
   b. Contact adjacent teeth, be crimped with crimping pliers to fit snugly, and be sealed at the margins
   c. Contact adjacent teeth and be sealed at the margins
   d. Contact adjacent teeth, be crimped with crimping pliers to fit snugly, be sealed at the margins, and be made of metal for strength on posterior teeth
2. What are polycarbonate crowns primarily used for?
   a. Molars
   b. Anterior teeth and premolars
   c. For multiunit bridges
   d. For inlays
3. Which *one* of the following statements is most complete and correct? If the provisional restoration does not fit the tooth properly:
   a. Food impaction and periodontal irritation may occur
   b. Periodontal irritation and tooth migration may occur
   c. Food impaction, periodontal irritation, and hypersensitivity of the prepared tooth may occur
   d. Food impaction, periodontal irritation, hypersensitivity of the prepared tooth, and tooth migration may occur
4. Important physical properties of provisional materials used for posterior teeth include the following:
   a. Strength
   b. Tissue compatibility
   c. Ease of handling
   d. All of the above
5. Appropriate choices for extracoronal provisional restorations include:
   a. Stainless-steel crowns
   b. Acrylic and/or composite customized provisionals
   c. A and B
   d. None of the above
6. You will need to obtain a prepreparation template of the tooth before fabricating what type of provisional?
   a. Intracoronal provisional restorations
   b. Aluminum crown provisionals
   c. Polycarbonate crown provisionals
   d. Custom provisional restorations
7. What is the first step in fitting a stainless-steel crown?
   a. Determining occlusal/incisal-to-gingival dimensions
   b. Determining mesial/distal dimensions
   c. Determining the contour of the finish line
   d. Determining occlusal height
8. Which of the following materials is NOT used to customize the internal fit of a preformed crown?
   a. Self-cured composite resin provisional material
   b. Acrylic provisional material
   c. Dual-cured composite resin provisional material
   d. Zinc phosphate cement
9. Provisional *custom* crowns placed on prepared teeth may be constructed of:
   a. Celluloid
   b. Acrylic
   c. Stainless steel
   d. Polycarbonate
10. With intracoronal provisional restorations, place the cement and:
    a. Wipe the cement toward the margin
    b. Wipe the cement away from the margin
    c. Wipe the cement toward the matrix band
    d. Allow the cement to harden before sealing the margins
11. Criteria for an intracoronal cement provisional restoration include all of the following *except:*
    a. Marginal ridges at the same height as adjacent teeth
    b. Sufficient contact with adjacent teeth
    c. Detailed occlusal anatomy
    d. Reproduction of the gingival embrasure
12. Which *one* of the following statements regarding cementation of custom provisional crowns is true?
    a. The crown should be completely filled with cement to assure a good seal of the crown margins after seating it.
    b. After cementation, some excess cement can be left in the gingival sulcus to help with the retraction process for a separate impression appointment if bleeding has been a problem.
    c. Placing a thin coat of lubricant around the cervical portion of the crown will make cleaning up the provisional crown easier after cementation.
    d. A thick mix of the cement is preferred for luting for added strength.

For answers to Review Questions, see the Appendix.

Case-Based Discussion Topics

1. How would each of the following situations be best handled?
   a. *A patient has a badly fractured central incisor. The preparation is close to the pulp. Which provisional material and technique would be most appropriate?*
   b. *A custom composite provisional crown is deficient at the gingival margin of the facial surface. How would you correct this problem?*
   c. *Your patient is concerned about the color match and smoothness of provisional crowns. Which provisional material and technique would be most appropriate?*
   d. *A patient is scheduled for a three-unit posterior bridge preparation. The patient has a limited opening because of temporomandibular joint pain. Which provisional material and technique would be most appropriate?*

BIBLIOGRAPHY

3M ESPE: A comprehensive guide to achieving the best results with *Prefabricated crowns*. Available at https://multimedia.3m.com/mws/media/597973O/3m-espe-crowns-folder-ebu.pdf.

Bird DL, Robinson DS: *Modern dental assisting*, ed 13, St. Louis, 2021, Elsevier.

Brinker SP: A modern guide to temporization materials and techniques, *Inside Dental Assisting* 8(4), 2012. Available at https://www.aegisdentalnetwork.com/ida/2012/08/modern-guide-to-temporization-materials-and-techniques.

Comisi JC: Provisional materials: advances lead to extensive options for clinicians, *Compendium Dent Educ Dent* 36(1), 2015. Available at https://www.aegisdentalnetwork.com/cced/2015/01/provisional-materials-advances-lead-to-extensive-options-for-clinicians.

Gottlieb M: Using an old technique with modern materials to fabricate esthetic temporary restorations, *J Am Dent Assoc* 130:99–100, 1999.

Hester RE: Fabricating high-quality provisional restorations for indirect inlays, onlays or crown preparations, *J Am Dent Assoc* 130((7):1093–1094, 1999.

Kurtzman GM: Crown and bridge temporization part 1: provisional materials, *Inside Dent* 14((8), September 2008. Available at https://www.aegisdentalnetwork.com/id/2008/09/crown-and-bridge-temporization-part-1-provisional-materials

Kurtzman GM: Crown and bridge temporization part 2: provisional cements, *Inside Dent* 14((9), October 2008. Available at https://www.aegisdentalnetwork.com/id/2008/10/crown-and-bridge-temporization-part-2-provisional-cements.

Leggat PA, Kedjarune U: Toxicity of methyl methacrylate in dentistry, *Int Dent J* 53(3), 2003. 126–13

Schwedhelm ER: Direct technique for the fabrication of acrylic provisional restorations, *J Contempor Dent Pract* 7(1):157–173, 2006.

Strassler HE: In-office provisional restorative materials for fixed prosthodontics part 1: polymeric resin provisional materials, *Inside Dent* 5(4), 2009. Available at https://www.aegisdentalnetwork.com/id/2009/04/in-office-provisional-restorative-materials-for-fixed-prosthodontics

Strassler HE: In-office provisional restorative materials for fixed prosthodontics part 2: preformed crown forms, *Inside Dent* 5(8), 2009. Available at https://www.aegisdentalnetwork.com/id/2009/09/in-office-provisional-restorative-materials-for-fixed-prosthodontics-part-1-polymeric-resin-provisional-materials

Strassler HE, Lowe RA: Chairside resin-based provisional restorative materials for fixed prosthodontics, *Compendium Contin Educ Dent*, 2011. Available at https://cced.cdeworld.com/courses/4552-Chairside_Resin-Based_Provisional_Restorative_Materials_for_Fixed_Prosthodontics.

Strassler HE, Morgan RJ: Provisional–temporary cements, *Inside Dental Assist* 8(4), 2012. Available at https://www.aegisdentalnetwork.com/ida/2012/08/provisional-temporary-cements.

Dental Cement

16

http://evolve.elsevier.com/Eakle/materials/

Chapter Objectives

On completion of this chapter, the student should be able to:

1. Compare the various types of cements for:
   Pulpal protection
   Luting
   Restorations
   Surgical dressing
2. Describe the properties of cement and explain how these properties affect selection of cement for a dental procedure.
3. Identify the components of the various dental cements and how those components affect the properties of the cement.
4. Compare the advantages and disadvantages of each cement.
5. Describe the manipulation considerations for mixing cements.
6. Describe the procedure for filling a crown with luting cement and removing excess cement after cementation.
7. Apply the mixing technique for each type of cement.

KEY TERMS

Cavity Varnish a thin layer of resinous material placed on the floor and walls of the preparation to seal the tubules and minimize microleakage

Liner a thin layer of material placed to protect the pulp from the chemical components of dental materials, from oral fluids and microorganisms associated with microleakage, to stimulate reparative dentin, or to act as a pulp capping

Base a thick layer of cement used to protect the tooth from chemical and thermal irritation and to support restorations in deep cavity preparations

Secondary Consistency thick, putty-like, condensable physical state of a material that can be rolled into a ball or rope, suitable for use as a base

Buildup a thick layer of cement or restorative material used to replace missing tooth structure in a badly broken-down tooth and to act as support for a restoration such as a crown

Luting cementing two components together such as an indirect restoration cemented on or in a tooth, including inlays, crowns, bridges, veneers, orthodontic brackets and bands, and posts and pins

Permanent lasting indefinitely

Temporary/Provisional referring to materials expected to last from a few days to a few weeks

Intermediate referring to materials expected to last from a few weeks to a year

Sedative soothing; acting to relieve pain

Primary Consistency less viscous, easily flowing state of a material which can be drawn out to a 1-inch string with a spatula lifted from the center of the mass, suitable for luting

Adhesion the attractive forces of atoms or molecules that join two surfaces together

---

Few materials in dentistry are used as frequently or with as many applications as dental cements. There are numerous dental cements available, and each may have specific or multiple uses. No single cement is universally acceptable for all applications; rather, various cements are available whose properties and manipulation make them an appropriate choice for a given application. There are cements specifically targeted for use in orthodontics, endodontics, surgery, and implants. Many dental cements have inferior strength and high solubility when compared with other restorative materials and, with the exception of resin and glass ionomer cements, have little or no adhesive properties.

The clinical demands of different types of prosthetic restorations, ranging from gold crowns, porcelain-fused-to-metal crowns, all-ceramic crowns, and indirect composite resins have made the selection of cements more challenging. With the multitude of cements available, it is easy to become confused about which cement should be selected for a given situation. In most cases, the dentist will select the cement for a procedure on the basis of mechanical as well as biological factors. It becomes the dental auxiliary's responsibility to manipulate the cement to the proper consistency within the recommended mixing time. Many expanded function auxiliaries are also placing the cement, seating the crown, and removing the excess at the end of a procedure. The dental hygienist may be placing and removing cements and instrumenting against the cement surface during periodontal procedures. It is important that the oral health practitioner have a thorough understanding of cement uses, properties, limitations, and manipulation to effectively use and work around these materials.

DENTAL CEMENTS

Cement can be defined as a substance that binds two surfaces together rigidly. In dentistry, cement is a hard, brittle material when set with a wide range of applications such as:
- Lining a cavity preparation
- A temporary or permanent filling
- Securing a crown in place

Typically cement is formed by mixing two components together, often a powder and liquid or two pastes, that becomes a viscous liquid or mass that hardens. Luting agents are cements used as adhesives to secure indirect restorations to the tooth.

CLASSIFICATION

Dental cements have been classified by their uses and properties into three categories by the International Standards Organization and the American Dental Association.

Type I Cements. These cements are luting agents that glue crowns, bridges, onlays and inlays to the tooth or cement or bond orthodontic bands or brackets in place. These cements can be permanent (long term) or provisional (temporary).

Type II Cements. These cements are used for provisional or intermediate restorations or long term in the case of glass ionomer cements. Cements used as dental sealants are also in this group.

Type III Cements. These cements are used for bases or liners for cavity preparations.

USES OF DENTAL CEMENTS

Dental cements have a variety of uses (Table 16.1). These include:
- Pulpal protection and sedation
- Liners
- Bases
- Luting of indirect restorations
- Provisional restorations
- Intermediate intracoronal restorations
- Root canal sealers
- Surgical dressings

Pulpal Protection

The bacterial effects of caries, the biological response to chemicals contained in restorative materials, and even the cutting of tooth structure may cause pulpal irritation. Pulpal irritation can also occur as the result of thermal conductivity of metal restorations placed near the pulp, and when the dentin remaining over the pulp is too thin to withstand compressive, tensile, and shearing stresses. Many of the chemicals contained within the materials used to restore teeth have the potential to cause irritation. Older amalgam

Table 16.1 Uses of Dental Cements

USES OF CEMENTS	CEMENT
Cavity liner/pulpal cap	Calcium hydroxide
Pulpal medicament/low-strength base	Zinc oxide eugenol
High-strength bases	Reinforced zinc oxide eugenol, zinc phosphate, zinc polycarboxylate, GIC, RMGIC, resin-based cements
Crown buildups	RMGIC, composite resins
Permanent cementation	
Cast crowns, inlays/onlays, and bridges	Zinc phosphate, zinc polycarboxylate, GIC, RMGIC, resin-based
Porcelain, ceramic or composite veneers, inlays, onlays, and all-ceramic crowns High-strength ceramics	Resin cements, self-adhesive resin cements RMGIC, adhesive resin, self-adhesive resin
Endodontic posts	Zinc phosphate, GIC, RMGIC, adhesive resin, and self-adhesive resin
Orthodontic bands	Fluoride-added zinc phosphate, polycarboxylate, GIC, RMGIC
Orthodontic brackets	GIC, RMGIC, resin
Provisional cementation	Zinc oxide eugenol or noneugenol, zinc polycarboxylate, resin provisional cement
Provisional restorations	Reinforced zinc oxide eugenol, polycarboxylate, zinc phosphate, GIC, RMGIC
Surgical dressing	Zinc oxide noneugenol

GIC, Glass ionomer cement; *RMGIC*, resin-modified glass ionomer cement.

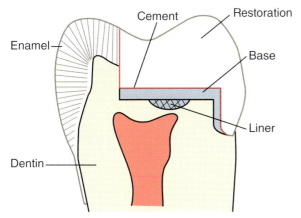

FIG. 16.1 Line drawing of layers of cement, base and liner, under a restoration.

formulations were prone to more corrosive products leaking into the tubules of the tooth structure resulting in discoloration. Cavity varnishes, liners, and bases act as protective layers between the dentin and the restorative material (Fig. 16.1). There has been a dramatic reduction in the use of pulpal protection materials as resin bonding technologies and high-copper amalgams have replaced these older types of restorations.

Cavity Varnish. Cavity varnish is not cement, but it acts as a protective barrier between the tooth preparation and restoration (see Chapter 11), varnish formulations are solutions of natural resins (copal) or synthetic resins dissolved in a solvent such as alcohol, ether, or chloroform.

Liners. A liner is a thin layer of protective material that is placed over the dentin to seal the tubules from chemical or bacterial irritants.

Calcium hydroxide is used as a liner in cavity preparations in which the remaining dentin over the pulp is minimal. When close to the pulp or very small exposures are suspected, this material is used as an indirect or direct pulp-capping agent or as a dressing after vital pulpotomy procedures on primary teeth. Components of a popular two-paste system include calcium hydroxide, zinc oxide, and glycol salicylate. A light-cured form of the paste-paste system is also available and, due to its resin content, it is a bit stronger than the other liners. With paste-paste systems, equal amounts of catalyst and base are mixed to a creamy consistency. Calcium hydroxide powder in an aqueous suspension is another form of the material used for pulp capping or vital pulpotomies.

Mixing Calcium Hydroxide (Dycal) for Cavity Liner

Mix: Equal lengths of base and catalyst pastes on paper pad for 10 seconds to a uniform color
Working time: 2 minutes 30 seconds
Setting time: 3 minutes 30 seconds

Calcium hydroxide has an alkaline pH about 11 and can neutralize some acids. The alkali stimulates secondary dentin when in direct contact with the pulp, providing a barrier between pulp and restoration. It has some antimicrobial activity, limited thermal insulating properties, and provides minimal strength to support the forces of condensation. Under amalgam restorations calcium hydroxide paste slowly leaches out over time, as it is water soluble.

Bases. A base is cement that is applied in a 1 to 2mm thick layer over the dentin to provide thermal and chemical insulation to the pulp and provide support to restorations in deep cavity preparations. Some bases may act as a pulpal medication as well. Bases may be classified as low strength or high strength.

Low-Strength Base. Zinc oxide eugenol (ZOE) is considered a low-strength base material. Unless it is reinforced with other materials such as PMMA fibers (acrylic) to make it stronger, it typically will not be used to support a restoration. The eugenol in ZOE does have some soothing effects on the pulp. An unreinforced ZOE base is often used more like a liner and is placed in a thin layer, which as a consequence will provide little thermal insulation. ZOE is supplied as:
- powder (zinc oxide) and liquid (eugenol)
- paste-paste formulation

Equal lengths of the two pastes are extruded from tubes, mixed to a uniform consistency, and applied in a thin layer over the desired area. ZOE will be discussed in detail later in the chapter.

High-Strength Base. High-strength bases have approximately four times the compressive strength of low-strength bases and liners. They have the strength needed to support restorations in deep preparations. Cements used as bases are mixed to secondary consistency—a thick putty-like consistency that is condensable and can be rolled into a ball or rope. Bases placed at a thickness of 0.75mm or greater provide protection from the thermal conduction of metallic restorations and galvanic shock. When the cavity preparation is so deep that there is 2mm or less of remaining dentin over the pulp, many clinicians will choose to provide mechanical support for the restoration by first placing a cement base. The restorative material is placed after the initial set of the base has occurred.

Packaging. Some high-strength bases are provided as hand-mixed powder and liquid or premeasured capsules of powder and liquid that are mixed by trituration. Others are provided as paste-paste systems in tubes with automixing tips.

Examples of cements used for high-strength bases include:
- reinforced ZOE
- zinc phosphate
- zinc polycarboxylate
- glass ionomer
- resin-modified glass ionomer
- resin

Zinc phosphate cement is acidic, so a liner or varnish may be needed under it to protect the pulp in deep preparations. Resin-modified glass ionomer cement is one of the most popular materials used as a base material because it is not irritating to the pulp, bonds to tooth structure, releases fluoride, and is strong. When placed in a thin layer, resin-modified glass ionomer cement can also be used as a liner.

 Do You Recall?

When would a cement be used for pulpal protection?

 Clinical Tip

Because of their fluoride release and low solubility, light-cured resin-modified glass ionomer cements are a popular choice as general cavity liners or bases. Some of the new bioactive formulations release calcium ions to promote hydroxyapatite and secondary dentin growth.

Mixing Reinforced ZOE (Intermediate Restorative Material) for a Base

Mix:
- Dispense a ratio of 1 level scoop to 1 drop of liquid on a paper pad or glass slab
- Use a stiff spatula to mix ½ the powder into the liquid, then add the remaining powder in one or two increments
- Spatulate thoroughly to produce a thick mix
- Wipe the mix with the spatula vigorously 5 to 10 seconds to produce a smooth, stiff mix
- Total mixing time is about 1 minute

Working time:
- Three and a half to 4 minutes

Setting time:
- Five minutes from the start of mix
- Setting time is accelerated by increased temperature, humidity, and powder/liquid ratio

Buildup

A **buildup**, much like a high-strength base, provides mechanical support for a restoration when an excessive amount of tooth structure is missing. The remaining tooth structure first needs to be rebuilt to better support the restoration material or to act as a foundation before crown preparation. With placement of a cement buildup, the compromised tooth is reinforced (Fig. 16.2).

Resin-modified glass ionomer and resin cements are the strongest of the cements. Typically, resin cement is not used in thick layers as a buildup, but composite resin restorative material serves this purpose well. Resin-modified glass ionomer cement is frequently used as a buildup material when only a portion of the coronal tooth structure is missing so that there is still remaining sound tooth structure to support the crown. Desirable features of resin-modified glass ionomer are:
- Its strength (compared to the conventional cements)
- Chemical bond to the mineral component of enamel and dentin

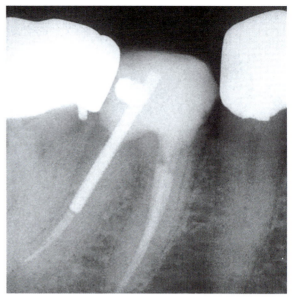

FIG. 16.2 Radiograph of a cement buildup over endodontically treated tooth 30 to reinforce the remains of the tooth in preparation for crown placement. (Courtesy Steve Eakle, University of California, San Francisco, San Francisco, California.)

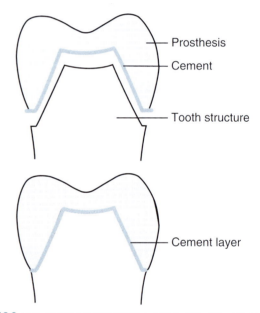

FIG. 16.3 Line drawing of cementing a crown. *Top:* crown lined with cement. *Bottom:* seated crown with cement filling the restoration/tooth interface.

- Good seal to the tooth
- Fluoride release

Luting of Indirect Restorations

A luting agent is a material with low viscosity that is placed between the prepared tooth and restoration, sets, and firmly attaches the restoration to the tooth (Fig. 16.3).

Orthodontic Bands and Brackets

Orthodontic bands and brackets are retained on teeth for several months or years. Brackets are usually

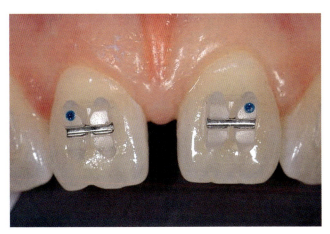

FIG. 16.4 Orthodontic brackets bonded directly to enamel with resin cement. (From Powers JM, Wataha JC. *Dental Materials: Properties and Manipulation*. 10th ed. Mosby, 2013:87.)

bonded directly to the enamel with resin cements (Fig. 16.4; Procedure 16.1), whereas bands are cemented without bonding.

The cement must adhere tenaciously to the enamel and the orthodontic band to provide leverage for tooth movement and when the band is removed have minimal effect on the tooth surface. Demineralization of the tooth surface due to solubility of cements and resultant leakage of bacteria between the bands and the tooth surface has often led to white spots on the enamel or early caries. This concern has been minimized to some extent with fluoride releasing, anticariogenic glass ionomer and resin-modified glass ionomer cements.

Metal, plastic, and ceramic brackets can be bonded to the enamel with resin cements. To ramic brackets can be bonded to the enamel with resin cements. To bond brackets the enamel is:
- Treated with phosphoric acid
- Rinsed
- Dried before application of the bonding agent
- Resin cement is applied to the bracket
- Then seated on the primed enamel

Self-etching primers could be used as well, but some of these do not etch the enamel as well as phosphoric acid. Self-, light- and dual-cured cements are available. It is possible to use light-cured cement under metal brackets by positioning the curing light at 45 degrees to the bracket from all angles on the facial, then curing with the high intensity light from the lingual as well.

Cements as Restorative Material

Permanent Restorations. Because of their lower strength and wear resistance and higher solubility, cements are not frequently chosen as **permanent** restorations. The exceptions are glass ionomer cement (GIC) and resin-modified glass ionomer cement (RMGIC). Due to their release of fluoride and chemical bond to tooth structure they are used for class V restorations of root caries in adults and restoration of primary teeth (see Chapter 9). The formulations of glass ionomer cement and resin-modified glass ionomer cement as restorative materials are different and much thicker than the luting cements. The luting cements must have a low film thickness to allow the restoration to seat fully.

Provisional and Intermediate Restorations. As **provisional (also called temporary)** and **intermediate** restorations, dental cements are mixed to secondary consistency (Procedure 16.2). The choice of cement for this type of restoration is largely based on the particular clinical situation. Provisional restorations are used for:
- Emergency situations
  - When appointment scheduling does not allow sufficient time to place a permanent restoration
- A tooth that is symptomatic or when deep caries removal is required
  - By placing a **sedative** provisional restoration, the dentist is able to evaluate the response of the pulp before reappointing for a permanent restoration
- Restoration of teeth awaiting treatment
  - Such as inlays, between endodontic appointments, or when extensive treatment plans require several weeks or months of coverage before treatment can be completed

See Chapter 15 for a discussion of provisional luting and intracoronal cement provisionals.

Root Canal Sealers

There are many types of cement that can be used along with gutta percha or without it to seal the canal space when doing root canal therapy. The sealers are available as two pastes that can be packaged in syringes or premeasured capsules or powder and liquid which are hand mixed on a pad or glass slab. The sealer materials may encompass a wide range of components such as:
- Calcium hydroxide
- Zinc oxide with eugenol or non-eugenol substitute
- Resins
- Glass ionomer
- Calcium silicate
- Mineral trioxide aggregate

Some of the materials are also used for vital pulpal therapy. They all have different properties, handling characteristics, working and setting times. Manufacturers' specifications must be followed carefully.

Surgical Dressings

As surgical dressings, cements are used to provide protection and support for the surgical site, to provide patient comfort, and to help control bleeding. Surgical dressing is a two-paste system—base and catalyst. The base contains zinc oxide as the main component with oils as plasticizers (make it flexible), gums to give it body for handling, and lorothidol as a fungicide. The catalyst paste contains coconut fatty acids that are thickened with rosin and chlorothymol as an antibacterial agent. It is available in regular and fast-set and hard-set formulations. It also comes as manual mix or automix delivery (Fig. 16.5). A non-eugenol version is also available.

CHAPTER 16 Dental Cement

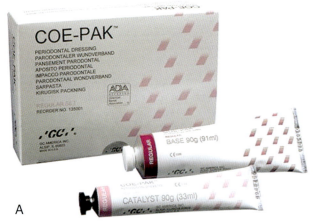

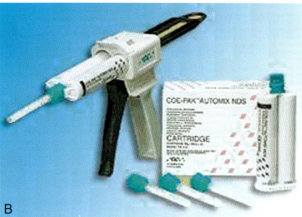

FIG. 16.5 Surgical dressing in two-paste systems. **(A)** Tubes of hand-mixed material. **(B)** Pastes in automix system. (Courtesy Coe Pak, GC America.)

Preparing the Surgical Dressing

For the hand-mixed dressing, equal lengths of base and catalyst pastes are dispensed onto a nonporous paper pad. They are mixed with a tongue depressor (disposable) or spatula to a soft putty-like consistency of uniform color. The setting time can be accelerated by immersing the mixed putty-like material in warm water. When the mix is no longer tacky, it can be shaped into two ropes about the width of a little finger. These materials tend to stick to gloves, so a lubricant such as K-Y Jelly, petroleum jelly, or water should be applied to the gloves before handling. Starting at the distal of the surgical site a rope is spread over the tissues on the facial and lingual and pressed into the interproximal areas with a plastic instrument or other suitable instrument. The dressing is mechanically retained by gently forcing the material into the embrasure spaces and under the contacts (Fig. 16.6 D). The material should not extend more than 2 mm beyond the surgical site. If needed, the patient (or the clinician if the patient is too numb) should move the cheeks, lips, and tongue in a range of motions to shape the edges of the dressing (a process called *muscle trimming* or *molding*). This process helps to prevent the hardened material from irritating tissues and dislodging the dressing after it has set. The occlusion should be checked to assure that the dressing is not interfering. Use a plastic instrument or other suitable instrument to keep the dressing from extending above the height of contour of the teeth. Some materials become hard and others remain somewhat flexible depending on their formulation.

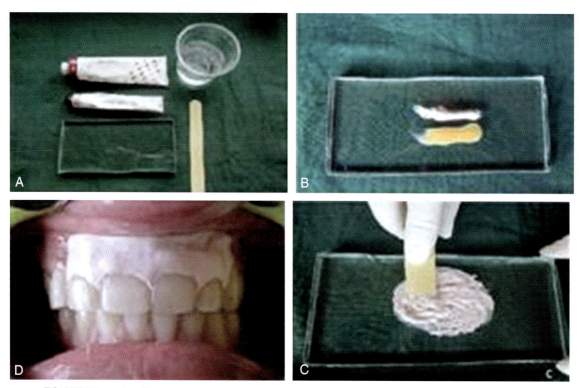

FIG. 16.6 Mix and application of surgical dressing (Coe Pak, GC America). Clockwise: **(A)** Tubes of material, mixing slab, and disposable spatula. **(B)** Base and catalyst pastes dispensed on a slab. **(C)** Mixed pastes. **(D)** Dressing applied to the surgical site. (From Kathariya R, Jain H, Jadhav T. To pack or not to pack: the current status of periodontal dressing. *J Appl Biomater Funct Mater*. 2015;13(2):e73–e860.)

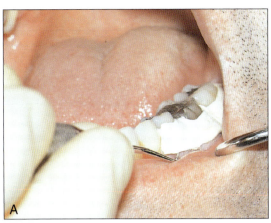 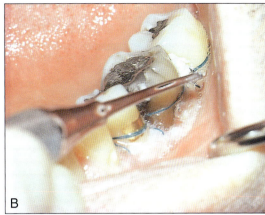

FIG. 16.7 Removal of surgical dressing. **(A)** Instrument under the edge of the dressing to loosen it. **(B)** Use an instrument to remove pieces of the dressing from the interproximal spaces. (From Robinson DS, Bird DL. *Essentials of Dental Assisting*. 6th ed. Elsevier; 2017.)

> **Clinical Tip**
>
> When mixing surgical dressing material use a wooden tongue depressor. It can be discarded when done. The material is sticky and can be difficult to remove from a spatula.

Removing the Dressing

After the tissues have healed, it is time to remove the dressing. A blunt instrument is used under the edge of the dressing with gentle lateral pressure to loosen the pack. The clinician must be aware of the location of sutures and avoid breaking the sutures away with the dressing. Large pieces of the dressing are lifted with cotton forceps and the surgical site is cleaned with a dilute solution of hydrogen peroxide or sterile water (Fig. 16.7). Occasionally, all or part of a dressing will come off prematurely and need to be reapplied.

Criteria for a Well-Placed Dressing

- Does not dislodge or disturb the placement of any surgical sutures
- Smooth, with as little bulk as possible
- Covers the surgical site with minimal overextension
- Interlocked interdentally to provide stability

> **Do You Recall?**
>
> What type of cements are considered the strongest cements and should be used for buildups?

TYPE I CEMENTS: LUTING AGENTS

Luting cements can be placed into two broad categories:
- Nonadhesive
- Adhesive cements

Nonadhesive cements: Retention of the restoration is enhanced by filling the interface between the restoration and the prepared tooth with a hard setting cement.

Adhesive cements: Stronger than nonadhesive cements, adhesive cements fill the interface and provide micromechanical and/or chemical retention between the tooth substrate and restorative materials.

PROPERTIES OF LUTING CEMENTS

Properties of luting cements differ from one type of cement to another. No cement is ideal for every clinical situation. Although one type of cement may be appropriate for a single crown, it may not be ideal for a multiple-unit bridge; some cements work well on metal surfaces, but others are more appropriate for ceramic or porcelain surfaces. Ideally, the cement should adhere to the tooth structure as well as the restoration. The clinician must consider both physical and biological properties when selecting cement for a specific dental procedure. The most important properties are as follows (Table 16.2):

- Strength
- Solubility
- Viscosity (affecting film thickness)
- Biocompatibility
- Anticariogenic properties
- Retention
- Esthetics
- Radiopacity
- Ease of manipulation

Ideal Properties of a Luting Agent

- Adhesion to tooth structure
- Adhesion to restorative material
- Adequate strength to resist functional forces
- Not soluble in oral fluids
- Ability to achieve low film thickness
- Biocompatibility with oral tissue
- Anticariogenic properties
- Radiopacity
- Ease of manipulation
- Esthetics and color stability

Table 16.2 Properties of Luting Cements

PROPERTY	GIC	RMGIC	RESIN	ZINC PHOSPHATE	ZINC POLYCARBOXYLATE	ZOE
Strength	Moderate	Moderate	High	Low	Low	Low
Solubility	Moderate	Low	Very low	High	High	High
Film thickness	Low	Low	Low	Low	Low, medium	Low, medium
Postoperative sensitivity	Moderate	Low	Low	Moderate	Low	Low
Fluoride release	High	High	None	None	None	None
Adhesion	Moderate	Moderate	High	None	Moderate	None
Esthetics	Good	Good	Good	None	None	None
Manipulation[a]	Moderately easy	Easy	Moderate	Difficult	Moderately easy	Easy

GIC, Glass ionomer cement; *RMGIC*, resin-modified glass ionomer cement; *ZOE*, zinc oxide eugenol cement.
[a]Encapsulated and automix forms are easy to manipulate.

Strength

Cement's resistance to deformation or fracture under an applied force is a measure of its mechanical properties. Cements must be strong enough to resist the forces of mastication and the dynamics of the patient's mouth and occlusion. Compressive, tensile, and flexural strengths are important considerations for differing cement applications. Bond strength is important in high-stress areas.

Caution

Cements are brittle materials with good compressive but more limited tensile and flexural strength.

The strongest cements are resin cements, and the weakest is zinc oxide eugenol. Cements used for permanent luting and high-strength bases need good compressive, tensile and flexural strength. As can be seen in Table 16.2, resin-based cement is high in mechanical strength and fracture toughness, and polycarboxylate cement is low in both. Many cements consist of a combination of powder and liquid; their ratio determines many of their properties. The strength of cement is controlled primarily by the amount of powder used in the prepared mix. In general, an increase in the powder-to-liquid ratio increases the strength of the cement. However, excessive powder or liquid can weaken the cement.

Solubility

One of the greatest challenges for dental cements is the tendency to dissolve in oral fluids, leading to marginal ditching, microleakage, recurrent caries, and failure of the restoration. Solubility is important whenever the cement is expected to remain exposed to mouth fluids for prolonged periods. Many cements will disintegrate in the oral environment over time. Increasing the amount of powder incorporated into the liquid can reduce the solubility of the cement. However, there are limits since it may increase the viscosity and film thickness. High resistance to oral solubility helps to maintain the marginal seal. Bonded, resin-containing cements are nearly insoluble.

Viscosity and Film Thickness

The consistency, or viscosity, of mixed cement refers to its thickness and ability to flow. Cements used for permanent or temporary luting of fixed prostheses, other indirect restorations, and endodontic posts must be able to flow to a thin film thickness to allow the restoration to seat properly and completely. On the inside of a crown a small space is created in the laboratory to allow room for the cement. Without this space the crown would not seat fully. Also, if the film thickness is too thick, the restoration will not seat fully, leaving cement exposed at the margins. This will result in the need for excessive occlusal adjustment and the increased likelihood of cement washing away at the margins leading to tooth sensitivity, recurrent decay, and staining.

For primary consistency, also known as *luting consistency*, cements should be able to be mixed thin—to about the consistency of honey with a film thickness of 25 μm or less (Procedure 16.3).

Clinical Tip

Low film thickness is critical to fully seating and retaining indirect restorations.

The cement must be able to flow easily and completely throughout the interface between the restoration and preparation. To be considered an effective luting cement, American Dental Association (ADA) specifications require the cement be able to flow to a film thickness of 25 μm or less. As a comparison, a human hair is about 20 to 50 μm. Resin-based cements and resin-modified glass ionomer cements are thixotropic, meaning they will flow under pressure. When cementing with any of these cements the patient should be instructed to bite down on a stick during initial set to force the material into all intracoronal areas.

Mixing cement to secondary consistency requires the addition of powder to increase strength and bring the cement to a thick, putty-like consistency (see Procedure 16.2). Cements mixed to secondary consistency are used as bases and restorations, provisional or permanent.

Several factors influence the consistency of mixed cement. Temperature has a great effect; a lower temperature will slow the setting reaction, giving the clinician more working time and allowing incorporation of more powder into the liquid.

Do You Recall?

Why are viscosity and film thickness important when cements are utilized as a luting agent?

Caution

Although the amount of powder incorporated into the mix has a direct relationship to strength and solubility, it may substantially increase the viscosity of the mixed cement, making it unsuitable for cementation of a restoration.

Biocompatibility and Anticariogenic Properties

Cements must be safe to use on patients. Where a specific type of cement may be appropriate in one circumstance, it may be inappropriate in another. Cement may be suitable for use in a conservative preparation, but then cause sensitivity and even pulpal necrosis in a deep preparation. Some cements are composed of a combination of zinc oxide powder or powdered glass mixed with an acid. The pH of the acid both at placement and after complete setting is a matter of concern due to postoperative pulpal sensitivity associated with the acid exposure. Other causes of pulpal sensitivity include:
- Unsealed dentinal tubules
- Trauma to the pulp during preparation
- Bacterial leakage under the provisional restoration

To minimize sensitivity from cements, careful attention should be taken with:
- powder-to-liquid ratios
- dispensing technique
- mixing recommendations

Cement with low risk for postoperative sensitivity should be selected when susceptibility to sensitivity is a concern. Eugenol, found in the liquid of zinc oxide eugenol cements, has an obtundent (i.e., soothing, sedative) effect on the pulp due to its good sealing ability, antibacterial properties, and neutral pH.

Clinical Tip

Many products include fluoride in their formulations; it is important to distinguish between fluoride release and fluoride-containing products. Fluoride released from powdered glass formulations found in glass ionomer cements has an anticariogenic property for reducing secondary caries. Products that do not release fluoride do not have an anticariogenic effect.

Retention and Adhesion

Good adhesion is a critical component of restorative dentistry, as good adhesion helps to increase retention of the restoration and minimize microleakage. **Adhesion** is the bonding of dissimilar materials by the attractive forces of atoms or molecules and includes two types of adhesion:
- *Mechanical adhesion*:
  - Mechanical adhesion is based on the interlocking of one material with another; an excellent example is Velcro.
- *Chemical adhesion*:
  - Chemical adhesion occurs at the molecular level, when atoms of the two materials swap electrons (ionic bonding) or share outer electrons (covalent bonding).

In many dental applications, chemical adhesion and mechanical adhesion occur together. The most recently developed dental cements, using resin adhesive technologies, strive to achieve a micromechanical and chemical bond between the tooth and the restoration.

Several things may weaken the adhesion between two materials, including:
- Differences in the coefficient of thermal expansion of the two materials
- Dimensional changes that occur during setting of the adhesive agent
- Contamination of the substrates by water and saliva and/or by residual enamel and dentin cutting debris from tooth preparation, known as the "smear layer"

Clinical Tip

Good adhesion will not occur unless there is a good fit between the restoration and the tooth preparation.

There are three possible reasons for failure of an adhesive:
- Structural
  - Structural failure occurs as a result of internal failure within the tooth structure; the tooth itself breaks away from the restoration, leaving the restoration intact.
- Adhesive
  - Adhesive failure is a failure of the bond, and it occurs when the adhesive cement separates from the tooth structure, causing the restoration to dislodge from the tooth.
- Cohesive failure
  - Cohesive failure is a measure of the strength of the bonding material itself, and it occurs when there is failure within the adhesive layer; this may also result in dislodging of the restoration with the cement layer still present in the restoration and on the tooth preparation (Fig. 16.8).

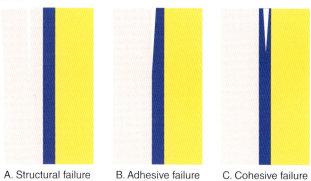

A. Structural failure   B. Adhesive failure   C. Cohesive failure

FIG. 16.8 Failure mechanisms of adhesive bonding. The blue line is the adhesive, to the left is tooth structure and to the right is the restoration. **(A)** Structural failure occurs within the tooth structure (or the restoration). **(B)** Adhesive failure occurs between the adhesive and the tooth structure (or the adhesive and the restoration). **(C)** Cohesive failure occurs within the adhesive itself.

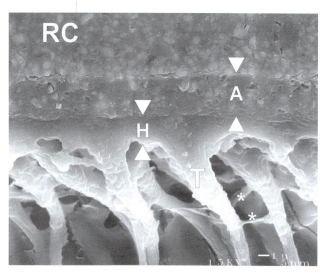

FIG. 16.9 Scanning electron micrograph of tooth-restoration interface bonded with dental adhesive. *A*, adhesive layer. *H*, hybrid layer with *T*, resin tags. *RC*, resin composite restoration. (From Frankenberger R, Perdigão J, Rosa BT, et al: "No-bottle" vs "multi-bottle" dentin adhesives—a microtensile bond strength and morphological study. *Dent Mater*, 17:373–380, 2001.)

Failure of the adhesive can result in failure of the restoration, leakage occurring between the tooth structure and restoration, and the formation of secondary caries.

The acid-etch bonding system is the basis of today's adhesive dentistry. In this process, the main mineral component of enamel and dentin, hydroxyapatite, is removed from the surface of the tooth structure with an acid etchant to create roughness and micropores. When resin bonding agents or self-adhesive cements are applied to the etched surfaces resin monomers of the bonding agent or cement fill the micropores and roughness to create resin tags that micromechanically lock the substrate to the restoration (Fig. 16.9).

 Caution

A bond will not occur if the surfaces being bonded are not completely clean and dry. Enamel should be dry and dentin free of excessive moisture or saliva. Over-drying of the dentin can cause sensitivity and a weaker bond in some techniques.

Esthetics

Cements are available in a variety of shades and opacities. Typically, resin cements are used for bonding porcelain veneers, ceramic or composite inlays and onlays, and ceramic full crowns.

Radiopacity

Radiopacity is an important property in the measure of the success of a cement. High radiopacity will allow the cement to show when examined with x-rays so that it will not be mistaken for caries or a void. Good radiopacity will also make excess cement easier to see. This is particularly important in the case of implants and in restorations with deep subgingival margins.

SELECTING A LUTING CEMENT

When choosing a luting cement, the clinician must consider which of the following indirect restorations are being used:
- Metal and metal-based restorations
  - Crowns, bridges, inlays, or onlays
- Glass-ceramic restorations
- High-strength ceramic restorations
- Indirect composite restorations

The restorative material itself may be the primary determinant for the cement selection. For example, some glass-ceramic restorations need to be bonded to the tooth to enhance their strength, but a high-strength ceramic such as zirconia can be cemented with non-adhesive cement. Other considerations include the amount of mechanical retention from the form of the preparation and whether the patient has parafunctional habits (i.e., bruxing). In order for the cement to be successful, the tooth preparation must have adequate retention and resistance form. While adhesive cements can enhance retention of the restoration, they cannot overcome the negative influence of an overtapered, nonretentive preparation and extreme bruxing forces.

CLASSIFICATION OF LUTING CEMENTS

Luting cements not only serve to retain a restoration to the tooth but also help to prevent microleakage by sealing the interface between the tooth and the restoration. Retention of the restoration to the tooth can be by:
- Mechanical means
- Chemical interaction with the tooth
- A combination of the two

Luting cements may be chosen as permanent cements or provisional (temporary) cements depending on the clinical need. Luting cements can be classified according to their composition. That is:
- Water-based
- Resin based
- Oil based

Functions of Luting Cements

The two main functions of luting cements are:
1. To seal the interface between the tooth preparation and the restoration
2. To increase the retention of the restoration

WATER-BASED LUTING CEMENTS

Water-based cements undergo an acid–base setting reaction. The cements are typically:
- A liquid
  - The acid
- A powder
  - The base

When the liquid and powder are mixed together, they undergo a chemical reaction that neutralizes the acid and base. The cation (H^+) of the acid and the anion (OH^-) of the base combine to form water and the remaining components form a salt. It may take several hours for the setting reaction to reach completion and the acidity to become neutral.

Zinc Phosphate Cement

Zinc phosphate, the oldest of the cements, has produced problems with postcementation hypersensitivity due to its acidic nature. These cements are also soluble and, among the cements in use today, are weaker cements. For these reasons, zinc phosphate cements are not widely used. If used, they are applied as permanent luting agents under metal-based indirect restorations and for cementation of orthodontic bands. The incorporation of additional powder into the mix makes them strong enough for high-strength bases, and they provide thermal insulation for the pulp.

Composition. Zinc phosphate cement is composed of:
- Powder
  - Zinc oxide (90%)
  - Magnesium oxide (10%)
  - Fluoride is added by some manufacturers to aid in the prevention of caries under orthodontically banded teeth
- Liquid
  - Phosphoric acid
  - Water

When the cement powder is incorporated into the liquid, an exothermic chemical reaction occurs (heat is produced). Attention to proper mixing technique is required to minimize this reaction. The setting and exothermic reactions of zinc phosphate cement are controlled by time and temperature. Incremental incorporation of the powder into the liquid allows for controlled dissipation of heat. Mixing over a large area of a cooled glass slab also dissipates the heat. The glass slab should be cooled to be effective in dissipating heat, but not to below the dew point (approximately 18°C [65°F]), at which water condensation would shorten the setting time. Use of a frozen slab can greatly increase the incorporation of powder and can increase the working time, which is helpful when several orthodontic bands are cemented.

Properties. Initially, the acidity (pH about 2.5) of zinc phosphate cement is low and becomes neutral within 24 to 48 hours. The initially low acidity may irritate the pulp in deep preparations (usually those with less than 1 mm of remaining dentin over the pulp) resulting in post-cementation hypersensitivity or, in rare occasions, even pulpal necrosis. Pulpal protection in deep cavity preparations is recommended with cavity varnish, liners, bases, or dentin bonding systems.

Strength, solubility, and film thickness are important properties. The internal surface of indirect restorations such as PFM or gold crowns, inlays, and onlays are sandblasted to enhance retention. The cement flows into irregularities in the roughened surface of the restoration and onto the prepared tooth surface, locking the two together. The low film thickness of properly mixed cements allows for the intimate contact necessary for good retention. Zinc phosphate cement has adequate strength and rigidity for cementation of single-unit and long-span bridges, but it is weaker than resin or hybrid ionomer cements. Ceramic restorations are not cemented with zinc phosphate cement, because it does not bond the ceramic to the tooth and thus puts the brittle ceramic restoration at risk of fracture. Zinc phosphate cement's solubility is clinically acceptable but greater than that of most other cements. This greater solubility has made it less favorable with clinicians for the cementation of orthodontic bands.

Zinc Phosphate

ADVANTAGES
- Low film thickness
- Inexpensive
- High rigidity

DISADVANTAGES
- Initial pulpal irritation and postoperative sensitivity
- Mechanical bond only
- Technique-sensitive proportioning and mixing
- Relatively high solubility
- Weaker than most other cements

Manipulation. Zinc phosphate cements are handled as follows:
- Packaged in a powder/liquid system
- Mix on a cooled glass slab with a metal cement spatula
- Shake powder before dispensing
- Separate powder into four to six portions on one end of the slab
- Dispense liquid in drops at the other end of the slab
- Add powder added slowly in small increments to the liquid
  - With smaller initial increments the acidity is reduced and the reaction is slowed
- Mix each increment for 10 to 15 seconds for a total of 60 to 90 seconds
- Mix cement in a figure-eight motion over a large area of the cooled slab to absorb the heat of the exothermic reaction, neutralize the acid, and allow more powder to be incorporated
- Achieve a proper luting consistency when the mixed cement strings 1 inch above the slab from the mixing spatula (see Procedure 16.3).

Excess cement should be removed from interproximal areas before the cement sets. A knotted strand of dental floss is a helpful tool when dragged back and forth across the restoration margins several times. The excess at accessible margins should be allowed to set before removing it. Ideally, varnish or another surface sealer should be applied to the margins after the excess cement is removed to allow maturation of the set and decrease solubility.

> **Clinical Tip**
> Zinc phosphate cements are difficult to remove from mixing surfaces; glass slabs and spatulas should be wiped clean before the cement sets. Set cement may be removed with the use of ultrasonic cleaners or a solution of baking soda and water.

Mixing Zinc Phosphate Cement for Luting

Mix: On a cool glass slab, mix four to six small increments of powder into liquid over a large area to dissipate heat for 10 to 15 seconds for each increment. Mix for a total of 60 to 90 seconds until smooth and creamy. It should string 1 inch from the spatula.
Working Time: 2 minutes
Setting Time: 5.5 minutes

Zinc Polycarboxylate Cement

Zinc polycarboxylate cement was the first cement developed with an adhesive bond to tooth structures. This cement has been used for final cementation of indirect restorations; today it is used primarily as a long-term temporary cement.

Composition. Zinc polycarboxylate cement is supplied as:
- Powder
  - Zinc oxide with magnesium oxide
  - Bismuth
  - Aluminum oxide
- Liquid
  - Aqueous solution of polyacrylic acid

Zinc polycarboxylate cement sets through an acid–base reaction. The polyacrylic acid produces minimal irritation to the pulp. Some manufacturers are supplying premeasured capsules for mixing the material in a triturator.

Properties. The viscosity of zinc polycarboxylate cement is higher than that of most other cements. However, with vibratory action on the restoration during seating the cement flows to an appropriate film thickness. The liquid of this cement should not be dispensed before mixing time, as the loss of water by evaporation can make the material more viscous.

These cements have lower compressive strength (55 MPa) and higher solubility when compared with glass ionomer and resin cements. Zinc polycarboxylate cement causes little irritation to the pulp, even when the remaining dentin layer is as thin as 0.2 mm. It is useful for cementing:
- Indirect restorations
- Bases
- Liners
- Temporary fillings

It is radiopaque, so excess interproximal cement can be seen on an x-ray.

Retention of polycarboxylate cements is both chemical and mechanical, making this cement useful for retention of indirect restorations. The chemical adhesion to the tooth is created by free carboxylic acid groups interacting (chelating) with calcium ions in the tooth structure. The bond is achieved only if the cement still exhibits a glossy appearance when the restoration is seated. The bond is not as strong as that obtained with resin cements combined with bonding agents. The working time can be extended with the use of a cooled glass slab.

Zinc Polycarboxylate

ADVANTAGES
- Adheres to tooth structures
- Nonirritating to the pulp
- Inexpensive

DISADVANTAGES
- Higher solubility
- Lower strength
- Shorter working time
- Early increase in film thickness can inhibit seating of the restoration

Manipulation. Polycarboxylate cements are handled as follows:
- Packaged in a powder/liquid system
- Mix on a glass slab or a nonabsorbent paper pad with a metal cement spatula
- Dispense powder with the manufacturer-supplied scoop
- Dispense the viscous liquid with a dropper or a unit-marked syringe
  - Never increase the amount of liquid, as this will dramatically reduce the strength of the cement.
- Add the powder to the liquid
- Mix for 30 seconds until the mix is creamy

The cement must be used immediately because of the short working time. The cement is no longer usable when it loses its gloss and becomes stringy (Procedure 16.4).

Do You Recall?

What cement is the most acidic but neutralizes in the first 24 to 48 hours?

Mixing Polycarboxylate Cement for Luting

Mixing: Mix all powder into liquid at once for 30 seconds until creamy
Working Time: 2.5 minutes. Do not use when it loses its gloss and becomes stringy
Setting Time: Regular set—10 minutes; Fast set—5 minutes

Clinical Tip

As with other cements, cleanup of mixing surfaces and spatula should be done while zinc polycarboxylate cement is still soft.

Glass Ionomer Cements

Glass ionomer cements were derived from silicate cements and polycarboxylate cements. Originally developed as an alternative to silicate cements for esthetic restoration of anterior teeth, glass ionomer cements have become one of the most versatile cements used today. Similar to the polycarboxylate cements, these cements chemically bond with tooth structures through chelation with calcium ions, although retention is primarily through micromechanical retention. Glass ionomer cements also contain aluminum fluorosilicate glass, giving them the ability to release and replenish fluoride. Glass ionomer cements are used as permanent luting agents for:
- Indirect restorations
- Luting of orthodontic bands
- Restorative materials (see Chapter 9)
- High-strength bases
- Core buildups

Although the cement is able to chemically bond to metals such as noble, non-noble, and stainless steel

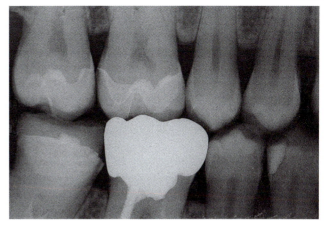

FIG. 16.10 Radiograph of the interface between restorations and teeth filled with radiopaque cement in upper-right molars.

and tooth substrate, it is not able to bond to glazed porcelain. In many instances, the same product can be mixed to different viscosities for different uses. This simplifies product selection and inventory control.

Traditional Glass Ionomer Cements

Composition. The cement is supplied as:
- Powder
  - Aluminum fluorosilicate glass
  - Barium glass
    - Added for radiopacity (Fig. 16.10)
- Liquid
  - Polyacrylic acid copolymer in water

When the powder and liquid are mixed, the polyacrylic acid attacks the glass to release fluoride ions. Fluoride improves the translucency of the otherwise opaque material and improves the material's strength.

Properties. Glass ionomer cements (GIC) are biologically compatible with the pulp when manipulated properly. Mild to severe postoperative sensitivity has been reported. Overdrying of the preparation, moisture contamination during the first 24 hours of setting, and hydrostatic pressure on fluid in the dentinal tubules when seating a crown have all been indicated as possible sources of this sensitivity. Fluoride release during the life of the cement is bacteriostatic, may have an anticariogenic effect, and may act to remineralize tooth structure attacked by bacterial acids. GIC acts as a fluoride reservoir. It can release fluoride but can also absorb fluoride from oral sources such as fluoride-containing toothpaste or mouthrinse and release it at another time. Strength, solubility, and film thickness are comparable with other permanent cements. Its compressive strength is over 100 MPa (14,503 pound/sq in.) but its brittle nature causes it to be weak in tension, about 6 MPa (870 psi).

An increase in solubility has been demonstrated with moisture contamination during the first 24 hours. Teeth restored with glass ionomer restorations, bases, and core buildups must be properly isolated for the 6- to 8-minute setting time. The margins of the cemented crown must be coated with the supplied coating agent or varnish until the initial set is achieved. Faster-setting materials are less sensitive to the solubility issue. The best bond to enamel and dentin can be achieved for GIC and RMGIC by first removing the smear layer created by cavity preparation debris. To remove the smear layer, mild acid such as 10% polyacrylic acid is applied to the preparation for 5 to 10 seconds and rinsed off. Leaving the acid on longer will begin to remove mineral from the tooth surface and weaken the bond since the glass ionomer cement bonds to mineral.

Traditional Glass Ionomer Cements

ADVANTAGES
- Chemical adhesion to tooth and metal
- Fluoride release
- Easy to mix
- Moderate strength

DISADVANTAGES
- History of postoperative sensitivity
- Sensitive to moisture or drying during setting
- Does not bond to glazed porcelain
- Marginal solubility

Manipulation. Glass ionomer cements are:
- Dispensed in a powder/liquid system or in premeasured capsules.
  - Premeasured capsules are very popular because of their ease of use and consistency of mix (Fig. 16.11)
  - When using the premeasured capsules, follow the manufacturer's directions on activating the capsule and mixing in the triturator
  - After mixing, the capsule is mounted in a gun-type applicator and has a delivery tip for dispensing of the mixed cement
    - The mix should be used right away and mixes that become thick or lose their glossy appearance should be discarded.

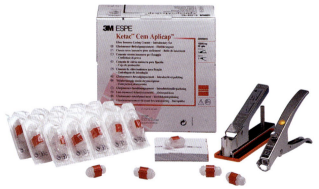

FIG. 16.11 Glass ionomer cement kit with premeasured capsules, activator, and delivery gun. (Ketac Cem Aplicaps, Courtesy 3 M ESPE.)

- The mixing time is typically around 20 seconds (depending on manufacturer) with a working time of 2.5 minutes and a setting time of 2 minutes and 50 seconds.

Glass ionomer luting cements are self-curing (Procedure 16.5).

Mixing Glass Ionomer Cement for Luting

Mix:
1. Premeasured capsules: mix in triturator according to manufacturer's instructions
2. Powder-liquid: mix level scoop to one or two drops (varies by manufacturer) incorporating all of the powder into the liquid until smooth mix is achieved.

Working Time: About 3 minutes depending on product
Setting Time: minutes, depending on product
Note: *If the mix loses its glossy appearance, do not use it.*

Resin-Modified Glass Ionomer Cements

Resin-modified glass ionomer cements (also called *hybrid glass ionomer cements*) are traditional glass ionomer cements with resin added to them to help improve their properties. For luting they can be used for:
- Metal-based restorations
- Endodontic metal posts
- Orthodontic bands and brackets
- Stronger ceramics
  - Such as zirconia or lithium disilicate

Composition. The composition of resin-modified glass ionomer cement (RMGIC) is similar to that of traditional glass ionomer cement, but it is modified by the addition of resin. The cement is supplied as a:
- Paste-paste formulation
- Powder and liquid
  - The powder is similar to traditional GIC but has chemicals added to catalyze the light-cure or chemical-cure reaction of the resin component.
  - The liquid contains water-soluble methacrylate monomers, tartaric acid, water, and 2-hydroxyethyl methacrylate (HEMA) as well as initiators for light curing.

The set of the material occurs by two mechanisms: an acid-base reaction and a resin polymerization reaction that can be light cured, chemical cured, or both (dual cured). The polymerization reaction occurs first and can be initiated by exposure to a curing light, or where light can't reach it, occurs by self-cure of the resin. The acid-base reaction is slower and continues for some hours after the material has hardened.

Properties. The addition of resin helps to improve the compressive and tensile strength and to decrease solubility. These cements do not have the susceptibility to early moisture contamination that traditional glass ionomers have because of the resin component. They have excellent film thickness. Fluoride release is the same as that of traditional glass ionomer cements. RMGIC expands as it absorbs moisture after setting. The expansion is greater in some RMGICs than others, and some non–high-strength all-ceramic restorations fractured after they were cemented with RMGIC because of excessive expansion.

Resin-Modified (Hybrid) Ionomer Cements

ADVANTAGES
- Good strength
- Fluoride release
- Insoluble
- Chemical adhesion to tooth
- Less postoperative sensitivity
- Excellent film thickness

DISADVANTAGES
- Recommended for luting only high-strength all-ceramic restorations or metal-based restorations

Manipulation. With the powder and liquid formulation, the material can be hand-mixed. The two-paste systems come in two varieties: One system has a cartridge that delivers each paste separately to be hand mixed and the other system has a cartridge with an automixing tip making mixing and dispensing easy and convenient. The most popular version comes in a premeasured capsule and is mixed as follows:
- The capsule is activated to allow powder and liquid to join
- Mixed in a triturator as specified by the manufacturer (see Procedure 16.5)
- The capsule has a dispensing tip
  - To allow for placement directly into a crown
  - To allow for placement directly into the preparation if being used as restorative material
  - When handling the glass ionomer cement a no-touch technique is mandatory since the liquid contains HEMA, a known contact allergen

The typical working time is 2 minutes 15 seconds and setting time in the mouth is 4 minutes 30 seconds.

Do You Recall?

What type of cement(s) can be used as a permanent restoration?

Clinical Tip

To avoid postoperative dentin hypersensitivity when using a RMGIC, it is important ***not*** to over-dry and desiccate the preparation before cementation.

RESIN-BASED LUTING CEMENTS

Resin cements are essentially composite resins modified to have lower viscosity. They are used for bonding of ceramic restorations, conventional crowns and bridges, and for direct or indirect bonding of orthodontic brackets. Low-strength ceramic restorations (especially porcelain-based materials) must be bonded to the tooth with resin cements to reduce their risk of fracturing under functional stresses. However, high-strength (zirconia and some lithium disilicate) crowns are very strong and can be cemented with RMGIC. Resin cements help increase retention of crowns placed onto clinically short teeth or teeth with less than ideal preparation taper.

Composition

Resin-based cements have several features:
- Similar in composition to composite restorative materials.
- Filler particle size is kept very small.
  - Similar to microfills, microhybrids, or nanohybrids (see Chapter 8)
- Initiators of polymerization are added to change the setting mechanism.
- Pigments are added to aid in tooth color matching.

Properties

Resin cements are virtually insoluble in the oral cavity. They have superior bond strength to enamel and dentin, wear resistance at exposed margins, and high compressive strength.

Methods of Cure

Polymerization (curing) of resin cements occurs by three possible mechanisms:
- Chemical cure (self-cure)
  - The set is initiated when the components are mixed together
  - Useful where light curing is not possible as with thick or opaque ceramic restorations, metal restorations, or endodontic posts
  - Limited number of shades and translucencies are available
  - They are more radiolucent than the other types of resin cements making it difficult to detect excess cement on radiographs
  - Careful removal of excess cement should be done before the cement reaches its final set
- Light cure
  - Require a light of a certain wavelength to activate photoinitiators that start the polymerization process
  - Allow the clinician to have extended working time and decide when to initiate curing
  - When removing excess cement some clinicians use a "wave" technique (also called *tack cure*) whereby they wave the curing light over the resin margins

for a few seconds to cause the resin to gel but not reach its final set
- This "tacks" the restoration in place and allows for easier cleanup of the excess cement
- Popular for thin porcelain veneers or in easily accessible parts of the mouth
- Does not work well when the restoration is too opaque or too thick to allow the light to transmit to all of the cement
- The most color stable compared to chemical- or dual-cured cements
- Dual cure
  - Use both light-curing and self-curing methods
  - The chemical curing is slow to allow for adequate working time and the light initiates the cure
  - In areas where the light cannot reach, the chemical curing will take the set to completion
  - Are very popular but have the drawback of potentially discoloring over time because of chemicals called aromatic amines that help in the setting process
  - The highest degree of polymerization occurs when light curing is used to initiate the setting process

Categories of Resin Cements

Resin cements can be categorized into four main groups:
- Esthetic resin cements
- Adhesive resin cements
- Self-adhesive resin cements
- Provisional resin cements

Esthetic Resin Cements. Esthetic resin cements are low-viscosity resins derived from composite resin. They are only lightly filled with very small particles and are mostly low-viscosity resin to maintain a low film thickness. They are strong, radiopaque, and have good bond strength to tooth and restoration when proper surface preparation is performed.

Some of these esthetic cements are manufactured as a single paste that is light cured. They are used extensively for cementation of porcelain veneers and for ceramic and indirect composite resin restorations that are somewhat translucent. Because of their translucency, the final color of the restoration can be impacted by the color of the underlying cement. These light-cured cements provide the clinician with almost unlimited working time to seat and position multiple veneers at one time. They are, however, rather light sensitive so the overhead operatory light or loupe head lamps should be positioned away from the mouth or turned off once the veneers have been seated. Esthetic resin cements can also be used for bonding of orthodontic brackets.

Other esthetic resin cements are manufactured as two-paste systems (base and catalyst) that come in dual-barrel syringes with automixing tips. These cements are dual cured and that assures a final cure in all aspects of the restoration, especially in those restorations with thicker or opaque parts that the curing light cannot penetrate.

Esthetic resins are not adhesive in nature. Hence, they require the use of enamel and dentin bonding agents on the tooth and silane coupling agents or special primers on the ceramic or composite restoration to bond the restoration to the tooth. The enamel and dentin is usually prepared by the etch-and-rinse technique before bonding agents are applied. Internal surfaces of ceramic restorations are etched with hydrofluoric acid or sandblasted before the application of silane or primers.

When esthetic cements are used to cement porcelain veneers, the surface to which they are being bonded is mostly enamel and the etch-and-rinse technique is preferred. Acidic (self-etching) primers are easier to use by eliminating etch and rinse steps, but they do not etch enamel as well as the etch-and-rinse technique (see Chapter 7).

Esthetic resins are made in a variety of tooth colors and translucencies to aid in achieving a desirable esthetic outcome. Usually, a shade is chosen to approximate the shade of the restoration, so that the appearance of the restoration is not altered by the underlying cement as light passes through the restoration and reflects off the cement. On occasion, it is necessary to mask the color of the dentin, especially if it is discolored. In this situation, an opaque cement of the appropriate shade is selected.

Many manufacturers provide try-in paste. This water-soluble, nonsetting paste is matched to the base shade of the cement and is used to temporarily hold the restoration in place while the clinician confirms the shade of the final product (Fig. 16.12).

Clinical Tip

Try-in paste is used to confirm the final shade of the restoration and to hold the restoration in place while the dentist and the patient inspect its form and esthetics.

Adhesive Resin Cements. Adhesive resin cements have wide applications for luting metal, ceramo-metal, and all-ceramic restorations but are not used for porcelain veneers. They are strong, radiopaque cements with low film thickness and strong bonds to properly prepared tooth and restoration surfaces. Adhesive resin cements when used with bonding agents have the capability of bonding to metal as well as ceramic restorations. Ceramic restorations are prepared for bonding by either sandblasting or etching with hydrofluoric acid, and then silane is applied. Internal surfaces of metal restorations are sandblasted. A special primer is used on the metal or ceramic. The adhesive cement is typically a dimethacrylate resin (with glass filler particles) which bonds to the primer. It is formulated in self-cure or dual-cure modes.

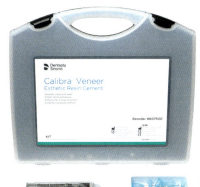

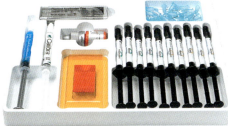

FIG. 16.12 Esthetic resin kit for luting ceramics such as porcelain veneers. Kit contains etchant, bonding agent, and several colors of try-in paste and resin cement. (Calibra Esthetic Resin Cement, Courtesy Dentsply Sirona.)

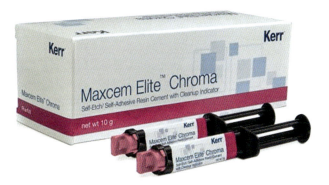

FIG. 16.13 Self-adhesive resin cement with a dual-barrel syringe to which an automixing tip can be attached. (MaxCem Elite Chroma, Courtesy Kerr Dental.)

Adhesive resin cements are available in:
- universal
- translucent
- opaque colors

Adhesive resin cements are formulated in paste-paste automix systems.

While the use of self-etching primers greatly simplify the bonding process by reducing the number of steps and potential clinician errors compared to the etch-and-rinse technique, it is still vitally important to carefully follow manufacturer's instructions. Do not mix and match primers and adhesive resins from different manufacturers, because there may be incompatibility that will weaken the bond or inhibit full setting.

> **! Caution**
> Carefully follow manufacturer instructions for use of resin cements and bonding agents. Do not use bonding agents from one manufacturer with resin cement from another manufacturer. There may be incompatibility of materials that prevent full setting of materials or weaken the bond.

Self-Adhesive Resin Cements. While adhesive resin cements require separate bonding agents to bonding to tooth or restoration surfaces, self-adhesive resin cements eliminate the need for separate etching and priming for bonding. This is achieved by combining acidic monomers with the adhesive diacrylate resin. The acidic monomers have a low pH and etch the tooth. The negatively charged acidic monomers form ionic bonds with positively charged calcium ions in the tooth. During setting of the self-adhesive resin the acidic monomers undergo a change in pH from very acidic (pH 2) to less acidic (pH 5 to 6) as glass filler particles react with the acidic monomer and fluoride is released. The smear layer is incorporated into the cement rather than being dissolved and rinsed away as with the etch-and-rinse technique. The cement must be completely cured, because uncured resin will be acidic and irritate the pulp. The advantage for the clinician is a reduction in the number of clinical steps required. There is no need for etching, rinsing, or drying the tooth structure. This also reduces the risk of over- or under-drying the dentin and reduces post-cementation sensitivity.

The disadvantage of self-adhesive resin cements is that they do not achieve bond strengths as great as esthetic or adhesive resin cements. The bond to dentin is of moderate strength, but the bond to enamel is not as good. Self-adhesive resin cements should not be used where a strong enamel bond is needed as with cementation of orthodontic brackets or porcelain veneers unless a separate selective acid etching of enamel is also used. With selective enamel etching, phosphoric acid is applied to enamel only for 10 to 20 seconds before the self-adhesive resin is applied. Phosphoric acid should be kept off the dentin because etching it lowers the bond strength of self-etching resins to dentin.

The application of the mixed cement is very simple. It takes only a single step, much like the application of zinc phosphate cement: mix and apply. These materials are supplied as dual-cured formulas. They are packaged in automix syringes with two pastes or capsules with dispensing tips (Fig. 16.13). A new self-adhesive resin cement has been introduced that is called a *universal cement*, because it has incorporated two monomer technologies that allow it to bond to glass-based ceramics without etching and applying silane and to nonglass ceramics without the need for a separate special primer.

Types of Restorations and Methods of Curing

LIGHT CURED
- Porcelain veneers less than 1.5 mm thick
- Orthodontic retainers not containing metal
- Periodontal splints not containing metal

DUAL CURED (LIGHT ACTIVATED AND CHEMICALLY ACTIVATED)
- Ceramic or indirect resin inlays, onlays, crowns, and bridges

CHEMICAL CURED (SELF-CURED)
- Metal-based inlays, onlays, crowns, and bridges
- Full metal crowns and bridges
- Endodontic posts
- Ceramic or indirect resin inlays, onlays, crowns, and bridges

 Caution

Light-cured and dual-cured resin cements should be protected from ambient light in the operatory as it may initiate the curing process.

Cementation of Ceramic Restorations with Resin Cement

Try-In of Ceramic Restoration. Before cementation the ceramic restoration is tried on the prepared tooth (crown/inlay/onlay) to confirm esthetics and adjust the fit as needed. The internal surface of the restoration will be contaminated after try-in and must be cleaned. Additionally, the surface of the ceramic must be prepared for bonding. Some clinicians use a solution of acid (typically hydrofluoric acid) for ceramics or sandblasting depending on which ceramic system is used. Some ceramics should not be acid treated but require special primers (see Chapter 10). If the laboratory has pre-etched the ceramic restoration, do not re-etch it after try-in. Use alcohol or a commercial ceramic cleaner.

Removal of Excess Resin Cement. Dental auxiliaries may be asked to remove excess cement from crown margins after seating. It is important to be familiar with the proper consistency recommended for each type of cement intended for removal. Check the manufacturer's recommendations.

When cementing permanent ceramic restorations, excess resin cement should be removed as soon as seating is completed and before the chemical set or light cure is complete (Procedure 16.6). Excess cement is removed by going from restoration to tooth or parallel to the margins. Avoid moving from tooth to restoration as cement may be pulled away from the margins, leaving an opening (Procedure 16.7).

Some clinicians prefer to "tack-cure" the resin cement to aid in removal. The tack-cure is best used for translucent restorations, because the light can penetrate the restoration and the gel set will be the same inside and outside the restoration. That way cement will not be pulled from under the margins when removing the excess. Once the excess cement has been removed, light curing is completed.

Self-cured resin cements are best used for metal or opaque ceramic restorations. Remove the excess cement when it just begins to stiffen. The resin under the margins will be partly set to the same degree as the excess outside the restoration. Removal of the excess at this stage will avoid pulling cement from under the margins.

The set of some resin cements is more strongly inhibited by oxygen, so the manufacturer recommends coating the margins with glycerin or another gel to exclude oxygen during the set. Knotted floss can be used interproximally to remove excess cement before it sets. It is possible that all excess cement will not be removed before it sets. Having a good knowledge of the tooth morphology is helpful in knowing where to look for residual cement, because concavities on the crown/root or root furcations can tend to retain excess cement. Explorers, scalers, and curettes are helpful in removing excess cement. A good, solid finger rest and short strokes are a must when using a sharp bladed instrument for cement removal to avoid slippage and soft tissue trauma. Residual excess cement will act as a plaque trap with risks of recurrent caries, gingival inflammation, or periodontal infection with bone loss. Some clinicians prefer to take a radiograph after cementation if excess cement is suspected. Many resin cements are radiopaque and can be seen on the radiograph. Cement on the proximal surfaces is easier to detect on the radiograph than buccal and lingual surfaces, because radiographs are two-dimensional images of a three-dimensional object where the bulk of the tooth structure can hide the cement from view.

 Clinical Tip

It is important to pay attention to the manufacturer's directions regarding bonding of the tooth surface and preparation of the restoration surface to achieve a strong bond and to eliminate postoperative sensitivity.

 Caution

Removal of excess resin cement is difficult if the material is allowed to set completely; follow the manufacturer's directions for removal. Excess cement is easy to remove after a few seconds of exposure to a curing light, but difficult to clean up if cured too long.

Provisional Resin Cements

Provisional resin cements are used to temporarily retain provisional crowns, bridges, or other indirect provisional restorations. They are formulated to have low compressive and tensile strengths, so the provisionals can readily be removed. Some provisional resin cements are formulated to have higher compressive strength for cases where longer-term provisionals are needed. They are not bonded so cleaning of the prepared tooth for cementation of the final restoration is simple. Because they shrink on setting, microleakage is slightly greater than with other provisional cements. They eliminate the problem associated with eugenol from ZOE provisional cements. Residual eugenol from provisional crowns cemented with zinc-oxide/eugenol can adversely affect the set of resin cements used for the final restoration.

Resin-Based Cements

ADVANTAGES
- High strength
- Insoluble
- Low wear
- Excellent adherence to tooth structure
- Can bond all-ceramic restorations
- Esthetic shades available
- Low chance of postoperative sensitivity

DISADVANTAGES
- The introduction of water or oral fluids at any point during the bonding procedure can lead to lowered bond strength
- Self-adhesive resin cements should not be applied on exposed pulp or dentin that is close to the pulp
- Requires additional steps in preparation of internal restoration surfaces
- Removal of excess cement may be difficult

Provisional resin cements are composed mostly of dimethacrylate resin with glass filler particles. They are compatible with other resin systems such as bonding agents, composites, and resin buildup materials. They are available in paste-paste systems in cartridges or syringes with automixing tips, so mixing and dispensing is easy (Fig. 16.14). They come with the following curing capabilities:
- Self
- Light
- Dual

Some of the self-cure cements are available in regular or fast-set modes.

Compomer Cements

Compomer cements are considered to be a subset of resin cements. Compomer cement are somewhere between resin cements and glass ionomer cements in their composition since they contain some of the components from each type. Compomer is a composite modified by polyacid, so that it releases fluoride like GIC (but to a lesser extent) and is strong and wear resistant like composite. It has both the slow acid-base reaction similar to GIC and the polymerization reaction of resin.

Compomer cements can be:
- Self-cured
  - Occurs in about 3 minutes in the mouth
- Light cured
- Dual cured

The luting compomer comes in a powder-liquid formulation or a two-paste system. Some versions are not adhesive to the tooth structure like glass ionomer. Compomer luting cements are not widely used.

OIL-BASED LUTING CEMENTS

Zinc Oxide Eugenol

Zinc oxide eugenol cements, commonly referred to as ZOE cements, have been widely used for many years. Generally, ZOE cements do not have the strength needed to serve as permanent cements or high-strength bases. So, they are mainly used for:
- Provisional cementation
- Provisional and intermediate restorations
- Low-strength bases
- Root canal sealers
- Periodontal dressings

Composition. Various ZOE cements are available in:
- Powder/liquid (Fig. 16.15)
  - The principal ingredient of the powder is zinc oxide
    - It can contain up to 8% other zinc salts which act as accelerators
  - The liquid, eugenol, has the distinct smell of cloves
    - Is a derivative of oil of cloves
    - It is a weak acid and up to 2% acetic acid may be added as an accelerator

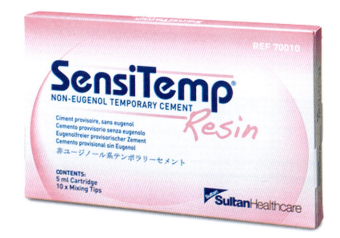

FIG. 16.14 Provisional resin cement kit containing cartridge of resins (base and catalyst), automixing tips, and mixing/dispensing gun. (SensiTemp Resin, Courtesy Sultan Healthcare.)

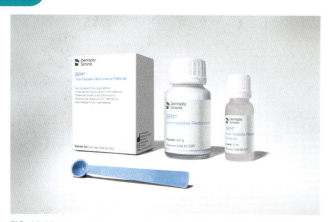

FIG. 16.15 Zinc oxide eugenol hand-mixed powder/liquid (*IRM, intermediate restorative material*). It has resin fibers added to increase strength and wear resistance and is used as an intermediate restoration. (Courtesy Dentsply Sirona.)

Because eugenol can interfere with the set of resins, ZOE should not be used as a base or provisional cement if composite resin or resin bonding agents will be used. However, if the surface of the enamel or dentin is cleaned thoroughly before bonding, the effect of the eugenol may be removed. After the provisional crown and excess cement is removed, cleaning the preparation with flour of pumice and a prophy cup or brush is an effective way of removing the small bits of residual ZOE cement.

Formulations are made without eugenol and are called *non-eugenol zinc oxide cements*. They are used as provisional cements for provisional crowns when resin cement is planned for the permanent restoration.

Properties. Eugenol has long been known for its sedative effect on the pulp, largely caused by its antibacterial effects and its good marginal seal. It can be irritating when in direct contact with oral mucosa or pulp. The mixed ZOE has a neutral pH of 7, which makes it very biocompatible with tooth structure.

ZOE cements are not as strong as other permanent luting agents and are rarely used for this purpose. Thus they are ideally suited for provisional cementation. Their weaker tensile strength allows them to be easily removed at a second appointment, when a permanent restoration is to be placed. ZOE cement has a compressive strength of 26 MPa which falls below the ISO 3107 standard of 35 MPa for permanent luting cements. When EBA (2-ethoxybenzoic acid) is added to the eugenol in a 2:1 ratio and 30% alumina is added to the powder to reinforce it, much more powder can be incorporated into the liquid and the resultant mix is much stronger (72 MPa compressive strength). Resin fibers (20% polymethyl methacrylate [PMMA]) are also added to increase strength and wear resistance making them suitable for intermediate restorations and high-strength bases.

The film thickness of ZOE cements is between 16 and 28 μm and when alumina is present it approaches 57 μm (25 μm and below are more ideal for luting). ZOE cements are susceptible to hydrolysis and a significant amount of its volume can be lost in a 6-month period. This factor does not allow them to serve well for long-term provisional restorations. Glass ionomer and resin-modified glass ionomer cements perform much better as long-term provisional restorations.

 Caution

Cements that contain eugenol should not be used under composites or as provisional cements before final cementation with resin-modified glass ionomer or resin cements, because eugenol may inhibit the set of the resin. Non-eugenol zinc oxide cements are preferred in these clinical situations.

Powder/liquid and paste/paste systems are easily manipulated. The set, strength, and viscosity are controlled by the incorporation of powder into the liquid or, in the paste/paste system, by a change in the ratio of base to catalyst.

Zinc Oxide Eugenol

ADVANTAGES
- A wide variety of uses
- Sedative to the pulp
- Easily manipulated
- Low cost

DISADVANTAGES
- Low strength
- High solubility
- Unable to be used under composite restorations and indirect restorations cemented with resin or RMGICs

Manipulation. Paste-paste system:
- Equal lengths of accelerator and base pastes are placed on a paper mixing pad or glass slab.
- Materials are mixed until a uniform color is achieved.

Powder-liquid system:
- The powder bottle is shaken.
- The powder is measured with the manufacturer-supplied scoop.
- The liquid is dispensed in the corresponding number of drops.
- The powder is incorporated into the liquid until the desired consistency is achieved.
- Heavy spatulation with a metal spatula allows for the incorporation of more powder; this additional powder will greatly enhance the strength of the cement (see Procedure 16.2).

Clinical Tip

ZOE cements are difficult to remove from mixing surfaces; glass slabs and spatulas should be wiped clean before the cement sets. Set cement may be removed with alcohol or orange solvent.

BIOACTIVE CEMENTS

Bioactive cements are a relatively new category of cements. They are called bioactive because they stimulate living tissues. In dentistry the test for bioactivity is for them to form an apatite-like substance on their surface when left in a simulated body fluid for a specified length of time. The bioactive cements used in dentistry can stimulate the pulp to produce a reparative dentin bridge or they can stimulate the process of remineralization of demineralized dentin. The bioactive materials can be divided into two groups:
- Calcium silicates
- Calcium aluminates

They both have acid–base setting reactions and produce an alkaline by-product that raises the pH significantly.

Calcium silicates have been useful in pulp capping and vital pulpotomies. The first of these materials to be widely used in endodontics is mineral trioxide aggregate (MTA). It has a number of properties that contribute to wound healing:
1. It is alkaline in nature because it forms calcium hydroxide as it sets creating an antibacterial environment
2. It releases calcium ions that help repair dentin
3. It bonds and seals the area
4. It stimulates formation of secondary dentin and hydroxyapatite

The shortcomings of MTA are that it is difficult to handle, has a very long setting time, and a low compressive strength (about 50 MPa). Newer improved materials have emerged with new applications as liners and bases under direct restorations to stimulate dentin repair.

Calcium aluminate cements are usually hybrid materials containing calcium aluminate and glass ionomer. The calcium aluminate portion is responsible for the development of:
- A high pH during setting
- Strength
- Reduced microleakage
- Stability

The glass ionomer portion is responsible for its:
- Viscosity
- Early setting time
- Early strength

Due to their strength (compressive and shear bond), retention, low solubility, and low film thickness (about 15 μm), they make excellent permanent luting agents for all metal, ceramo-metal, or high-strength ceramic crowns and bridges. They do not require surface treatment of the tooth such as etching, priming, or conditioning. They are available in premeasured capsules with delivery tips.

Do You Recall?

What type of cements stimulate living tissues?

HANDLING OF CEMENTS

STORAGE

Cements should not be stored in warm or humid areas of the dental office. If you are refrigerating your cement, it should be taken out of the refrigerator at least 1 hour prior to use to allow it to reach room temperature.

PRE-CEMENTATION CHECK

Prior to mixing the cement the crown or other indirect restoration should be tried in/on the prepared tooth. In many states the dental auxiliary licensed or certified in expanded functions can prepare the restoration for cementation by performing many of the following procedures:
1. If the crown is not immediately seating all the way, the first thing to check and adjust is the proximal contacts.
2. If it is still not seating completely, the inside of the crown should be checked (using a variety of materials and techniques for marking spots that bind on the preparation) and adjusted.
3. Next, the margins should be checked with a fine-tipped explorer to see that they are flush with the prepared margins of the tooth. If they are not flush, then recheck the contacts and interior of the crown. If no problems are found with the fit, the discrepancies may be caused by a poor impression or a lab error (which would necessitate starting with a new impression).
4. Then, check and adjust the occlusion.
5. Confirm that the patient is happy with the appearance of the crown and the bite feels comfortable.
6. Repolish as needed and clean the interior of the crown in preparation for cementation.

MIXING

It is important that cements be mixed to their appropriate consistency in accordance with manufacturers' recommendations, with meticulous attention to detail. Cements that are mishandled may lead to difficulties in:
- Seating
- Retaining the restoration
- Pulpal sensitivity

Cements may be hand-mixed or may come in premeasured capsules mixed in a triturator or mixed as material is extruded through automixing tips attached to dual-barrel syringes.

Even skilled hand-mixing may incorporate air that is thought to lead to the reduction of bond strength between the restoration and the tooth substrate. Also, inaccurate ratios of powder and liquid can be dispensed from scoops and liquid droppers. If hand-mixing is chosen, the amount of time taken to mix the cement must be carefully monitored as too much mixing time may make the cement too viscous while too little time may cause the cement not to be mixed thoroughly. Cements mixed in capsules or via automix systems provide the following advantages:

- Consistent mix
- Reduced cleanup
- Reduced cross contamination
- Avoids incorporating air in the mix

Advantages and disadvantages of each delivery system are listed in Table 16.3.

Clinical Tip
There are many types of cement available and each one has multiple uses and differences in mixing techniques so that it is very important to **ALWAYS** follow the manufacturer's instructions for storage, mixing, and handling.

Caution
Light-cured cements may not be appropriate for deep preparations: the ultraviolet (UV) light may fail to activate some of the material, leaving part of the cement unset. Dual-cured products help to eliminate this problem.

WORKING AND SETTING TIMES

Working time and setting time are considerations in the choice of cement and mixing mechanism. A longer working time is needed for cementation of longer span bridges versus single crowns and a shorter setting time is desirable for difficult-to-isolate areas. Patient considerations and the dental team's mixing and delivery skills play a part in the selection of appropriate cement. The dental auxiliary is responsible for delivering the cement at the proper consistency within very definite time frames. A skilled auxiliary must be able to routinely mix a variety of cements rapidly to their proper consistency.

Cement Manipulation Considerations for Cements in Powder and Liquid Form

1. Keep powder and liquid separated when dispensing
2. Fluff powder before dispensing by gently rolling the container in your hand to aerate
3. Use scoop provided by the manufacturer and ensure scoop of powder is level, not heaping
4. Section the powder into increments according to the manufacturer's directions; when increment size varies, the smallest increments are mixed first
5. Dispense the liquid by holding the dispenser vertically before squeezing to obtain uniform drops
6. Close caps of powder and liquid containers immediately after dispensing to avoid evaporation or contamination
7. Incorporate powder and liquid thoroughly when mixing. If incremental mixing is used, each increment must be completely incorporated before the next is added
8. Use moderate pressure on the spatula when mixing
9. Use both sides of the spatula blade
10. Mix cement in a "stropping" motion
11. Gather all the material together to test the viscosity

Caution
Light-cured cements should not be used if there is a potential for incomplete set of the cement under a dental prosthesis because the curing light cannot reach the cement to activate curing.

Table 16.3 Advantages and Disadvantages of Delivery Systems

HAND-MIXING	AUTOMIXING	PREDOSED CAPSULES
Advantages		
Vary viscosity	Consistent mix	Consistent mix
Vary volume of material mixed	Vary volume of material used	Convenience
No extra equipment	Convenience	Disposable, less asepsis
Less expensive		Less cleanup required
Can mix shades if needed	No air voids incorporated in the mix	No air voids incorporated in the mix
Disadvantages		
Inconsistent mix	Unable to vary viscosity	Unable to vary viscosity
Air voids incorporated in the mix		
Less convenient	Additional equipment needed	Volume of capsule is fixed
More cleanup required	Cannot blend shades, more expensive	Cannot blend shades, requires extra equipment, more expensive

LOADING THE RESTORATION

The dental auxiliary may be responsible for filling the crown with a luting cement before transferring it to the dentist. The techniques described in the accompanying box ("Loading a Custom-Made Crown for Cementation") will ensure that the cement is evenly loaded in the crown, and that the margins are coated internally.

Loading a Custom-Made Crown for Cementation

1. Gather cement from the mixing surface with the blade of the spatula or a plastic instrument.
2. Wipe the blade against the margin of the crown (Fig. 16.16).
3. Cover all the interior walls of the crown with a thin, even coating of cement, making sure it is free of air bubbles (Fig. 16.17).
4. Do not fill the prosthesis to more than one-quarter the inner volume; overfilling the prosthesis may prevent complete seating.
5. Transfer the crown cement-side down on the palm of the hand for the dentist to pick up and seat.

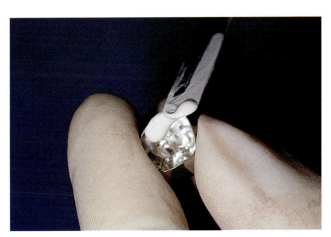

FIG. 16.16 Loading a crown—wipe the blade of the spatula against the margin of the crown.

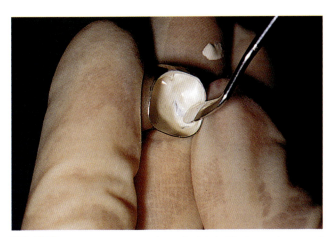

FIG. 16.17 Loading a crown—using a flat-bladed instrument, cover all the walls with a thin, even coating of the cement.

Reasons Cement May Keep a Crown from Seating Fully

1. The crown is overfilled with cement and hydraulic pressure does not allow excess cement to flow out.
2. The cement mix is too thick (viscous) and the cement does not flow readily.
3. The cement is starting to set and will not flow.
4. Cement was selected with a film thickness that is too great for luting.

Caution

Crowns that have long walls and a narrow diameter, such as crowns for lower incisors or for premolars, should not be filled with too much cement. Only a thin layer of cement should be applied to the walls of the restoration's interior (intaglio) to allow cement to flow out when the crowns are seated. With too much cement, hydraulic pressure may prevent the cement from flowing out and the crown from seating completely.

REMOVAL OF EXCESS CEMENT

Some cements should not be removed until completely set, such as zinc phosphate cement; others may be best removed when the cement reaches a rubbery or gel consistency, such as resin-modified glass ionomer cement; and others when the cement is tack cured, that is, light-cured resin cement. (Removal of excess resin cement was previously discussed.) Follow the manufacturer's directions for appropriate consistency of cement at removal. Cement consistencies vary from rock hard to rubbery.

Remove cement in bulk, when possible, utilizing the following steps:

1. Use a piece of knotted floss to remove cement from interproximal areas before it sets. Draw the floss out under the contacts rather than coming back up through the contact, which might dislodge the crown.
2. Use a scaler or curette followed by an explorer to remove excess cement from subgingival surfaces, taking care to not scratch the surface of the restoration or gouge the margins where the tooth and restoration meet.

Timing of Excess Cement Removal after Luting a Crown

(Follow the manufacturer's directions for appropriate consistency at removal). Remove interproximal cement before set.

In general:
- Zinc phosphate
  - Let cement set completely
- Zinc polycarboxylate
  - Let cement set completely. Do not try to remove when rubbery

Continued

- Zinc oxide eugenol
  - Let cement set completely
- Glass ionomer cement
  - Some versions can be removed at the gel stage
- Resin-modified glass ionomer cement
  - Expose excess to curing light for 1 second, then remove at gel stage or let it self-cure and remove at gel stage
- Resin cements
  - Remove excess *before* they set completely, often after 1 second tack cure

 Clinical Tip

When removing excess cement before it is fully set, be sure to secure the crown against the tooth so your manipulation does not lift the crown.

CEMENT-ASSOCIATED PERI-IMPLANT DISEASE

Excess cement remaining after placement of an implant is positively associated with peri-implant disease. Biofilm-related infections can result in the removal of the implant in severe cases. There are several factors associated with these infections, including cement residue. Radiographs do not always reveal this residual cement, especially on buccal/lingual surfaces. Margins that are subgingival exhibit a greater amount of undetected cement. Cement-related bone loss may occur quickly or be delayed for several years (Fig. 16.18).

At the time of the cementation of the implant restoration, a titanium scaler or curette should be used for removal of excess cement. Titanium instruments are strong enough to remove the set cement but are soft enough to avoid scratching the implant surface. Plastic or graphite are not recommended as the instruments may leave tiny bits of their material embedded in rough surfaces of the implant that may themselves contribute to peri-implantitis. The dental hygienist should evaluate each implant carefully to monitor probe depths, clinical and radiographic signs of inflammation, and/or the presence of cement residue.

 Caution

Complete removal of excess cement is essential to maintain gingival health.

CLEANUP, DISINFECTION, AND STERILIZATION

The removal of cement before it is set provides for easier cleanup of mixing slabs, spatulas, and delivery instruments. Instruments and equipment that come in contact with cement should be cleaned as soon as is reasonably possible using alcohol-saturated gauze squares or orange solvent when warranted. If immediate cleanup is not possible, use an ultrasonic cleaner with cement removal solution. If barriers have not been used, equipment such as triturators, cement activators, the outside of cement bottles, and dispensing scoops and syringes must be properly disinfected. Sterilization of mixing and delivery instruments is necessary. Glass and plastic mixing slabs are recommended because they can be sterilized in heat sterilizers. Paper pads, although convenient, are a source of contamination. There is no reliable way to combat this other than using only one sheet at a time, which can be very difficult to mix on. Porous paper pads absorb some of the cement liquid and alter the powder to liquid ratio.

CARE AROUND MARGINS

Proper instrumentation during prophylactic procedures and appropriate delivery of some therapeutic agents such as fluoride are important considerations for the continuing care of the fine line of cement at margins of indirect restorations. Care must be taken to avoid gouging or ditching the cement during hand instrumentation. Although the cement margin may be very small (25 μm), even minute breaks are a place for biofilm to form and initiate microleakage and secondary caries. Ultrasonic and sonic scalers should be avoided on margins of cemented restorations whenever possible because they may cause fracturing of the cement. Air polishers may abrade cement at restoration margins. Fluoride application on glass ionomer and resin-based cement margins should be limited to neutral sodium fluoride, because acidulated fluoride products may degrade the cement.

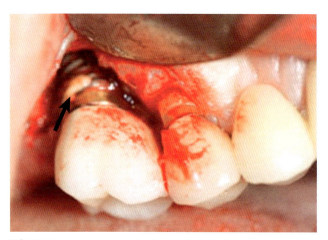

FIG. 16.18 Excess cement remaining subgingivally has become a chronic bacterial plaque trap causing bone loss around the dental implant. See cement on the distal surface wrapping around to the facial surface. (Courtesy Drs. Nick Shumaker and Leslie Paris; Slim L: Cement-associated peri-implantitis. *RDH Mag.* 2013;33(12).)

> **KEY POINTS**
>
> Cement Classification and Uses
> 1. Used frequently and for a variety of purposes
> 2. Classified by use and properties
>   - Type I – luting agents
>   - Type II – provisional and intermediate restorations
>   - Type III – bases and liners
> 3. Used for various applications
>   - Pulp protection
>   - Cavity varnish
>   - Liners
>   - Bases
>   - Buildups
>   - Luting restorations
>   - Bonding brackets
>   - Permanent restorations
>   - Glass ionomer or RMGI
>   - Temporary restorations
>   - Root canal sealers
>   - Surgical dressings

SUMMARY

A restoration may be esthetically pleasing and functional at the time of cementation, but if problems occur with retention, postoperative sensitivity, and recurrent caries, patients will most likely ask questions as to why the treatment failed and how good the dentist's skills are. No single cement satisfies all dental purposes. Cements are chosen to match the physical properties of the restorative material being used, and the requirements of each clinical situation. The dental auxiliary is responsible for handling, mixing, and delivering the cement to the dentist. Proper cement manipulation is important in determining the quality of a cement's physical properties. In addition, the use of instruments on a cement margin can directly affect a restoration's longevity. Procedures for placement of provisional restorations are important to the success of future permanent restorations. It is essential the auxiliary is knowledgeable in the uses, properties, handling characteristics, and precautions for all cements used in the dentist's office.

INSTRUCTIONAL VIDEOS

See the Evolve Resources site for a variety of educational videos that reinforce the material covered in this chapter.

Procedure 16.1   Bonding Orthodontic Brackets

See Evolve site for Competency Sheet.

Consider the following with this procedure: *safety glasses are recommended for the patient, personal protective equipment (PPE) is required for the clinician, ensure appropriate safety protocols are followed, and check local state guidelines before performing this procedure.*

EQUIPMENT/SUPPLIES (FIG. 16.19)

- Basic setup
- Low-speed handpiece, prophy angle, rubber cup, and slurry of pumice
- Etchant (37% phosphoric acid), light-cured bonding resin
- Curing light, lip retractors
- High-volume evacuator tip, cotton rolls
- Orthodontic brackets, bracket placement pliers, scaler

PROCEDURE STEPS

1. Inform the patient of the procedures to be done. Clean the facial surfaces of the teeth to be bonded with pumice slurry in a rubber cup.
   NOTE: Pumice removes adherent plaque and organic pellicle that might interfere with proper etching and bonding.
2. Place lip retractors or cotton rolls to isolate the anterior teeth for bracket placement.

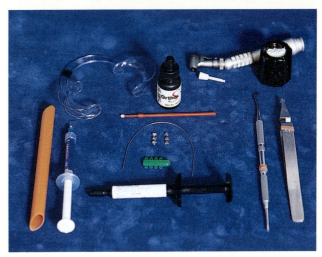

FIG. 16.19

NOTE: Moisture from the lip mucosa will interfere with bonding.

3. Apply etching solution or gel for 30 seconds to that portion of the enamel that will receive the bracket.
4. Rinse the etchant off with water and thoroughly dry the enamel (Fig. 16.20).
   NOTE: Properly etched enamel should appear frosty or chalky white. Because no dentin is involved, the enamel is dried thoroughly.

Continued

Procedure 16.1 Bonding Orthodontic Brackets—cont'd

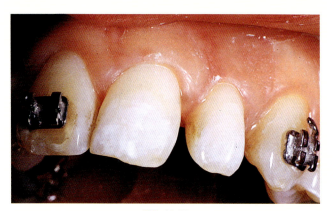

FIG. 16.20

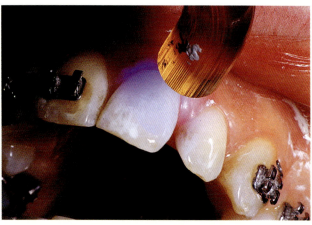

FIG. 16.21

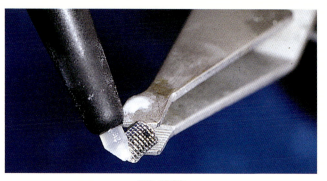

FIG. 16.22

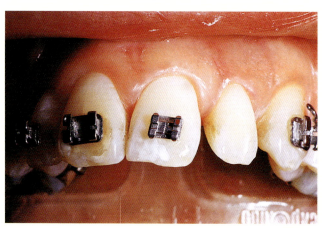

FIG. 16.23

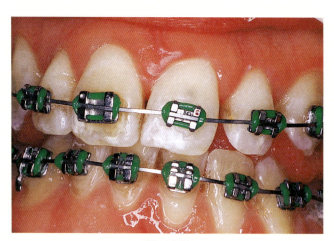

FIG. 16.24

5. Apply a thin coating of liquid bonding resin to the etched enamel and light cure for 20 seconds (Fig. 16.21).
   NOTE: This bonding resin acts to prepare or prime the enamel to allow adhesion of the resin adhesive paste that holds the bracket in place. The bonding resin and the adhesive resin chemically bond to each other.
6. Apply light-cured adhesive resin to the metal mesh on the back of the bracket (Fig. 16.22), and place the bracket in the location prescribed by the dentist, using bracket placement pliers. An orthodontic scaler can be used to adjust the position of the bracket and remove excess resin.
   NOTE: The resin adhesive does not chemically bond to the bracket, but it will physically lock into the mesh on the back of the bracket. Some brackets are manufactured with the adhesive applied at the factory and are covered with a plastic cover that is stripped away at the time of placement.
7. Light cure the adhesive resin for 40 to 60 seconds, directing the light from mesial, distal, incisal, cervical, and lingual toward the bracket.
   NOTE: Although the metal of the bracket blocks penetration of the light directly, the translucency of the enamel allows light to transmit through it to cure the resin underlying the bracket. High-intensity curing lights may alter the curing times.
8. Repeat the procedure to complete the placement of all of the brackets (Fig. 16.23).
   NOTE: Typically, the six anterior teeth are all etched and primed at the same time. Brackets may be bonded individually or placed together and light cured individually.
9. The archwire and elastic or wire ligatures can be placed after all brackets are bonded (Fig. 16.24).

Dental Cement CHAPTER 16 359

Procedure 16.2 Zinc Oxide Eugenol Cement (ZOE): Primary and Secondary Consistency

See Evolve site for Competency Sheet.

Consider the following with this procedure: safety glasses are recommended for the patient, PPE is required for the clinician, ensure appropriate safety protocols are followed, and check local state guidelines before performing this procedure.

EQUIPMENT/SUPPLIES (FIG. 16.25)
- Cement paste/paste or cement powder/liquid and dispensers
- Paper mixing pad or glass slab
- Flexible cement spatula

PROCEDURE STEPS: PRIMARY CONSISTENCY

1. Dispense the recommended amount of base paste and accelerator paste onto a mixing pad.
   NOTE: One-half inch of each is usually enough for a single crown restoration.
2. Mix the materials, using both sides of the flat blade of a cement spatula in a "stropping, pushing" motion.
3. The mix is in primary consistency when it is smooth and creamy and after gathering together lifts 1 inch off the mixing surface (Fig. 16.26).
4. Whenever possible, immediately clean the spatula with gauze.

PROCEDURE STEPS: SECONDARY CONSISTENCY (FIG. 16.27)-EQUIPMENT & SUPPLIES

1. Fluff the powder and measure onto one end of the mixing surface.
   NOTE: Aerated powder provides for a more accurate measurement.
2. Shake the liquid, and dispense at the opposite end of the mixing surface.
   NOTE: Hold the dispenser vertical while dispensing to obtain uniform drops.
3. Incorporate the powder into the liquid in two increments or all at once according to the manufacturer's directions (Fig. 16.28).
   NOTE: Incorporate as much powder as possible into the liquid (Fig. 16.29).
4. Mix the materials, using both sides of the flat blade in a "stropping, pushing" motion.
5. The cement will be in secondary consistency when it can be rolled into a ball and is no longer tacky (Fig. 16.30).
6. Whenever possible, immediately clean the spatula with moist gauze.

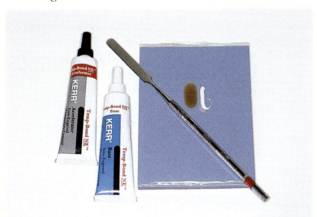

FIG. 16.25

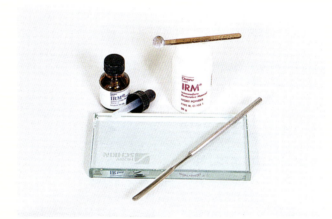

FIG. 16.27

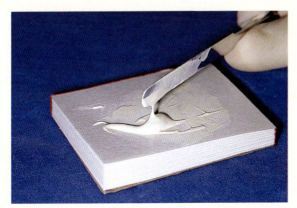

FIG. 16.26

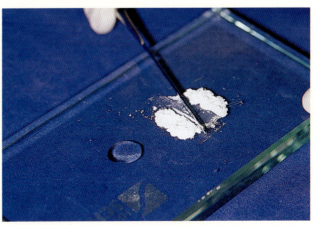

FIG. 16.28

Continued

Procedure 16.2 Zinc Oxide Eugenol Cement (ZOE): Primary and Secondary Consistency—cont'd

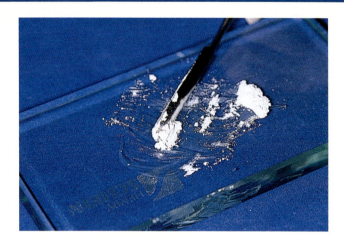

FIG. 16.29

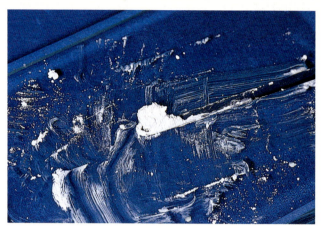

FIG. 16.30

Procedure 16.3 Zinc Phosphate Cement: Primary Consistency

See Evolve site for Competency Sheet.

Consider the following with this procedure: safety glasses are recommended for the patient, PPE is required for the clinician, ensure appropriate safety protocols are followed, and check local state guidelines before performing this procedure.

EQUIPMENT/SUPPLIES (FIG. 16.31)
- Cement powder
- Cement liquid and dispenser
- Cool glass slab
- Flexible cement spatula

PROCEDURE STEPS
1. Obtain a cooled glass slab.
   NOTE: The frozen slab method may be used for multiple orthodontic bands or long-span bridges.
2. Fluff the powder, and dispense the recommended amount onto one end of the slab.
3. Divide the powder into four to six increments to include smaller and larger increment sizes.
   NOTE: Smaller increments are incorporated first.
4. Shake the liquid and dispense the recommended amount at the opposite end of the slab.
   NOTE: Hold the dispenser vertical while dispensing to obtain uniform drops (Fig. 16.32).
5. Incorporate the first increment into the liquid.
   NOTE: Hold the spatula blade flat against the mixing surface. Use both sides of the spatula in a sweeping "figure-eight" motion over a large area of the slab (Fig. 16.33).
6. Each increment of powder is completely incorporated and is mixed for 20 to 30 seconds, beginning with the smallest and progressing through the largest.

FIG. 16.31

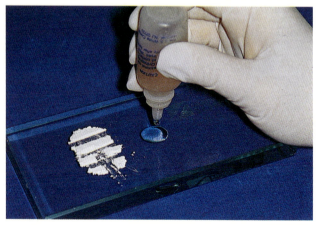

FIG. 16.32

Procedure 16.3 Zinc Phosphate Cement: Primary Consistency—cont'd

NOTE: Adding increments of powder and completely incorporating each into the mix will help to neutralize the acid, control the setting time, and allow for completion of the exothermic reaction before use (Fig. 16.34).

7. Place the spatula blade at a 45-degree angle to the slab, and gather the mass together to test the consistency.

NOTE: For primary consistency, the material should be smooth and creamy. Draw the spatula up from the mix; the cement should follow the spatula, breaking after 1 inch (Fig. 16.35).

8. Clean the spatula and slab with moistened gauze and disinfect or sterilize.

NOTE: If the cement is allowed to harden on the slab or spatula, it may be removed in an ultrasonic cleaner or by soaking in a solution of baking powder.

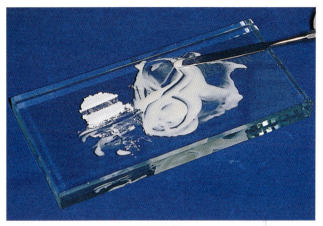

FIG. 16.34

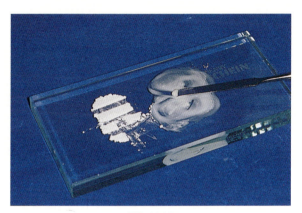

FIG. 16.33

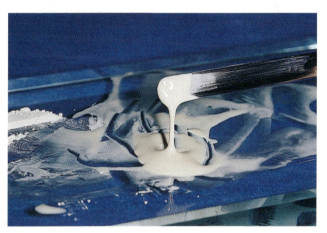

FIG. 16.35

Procedure 16.4 Zinc Polycarboxylate Cement: Primary Consistency

See Evolve site for Competency Sheet.

Consider the following with this procedure: safety glasses are recommended for the patient, PPE is required for the clinician, ensure appropriate safety protocols are followed, and check local state guidelines before performing this procedure.

EQUIPMENT/SUPPLIES (FIG. 16.36)
- Cement powder and dispenser
- Cement liquid and dispenser
- Paper mixing pad or glass slab
- Flexible cement spatula

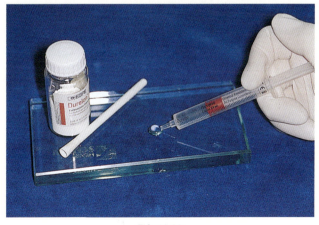

FIG. 16.36

Continued

Procedure 16.4 Zinc Polycarboxylate Cement: Primary Consistency—cont'd

PROCEDURE STEPS

1. Fluff the powder, and measure onto one end of the mixing surface.
   NOTE: Aerated powder provides for a more accurate measurement.
2. Shake the liquid and dispense at the opposite end of the mixing surface.
   NOTE: Hold the dispenser vertical while dispensing to obtain uniform drops, or, if using a syringe dispenser with lines marking calibrated doses, be careful to note the number of lined increments to dispense.
3. Incorporate the powder into the liquid in two increments or all at once according to the manufacturer's directions.
4. Mix the materials, using both sides of the flat blade in a "stropping, pushing" motion.
5. The mix is in primary consistency when it is smooth and creamy and after gathering together it lifts 1 inch off the mixing surface.
   NOTE: The consistency is somewhat thicker than that of other cements and appears glossy (Fig. 16.37). The cement is too thick and starting to set if it produces thin, stringy "cobwebs" when lifted off the mixing surface (Fig. 16.38). Do not use the mix if it loses its glossy appearance.
6. Whenever possible, immediately clean the spatula with moist gauze because the cement sticks tenaciously to metal.

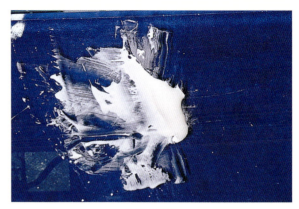

FIG. 16.37

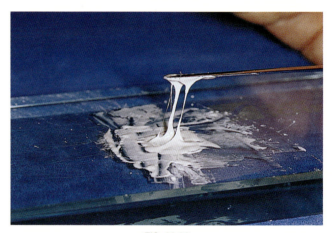

FIG. 16.38

Procedure 16.5 Glass Ionomer Cement: Pre-Dosed Capsule

See Evolve site for Competency Sheet.

Consider the following with this procedure: safety glasses are recommended for the patient, PPE is required for the clinician, ensure appropriate safety protocols are followed, and check local state guidelines before performing this procedure.

EQUIPMENT/SUPPLIES (FIG. 16.39)

- Premeasured capsule of cement
- Cement activator
- Triturator
- Cement dispenser

PROCEDURE STEPS

1. Place the premeasured capsule into the cement activator and press down on the handle.
   NOTE: The activator breaks the seal between the powder and the liquid in the capsule, allowing the materials to meet. Make sure you use sufficient pressure to feel the seal break (Fig. 16.40).

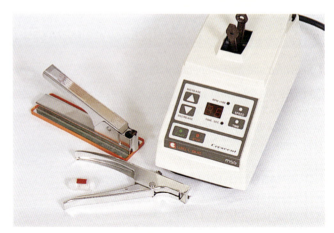

FIG. 16.39

2. Place the capsule into the triturator and set for the recommended amount of time, usually 10 to 15 seconds.
   NOTE: The capsule is similar to an amalgam capsule and needs to be secured in the arms of the triturator before mixing (Fig. 16.41).

Procedure 16.5   Glass Ionomer Cement: Pre-Dosed Capsule—cont'd

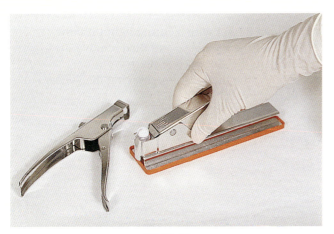

FIG. 16.40

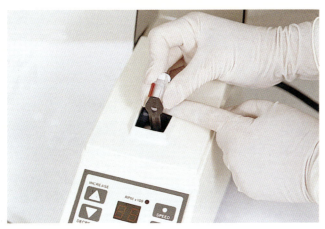

FIG. 16.41

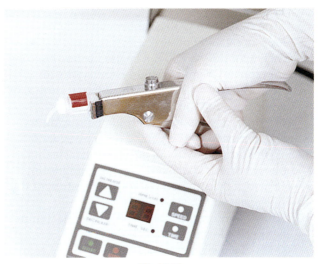

FIG. 16.42

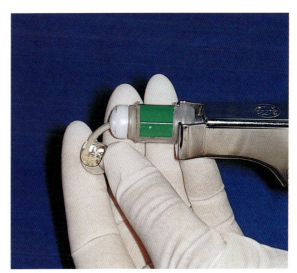

FIG. 16.43

3. Remove the capsule from the triturator and immediately place into the cement dispenser; advance the mixed cement to the end of the dispensing tip (Fig. 16.42).
4. Load the crown directly from the dispenser (Fig. 16.43). Use a flat-bladed instrument to carefully coat the wall and margins of the crown with a thin layer of cement Remove any excess cement.
5. Discard the capsule and disinfect the activator and triturator. The dispenser may be sterilized.

Procedure 16.6   Resin-Based Cement for Indirect Restorations: Ceramic, Porcelain, Composite

See Evolve site for Competency Sheet.

Consider the following with this procedure: safety glasses are recommended for the patient, PPE is required for the clinician, ensure appropriate safety protocols are followed, and check local state guidelines before performing this procedure.

EQUIPMENT/SUPPLIES

- Tooth conditioner (etchant)
- Primer/bond (universal) adhesive
- Disposable applicator
- Dispensing dish
- Cement/adhesive
- Blunt instrument

PROCEDURE STEPS

1. Clean preparation of all provisional material.
   NOTE: Eugenol-containing materials should not be used in provisional coverage.

Continued

Procedure 16.6 Resin-Based Cement for Indirect Restorations: Ceramic, Porcelain, Composite—cont'd

2. Clean the dentin with a rubber cup and non-fluoride cleaning paste.
   NOTE: Fluoride should not be used before bonding.
3. Rinse preparation thoroughly and lightly air dry.
4. Clean and dry and prepare the internal surface of the final restoration.
   NOTE: Organic debris accumulated during try-in must be removed; this can be done by several means, including the use of an ultrasonic cleaner and phosphoric acid etchant. Microetching (with 9% HF acid) is recommended for preparation of the internal surface of the restoration.
5. Apply tooth conditioner according to the manufacturer's directions.
   NOTE: The use of a fine needle tip attached to the syringe of the conditioner will allow control of the conditioner to prevent etching of areas prone to postoperative sensitivity.
6. Rinse and blot dry, leaving a moist glistening surface.
   NOTE: Blot drying provides the correct amount of "wetness" on the tooth surface while avoiding desiccating the tooth surface.
7. Isolate the area to prevent saliva contamination.
   NOTE: If saliva contamination occurs, repeat steps 5 and 6.
8. Apply primer/bond adhesive agent to the tooth and internal surface of the restoration according to the manufacturer's directions. Fig. 16.44 shows the etch-and-rinse procedure to maximize bond strength with a significant amount of enamel remaining in the preparations for these veneers.
9. The universal adhesive is applied to the teeth and scrubbed for 20 seconds with a microtip (Fig. 16.45).
10. Dispense the desired shade of cement base paste into the restoration and seat the restoration.
11. Initiate the set with a curing light until the cement reaches the gel phase and then remove the excess cement (Fig. 16.46).
12. Review the final results, showing the veneers in place (Fig. 16.47).

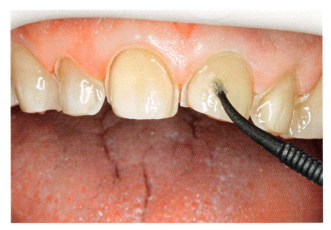

FIG. 16.45

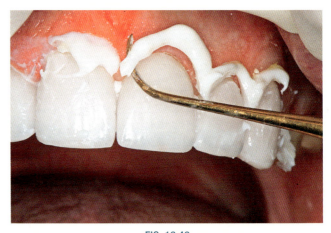

FIG. 16.46

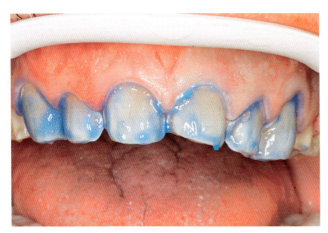

FIG. 16.44

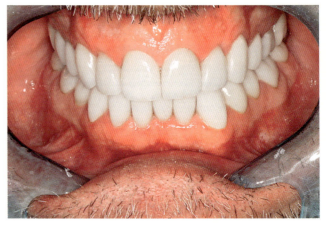

FIG. 16.47

Figures 16.44–16.47 from Blank JT: 3M ESPE's RelyX Ultimate Adhesive Resin Cement: A cement for nearly any indirect indication, www.dentalproductsreport.com.

Procedure 16.7 Self-Adhesive Technique for Indirect Restorations: Ceramic, Porcelain, Composite

See Evolve site for Competency Sheet.

Consider the following with this procedure: safety glasses are recommended for the patient, PPE is required for the clinician, ensure appropriate safety protocols are followed, and check local state guidelines before performing this procedure.

Shown is the cementation of a ceramic crown with a self-adhesive resin cement.

EQUIPMENT/SUPPLIES
Matrix
Self-adhesive resin cement (Fig. 16.48).
Light-cure delivery system
Floss; explorer or scaler

PROCEDURE STEPS

1. Follow steps 1–3 in Procedure 16.6.
   NOTE: When using self-adhesive cements the etching and bonding steps are not done (Fig. 16.49).
2. Try in the crown and confirm fit at margins, contact areas, and bite (Fig. 16.50).
3. Prepare the internal surface of the crown by sandblasting (Fig. 16.50).
4. Rinse thoroughly and dry the crown (Fig. 16.51).
5. Place the mixing and delivery tips on the cement cartridge. Express cement and coat the walls of the crown with a thin layer of cement and fully seat the crown with finger pressure or have patient bite on a cotton roll (Fig. 16.52).
   NOTE: Do not overfill the crown with cement. Hydraulic pressure may prevent the crown from seating fully.
6. The cement is dual cured, so wave the curing light over the margins of the crown for 2 seconds to gel the cement. Remove the excess cement with a scaler or explorer. Use knotted floss to remove excess cement from the interproximal area (Fig. 16.53).

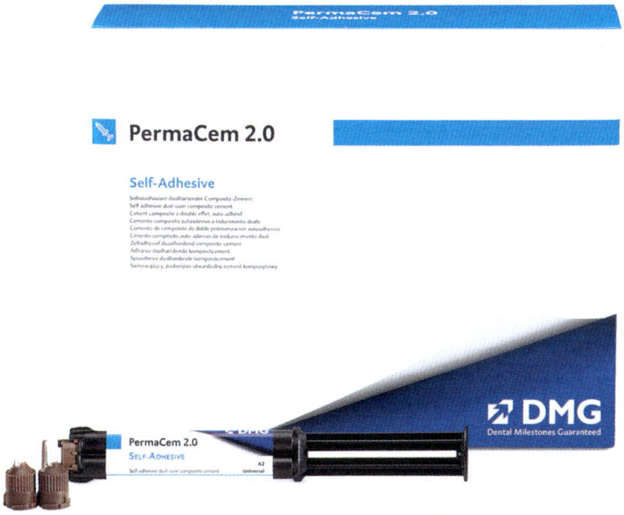

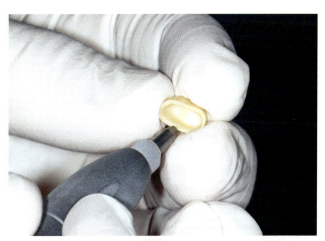

FIG. 16.50

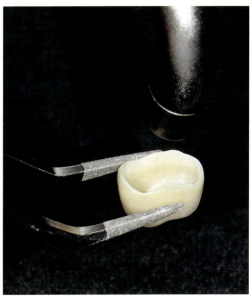

FIG. 16.51

FIG. 16.48

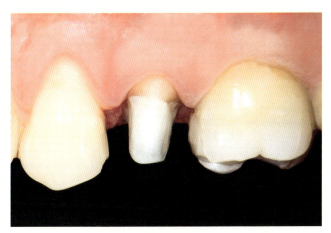

FIG. 16.49

Procedure 16.7 Self-Adhesive Technique for Indirect Restorations: Ceramic, Porcelain, Composite—cont'd

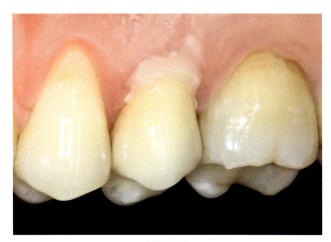

FIG. 16.52

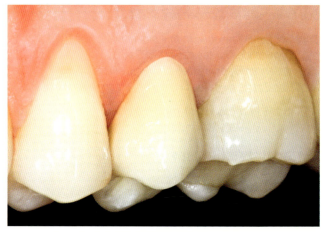

FIG. 16.54

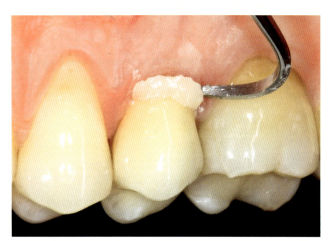

FIG. 16.53

NOTE: The removal of excess cement before curing is necessary; a short light cure to cause the cement to gel allows for easier removal. Pay special attention to interproximal areas, using knotted floss to remove excess cement. Once the cement has fully set it is very difficult to remove, especially from interproximal areas.

Figures 16.48–16.54 Courtesy DMG America, Englewood, New Jersey.

7. Check the cure marginal fit, contact areas and adjust occlusion as necessary (Fig. 16.54).
8. Check the radiograph to confirm seating and cement removal.
9. Finish and polish any areas that have been adjusted.

TRY-IN OPTION: BEFORE PREPARATION OF THE TOOTH FOR BONDING

1. Dispense the appropriate shade of try-in paste onto a mixing pad. Load the restoration and seat onto the preparation.
   NOTE: Try-in paste is matched to the cement base material and is used to obtain the correct shade of cement. Restoration "try-in" particularly for anterior crowns is recommended before final cementation to ensure acceptance of restoration esthetics.
2. Once the restoration fit and esthetics are verified, the try-in paste is removed from the preparation and the restoration is cemented, using one of the techniques already described.

Review and Discussion

Review Questions

Select the one correct response for each of the following multiple-choice questions.

1. Cements mixed to primary consistency are used for:
   a. High-strength bases
   b. Luting
   c. Core buildups
   d. Surgical dressings
2. In which situation may it be necessary to place an insulating base under restorations?
   a. Encourage sclerotic dentin formation
   b. Protect the pulp from sudden temperature changes
   c. Reduce acidity
   d. Calcify the dentinal tubules
3. The test for a properly mixed zinc phosphate luting cement is:
   a. Putty consistency
   b. Granular consistency
   c. Checking whether cement will break and form a drop at the end of the spatula
   d. Checking whether cement will hold a thin string, breaking when the spatula is raised an inch
4. Which cement should *not* be used for temporary cementation of crowns to be permanently cemented with resin cements?
   a. Zinc polycarboxylate
   b. Zinc phosphate
   c. Zinc oxide eugenol
   d. Any cement is appropriate
5. Which cement exhibits an exothermic reaction during mixing?
   a. Glass ionomer
   b. Zinc phosphate
   c. Resin cement
   d. Calcium hydroxide
6. Which dental cements use the bonding procedure before placement of the dental cement?
   a. Zinc phosphate and polycarboxylate
   b. Zinc oxide eugenol and glass ionomer
   c. Resin
   d. Calcium hydroxide and zinc oxide eugenol
7. When luting a crown, it is important to:
   a. Have a film thickness that allows for complete seating
   b. Have a film thickness that provides proper insulation
   c. Have a film thickness for complete filling of the crown
   d. None of the above
8. Why should many cements *not* be dispensed until ready to mix?
   a. Dehydration can occur from exposure to air
   b. Contamination can occur from moisture in the air
   c. Components of the cement might come in contact with each other
   d. All of the above
9. Which dental cement bonds to dentin, is "kind" to the pulp, and resists recurrent decay?
   a. Zinc oxide eugenol
   b. Polycarboxylate
   c. Calcium hydroxide
   d. Glass ionomer
10. Why is zinc phosphate cement mixed over a large area of the glass slab?
    a. Helps lengthen the working time
    b. Helps neutralize the chemicals
    c. Helps dissipate the exothermic reaction
    d. All of the above
11. Proper instrumentation at cement margins includes:
    a. Avoiding gouging or ditching cement margins
    b. Using ultrasonic scalers to remove deposits on resin-based cement margins
    c. Using air polishing on resin-based cement margins
    d. All are correct
12. Light-cured cements may be used for luting which of the following?
    a. Nonmetal orthodontic retainers
    b. Porcelain veneers less than 1.5 mm thick
    c. Porcelain or gold inlays
    d. A and B
13. Which cement should *not* be used under a composite restoration because of the oil content of the liquid?
    a. Zinc phosphate
    b. Glass ionomer
    c. Calcium hydroxide
    d. Zinc oxide eugenol
14. Adhesion is molecular attraction between materials with:
    a. Similar molecules
    b. Dissimilar molecules
    c. Irregular surfaces
    d. None of the above
15. When should newly mixed polycarboxylate cement no longer be used for luting?
    a. The mix is shiny.
    b. The mix flows readily.
    c. The mix is creamy.
    d. The mix is stringy or weblike.
16. Adding resin to glass ionomer cement does all of the following *except* one. Which one?
    a. Increases the fluoride release
    b. Increases compressive strength
    c. Decreases solubility
    d. Increases tensile strength
17. Failure to remove all excess cement from subgingival margins may cause all of the following *except* one. Which one?
    a. Aphthous ulcers
    b. Periodontal infection
    c. Bone loss
    d. Recurrent caries

For answers to Review Questions, see the Appendix.

Case-Based Discussion Topics

1. A 22-year-old administrative assistant is scheduled for a gold crown preparation. They have been seen in your office previously for a crown and experienced some difficulty with sensitivity while the provisional crown was in place.

Which cement would be the best choice for luting the temporary crown, and why?

Continued

Review and Discussion—cont'd

2. A 40-year-old accountant is scheduled for cementation of an all-ceramic crown on tooth 5. The provisional crown has been cemented with a non-eugenol zinc oxide cement.

Why was this cement chosen for the provisional coverage, and which cement would be the best choice for the permanent crown?

3. A 9-year-old is scheduled for cementation of orthodontic bands.

Which cement would be the best choice, and why?

4. You are asked to mix a final luting cement and fill a crown with it in preparation for seating. Although the crown seated completely on try-in, when the dentist attempts to seat the cement-filled crown, the margins remain open and the crown is high.

What might be the explanation for this situation?

5. Your office is considering going to a premeasured cement system.

What situations can you foresee in which this system may be problematic?

BIBLIOGRAPHY

Bezawada N, Bali S, Aggarwal S: Niveditha Reddy. Periodontal dressing: a review, *Santosh Univ J Health Sci* 6(1):5–9, 2020.

Cao Y, Bogen G, Lim J, Shon WJ, Kang MK: Bioceramic materials and the changing concepts in vital pulp therapy, *J Calif Dental Assoc* 44(5):278–290, 2016.

Croll TP, Nicholson JW: Glass ionomer cements in pediatric dentistry: review of the literature, *Pediatr Dent* 24(5):423–429, 2002.

Fruits TJ, Coury TL, Miranda FJ, Duncanson Jr., MG: Uses and properties of current glass ionomer cements: a review, *Gen Dent* 44(5):410–422, 1996.

Ghodsi S, Arzani S, Shekarian M, Aghamohseni M: Cement selection criteria for full coverage restorations: A comprehensive review of literature, *J Clin Exp Dent* 13(11):e1154–e1161, 2021.

Gutkowski S: Minimal intervention: making it stick: cements in dental hygiene, *RDH Mag* 28:36–37, 2008.

Heboyan A, Vardanyan A, Karobari MI, Marya A, Avagyan T, Tebyaniyan H, Mustafa M, Rokaya D, Avetisyan A: Dental luting cements: an updated comprehensive review, *Molecules* 28:1619, 2023.

Jeffries SR: Bioactive dental materials, *Inside Dent* 12(2), 2016. https://www.aegisdentalnetwork.com/id/2016/02/bioactive-dental-materials.

Jivraj SA, Reshad M, Donovan T: Selecting luting agents, *Inside Dent* 9(2), 2013.

Kathariya R, Jain H, Jadhav T: To pack or not to pack: the current status of periodontal dressing, *J Appl Biomater Funct Mater* 13(2):e73–e86, 2015.

Poli PP, Cicciu M, Beretta M, Maiorana C: Peri-implant mucositis and peri-implantitis: A current understanding of their diagnosis, clinical implications, and a report of treatment using a combined therapy approach, *J Oral Implantol* 43(1):45–50, 2017.

Sakaguchi RL, Ferracane J, Powers JM: *Craig's Restorative Dental Materials*, ed 14, St. Louis, 2019, Elsevier.

Shen C, Rawls H, Esquivel-Upshaw JF: *Phillips' Science of Dental Materials*, ed 13, St. Louis, 2022, Elseviers.

Strassler HE, Morgan RJ: Cements for PFM and all-metal restorations, *Inside Dentistry* 9(11), 2013. https://www.aegisdentalnetwork.com/id/2013/11/cements-for-pfm-and-all-metal-restorations?page_id=297.

Strassler HE, Morgan RJ: Cements for today's all-ceramic materials, *Inside Dent* 9(12), 2013. https://www.aegisdentalnetwork.com/id/2013/12/cements-for-all-ceramic-materials.

Strassler HE, Morgan RJ: Provisional–temporary cements: techniques to facilitate placement of provisional restorations, *Inside Dental Assist* 8(4), 2012. https://www.aegisdentalnetwork.com/ida/2012/08/provisional-temporary-cements.

Abrasion, Finishing, Polishing, and Cleaning

17

http://evolve.elsevier.com/Eakle/materials/

Chapter Objectives

On completion of this chapter, the student should be able to:
1. Define abrasion, finishing, polishing, and cleaning.
2. Discuss the purpose of finishing, polishing, and cleaning of dental restorations and tooth surfaces.
3. Identify and discuss the factors that affect the rate and efficiency of abrasion.
4. Compare the relative ranking of abrasives on restorations and tooth structures.
5. List methods by which dental abrasives are applied.
6. Describe the contraindications to the use of abrasives on the tooth structure and restorations.
7. Describe the clinical decisions made to determine which abrasive to use when finishing, polishing, or cleaning dental restorations or tooth structures.
8. Identify the abrasives and the procedures used for finishing and polishing metals, composite, and porcelain.
9. Describe the abrasives and the procedures used for polishing and cleaning metals, composite, ceramic, and gold alloys as part of oral prophylaxis.
10. Describe the safety and infection control precautions taken by the operator when using abrasives.
11. Relate the instructions given to patients to prevent and remove stain from tooth surfaces and restorations.
12. Finish and polish a preexisting amalgam restoration.
13. Polish a preexisting composite restoration.

KEY TERMS

Finishing a procedure used to remove excess restorative material to develop appropriate occlusion, contour, and functional form; usually done with rotary cutting instruments. Finishing removes surface blemishes and produces a smooth surface

Polishing a procedure that produces a smooth, shiny surface by eliminating minor surface imperfections, fine scratches, and surface stains using mild abrasives frequently found in the form of pastes or compounds. Polishing produces little change in the surface

Mohs Hardness a measure of hardness on a scale of 1 to 10, where 1 is a very soft material and 10 is the hardest material

Cleaning a procedure that is primarily meant to remove soft deposits from the surface of restorations and tooth structures. Polishing and cleaning are done to remove surface stains and soft deposits from the clinical crowns and exposed root surfaces of teeth after all hard deposits are removed

Abrasive a material composed of particles of sufficient hardness and sharpness to cut or scratch a softer material when drawn across its surface

Hardness is the ability of a material to resist abrasion

Grit the size of the abrasive particles, typically classified as coarse, medium, fine, and superfine

Margination a procedure for removal of excessive restorative material from the margins of restorations

Flash feather-like excesses of material present at the margins of a restoration typically on occlusal and proximal surfaces

Overhang excessive material present at the cervical cavosurface margin

Supragingival Air Polishing the process of polishing or finishing the clinical crown (portion of the crown located above the gingiva) using fine, soft particles under air pressure to remove biofilm and stain from enamel surfaces and in pits and fissures; an alternative to prophy pastes

Subgingival Air Polishing the process of polishing the anatomical crown (portion of the crown located below the gingiva) and clinical root surface using fine, soft particles under air pressure to remove biofilm subgingivally

Air Abrasion or Microabrasion like air polishing, but using greater air pressure and harder particles. Used to cleanse cast appliances before cementation, repair porcelain and composite restorations, prepare tooth surfaces before bonding, and cut the tooth structure for restorative preparations

Proper finishing, polishing, and cleaning of tooth structures and restorative materials is clinically relevant because this improves esthetic and tissue health, while increasing the longevity of the restorative material. Patients are increasingly requesting whiter and brighter teeth. Dental manufacturers have responded with a multitude of products, both in-office and over-the-counter, to meet this demand. The dental auxiliary must carefully evaluate the clinical procedures used for the removal of stains and soft deposits with the use of abrasives. First, the needs of the individual patient are considered, and the types of stains and restorative materials present are properly identified. Then, procedures, if needed, are selected based upon the evaluation. For example, the routine polishing of teeth with abrasive prophylactic (prophy) paste after scaling and root planing is not recommended. The clinician must critically evaluate the potential negative effects of the coronal polish procedure against the benefits.

The goal of finishing and polishing restorations, intraoral appliances, and tooth structure is to remove excess material, smooth roughened surfaces, and produce an esthetically pleasing appearance with minimal trauma to hard and soft tissues. The finishing and polishing of a surface involves removing marginal irregularities, defining anatomic contours and occlusion, removing the surface roughness of the restoration, and producing a mirror-like surface luster. Many benefits are derived from smooth tooth surfaces, restorations, or appliances in the oral environment. A smooth surface resists accumulation of soft deposits and stains, is less irritating to the gingival or mucosal tissue, and is esthetically pleasing because it is shiny. A smooth and polished tooth surface can help to motivate the patient to maintain these positive results with better self-care procedures. A highly polished smooth restorative surface is more resistant to the effects of corrosion and surface breakdown. A properly finished and polished surface will contribute to the appearance and longevity of the restoration or appliance and the health of the surrounding oral tissues (Fig. 17.1).

Clinicians who perform finishing and polishing procedures must have a clear understanding of the factors that cause and control abrasion. Improper use of abrasives can lead to roughening and over-reduction of tooth and restorative surfaces. The clinician must be able to recognize that different types of tooth structures and restorative surfaces abrade differently and must use the proper protocol for finishing, polishing, or cleaning each surface. It is also the clinician's responsibility to teach the patient how to properly care for tooth and restorative surfaces with home care devices and how to prevent habits that produce stains and diminish their appearance (see Chapter 2).

FINISHING, POLISHING, AND CLEANING

The process of finishing and polishing involves using a sequence of abrasives on a surface to first contour, then smooth, and finally bring a luster to the surface. The sequence moves from coarse to fine abrasive particles or disks. Contouring by cutting or grinding away excessive materials with rotary instruments may be required first to produce the desired anatomic form.

Finishing removes excess material to develop the surface morphology and functional form. Contouring of the restoration is most often done with rotary instruments in high- and low-speed handpieces.

Gross finishing is done first:
- Removing large excesses of restorative material
- Using coarse or medium grit
  - Diamond burs
  - Abrasive discs and strips
- Using carbide finishing burs

Fine finishing uses medium and fine versions of the gross finishing instruments to refine the anatomic morphology including:
- Occlusal surfaces and occlusion
- Embrasure spaces
- Marginal ridge form
- Facial and lingual contours
  Fine finishing prepares the surface for polishing.

Polishing is the process of:
- Removing scratches from the surface of a restoration with a series of abrasive particles
- Moving in a sequence from coarse to fine abrasives
- Producing a smooth, glossy surface

A smooth surface is necessary for multiple reasons that include:
- Esthetically pleasing
- Tolerated well by soft tissues
- Resistant to biofilm adhesion

When finishing is done properly, polishing produces little change in the surface. Polishing may have to be repeated periodically during the life of the restoration if scratches, tarnish or stains develop. Polishing requires materials with a **Mohs' hardness** of only one to two units above the substrate being polished. In other words, the abrasive agent needs only to be a little harder than the material it is polishing. Finishing and polishing are intended to produce selective and controlled wear of the surface being manipulated.

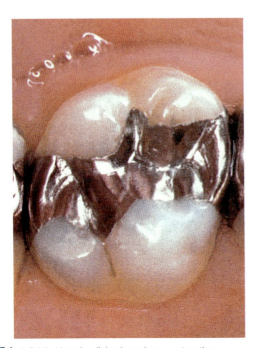

Fig. 17.1 A finished and polished amalgam restoration.

Cleaning does not produce scratches or wear and is primarily used for the removal of biofilm. Polishing and cleaning are done to remove surface stains and soft deposits from the clinical crowns and exposed root surfaces of teeth after all hard deposits are removed. Aside from abrasives, there are also chemical cleaning products that are primarily used for removable appliances. There is no single type of abrasive that can be used safely and effectively on all types of dental materials and structures of the tooth.

FACTORS AFFECTING ABRASION

Understanding the properties of **abrasives** and the factors that control the rate or efficiency of abrasion will help the clinician or auxiliary make appropriate clinical decisions. The rate of abrasion is determined by the abrasive being used and the surface being abraded (the *substrate*). The abrasiveness of particles is determined by:
- Size
- Irregularity
- Hardness
- The number of particles contacting the surface
- The pressure and speed at which they are applied

The rate of abrasion is also dependent on the surface being abraded; a hard substrate such as enamel is much more resistant to abrasion than softer cementum. An understanding of these factors will assist the clinician and auxiliary in making appropriate clinical decisions for the indications, contraindications, and control of abrasion.

Do You Recall?

Why is there not one single type of abrasive that can be used on all types of dental materials?

Size, Irregularity, and Hardness of Abrasive Particles

The size, irregularity, and hardness of the abrasive particle determine the depth of the scratches in the material being abraded and therefore the amount of material potentially removed. **Hardness** is the ability of a material to resist abrasion. If the surface being abraded is harder than the abrasive, there is little to no effect.
- It is important that the clinician have an appreciation for the relative hardness of various intraoral natural and restorative materials and the abrasives used on these materials.
- The Mohs scale of hardness ranks materials by their relative abrasion resistance.
- The Knoop hardness test is based on the ability of materials to resist indentation.
- In both of these tests the softer the substrate and the harder the abrasive, the more effective is the abrasive process.

See Table 17.1 for hardness ratings of materials and tooth structure.

Table 17.1 Mohs and Knoop Hardness Scales

	MOHS	KNOOP
Diamond	10	7000–10,000
Silicon carbide (carborundum)	9–10	2500
Tungsten carbide	9	1900
Aluminum oxide (corundum), emery	7–9	2100
Sand (quartz)	7	820
Zirconium silicate	6.5–7.5	
Silicon dioxide (Silex)	6–7	
Flour of pumice	6–7	460–560
CAD/CAM ceramic	6–7	
Porcelain (ceramic)	6–7	560
Tin oxide	6	
Perlite	5.5–7	
Enamel	5.5–6	340–431
Composite	5–7	30–55
Rouge	5–6	
Amalgam	5–6	90
Gold type IV alloy	3–4	220
Dentin	3–4	70
Cementum	2–3	40
Denture base resin (acrylic)	2–3	20
Calcium carbonate	3	
Aluminum trihydroxide	2.5–4	
Sodium bicarbonate	2.5–3	
Glycine	2	
Potassium and sodium	0.04–0.05	

Tooth structure in shaded rows. *CAD/CAM*, Computer-assisted design/computer-assisted machining.

It is important to note that porcelain is harder than enamel and dentin. Abrasive wear of tooth structures in contact with porcelain restorations is a problem for many patients. The greater the difference in hardness between the abrasive and the surface it is abrading, the faster and more effective the abrasive action. A particle must be harder by 1 to 2 Mohs units than the surface it is polishing to be effective.

Cleaning, when no abrasion is indicated, requires a substance 1 Mohs unit less than or equal to the surface on which it is intended to clean.

Clinical Tip

It is important that patients are provided with instructions to use only approved denture cleaners for their home care; even toothpaste may be too abrasive for acrylic intraoral appliances such as dentures and partials.

The size and shape of the particles must be considered in manipulating an abrasive. Particles that are large and irregular, with jagged edges, will cut more efficiently. The sharpness, or efficiency, of the particles is usually lost with use as the jagged edges break down and become rounder and the particles no longer "grab" the surface. Unlike the shape of the particles, the size of the particles does not always change significantly with use.

Abrasive particles are classified from coarse to fine, based on their size measured in micrometers (also called *microns* [symbol, μm]). One micrometer is equal to one-thousandth of a millimeter (1 mm = 1000 μm).

Abrasives are classified as
- Coarse (particles 100 μm and above)
- Medium (20–100 μm)
- Fine (20 μm to submicron particle sizes)

Manufacturers use the term **grit** to refer to the size of abrasive particles. Particles are passed through a standardized filter that allows a specific size of particles to pass, categorizing them from coarse through superfine. Prophylactic polishing pastes are commonly manufactured in various degrees of coarseness, as are abrasive disks and rotary diamonds (Fig. 17.2).

If too hard an abrasive with large particles is used, the result will be deep scratches in the surface that cannot be finished or polished out. The clinician must make decisions as to the coarseness of the abrasive and the application method needed for each procedure.

Number of Particles That Contact the Surface

The more concentrated the particles that contact the surface, the more quickly the surface will be abraded. If a lubricant is used to dilute the concentration of the particles, the abrasiveness of the material is reduced. Water and saliva are lubricants commonly used to dilute the effects of abrasion. When using an abrasive, the clinician has control of how much lubricant to add to the material, whether this is done before it is placed in the mouth or while it is being used intraorally as it picks up saliva. Pumice (Fig. 17.3) is manufactured as a powder or paste which allows the clinician the opportunity to further dilute this abrasive. Rotary cutting instruments such as abrasive disks and stones will lose effectiveness as particles break away from their surface or debris clogs the surface. Many rotary cutting stones and diamonds use the water from the handpiece or three-way syringe to assist in the removal of debris from the cutting edge and act as a surface coolant, thus allowing the surface to maintain its abrasive action much longer.

Speed and Pressure

Increasing the speed and pressure at which an abrasive is applied will increase the rate of abrasion. Increased speed alone can produce undesired effects if it results in a lack of control. Increased pressure will produce deeper scratches, as well as several other possible results:
- Less control of the amount of material being removed
- Decreased clinician's tactile sensitivity, possibly leading to an undesired overabraded surface
- Reduced cutting efficiency of the abrasive, the result of decreased instrumental torque

Increased speed and pressure also result in frictional heat, which may have a detrimental effect on the tooth structure, the pulp, and on patient comfort. Heat generated from rotary instruments can bring mercury to the surface of an amalgam restoration and degrade its properties. Polishing that is done dry with continuous application produces the highest temperature increase on the surface of the restoration. If polishing needs to be done dry, then intermittent application with light pressure should be used.

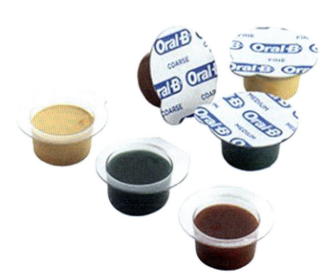

Fig. 17.2 The grit in prophy paste (available as single-dose units in holders) comes in various sizes. (Courtesy Proctor & Gamble.)

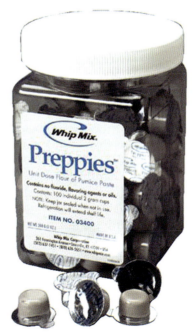

Fig. 17.3 Pumice delivered in a single dose of premixed paste. (Copied from smartpractice.com.)

> **Caution**
> Care must be taken to control the amount of pressure and speed with which abrasives are applied to avoid generating heat or abrading the restoration too much. For most applications a light intermittent touch is recommended.

When has polishing been accomplished?
- Patients can detect surface roughness on restorations with their tongue.
- The tongue can sense a surface roughness of less than 1 μm.
- Roughness greater than 1 μm may lead to breakdown of the restoration surface due to biofilm accumulation and corrosion.
- Gloss and/or luster are produced when the scratches on the restoration surface are smaller than the wavelength of visible light (<0.5 μm) resulting in a shiny surface that reflects light.
- The clinician must be able to determine if the surface of the restoration is smooth to properly determine the amount and rate of abrasion needed to polish the surface.
- When the surface of a restoration is rough, polishing should be completed to smooth the surface.

Selective Polishing
The clinician will select the appropriate type of material to polish the surface without causing excessive damage; this is known as selective polishing. Determining the amount and rate of abrasion is an important consideration when clinical decisions are made regarding what type of material to be abraded, how much material is to be removed, and the desired outcome.

> **KEY POINTS**
> **FINISHING, POLISHING, AND CLEANING**
> 1. Finishing
>   - Intended to remove excess material to develop proper dental anatomy and functional form of the tooth
> 2. Polishing
>   - Intended to remove scratches on the tooth or restoration surface
> 3. Cleaning
>   - Intended to remove stains and surface debris such as biofilm

MODE OF DELIVERY OF ABRASIVES
Dental abrasives are supplied in a number of forms (Fig. 17.4):
- Two-body abrasives, including:
  - Bonded abrasives
  - Coated abrasives
- Three-body abrasives, including:
  - Paste abrasives
  - Loose abrasives
- Microparticle (or hard-particle) abrasives, delivered by air pressure

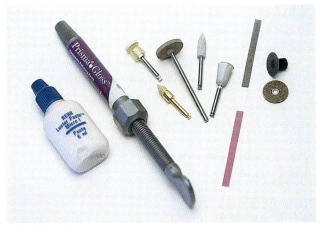

Fig. 17.4 Various delivery designs for abrasives: Paste, bonded, and coated.

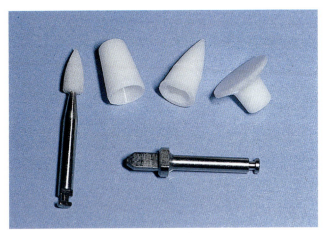

Fig. 17.5 Bonded abrasives: reusable point on mandrel, and disposable cup, point, and disk with sterilizable mandrel.

Two-Body (Direct Contact) Abrasives
Two-body abrasives, also known as direct contact abrasives, include abrasive agents that are fixed on an abrasive instrument such as on sandpaper disks, strips, or burs. Tooth-to-tooth contact, known as attrition, is an example of two-body abrasion.

Bonded Abrasives
Bonded abrasives are attached to rotary instruments; the abrasive particles are uniformly incorporated in a binder and bonded to the device. The devices vary in the available shape, such as points, disks, cups, brushes, and wheels. These devices are frequently used for intermediate finishing and initial polishing of restorations (Fig. 17.5).

Coated Abrasives
Coated abrasives are supplied on rotary disks and handheld finishing strips. The abrasive particles are secured to one side of a flexible backing with an adhesive. Devices with coating on only one side protect the adjacent tooth from the abrasive and are referred to as *safe-sided*. Flexible backing, such as paper or plastic, gives such devices the advantage of flexibility but eliminates their ability to be sterilized. Abrasive

coated rotary devices are typically attached to an autoclavable shaft or mandrel, for convenience and cost-effectiveness (Fig. 17.6). Sof-Lex spiral finishing and polishing wheels (3M ESPE) (Fig. 17.7) are an alternative to points, cups, discs and brushes.

Three-Body Abrasives
Three-body abrasives are those that are free to rotate between the delivery device and the surface being polished. Prophy paste in a rubber cup is an example of a three-body abrasive.

Paste Abrasives
Paste abrasives are found in the form of prophy paste and toothpaste. A more complete discussion of both follows in the section "Preparations Used for Abrasion".

Loose Abrasives
Loose abrasives are manufactured as powders and pastes and are classified by their grit or particle size. Grits of coarse, medium, fine, and superfine are available for finishing, polishing, and cleaning surfaces. These may be applied with wheels, brushes, cups, or soft pads. The concentration of particles that contact the surface is clinically controlled. If the clinician uses a coarse, thick paste, rapid removal of surface material will result, along with possible pulpal damage due to excessive frictional heat. However, if a superfine, highly diluted paste is used, little or no material may be removed. The proper grit and dilution of the loose abrasive must be considered to obtain the best results in finishing and polishing a given surface.

MICROPARTICLE ABRASIVES
Microparticle abrasives are those that are forced against the substrate by air pressure. This technique, called *air polishing* (with a ProphyJet, Dentsply) or *air abrasion* depending on the particles and air pressure used, is an example of the use of hard-particle abrasive particles. See the section "Air Polishing and Air Abrasion" later in the chapter for a detailed discussion.

Abrasives are manufactured for use at chairside and in the laboratory. Some may be used for either purpose. Regardless of how the abrasive material is supplied, the clinician must control the rate of abrasion.

MATERIALS USED IN ABRASION
Many types of natural and synthetic (human-made) materials are available for use in dentistry. See Table 17.2 to identify materials in order from most to least abrasive.

Prophylaxis (Prophy) Paste
Prophylaxis (prophy) paste is not listed independently in the table above because the paste is a mixture of 50% to 60% abrasive materials such as pumice and tin oxide and lubricants. Prophy paste may be 20 times more abrasive to dentin and 10 times more abrasive to enamel than commercially prepared dentifrice. Preservatives, flavoring agents, coloring agents, and therapeutic agents are added to prophy paste. The abrasive powder is diluted with a lubricant to reduce the rate of abrasion and the amount of frictional heat produced. The lubricant also helps keep the preparation in a paste form by preventing hardening on exposure to air. Preservatives are included to prolong shelf life, and coloring and flavoring agents are added to increase patient acceptance. Fluoride is added to many preparations and is claimed to be a therapeutic agent in the prevention of caries, but studies have shown it not to be effective in the amount and concentration used.

Prophylaxis pastes are commercially prepared pastes supplied as coarse grit (5 µm) to superfine grit (2 µm) for polishing and cleaning of tooth structures. Coarse prophylaxis paste can produce scratches on polished surfaces of restorations such as gold, amalgam, and composite (see Fig. 17.14).

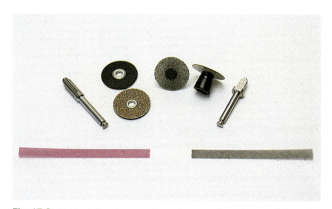

Fig. 17.6 Coated abrasives: various designs of sandpaper disk and mandrels and sandpaper strip.

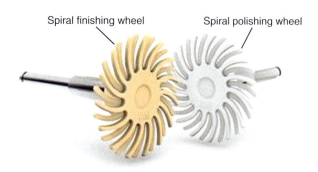

Fig. 17.7 Sof-Lex spiral finishing and polishing wheels use aluminum oxide as an abrasive. Its shape adapts to all tooth surfaces, making it an alternative to traditional points, cups, disks, and brushes. (Courtesy 3M ESPE, St. Paul, Minnesota.)

 Caution

Remember: Polishing materials should be harder (but by only one to two Mohs hardness rankings) than the surface to which they are applied. Cleaning materials should be equal to or less hard than the surface to which they are applied.

Table 17.2 Materials Identified in Order of Abrasiveness

MATERIAL	MOHS HARDNESS	DELIVERY METHOD	INFECTION CONTROL	IMPORTANT INFORMATION
Diamond	10	• Rotary cutting shanks, disks (Fig. 17.8) • Fine particle diamonds in a paste	Burs and disks sterilizable	Will efficiently abrade any substance. Fine particles used to polish composite and porcelain restorations.
Silicon carbide	9–10	• Coated disks, bonded rotary devices	Disks disposable, mandrel sterilizable	Used as a beginning step or finishing procedure for composites and ceramics.
Tungsten carbide finishing burs	Rank up to 9 (very hard material; harder than steel)	• Burs	Burs sterilizable	Do not dull quickly. 7–30 cutting flutes (blades on bur). More flutes equate to a finer finish (Fig. 17.9).
Aluminum oxide (Corundum), Emery	9	• White or tan powder for air abrasion • Bonded and coated rotary devices • Burlew wheels–impregnated rubber wheels	Powder and rotary disks should be discarded after use Burlew wheels may be autoclaved	Used to smooth enamel or finish metal alloys and ceramic materials. Used to polish highly filled and hybrid composite and porcelain restorations.
Sand (quartz and silica)	7	• Coated disks and handheld strips	Disks and strips disposable	Used in finishing process.
Silicon dioxide	6–7	• Prophy paste, rubberized cups and points	Paste discarded, rubberized cups and points may be reusable (follow manufacturer instructions)	Used for finishing and polishing composite restorations.
Pumice (volcanic silica)	6 (superfine, flour of pumice)	• Prophy paste	Paste discarded after use	Used to polish tooth structure and restorations. Fine, medium, and course pumice used in the laboratory, should not be used on natural tooth structures.
Tin oxide	6	• Powder (Fig. 17.10) mixed with water or glycine	Powder discarded after use	Used as final polishing agent for enamel and restorations.
Rouge	5–6	• Block form (Fig. 17.11)	Only use clean rag wheels to prevent cross-contamination–block cannot be sterilized	Used to polish precious and semiprecious metal alloys in the laboratory
Calcium carbonate (chalk or whiting)	3	• Prophy paste and dentifrice	Discard after use	Used to polish teeth, metal restorations, and plastic materials
Sodium bicarbonate	2.5–3	• Powder for supragingival air polisher (Fig. 17.12) and dentifrice	Discard after use	Used as cleaning agent
Glycine	2	• Powder for supra and subgingival air polisher (Fig. 17.13)	Discard after use	Used as cleaning agent
Potassium and sodium	0.4–0.5	• Toothpaste and desensitizing agents	Discard after use	Nonabrasive material used as cleaning agent or to occlude tubules

Polishing of tooth surfaces should remove soft deposits (biofilm) and polishable stains without damage to hard or soft tissues. No scientific proof shows how much enamel is removed during polishing or if it is removed at all as a result of the polishing process. These results led to the philosophy of "essential

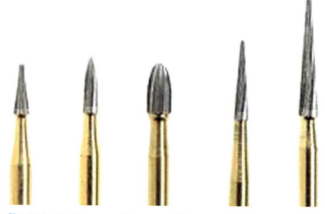

Fig. 17.9 Finishing burs. (Courtesy AXIS Dental Sàrl.)

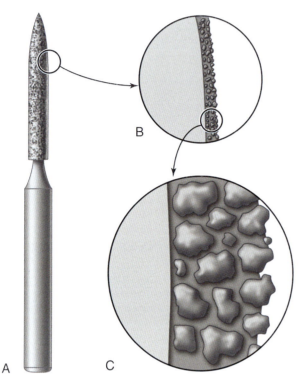

Fig. 17.8 Diamond particles attached to rotary instrument: **(A)** Diamond rotary instrument. **(B)** Diamond particles glued to the metal. **(C)** Magnification showing diamond particles bound in glue. (From Heymann H, Swift E, Ritter A: *Sturdevant's art & science of operative dentistry,* ed 6, St. Louis, 2013, Elsevier.)

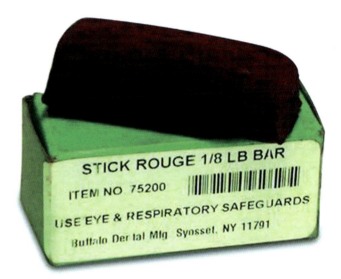

Fig. 17.11 Stick rouge to be utilized on a rag wheel in the dental laboratory to polish precious and semiprecious metal alloys. (Courtesy Buffalo Dental Manufacturing Co, Inc.)

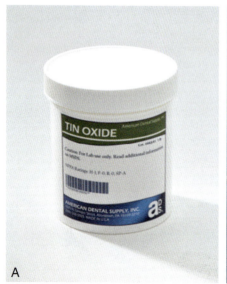
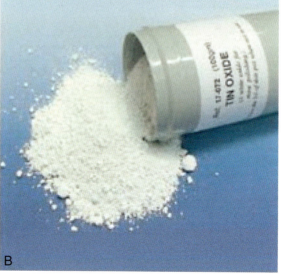

Fig. 17.10 Tin oxide. **(A)** image of external labelling of tin oxide container. **(B)** representation of tin oxide powder. ((A) Courtesy American Dental Supply, Inc. (B) Courtesy How to Clean Marble.)

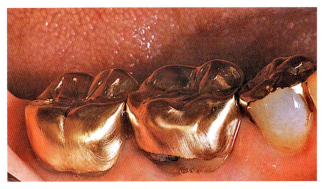

Fig. 17.14 The scratched surface of these gold crowns is due to inappropriate use of polishing agents.

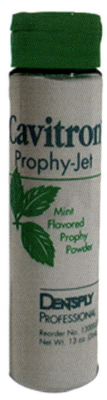

Fig. 17.12 Sodium bicarbonate utilized for supragingival air abrasion. (Courtesy Dentsply Sirona.)

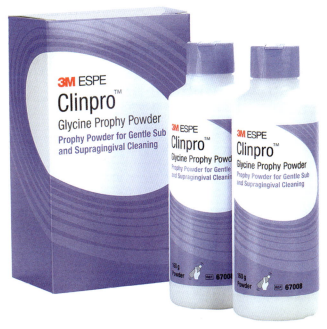

Fig. 17.13 Glycine powder utilized for supragingival and subgingival air polishing. (The photograph is reproduced herein the permission. © 3M 2020. All rights reserved.)

selective polishing," which is now regarded as the most appropriate approach in selecting a suitable polishing agent for the clinical situation.

All teeth stained or unstained may be polished; it is just a matter of selecting the appropriate agent to complete the polishing procedure for the specific teeth and surfaces. However, before a polishing or cleaning agent is selected, it is essential to evaluate:

1. The type of tooth structure (enamel, dentin, cementum)
2. The state of demineralization
3. The type of restorative material (metal, porcelain, composite) present

 Caution

A significant amount of roughening of composite, porcelain, and gold restorations is produced even by fine prophy pastes.

Which Prophy Paste to Select

When considering prophy pastes, select the least abrasive paste possible, or a nonabrasive paste, to remove existing stains and soft deposits. These abrasives should be applied as wet as possible with a light, intermittent touch and at low speed. Whenever coarse or medium paste is selected, it should be followed with a fine paste in a new or cleaned prophy cup. Unstained teeth should not be polished with abrasive agents but rather a nonabrasive cleaning paste.

Various prophy pastes have been developed with additives to assist in remineralization and to reduce tooth sensitivity.

- MI Paste (GC America) contains Recaldent (casein phosphopeptide-amorphous calcium phosphate), which allows teeth to remineralize and repair the very early stages of decay.
- NuCare (Sunstar Butler) with NovaMin (Sultan Healthcare) contains bioactive glass particles that release calcium, sodium, phosphate, and silica ions in the presence of water/saliva. These ions combine to form a hard and strong hydroxycarbonate apatite layer to occlude, and thereby desensitize, dentinal tubules.
- Use of these pastes before nonsurgical periodontal therapy may be indicated for those patients whose sensitivity to scaling is not profound enough to warrant the use of local anesthetics.

Specialty products are recommended for today's cosmetic restoration when the use of traditional paste will damage the surface, resulting in a less than ideal appearance.
- NUPRO Shimmer (Dentsply Sirona) is not designed for stain removal due to the particle size in the paste being so fine they are not coarse enough to remove stain; however, they do produce a high shine on the already polished restoration.
- Clinpro Prophy Paste (3M ESPE) uses abrasive variability in its formulation; this abrasive begins as a coarse material to remove stain and then quickly breaks down to a fine paste to provide luster.
- Soft Shine (Waterpik Technologies) is made from micron-fine particles that effectively polish all types of composite and ceramic restorations.
- Traditional prophy paste is not recommended for use on esthetic restorative materials; use agents that have been specially formulated for esthetic restorative surfaces.

Dentifrice (Toothpaste)

Similar to prophylaxis paste, toothpaste contains a mixture of abrasive materials to clean tooth structures and restorations to enhance resistance to discoloration and plaque accumulation. The commercial toothpaste preparations contain 20% to 40% abrasive, coloring, flavoring, and therapeutic agents. The abrasive agents improve the efficiency of the toothbrush in the removal of stains, food debris, and biofilm. Additionally, they increase light reflected by the enamel. The lowest possible abrasive rankings are desirable to prevent removal of softer tooth structures and restorations (Fig. 17.15).

The American Dental Association Seal of Acceptance on toothpaste products indicates that the abrasive particles in the dentifrice do not exceed the maximal acceptable abrasiveness, and that scientific data verify claims made by the manufacturer (Table 17.3). The US Food and Drug Administration regulates the amount and type of abrasive that is placed in dentifrice.

Benefits of Dentifrices

- Assist in the reduction of biofilm
- Assist in the reduction of stains

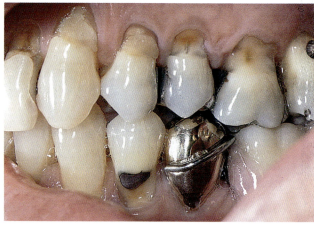

Fig. 17.15 Toothbrush abrasion; notice that the effects of abrasion are also seen on the amalgam restoration. (Courtesy Dr. Steve Eakle.)

- Assist in the reduction of dental caries
- Assist in the reduction of dentin hypersensitivity
- Assist in the remineralization of tooth structures
- Assist in the remoisturizing of dry mouth
- Assist in the reduction of calculus formation

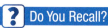 **Do You Recall?**

Why it is important to sequentially move from a course abrasive to a fine abrasive when polishing the tooth structure?

Factors Contributing to Dentifrice Abrasion

- Type of abrasive in the dentifrice
- Amount of abrasive used
- Stiffness of the toothbrush bristle
- Toothbrushing method used by the patient
- Frequency and duration of toothbrushing
- Amount of saliva present
- Type of restorations present
- Amount and location of exposed root surfaces present

Denture Cleansers

The use of a toothbrush or denture brush (preferred) with water and a mild cleaning agent (Fig. 17.16) is sufficient to remove most plaque, surface stains, and food debris from removable prosthetic appliances. Immersion of the prosthesis into commercially prepared denture

Table 17.3 Components of Prophy Paste and Toothpaste

PROPHY PASTE (%)	COMPONENT	TOOTHPASTE (%)
50–60	Abrasive	20–40
20–25	Humectant	20–40
10–20	Water	20–40
—	Foaming agent—SLS; removed from many dentifrices because of patient sensitivity	1–2
2–3	Flavoring/coloring agents	2–3
1–2	Therapeutic (fluoride)	1–2

SLS, Sodium lauryl sulfate.

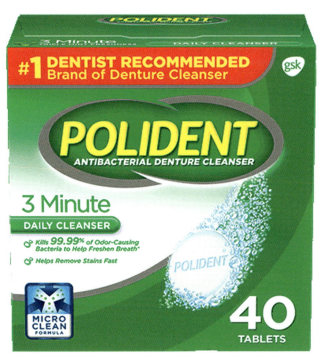

Fig. 17.16 Polident denture cleansing agent. (Courtesy GlaxoSmithKline.)

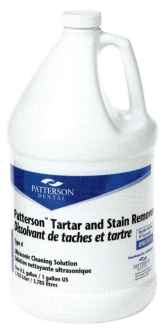

Fig. 17.17 In-office tartar and stain remover. (Courtesy Patterson Dental.)

cleansers that loosen stains and deposits then can be rinsed or brushed away is also appropriate. A dental ultrasonic agitating device may be used to improve the efficiency of a commercially prepared immersion agent. Commercially prepared stain and tartar agents are beneficial in the removal of calculus from the prosthesis.

> **Caution**
>
> A well-thought-out infection control protocol must be in place to prevent contamination of a removable prosthesis and ultrasonic cleaner.

Procedure for Cleaning a Removable Prosthesis in the Dental Office with an Ultrasonic Cleaner and Immersion Agent

1. Completely submerge the prosthesis in a sealed bag, such as a ziplock bag, or use an autoclavable beaker filled with an immersion agent (tarter and stain remover) (Fig. 17.17).
2. Follow the manufacturer's directions for correct dilution of the immersion agent, amount of time for immersion, and agitation in the ultrasonic, typically 10 to 15 minutes.
3. Remove the prosthesis and rinse thoroughly with water. Be careful to avoid contamination of the prosthesis and the liquid in the ultrasonic basin.
4. Remove loosened debris with a new denture brush, if needed.
5. Provide the denture brush to the patient for use at home.

Commercial denture cleansers should be nontoxic, nonabrasive, and harmless to the components of the prosthesis. Full acrylic prostheses can be soaked in dilute alkaline or acid commercial preparations. Prostheses with metal components should NOT be placed in dilute acid solutions or hypochlorites (bleach) because of the resultant corrosion to these metal components.

> **Clinical Tip**
>
> Patients should always be reminded to use products specifically developed for home care of removable prostheses and never to use regular toothpaste, powdered household cleansers, or bleach when cleaning their removable appliances at home, including dentures, partial dentures, orthodontic appliances, mouth guards, and whitening trays.

FINISHING AND POLISHING PROCEDURES

Finishing and polishing procedures follow a similar sequence. Sufficient amounts of material are removed to reproduce the anatomic contours of the restoration/prosthesis, and finer and finer cuts are then made into the material with diminishing abrasive agents until it takes on a smooth, shiny, mirror-like surface. The benefits of a properly finished and polished restoration/prosthesis include:

- Decreased biofilm retention
- Resistance to tarnish/corrosion
- Increased longevity of the restoration
- Decreased attrition of natural tooth surfaces during chewing
- Improved esthetics
- Improved health of surrounding tissues

It is important that the appropriate clinical decision be made regarding the choice of abrasive agents, the properties of the surface, and the order in which the abrasives are applied, and that attention be given to thorough removal of each abrasive agent before a finer one is used. If abrasive agents are left on structures or on delivery equipment, they continue to abrade even though a finer abrasive is currently being applied.

Some abrasive agents are designed for both finishing and polishing because of the presence of components with abrasive variability. One-step diamond micropolisher cups and points are appropriate for both finishing and polishing. The clinician must be careful of heat generated by the use of rotary instruments, controlling this by applying pressure and speed intermittently, and using water or air for cooling purposes.

In addition, care must be taken to consider the anatomic form of the tooth. The finished and polished restoration should have a smooth, continuous margin flush with the tooth surface. When restorative margins end at or near the root, instrumentation near or on this cavosurface margin may result in ditching or gouging of the softer cementum surfaces. Contours of teeth must be re-created and should not be flattened or overly rounded. The contact should not be polished. Polishing this area may remove material, resulting in an open contact that can lead to impaction of food, causing damage to the periodontium, or contributing to caries formation.

The provision of finishing and polishing procedures for tooth structures and restorative materials by the dental auxiliary is dependent on the scope of practice regulations established by each state.

> **⚠ Caution**
>
> Some intraoral finishing and polishing procedures are not allowed by the auxiliary under certain circumstances or with specific types of equipment according to state dental practice acts.

MARGINATION AND REMOVAL OF FLASH

Before finishing or polishing an amalgam or composite restoration, the clinician should check the integrity of the cavosurface margins for prematurities (overhanging margins) and deficiencies (Fig. 17.18). The detrimental effects of overhanging margins on hard and soft tissues are well documented. The overhanging margin catches biofilm that contains microorganisms that contribute to periodontal disease and caries, prevents the efficient use of dental floss, and increases inflammation.

The process of removing restoration prematurities to bring the restoration flush with the cavosurface

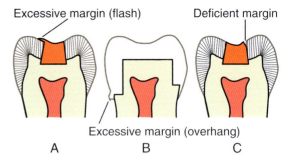

Fig. 17.18 Line drawing of **(A)** excessive occlusal margin (flash), **(B)** excessive proximal margin (overhang), and **(C)** deficient occlusal margin.

tooth structure is called **margination**. This process may vary from removal of feathered **flash** (thin, excess material extending beyond the preparation margin) to removal of **overhang** (ledges created by overhanging cervical margins). The decision to remove excessive material from a restoration is based on clinical and radiographic findings. Careful evaluation of the restoration is necessary to determine whether margination is indicated or the restoration needs to be replaced (see the accompanying box "Indications for Margination"). Margination may be indicated if the overhang is small, the contact is intact, and there is no indication of caries.

Margination is not generally within the scope of practice for the dental assistant, and although it is within the scope of practice for the dental hygienist in many states, it should not be considered a routine procedure. Careful consideration as to the type and amount of restorative material present must be made before completing this procedure.

> **Indications for Margination with Hand Instruments or a Slow-Speed Handpiece**
>
> Some state laws allow for assistant or hygienist to marginate restorations under these circumstances:
> - Overhang or flash is not extensive in size.
> - Tooth anatomy and contour can be improved.
> - Proximal contact is present.
> - Restoration is intact; fractures, open margins, or caries are not present.
> - The margin is accessible without damage to tissue or adjacent tooth structures.

The dental hygienist may use hand cutting instruments or an ultrasonic scaler to safely remove large overhanging margins. In some states, both auxiliaries can utilize slow-speed handpieces and rotary instruments to remove excess materials. Hand cutting instruments such as an amalgam knife, scalers and files, or rotary cutting diamonds burs and carbide burs, are used to remove overhangs. When using hand instruments for margination, use very sharp instruments and work apically to the margin of the restoration, using a shaving motion in diagonal overlapping strokes and keeping the instrument in contact with the tooth surface. Avoid trying to remove too much of the overhang, in a single stroke. An ultrasonic scaler, or slow-speed rotary handpiece with abrasive points and cups, may be used to remove overhanging margins as well. Follow this with hand cutting instruments and finish with abrasive strips, and then check the results with floss and an explorer.

Do You Recall?

How does the removal of flash contribute to the health of the oral tissues around a restoration?

! Caution

If it is determined that the overhanging margin or flash is too large for safe and effective removal by the auxiliary, the patient should be scheduled for an appointment with the dentist, who will perform this procedure or replace the restoration.

FINISHING AND POLISHING AMALGAM

It is generally recommended that amalgam restorations be polished no sooner than 24 hours after placement. The amount of finishing and polishing required depends on the care taken in carving and burnishing the amalgam at the time of placement and the effects of the oral environment on older restorations (Fig. 17.19).

PROCEDURES FOR FINISHING AND POLISHING AMALGAM RESTORATIONS

Polishing of amalgam should begin by evaluating cavosurface margins for excess material, and remove as indicated (Procedure 17.1). Finishing is next, using abrasive devices to remove severe scratches and surface defects. Bonded and coated abrasives greater than 25 μm in particle size or special multifluted finishing burs are used. Polishing that is accomplished with bonded, coated, or loose abrasives ranging in particle diameter from 20 μm to submicron-sized gives the amalgam restoration a mirror-like luster. Care must be taken whenever rotary instruments are used to avoid the generation of excessive heat and aerosols. The use of water through an air-water syringe or from the handpiece and proper evacuation are recommended.

FINISHING AND POLISHING COMPOSITE

Composite restorations are finished and polished in three steps as part of the restorative procedure (Procedure 17.2). Marginal and occlusal excesses are first removed in initial finishing with diamonds or multi-fluted carbide burs. Intermediate finishing is accomplished with flexible disks (Fig. 17.20), cups, and strips, beginning with coarse and sequentially proceeding to superfine. Final polishing is accomplished with a submicron aluminum oxide–based polishing paste applied with soft cups or felt pads (see the accompanying box, "Finishing and Polishing Composite Restorations").

Finishing and Polishing Composite Restorations

Initial finishing: Bonded and coated rotary abrasives, 100 μm or larger, or multi-fluted carbide or diamond finishing burs
Intermediate finishing: Bonded and coated rotary abrasives <100 μm but >20 μm
Final polishing: Bonded and coated abrasives or polishing paste from 20 to 0.3 μm to produce a final luster.

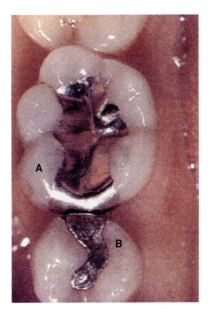

Fig. 17.19 **(A)** Polished amalgam restoration. **(B)** Unpolished amalgam restoration.

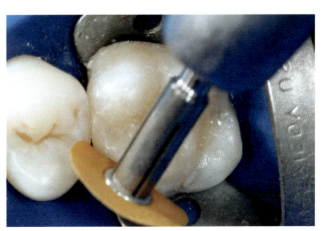

Fig. 17.20 Intermediate finishing with flexible disk. (From Heyman H, Swift E, Ritter A: *Sturdevant's art & science of operative dentistry*, ed 6, St. Louis, 2013, Elsevier.)

Traditional prophy paste, air polishing, and the use of ultrasonic scalers are not recommended for most esthetic restorations. If the composite has developed extrinsic staining, it may need to be polished after placement. Fine abrasives are used in progression from fine to finest, with care taken to change the delivery device and rinse thoroughly between each polishing. The procedure should remove only the outermost stained surface and should produce a lustrous finish.

FINISHING AND POLISHING GOLD ALLOY

Precious and nonprecious crowns, inlays, and onlays are finished and polished in the dental laboratory before they are delivered to the dental office for final fitting and cementation. In the process of final fitting, minor adjustments made with abrasive stones and diamonds may be necessary. It is important that the resultant scratches are removed before final cementation. Burlew wheels on a slow-speed handpiece are used, followed by rouge on a rag wheel (Fig. 17.11).

FINISHING AND POLISHING CERAMICS (PORCELAIN)

Ceramic restorations (including porcelain) achieve a glassy smooth surface from the glazing procedure at high temperatures (see Chapter 10). Occasionally, they need some adjustment and are finished and polished in the dental laboratory. Adjustments made chairside during the fitting of these restorations are done with fine-grit diamonds (diamonds leave a surface that is very rough and difficult to smooth). The resultant roughened ceramic surface after clinical adjustment has been shown to increase wear of opposing tooth structure. Clinicians must properly finish and polish ceramic restorations after making adjustments. Rubber polishing points and wheels designed for ceramics are used for finishing, and diamond polishing paste (Fig. 17.21) is used for the final polish of the restoration to an enamel-like luster.

> ⚠ **Caution**
> Heat generated during adjustment may also result in cracking of ceramic—always use low speed and low pressure to minimize heat generation and cracking.

Characteristics of a Properly Finished and Polished Restoration

- Smooth anatomic contours
- Contact areas intact with normal form
- Embrasures spaced correctly
- Refined margins
- Smooth surfaces
- Restored function
- Eliminate biofilm retention irregularities
- Restored gingival health

Chairside Adjusting and Polishing of Acrylic Denture Bases

After the placement of a new denture or partial denture, a patient may need to have a denture or partial adjusted due to sore spots or overextensions of the acrylic flanges into the vestibule or posterior of the mouth that makes the appliance hard to wear. The dentist will evaluate the denture for any necessary adjustments and make those adjustment at chairside. The first step is to trim any excess material with an acrylic bur (Fig. 17.22, far left). (See Chapter 14 for detection of sore spots with Pressure Indicator Paste or Colored Transfer Applicators.)

Once the appropriate amount of material has been removed, the dentist will polish the denture by using a series of abrasives and rubber points to eliminate the roughness caused by the burs and more abrasive points (see Fig. 17.22; points are in order by abrasiveness with blue as most abrasive to yellow as least abrasive). To ensure scratches are not left in the surface of the appliance that could harbor bacteria, the

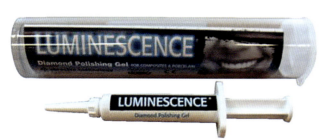

Fig. 17.21 Diamond polishing paste utilized for the final polish of ceramic restorations. (Courtesy Abrasive Technology, Inc.)

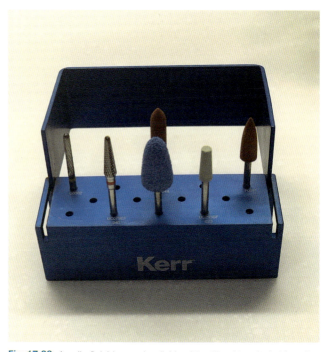

Fig. 17.22 Acrylic finishing and polishing kit utilized for chairside polishing of a partial or complete denture. (Courtesy Matt Crimaldi.)

dentist will incrementally move from the most abrasive material to the least abrasive material. This will leave a smooth surface on the appliance.

Additionally, when a patient loses weight or healing has occurred after surgical removal of the teeth, a denture or partial may require a reline procedure to ensure proper fit. This reline material may also require adjusting and polishing.

> **KEY POINTS: Finishing and Polishing of Various Materials**
>
> 1. Amalgam—clinicians must wait 24 hours before finishing and polishing with rotary instruments
>   - Finishing accomplished with carbide burs or stones
>   - Polishing completed in a sequence of brownies, greenies, and super greenies
> 2. Composite—can be finished and polished immediately after placement and proper polymerization
>   - Finishing accomplished with flexible abrasive disks or cups or multi-fluted finishing burs
>   - Polishing completed with aluminum oxide polishing paste
> 3. Gold—finished and polished in the dental lab, but requires additional finishing and polishing when the occlusion needs adjustment in the dental office
>   - Finishing accomplished with abrasive stones and diamond burs
>   - Polishing completed with burlew wheels and rouge on rag wheel
> 4. Ceramic—finished and polished in the dental lab, but requires additional finishing and polishing in the dental office when adjustments have been made
>   - Finishing accomplished with rubber polishing points and wheels
>   - Polishing completed with diamond polish paste
> 5. Acrylic—finished and polished in the dental lab; however, adjustments may be needed in the dental office to resolve sore spots for the patient
>   - Finish and polish with rubber points and slurry of pumice on rag wheel

POLISHING DURING ORAL PROPHYLAXIS (CORONAL POLISH)

Before the coronal polishing procedure is started, a careful tactile evaluation of tooth surfaces must be done to correctly identify and remove calculus. If a restoration is incorrectly identified as calculus and is aggressively scaled, the restoration may be removed or altered to the point of needing replacement. In addition, all restorative materials must be identified to prevent undesired removal, damaging of margins, or scratching of the surface by traditional, commercially prepared prophy paste (see Chapter 2 for identification of restorative materials). Adverse effects on the tooth surface with the use of prophy paste and the philosophy of selective polish are discussed earlier in this chapter (see the Caution box in the section "Prophylaxis (Prophy) Paste"); polishing must be a carefully considered part of the oral prophylaxis.

AMALGAM

Low-copper amalgam restorations will tarnish and corrode over the years (see Chapter 11). Polishing during oral prophylaxis may greatly benefit these restorations. Rubber cups or bristle brushes with commercially prepared prophy paste are used on occlusal and smooth surfaces and dental tape on proximal surfaces.

COMPOSITE

Composite restorations, which become stained after placement, may be polished as part of a regular maintenance appointment. The use of ultrasonic and sonic scalers and air-polishing devices should be avoided on or around these restorations because these instruments may damage the surface of the restoration. The use of traditional prophy pastes may cause excessive wear; typically these restorations should be polished with aluminum oxide polishing paste. It is important that composite restorations be polished only if stain is present, and that appropriate manufacturer's recommended materials are selected and used to avoid scratching or altering the surface of the softer composite materials.

Begin stain removal with the least abrasive products. If the stain is not easily removed with fine paste, proceed to more aggressive grits or rubber polishing points and finishing disks. Pay close attention to the restoration's contour and marginal integrity, always keeping the rotary instrument moving using a light, sweeping intermittent motion. Complete the polishing procedure using light pressure with a very wet, specialized polishing paste on a soft felt pad. Total polishing time should not exceed 30 seconds on any stained surface.

Remember to proceed sequentially from most abrasive to least abrasive polishing material, using a clean or new prophy cup at each step, to polish the restoration. Staining at the margins may also represent microleakage (see Chapter 8) that penetrates under the restoration. These stains cannot be polished away (Procedure 17.2). Have stains at the margins evaluated by the dentist if they cannot be polished away.

GOLD ALLOYS AND CERAMICS

Ceramics and gold alloys are extremely resistant to staining (see Chapter 10). If scratches or irregularities are present, they are usually due to instrumentation that has scratched the outer glaze of the ceramic or high polish of the gold. Regular prophy paste is not recommended for polishing ceramic restorations because of possible removal of the glaze layer. Specialty pastes are available that contain microfine particles that are not harmful for polishing porcelain veneers and crowns (Fig. 17.23).

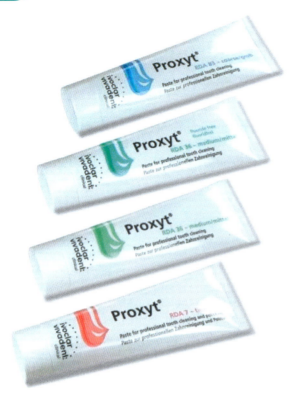

Fig. 17.23 Proxyt polishing paste. (Courtesy Ivoclar Vivadent.)

RESIN/CEMENT INTERFACE

Margins on resin-bonded ceramic restorations are more susceptible to staining because of the properties of resin cements. Stains accumulating at the ceramic/cement interface must be evaluated carefully for actual staining or microleakage.

IMPLANTS

The clinician must be careful not to abrade the surface integrity of titanium implants (see Chapter 13). Biofilm may be removed with special titanium hand instruments, and nonabrasive cleaning paste or tin oxide. Air polishing with glycine or erythritol is also appropriate for removal of soft deposits on implants.

AIR POLISHING AND AIR ABRASION

Air polishing and air abrasion have specific applications in the dental office. When used, clinicians should follow manufacturers' recommendations for precautions in safety and contraindications in individual clinical applications (see Table 17.4).

Supragingival Air Polishing

Supragingival air polishing uses several forms of powder:
- Sodium bicarbonate
- Aluminum trihydroxide
- Glycine
- Erythritol

Table 17.4	Indications and Contraindications for Air Polishing
INDICATIONS FOR AIR POLISHING	CONTRAINDICATIONS FOR AIR POLISHING
Patient with supragingival extrinsic stain	Patient with respiratory disease
Patients with biofilm accumulation	Patient with sodium restriction diets when sodium bicarbonate is powder of choice for stain removal
Patients with biofilm induced inflammation	Patient with limited swallowing
	Patient with difficulty breathing
	Patient with communicable infections
	Immunocompromised patients
	Patient taking potassium, antidiuretics, or steroid therapy

- Calcium sodium phosphosilicate
- Calcium carbonate

Additionally, there are flavoring agents, air, and water dispensed at a pressure of approximately 40 to 60 psi as a fast, effective, and efficient means of removing stains and soft deposits from enamel surfaces and in pits and fissures. Glycine and erythritol powders have been found to produce less surface damage on restoratives than sodium bicarbonate powders; however, glycine does not remove stain and is only effective in biofilm removal. Calcium sodium phosphosilicate powder has desensitizing results in cases of dentinal hypersensitivity, and aluminum trihydroxide powders contain harder particles that should not be used on most esthetic restorations.

Proper technique is essential to remove stain and biofilm while controlling contaminated aerosols and prevent soft tissue damage. The closer the tip of the air-polishing unit is to the tooth surface, the greater the amount of aerosols produced. The nozzle of the air-polishing unit should be kept in a constant circular motion 3 to 4 mm from the tooth surface, at an angle of 60 to 80 degrees on smooth surfaces and a 90-degree angle on occlusal surfaces. Most research continues to recommend caution near restorations, particularly composite, resin cement, and porcelain surfaces (Fig. 17.24).

Air polishing is less abrasive than traditional prophy paste, as the particles used in air polishing have a Mohs hardness ranking of 3 versus the ranking of 6 found in some traditional prophy pastes. Air polishing is not contraindicated for use on enamel and may be less damaging to cementum or dentin than traditional polishing. In addition, air polishing with glycine or erythritol can be safely used on titanium implants and orthodontically banded/bracketed teeth.

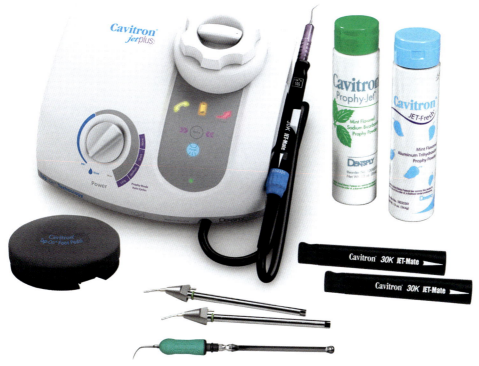

Fig. 17.24 Combined ultrasonic and supragingival air polishing unit. (Courtesy Dentsply International, York, Pennsylvania].)

> **? Do You Recall?**
>
> What type of air polishing powders are recommended for supragingival air polishing when stain removal is required?

Subgingival Air Polishing

Subgingival air polishing is the process of polishing the anatomical crown and clinical root surface using fine particles under air pressure of approximately 40 pounds per square inch to remove biofilm subgingivally. Subgingival air polishing improves periodontal health by detoxifying root surfaces in shallow to moderate or deep periodontal pockets. Glycine and erythritol (Mohs ranking of 2) may be used for subgingival air polishing. Other forms of powder (sodium bicarbonate, aluminum trihydroxide, calcium sodium phosphosilicate, or calcium carbonate) should not be used as they are more abrasive, which can cause damage to the tooth structure and the junctional epithelium.

As with supragingival air polishing, proper technique is essential with subgingival air polishing to prevent the spread of dental aerosols and air-polishing powders. A subgingival nozzle is required to reach the depth of the sulcus (Fig. 17.25). The nozzle is inserted into the sulcus parallel to the long axis of the root until resistance is met, then moved back from the base of the pocket about a 3 mm distance. At this time the tip is activated, dispensing powder (glycine or erythritol) and water under pressure to remove biofilm. The tip should not be activated for longer than 5 seconds per root surface.

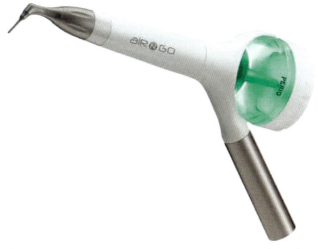

Fig. 17.25 Subgingival air polishing unit. (Courtesy Acteon Group.)

> **Clinical Tip**
>
> Air polishing has been shown to be very effective in the removal of stains and debris from pits and fissures. Debris in the fissures prevents adequate etching and penetration of sealant into the fissures. Air polishing eliminates this cause for many pit and fissure sealant failures.

Air Abrasion

Air abrasion, also known as *microabrasion*, uses greater compressed air pressure and a 27- or 50-μm aluminum oxide powder particle size with a Mohs hardness ranking of 9. This process is used for chairside cleaning of cast appliances before cementation, intraoral

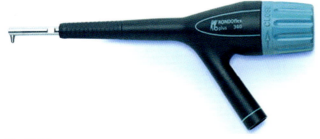

Fig. 17.26 Air abrasion tip. (Courtesy KaVo Dental, Charlotte, North Carolina.)

repair of ceramic and composite restorations, and preparation of tooth surfaces before bonding. Air pressure of 40 to 160 psi and a controlled adjustable-tip orifice allow aluminum oxide particles to strike a tooth or restoration with enough force to effectively abrade the surface. Cutting can be controlled to remove minimal amounts of tooth and restorative structure (Fig. 17.26).

 Caution

The use of appropriate clinician and patient safety equipment and control of aerosols with high-volume evacuation are critical for both air polishing and air abrasion.

LABORATORY FINISHING AND POLISHING

Some appliances and restorations such as complete and partial dentures and gold crowns must be polished after adjustments have been made to them. The adjustments can be made at chairside and some polishing devices are available for chairside use. However, many clinicians utilize rag wheels and/or felt tips or wheels on the dental lathe in the dental office laboratory to complete the final polishing of these appliances and restorations (prior to cementation) (Fig. 17.27).

RAG WHEEL

The rag wheel is a polishing device made of muslin or cloth clamped or sewn together in the shape of a wheel. They come in a variety of sizes that can be used with a laboratory handpiece or dental lathe. A polishing agent is added to the rag wheel and used for buffing or polishing acrylic appliances such as denture and partial denture bases (Figs. 17.28 and 17.29).

FELT CONES AND WHEELS

Felt cones and wheels are polishing devices made of felt in the shape of cones and wheels that can be used with a laboratory handpiece or dental lathe. The

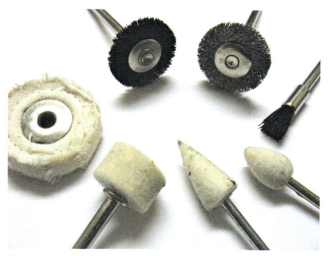

Fig. 17.27 Rag wheel (*left most*), felt tips (*bottom three*), and brushes (*top three*). (Courtesy T. Rand Collins, MD.)

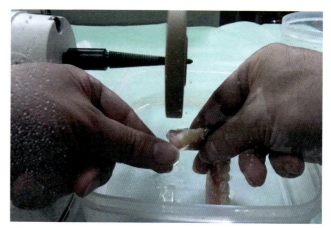

Fig. 17.28 Polishing acrylic on partial denture. (Courtesy Masanari Oshima.)

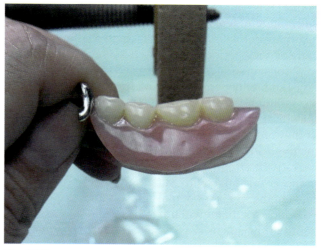

Fig. 17.29 Polished acrylic. (Courtesy Masanari Oshima.)

abrasive agent is added to the felt polishing device and used to smooth restorations and appliances (Fig. 17.30).

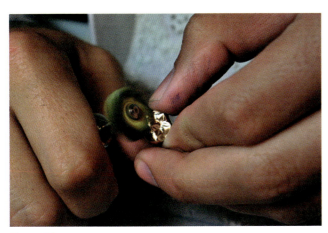

Fig. 17.30 Dental lab technician polishes a gold crown using polishing compound on a cloth wheel. (U.S. Air Force photo by Airman Nicole Sikorski/Released.)

SAFETY/INFECTION CONTROL

Aerosols are created whenever a rotary device and moisture are used, which can provide a means for disease transmission. The use of rotary devices may produce particulate matter and vapors from the substrate being abraded. More specifically, silica particles from restorations and mercury vapors pose potential health risks. In addition, splatter from abrasives can produce serious eye damage. These particles are released into the air and are hazards to dental personnel and their patients. The use of precautionary PPE, including a mask and eye protection, is essential for the dental team. Protective eyewear is highly recommended for the patient as well. The use of preprocedure antimicrobial rinses has been shown to reduce microbial aerosols, and high-speed evacuation is recommended instead of a saliva ejector.

Equipment utilized to adjust, finish, and polish restorations or appliances must be disinfected or sterilized between use with patients. All materials, such as burs, mandrels, rag wheels, and felt cones, must be cleaned of loose particles prior to being packaged for sterilization. Additionally, pumice should be replaced in the dental lathe between uses with patients to prevent cross-contamination.

> **⚠ Caution**
> - Maintain dental laboratory asepsis by sterilizing or disinfecting all wheels and rotary cutting devices
> - Use fresh, dry powders for each procedure, and remove contaminated portions of stick or block abrasives
> - Maintain adequate ventilation to efficiently remove particulates from the air

PATIENT EDUCATION

Composite restorations and resin-bonded ceramic restorations are particularly susceptible to staining. Effective oral hygiene techniques and awareness of dietary staining and stain-producing habits can prevent a certain amount of surface discoloration. Thorough removal of biofilm from restorative surfaces will prevent staining associated with bacterial accumulation.

Patient education on the effects of staining foods (colored beverages such as coffee, tea, soft drinks, and wine), and the result of tobacco stain on composite restorations and tooth surfaces, should be part of the original restorative procedure, as should regular recall appointments. Patients with exposed cementum and dentin are particularly susceptible to staining and the effects of abrasives. In an attempt to improve the color of their teeth, patients may use home remedies or excessively abrasive commercial products. The consequences often are toothbrush abrasion and wear of restorations and tooth surfaces. Patient education should include the use of approved abrasive agents.

The maintenance of esthetic restorations and tooth structure is a collaborative effort between the patient and the clinician. Good patient education and the evaluation of teeth and restorations for appropriate polishing and finishing will increase oral esthetics and patient satisfaction.

SUMMARY

The decision to abrade a surface to contour, finish, polish, or cleanse a structure requires careful consideration. The clinician must have knowledge of the properties of the material being abraded, the abrasive, and the factors that affect abrasion. The process of abrasion can produce undesirable effects if not carefully controlled. Appropriate use of abrasion can also produce a surface that will contribute to the esthetics and longevity of the restoration and the health of surrounding oral tissues.

INSTRUCTIONAL VIDEOS

See the Evolve Resources site for a variety of educational videos that reinforce the material covered in this chapter.

CHAPTER 17   Abrasion, Finishing, Polishing, and Cleaning

Procedure 17.1   Finishing and Polishing a Preexisting Amalgam Restoration

See Evolve site for Competency Sheet.

Consider the following with this procedure: safety glasses are recommended for the patient, personal protective equipment (PPE) is required for the operator, ensure appropriate safety protocols are followed, and check your local state guidelines before performing this procedure.

EQUIPMENT/SUPPLIES (FIG. 17.31)

1. Mirror and explorer
2. Air-water syringe
3. Articulating paper
4. Isolation materials
5. Slow-speed handpiece and attachment
6. Finishing burs, abrasive rubber points, disks, and cups
7. Dappen dish
8. Pumice or polishing paste
9. Disposable rubber cup and brush
10. Tin oxide

NOTE: Polish amalgam no sooner than 24 hours after placement to allow the amalgam to develop its maximal strength.

PROCEDURE STEPS

Examine the cavosurface margins of the entire restoration for excess material.
   NOTE: Remove excess material to prevent plaque accumulation or gingival irritation.
1. Check occlusion with articulating paper and clinically for premature occlusal contact; look for equal intensity of the articulating paper markings.
   NOTE: Premature occlusal contact can cause sensitivity and excessive wear on the restoration or opposing teeth; the dentist will need to adjust the occlusion.
2. Remove proximal cavosurface excesses with an amalgam knife or a similar sharp instrument, using short, overlapping strokes (Fig. 17.32).
3. Isolate the restoration with cotton rolls and saliva ejector.

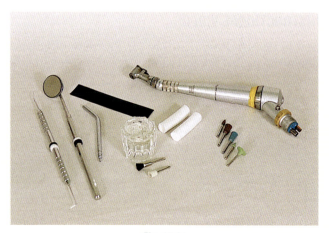

Fig. 17.31

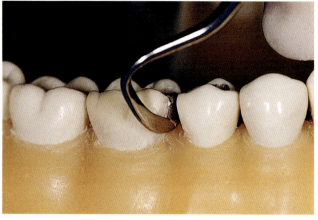

Fig. 17.32

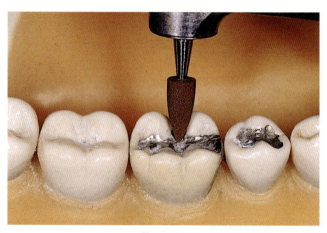

Fig. 17.33

4. Use rubber abrasive points or finishing burs for the occlusal surface and a disk or cup for smooth surfaces, beginning with the most coarse abrasive (i.e., a brown cup or "brownie") and then with finer abrasives ("greenies" and finally "super greenies") (Figs. 17.33 and 17.34). Adapt the side of the abrasive point to the restoration and tooth.
5. Use slow to low-moderate speed, always moving the abrasive from the tooth to the amalgam to prevent ditching the cavosurface margin.
6. Use a light sweeping intermittent motion while keeping the finishing instrument moving to avoid excessive heat and mercury vapor production. Maintain a wet environment to reduce heat.
7. Rinse the area thoroughly when changing abrasives to prevent the more abrasive particles from abrading the surface.
8. Use the rubber cup and brush with a slurry of pumice and then tin oxide (Fig. 17.35).
9. Keep the cup or brush in motion at all times, using light intermittent strokes and moderate speed.

Procedure 17.1 Finishing and Polishing a Preexisting Amalgam Restoration—cont'd

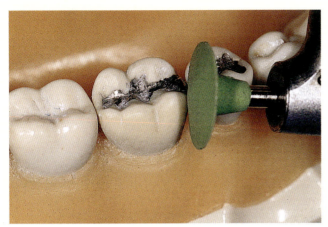

Fig. 17.34

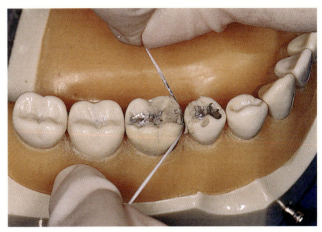

Fig. 17.36

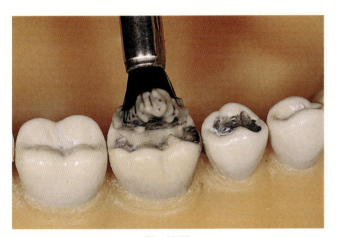

Fig. 17.35

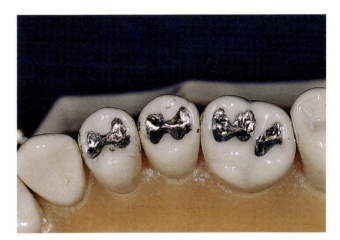

Fig. 17.37

10. Rinse thoroughly between the use of pumice and tin oxide.
11. Polish the proximal surfaces with a handheld finishing strip or pumice and dental tape.
12. Wrap the strip around the tooth contours to avoid flattening of proximal contours (Fig. 17.36).
13. Do not polish through the contact area. Polishing through the contact area can create a weak or open contact.
14. **NOTE:** The final product is shown in Fig. 17.37.

Procedure 17.2 Polishing a Preexisting Composite Restoration

See Evolve site for Competency Sheet.

Consider the following with this procedure: safety glasses are recommended for the patient, PPE is required for the operator, ensure appropriate safety protocols are followed, and check your local state guidelines before performing this procedure.

EQUIPMENT/SUPPLIES (FIG. 17.38)

1. Mirror and explorer
2. Air-water syringe
3. Isolation materials
4. Slow-speed handpiece and attachment
5. Abrasive finishing disks
6. Sterilizable mandrel
7. Abrasive flexible wheels and points
8. Polishing paste
9. Rubber cup

NOTE: Initial contouring, finishing, and polishing are done immediately after placement of the composite restoration.

Continued

Procedure 17.2 Polishing a Preexisting Composite Restoration—cont'd

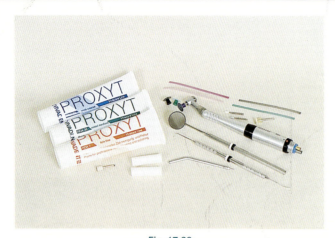

Fig. 17.38

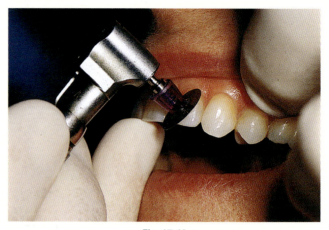

Fig. 17.40

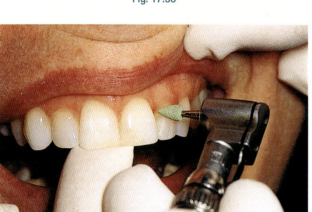

Fig. 17.39

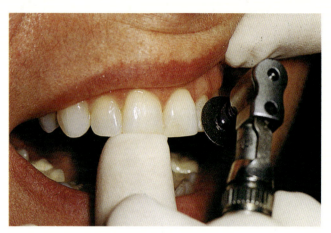

Fig. 17.41

PROCEDURE STEPS

1. Examine the restoration for staining.
   NOTE: Do not polish if stain is not present.
2. Isolate the area with cotton rolls and saliva ejector.
3. Remove cavosurface flash with a sharp scaler or a gold knife.
   NOTE: A gold knife, also called a finishing knife or amalgam knife, has a small, thin blade designed to carve restorative materials.
   NOTE: Avoid deeply scratching the restorative material. A shaving motion is used rather than bulk removal, as bulk removal may result in voids at the margins if excess composite is removed.
4. Use, in order, coarse to fine abrasive disks on a sterilizable mandrel or flexible wheels and rubber points, rinsing after each application (Figs. 17.39 and 17.40).
   NOTE: Rinse thoroughly to completely eliminate coarser particles before polishing with finer abrasive disks, to prevent overabrasion.
5. Use a light sweeping intermittent motion from enamel to restoration (Fig. 17.41).
   NOTE: This pattern of movement prevents ditching of restorations at the margins.
6. Keep the rotary device in motion at all times.
   NOTE: Smooth surfaces can be polished using cups and disks; occlusal surfaces are better reached with points (Fig. 17.42).
7. Complete the polish with sequentially applied abrasive paste on a rubber cup.
   NOTE: This must be an abrasive paste designed for polishing composites; begin with coarse and proceed through superfine.
8. Polish proximal surfaces with handheld polishing strips or polishing paste and dental tape (Fig. 17.43).
   NOTE: These strips must be very thin to prevent loss of the proximal contact.
9. Avoid flattening of proximal contours.
   NOTE: Keep the rotary polishing device or abrasive strip contoured to the shape of the tooth.
10. Rinse thoroughly and evaluate for smoothness and luster.

Procedure 17.2 Polishing a Preexisting Composite Restoration—cont'd

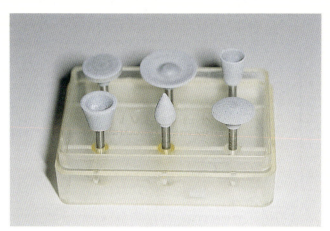

Fig. 17.42

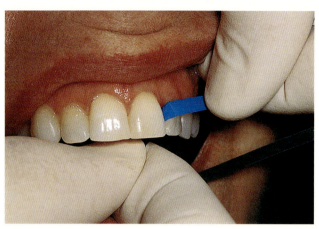

Fig. 17.43

Review and Discussion

Review Questions

Select the one correct response for each of the following multiple-choice questions.

1. The goal of finishing and polishing of restorations includes:
   a. The removal of excess material
   b. The smoothing of roughened surfaces
   c. The production of better esthetics
   d. All of the above
2. Cleaning of teeth is primarily meant to:
   a. Remove excess material
   b. Smooth roughened surfaces
   c. Remove soft deposits
   d. Recontour surfaces
3. The depth and space between cuts made by an abrasive are determined by:
   a. The properties of the abrasive
   b. The properties of the substrate being abraded
   c. The contour of the restoration
   d. Both a and b
4. Which of the following represents the correct hardness ranking, from hardest to softest?
   a. Gold, amalgam, composite, enamel
   b. Enamel, composite, amalgam, gold
   c. Composite, enamel, gold, amalgam
   d. Amalgam, enamel, composite, gold
5. All of the following will increase the rate of abrasion except:
   a. Increased pressure
   b. Decreased speed
   c. Use of larger abrasive particles
   d. Use of more abrasive particles than substrate
6. Which powder is best for subgingival air polishing practices?
   a. Sodium bicarbonate
   b. Aluminum trihydroxide
   c. Glycine
   d. Calcium carbonate
7. To control the numbers of abrasive particles that contact the surface:
   a. The operator should increase the speed
   b. The operator should decrease the pressure
   c. The operator should use a lubricant
   d. The operator should not use rotary instruments
8. Loose abrasives:
   a. Are safe sided
   b. Are embedded in cups and brushes
   c. Come in various shapes
   d. Use sterilizable mandrels
9. A substance used to prevent a dentifrice from drying is called a(n):
   a. Humectant
   b. Binder
   c. Detergent
   d. Alkaline peroxide
10. After polishing a patient's teeth, you notice scratches on a gold crown. The following most likely contributed to these scratches:
    a. Use of an inappropriate polishing agent
    b. Corrosion of the crown
    c. Improper toothbrushing
    d. None of the above would contribute to scratches on the crown

For answers to Review Questions, see the Appendix.

Case-Based Discussion Topics

1. Discuss how the operator uses knowledge of the factors that affect abrasion to control the polishing sequence of an amalgam restoration, a composite restoration, and a gold restoration.
2. Describe the process for using the subgingival air polisher to remove biofilm from a periodontal pocket, and identify which powders can be used subginvially.
3. List two materials used to polish stains from the coronal surfaces of teeth, and discuss the contraindications to using various abrasives on tooth surfaces.

A 30-year-old computer programmer comes to the dental office complaining of catching dental floss on a new Class II distal occlusal (DO) composite restoration on tooth #29. Examination reveals excess composite at the gingival margin and an overcontoured distofacial surface of this restoration.
Describe the instruments, materials, and techniques for correcting the problem and identify how this problem could have been prevented.

BIBLIOGRAPHY

Shen C, Rawls HR, Esquivel-Upshaw JF: *Phillips' Science of Dental Materials*, ed 13, St Louis, 2022, Elsevier.

Barnes CM: Polishing esthetic restorative materials, *Dimens Dent Hyg* 8(24):26–28, 2010.

Barnes CM: Shining a new light on selective polishing, *Dimens Dent Hyg* 10(3):42–44, 2012.

Barnes CM: *Air polishing: a mainstay for dental hygiene, ADA continuing education recognition program*, 2013, PennWell Publications. Available at https://www.yumpu.com/en/document/read/22671110/air-polishing-a-mainstay-for-dental-hygiene-ineedcecom.

Calley K: Maintaining the beauty and longevity of esthetic restorations, *Dimens Dent Hyg* 7:38–41, 2009.

Darby M: *An evidence-based approach to cleansing and polishing teeth*, 2012, The American Academy for Oral Systemic Health. Available at https://aaosh.org/evidence-based-approach-cleansing-polishing-teeth/.

Darby M, Walsh M: *Dental Hygiene Theory and Practice*, ed 4, Missouri, 2015, Elsevier.

Davis K: *Biofilm removal with air polishing and subgingival air polishing, ADA continuing education recognition program*, 2013, Pennwell Publications. Available at https://fliphtml5.com/jarv/ijwq/basic.

Davis K: Do you know about air-flow perio? *RDH Magazine*, Available at https://www.rdhmag.com/articles/print/volume-33/issue-1/coumns/glycine-powder-aids-in-periodontal-biofilm-removal.html, 2013.

Gomleksiz S, Gomleksiz O: *The effect of contemporary finishing and polishing systems on the surface roughness of bulk fill resin composite and nanocomposites* Available at. In *Wiley* 2021. https://onlinelibrary.wiley.com/doi/epdf/10.1111/jerd.12874.

Gutkowski S: The trek to positive polishing, mastering the challenge to actually use air polishers, *RDH Mag* 6:68–70, 2013.

Harmon J, Brame JL: *Air polishing for today's dental hygienist, a new addition to the biofilm management armamentarium, air polishing offers significant benefits to both patients and clinicians* Available at. In *Dimens Dent Hyg*, 2018. https://dimensionsofdentalhygiene.com/article/air-polishing-for-todays-dental-hygienist/.

Mopper K: Contouring, finishing, and polishing anterior composites, *Inside Dent* 7(3):62–70, 2011.

Mossman SL: Material selection and maintenance, *Dimens Dent Hyg* 12:63–67, 2014.

Pence S: Polishing basics, *Dimens Dent Hyg* 11(26):28, 2013.

Pence S: Polishing particulars, *Dimens Dent Hyg* 11(26):28, 2013.

Robinson DS: *Modern Dental Assisting*, ed 13, Philadelphia, 2023, Elsevier.

Sorensen JA: Finishing and polishing with modern ceramic systems, *Inside Dent* 2:10–16, 2013.

Vargas MA, Margeas R: A systematic approach to contouring and polishing anterior resin composite restorations: a checklist manifesto, *J Esthetic Restorat Dent* 33(1):20–26, 2020.

Wenzler J, Krause F, Bocher S, Falk W, Birkenmaier A, Conrads G, Braun A: Antimicrobial impact of different air-polishing powders in a subgingival biofilm model, *Antibiotics* 10(12): 1464, 2021.

Wilkins EM, Wyche CJ, Boyd LD: *Clinical Practice of the Dental Hygienist*, ed 13, Philadelphia, 2021, Wolters Kluwer.

18 Preventive and Desensitizing Materials

http://evolve.elsevier.com/Eakle/materials/

Chapter Objectives

On completion of this chapter, the student should be able to:

1. Describe the applications of fluoride in preventive dentistry.
2. Explain how fluoride protects teeth from caries.
3. Discuss the various methods of fluoride delivery.
4. Explain the benefit of using an antimicrobial rinse in conjunction with fluoride.
5. Describe the antimicrobial effects of chlorhexidine.
6. Apply topical fluoride gel, foam, varnish, or silver diamine fluoride as permitted by the state Dental Practice Act.
7. Describe how sealants protect pits and fissures from dental caries.
8. List the components of sealant material.
9. Apply sealants to teeth as permitted by the state Dental Practice Act.
10. Recite causes of tooth sensitivity.
11. Explain how desensitizing agents work.
12. List the types of materials used to treat sensitive teeth.
13. Apply desensitizing agents to sensitive teeth as permitted by the state Dental Practice Act.
14. Explain the remineralization process of enamel.
15. Describe how products for remineralization work.
16. Explain how resin infiltration of the early white spot lesion works.
17. Apply remineralizing products as permitted by the state Dental Practice Act.

KEY TERMS

Antimicrobial Mouthrinse liquid used to rinse the oral cavity to reduce or suppress bacteria associated with dental caries or periodontal disease

Cariogenic substances or microorganisms that promote dental caries

Demineralization action that removes mineral from the tooth, usually caused by acids

Dental Caries a disease process whereby bacteria in biofilm metabolize carbohydrates and produce acids that remove mineral from teeth and permit bacteria to invade the tooth and do further damage

Desensitizing Agent a chemical that seals open dentinal tubules to reduce tooth sensitivity to air, sweets, and temperature changes

Erosion loss of tooth structure caused by dietary or gastric acids, not by bacterial metabolism (caries process)

Fluorapatite tooth mineral that results when fluoride is incorporated into the tooth

Fluoride naturally occurring mineral that helps strengthen and protect tooth structure from dental caries

Fluorosis enamel condition caused by ingesting excessive levels of fluoride

Over-the-Counter (OTC) available in retail or drug stores without a doctor's prescription

Prevention/Preventive Aids chemicals, devices, or procedures that inhibit, reduce, or eliminate disease or tooth destruction in the oral cavity

Remineralization process that replaces mineral lost from the tooth by an acid attack

Sealant a protective resin that is bonded to enamel to protect pits and fissures from dental caries

Substantivity property of a material that has a prolonged therapeutic effect after its initial use

---

CAMBRA (caries management by risk assessment) is a common practice in many dental offices. Dental auxiliaries play important roles in assisting the dentist to prevent disease and maintain the health of patients. They can gather information about caries risk factors, educate patients about the disease processes, and the measures needed to prevent the disease. Materials needed to prevent dental diseases are widely used in the dental office. Fluorides, antimicrobial mouthrinses, silver diamine fluoride, and sealants are important preventive measures for caries management and are discussed in detail in this chapter. Patients often ask the dental auxiliary about the prescription or over-the-counter agents the dentist has recommended for the prevention of tooth decay and periodontal disease. Therefore they must have a working knowledge of these products. In addition, the auxiliary is often asked by the dentist to dispense, apply, or fabricate devices such as fluoride trays for home use and to deliver these prevention/preventive aids or devices to the patient. In many states, the dental auxiliary, when properly certified and/or licensed, can apply sealants and other preventive products prescribed by the dentist. The indications for sealants, application techniques, and troubleshooting guides are discussed. It is essential that all members of the dental team are familiar with the mechanism of action and application of these products. This chapter also presents information on desensitizing and remineralizing agents. Clinical and laboratory procedures for many of these topics are included.

FLUORIDE

Fluoride is a naturally occurring mineral found in many forms in the modern world. It may be found in well water, in food that has absorbed fluoride from the soil, and as an additive in many over-the-counter dental products or those prescribed by a healthcare professional. Consumption of excess fluoride during tooth formation may lead to a condition known as fluorosis. Severe fluorosis can cause brown staining and pitting of the enamel surface (called *mottled enamel*) (Fig. 18.1) and is found where high levels (more than 2 ppm) of fluoride occur naturally in the drinking water. Mild or moderate fluorosis may create opaque white spots or bands on the teeth. High levels of fluoride in the water supply usually cause fluorosis, but it may also be caused by children swallowing excess amounts of fluoride toothpaste or by iatrogenic (doctor-induced) factors such as overly prescribed fluoride drops or tablets.

TOPICAL AND SYSTEMIC EFFECTS

The enamel and dentin of the tooth are composed of millions of tiny mineral crystals (hydroxyapatite)

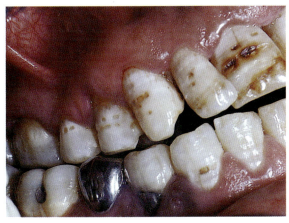

Fig. 18.1 Severe fluorosis. Note enamel defects and discolorations. (Courtesy Steve Eakle, University of California, San Francisco, San Francisco, California.)

within a protein-lipid matrix. Microscopic gaps or pores between these millions of crystals are filled with protein, lipid, and water. It is in these matrix gaps that small molecules such as lactic acid and ions such as hydrogen, calcium, and phosphate are allowed to pass. There is a constant interchange of mineral ions between the tooth surface and the saliva. Usually the minerals entering the surface balance the minerals coming out of the tooth surface.

The tooth crystals are not pure hydroxyapatite but contain inclusions of carbonate, which makes them much more soluble in acid. When bacteria in the plaque on the tooth surface metabolize cooked starches or sugars, they produce acids. The acids remove more mineral (demineralization) than the amount of mineral coming into the tooth from the saliva. When the acid attacks are repeated over time, the tooth surface becomes more porous and allows bacteria to enter the tooth. This is the start of the caries process.

Ingested fluoride that enters the developing tooth bud can come from multiple sources, such as:
- Drinking water
- Foods
- Beverages
- Fluoride supplements prescribed by the healthcare provider.

For years it has been thought that fluoride incorporated into the teeth at the time of development was the main reason for the decline of dental caries (tooth decay) rates seen in areas of water fluoridation. While fluoride incorporated into developing teeth does have a very important effect, work by Featherstone and others (1990) and epidemiological studies have shown that fluoride's greatest anticaries benefit is gained from topical fluoride exposure after the teeth have erupted. Fluoride in the saliva surrounding the teeth is incorporated into the surface of enamel crystals during remineralization (replacing minerals lost from the tooth surface) to form a surface veneer containing fluorapatite, which has a much lower solubility than the original tooth mineral. The pH (a measure of acidity) at which tooth mineral dissolves is 5.5 (7.0 is neutral pH—neither acid nor base). However, when the tooth mineral is converted to fluorapatite, the pH at which it dissolves is lowered to 4.5 (a lower number indicates that it is more acidic; e.g., stomach acid has a pH of less than 1.0). Therefore fluoride makes it more difficult for the acids produced by cariogenic (decay-causing) bacteria in plaque to demineralize the tooth structure and cause dental caries.

A study published in *The Journal of the American Chemical Society* (Loskill et al., 2013), researchers found yet another way in which fluoride helps to fight cavities. They tested how strongly *Streptococcus mutans* bacteria adhere to smooth hydroxyapatite before and after treatment with fluoride. They found that fluoride reduced the adhesive force of the bacteria to the hydroxyapatite surfaces.

Other than dietary sources, topical fluorides come from fluoride toothpastes and mouthrinses, and fluorides are applied in the dental office in the form of liquids, gels, foams, and varnishes. There is evidence that fluoride from drinking water, toothpastes, mouthrinses, and some foods remains in the saliva for several hours and has a prolonged topical effect. Some of the fluoride that is ingested returns to the mouth by way of the saliva.

PROTECTION AGAINST EROSION

Erosion is the loss of tooth mineral that can be caused by highly acidic foods and beverages such as citrus fruits, sodas, and wine. Erosion differs from caries as bacteria are not involved and most of the tooth mineral loss is on the surface. It is important to maintain a well-balanced diet to minimize excess acidic foods. Some medical conditions that cause stomach acid to enter the mouth can contribute to erosion of the teeth (Fig. 18.2). Examples are:
- Acid reflux (burping up stomach acid)
- Anorexia nervosa (body wasting from extreme dieting and forced vomiting to purge food and keep from gaining weight)
- Bulimia (chronic forced vomiting to control weight gain after binge eating)

By making the tooth structure less soluble in acids, fluoride provides some degree of protection against erosion, but repeated acid attacks will likely overcome the beneficial effects of fluoride.

BACTERIAL INHIBITION

Fluoride interferes with the essential enzyme activity of bacteria. Although the fluoride ion has been shown not to cross the bacterial cell wall, it can travel through it in the form of hydrofluoric acid (HF). As decay-causing bacteria produce acids during the metabolism of sugars and cooked starch, some of the fluoride present in the plaque fluid combines with hydrogen ions from the acid to become HF and rapidly diffuses into the cell. Once in the alkaline cytoplasm of the cell, the HF again separates into fluoride ions and hydrogen ions. These ions disrupt the enzyme activities essential to the functioning of bacteria and cause their death.

FLUORIDE AND ANTIBACTERIAL RINSES FOR THE CONTROL OF DENTAL CARIES

Studies have shown that fluoride alone is not as effective in managing dental caries as when it is used in conjunction with an antibacterial mouthrinse. Therapeutic mouthrinses help suppress bacteria associated with dental caries but are not meant to be substitutes for daily mechanical plaque removal.

Chlorhexidine gluconate is a bis-biguanide that is effective against a broad spectrum of microorganisms (Fig. 18.3). In several European countries, it is used at a concentration of 0.2%, but in the United States, the maximum concentration allowed in an oral rinse by the US Food and Drug Administration (FDA) is 0.12%. It is a prescription mouthrinse that is available commercially through several companies.

Chlorhexidine has several important features:
- One of the most effective agents for reduction of plaque (55%) and gingivitis (45%)
- Kills bacteria by binding strongly to the bacterial cell membrane, causing it to leak
- Binds very strongly on many sites (e.g., mucous membranes and plaque) and is released slowly, giving it a prolonged effect (called substantivity)
- Antibacterial effect from a single dose is greatest for several hours after use, but it may last for a few days
- Used in the management of many bacteria associated with periodontal disease
- Effective in suppressing *Streptococcus mutans* strains associated with dental caries

The current recommended rinsing regimen to control dental caries, as suggested by an organization of western US dental schools, is as follows:
- Rinse nightly for 1 minute with approximately 10 mL of 0.12% chlorhexidine for 1 week each month.
- Repeat the cycle monthly until the dentist, who is monitoring bacterial cultures of *S. mutans* strains and lactobacilli, determines that further rinsing is not needed.

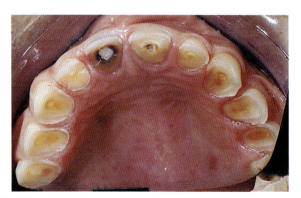

Fig. 18.2 Erosion from stomach acid. Note severe loss of enamel and dentin from the teeth due to chronic vomiting. (Courtesy Steve Eakle, University of California, San Francisco, San Francisco, California.)

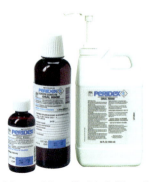

Fig. 18.3 Chlorhexidine oral rinse (Peridex). (From Darby ML, Walsh MM. *Dental Hygiene: Theory and Practice.* 4th ed. Elsevier; 2015.)

The side effects associated with chlorhexidine products are the formation of a brown stain on the teeth and tongue; on glass ionomer, compomer, and composite restorations; and on artificial teeth. Staining seems to be more rapid in some individuals. Diet and brushing habits are thought to play an important role in how rapidly staining occurs. More frequent professional teeth cleaning and polishing is usually necessary for patients who use these compounds routinely.

Chlorhexidine is known to have a bitter taste and may alter the taste of some foods. Some flavoring agents have been introduced in an attempt to offset the bitter taste. The solution contains alcohol, which might be harsh for individuals with sensitive mucous membranes. A nonalcohol version is available (Fig. 18.4).

The longest-used antibacterial mouthrinse agents are the phenolic compounds, also called essential oils. The best-known product is Listerine (Johnson & Johnson) (Fig. 18.5), which has received the American Dental Association (ADA) Seal of Acceptance. It is a combination of phenol-related essential oils (thymol, eucalyptol, and menthol) mixed in methylsalicylate in a 26.9% hydroalcoholic vehicle. The antibacterial action of these compounds is a result of their alteration of the bacterial cell wall. Listerine now has products on the market that do not contain alcohol and only contain essential oils (Fig. 18.6). These products are best for patients who cannot use alcohol products or have xerostomia as alcohol can further dry the oral tissues.

Clinical studies of Listerine have shown reduction of plaque scores by about 25% and gingivitis by 30% with the use of these compounds. In some patients, these compounds cause a burning sensation in the tissues and a bad taste. Flavoring agents have been added in an attempt to overcome the taste problem.

Do You Recall?

What are some side effects associated with chlorhexidine use?

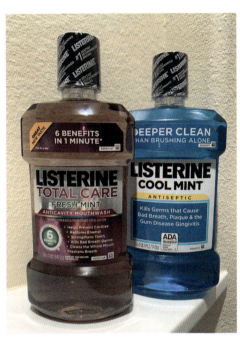

Fig. 18.5 Listerine antiseptic mouthrinse available over the counter.

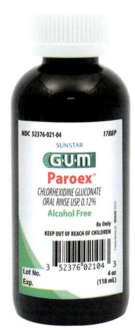

Fig. 18.4 Alcohol-free chlorhexidine oral rinse. (Courtesy Sunstar.)

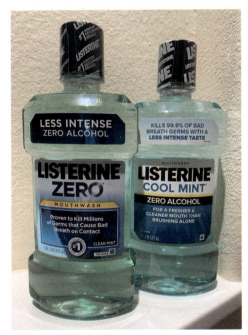

Fig. 18.6 Listerine Zero antiseptic mouthrinse without alcohol available over the counter.

METHODS OF DELIVERY

Dietary Fluoride Supplements

Fluoride may be obtained through drinking water, either naturally occurring or in fluoridated water supplies. In nonfluoridated communities, dentists and physicians may prescribe fluoride supplements for children in the form of tablets, drops, or lozenges (Fig. 18.7). Consideration should be given to the total fluoride exposure the child receives from other sources, such as:
- School rinse programs
- Toothpaste
- Prepared foods containing fluoride

There is a schedule that recommends daily doses of fluoride supplements based on the child's age and the fluoride content of the community water supply. Supplements should not be chosen when the community water supply has a fluoride content that is higher than 0.6 ppm. It is recommended that tablets and lozenges be allowed to dissolve slowly to gain a topical effect. A portion of systemically ingested fluoride, including that in drinking water, is returned to the oral cavity by way of saliva, thereby contributing to a topical effect.

In small communities where fluoridation of the water supply is not economically feasible, an alternative is to add fluoride to table salt. This type of fluoridation has been used for more than five decades in Switzerland and endorsed by the World Health Organization. Potassium fluoride and sodium fluoride are added to table salt at a concentration of 250 to 300 ppm. The salivary fluoride levels of the individuals using the fluoridated salt are similar to individuals drinking fluoridated water. This form of fluoridation can be used in areas of the world where other preventive measures for oral health are not available.

In-Office Fluoride Applications (Topical)

Children with newly erupted permanent teeth and any age group at high risk for caries are good candidates for professionally applied fluorides. The dental hygienist is most often the professional applying fluoride in conjunction with dental prophylaxis. In some states, properly educated dental assistants can also play this important role.

Silver Diamine Fluoride. Silver diamine fluoride (SDF) was approved in 2014 by the FDA for use in treating dentinal hypersensitivity. SDF has been used in other countries for over 80 years and silver alone has been used for over 100 years in health care. Fluoride has an anticariogenic effect, while silver has antimicrobial effects. The combination of fluoride and silver together as active ingredients in silver diamine fluoride produces a product that allows fluoride to strengthen and remineralize the tooth while the antimicrobial silver kills bacteria to prevent biofilm from forming on the tooth. This discovery has prompted many dental professionals to use SDF off-label for these benefits. Current evidence indicates SDF is effective in arresting caries in over 90% of lesions when applied two times annually.

SDF is supplied as a colorless or slightly tinted liquid or gel in an 8-mL bottle or unit dose container (Fig. 18.8). Both contain silver at 25%, fluoride at 5%, ammonia at 8%, and water at 65%. The label indicates the SDF is a 38% solution which is established by combining the silver, fluoride, and ammonia percentages. Ammonia is added to the solution to stabilize the high concentration of fluoride suspended in the water. The pH of SDF is very basic at 10 on the pH scale of 0–14. The average shelf life is 3 years. SDF is a trauma-free and inexpensive method to arrest dental caries in all populations. It is frequently used in children, geriatrics, and vulnerable populations (Table 18.1).

Application. One drop of SDF will treat up to five teeth. The solution should be applied using a microbrush and placed on the decayed area for 60 seconds (Fig. 18.9; Procedure 18.3). Good isolation is required as the silver in the solution will stain soft tissue and rough or unfinished margins of restorations such as

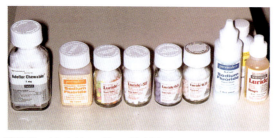

Fig. 18.7 Fluoride tablets. (From Bird DL, Robinson DS. *Modern Dental Assisting.* 12th ed. Elsevier; 2018.)

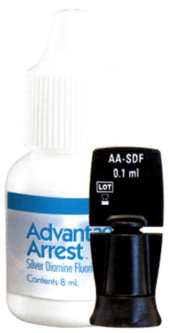

Fig. 18.8 Advantage Arrest silver diamine fluoride in bulk and single-dose containers. (Courtesy Oral Science.)

Table 18.1	Indications and Contraindications for Use of Silver Diamine Fluoride
INDICATIONS	**CONTRAINDICATIONS**
Active carious lesions	True silver allergy
Lack of access to dental care	Ulcerations or sores on soft tissues
Inability to tolerate conventional dental care	Concern for esthetics
Multiple lesions requiring extensive dental treatment over a period of time	Pregnancy

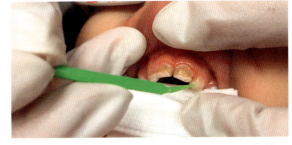

Fig. 18.9 Areas of decay on deciduous teeth being treated with silver diamine fluoride (SDF). (Courtesy Affiliated Children's Dental Specialists.)

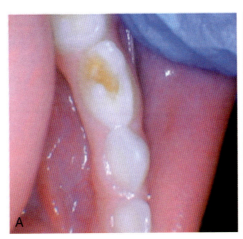 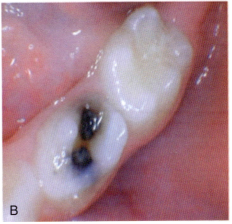

Fig. 18.10 **(A)** Area of decay. **(B)** Staining of tooth structure after application of SDF. (Courtesy Oral Science.)

composites and crowns. It should also be noted that the silver will stain surfaces, clothing, and skin. On applying SDF, the area of decay will turn dark brown or black in color (Fig. 18.10). It may take up to 30 minutes for the decay to darken after SDF application. Due to the discoloration of the decay as a result of the SDF application, it is recommended in posterior regions or on deciduous teeth where esthetics are not a concern. Some clinicians cover the area treated with SDF with a composite or glass ionomer to attempt to hide the darkness caused by the treatment.

There are no established guidelines for the number of applications or frequency of applications. The manufacturer recommends waiting 1 week between repeated applications. Research has evaluated effectiveness after one application versus two applications two times a year. After one application SDF effectively arrested more than 65% of active caries, while two applications annually resulted in a caries arrest rate above 90%.

Sodium Fluoride Varnish. Fluoride varnishes (Fig. 18.11) have become the most common form of fluoride application used in the dental office. These varnishes were introduced more than 30 years ago, their advantage being that they would hold the fluoride against tooth surfaces longer than other products. The FDA has approved varnishes for use in treating dentin hypersensitivity; however, they are primarily used worldwide as an in-office topical fluoride treatment applied directly onto the surface of teeth to prevent caries (Procedure 18.1). They are available as 5.0% sodium fluoride (22,600 ppm fluoride) in a resin carrier or as 1% difluorosilane (1000 ppm fluoride) in polyurethane. Fluoride varnish can remain on the teeth for 1 to 2 days if the patient brushes gently. Varnishes are particularly useful for direct application to early dental caries with the potential to remineralize. They supply a high concentration of fluoride to the porous demineralized enamel. They can be applied directly around orthodontic bands and brackets to help prevent the formation of white spots (evidence of demineralization) caused by inadequate plaque removal. Fluoride varnishes have replaced the use of foams and gels in the dental office because they can be applied rapidly and do not have the unpleasant side effects of nausea, vomiting, and gagging often seen with tray application of foam or gel. Fluoride varnish is an effective caries-preventive agent, with caries reduction of 18% to 77% depending on the frequency of application, home care practices, diet of the individual, and other factors.

Gels and Foams. Topical gels or foams (Fig. 18.12) that are applied for 4 minutes in disposable trays (Procedure 18.2) were historically the most commonly used fluorides in the dental office; however, varnishes have now taken their place. This is due to the quick

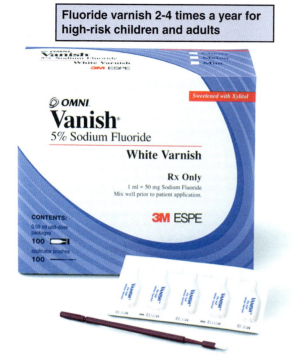

Fig. 18.11 Fluoride varnish with tricalcium phosphate. (From Darby ML, Walsh MM. *Dental Hygiene: Theory and Practice.* 4th ed. Elsevier; 2015.)

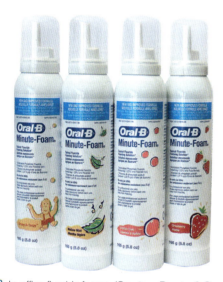

Fig. 18.12 In-office fluoride foams. (Courtesy Procter & Gamble.)

application of varnishes and the continual fluoride release over an extended period of time. Some manufacturers market topical fluorides suggesting they can be applied for only 1 minute. A 1-minute application is not recommended by the ADA. Evidence-based dentistry indicates the 1-minute application delivers approximately 85% of the fluoride that a 4-minute application delivers. However, a 1-minute application is appealing to clinicians managing small children with active tongues, excessive salivary flow, and patients who tend to gag easily. This is another reason varnishes have increased in popularity.

When used once or twice a year, topical fluoride treatments have been shown to produce 20% to 26% caries reduction. Before fluoride varnish became popular, acidulated phosphate fluoride (APF) was once used frequently with children because it contains 12,300 ppm fluoride and has good uptake in the enamel. Two percent neutral sodium fluoride (NaF) contains 9000 ppm fluoride and is used more often with adults because the phosphoric acid in APF tends to etch the surface of restorations made of porcelain, composite resin, glass ionomer, or compomer. The phosphoric acid will also worsen root sensitivity by dissolving plugs that block the dentinal tubules.

> **? Do You Recall?**
>
> Why should topical fluoride gels and foams be applied for 4 minutes rather than the manufacturer-recommended 1 minute?

Self-Applied Topical Gels and Pastes

Self-applied fluoride gels and pastes are recommended for:

- Individuals who are at high risk for dental caries.
- Orthodontic patients to prevent caries and decalcification around brackets and bands that cause permanent white spots and lines on the enamel.
- Elderly patients who take medications that dry up their salivary flow are at very high risk for caries, especially on exposed root surfaces, and can receive benefit from gels used at home.

Self-applied gels are available by prescription as 1.1% neutral sodium fluoride (5000 ppm fluoride), 0.2% sodium fluoride (900 ppm fluoride), (Fig. 18.13 - MI paste plus contains 0.2% sodium fluoride), or 0.4% stannous fluoride (900 ppm fluoride) (Fig. 18.14). Prescription rinses contain 0.2% sodium fluoride or 0.63% stannous fluoride.

Fluoride gels can be brushed on the teeth or applied in custom fluoride trays. Custom fluoride trays can be made with the same thermoplastic material as whitening trays (see Procedure 19.2). Four minutes of use in a custom tray is much more effective than 1 minute of brushing with the gel, because the tray prevents saliva from quickly diluting the gel and removing it from contact with the teeth. The custom trays, however, involve extra expense due to time and additional steps required to fabricate them. Gels are not recommended for children younger than 6 years of age due to swallowing risks. In place of a brush-on gel, some manufacturers have made prescription toothpastes containing 1.1% neutral sodium fluoride. The idea is that the prescription toothpaste will aid compliance because the patient will not have to brush their teeth first and then brush again with a gel, but can achieve both at the same time. Self-application by school-aged children has produced significant caries reduction (about 24%).

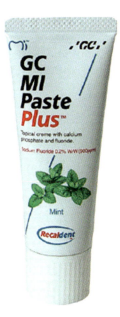

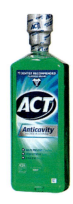

Fig. 18.15 Sample of over-the-counter fluoride rinse. (From Darby ML, Walsh MM: *Dental Hygiene: Theory and Practice.* 4th ed. Elsevier; 2015.)

Fig. 18.13 Sample prescription fluoride products. (From Darby ML, Walsh MM. *Dental Hygiene: Theory and Practice.* 4th ed. Elsevier; 2015.)

Over-the-Counter Fluoride Rinses

Over-the-counter (OTC) fluoride rinses have been demonstrated to provide 28% caries reduction when used in a daily rinse program. Rinses are available as 0.05% sodium fluoride (225 ppm fluoride) (Fig. 18.15).

Patients typically are instructed to:
- Rinse with 10 mL for 30 to 60 seconds
- Spit out the excess
- Not rinse, eat, or drink anything for at least 30 minutes
- Rinse with it just before bedtime so that a residue of fluoride can remain in the saliva during sleep

Parents should supervise children using fluoride-containing rinses to prevent the child from swallowing them.

Fluoride-Containing Toothpaste

The fluoride content of most toothpastes is about 1000 ppm. Children younger than 6 years of age should be supervised when brushing and should be given only a pea-sized amount of toothpaste once a day. Toothpaste made specifically with children in mind is available with much lower fluoride content. This is due to children's tendency to swallow the paste and run the risk of mild fluorosis of the permanent teeth if they ingest too much.

Fluoride-Containing Prophylaxis Pastes

Prophylaxis pastes contain pumice as an abrasive to remove surface stains and plaque/biofilm from the teeth. During the polishing process, they remove a small amount of the fluoride-rich enamel surface. It is thought that some of the lost fluoride can be regained by incorporating fluoride in the paste. The most common fluoride additive is 1.23% APF. These pastes have not received the ADA Seal of Acceptance as effective for caries prevention because studies have not shown them to be effective for this purpose. In some dental offices, polishing the teeth with prophy paste after prophylaxis is not routinely done to avoid removing

High concentration 5000 ppm fluoride toothpaste/gel for caries high-risk clients from age 6 years and older

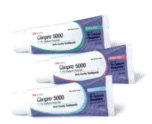
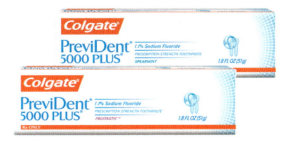

Fig. 18.14 MI paste, calcium and phosphate product with 0.2% Sodium Fluoride for home use. (From Darby ML, Walsh MM. *Dental Hygiene: Theory and Practice.* 4th ed. Elsevier; 2015.)

that fluoride-rich surface layer. Other methods such as air polishing may be implemented as an alternative to traditional polishing methods.

SAFETY

All fluorides should be used as directed and kept out of small children's reach for safety reasons. The lethal dose for a child weighing 20 lb is approximately 1800 to 1500 mg of sodium fluoride. Therefore it is recommended that prescriptions for dietary supplements of fluoride contain no more than 120 mg to avoid the risk of a fatal overdose. Dental auxiliaries should realize that overdoses causing acute illness can also occur from topical applications of fluoride. If it is determined that a child has consumed an excessive amount of fluoride, vomiting should be induced and milk of magnesia should be given to bind to the fluoride ions. Cow's milk could be given to slow absorption from the stomach. The child should be taken to the nearest hospital for emergency treatment. The most common reaction seen in the dental office or shortly after leaving the office when a child has swallowed fluoride gel is nausea and vomiting. The fluoride, particularly with the acidulated gel, irritates the stomach (see Procedure 18.2 for the clinical technique for in-office topical fluoride application). Table 18.2 lists common in-office and home-use fluoride products.

Table 18.2 Common In-Office and Home-Use Fluoride Products

USE	PRODUCT	FLUORIDE CONTENT (PPM)	COMMON BRANDS	FREQUENCY OF USE	PRECAUTIONS
In-office treatment	1.23% APF gel or foam	12,300	NUPRO APF Gel, Foam (Dentsply) DentiCare Gel, Foam (Medicom) Topex 60 Second Fluoride Gel, Foam (Sultan Healthcare)	Twice a year	Gastrointestinal upset, vomiting if swallowed; may etch esthetic restorations; not for children younger than age 3 years
	2.0% NaF	9000	Oral-B Neutra-Foam (Procter & Gamble) NUPRO Fluoride Oral Solution (Dentsply) DentiCare Foam (Medicom) Topex Neutral pH Fluoride Gel, Foam (Sultan Healthcare)	Twice a year	Gastrointestinal upset, vomiting if swallowed; not for children younger than age 3 years
	38% SDF	44,800	Advantage Arrest (Elevate Dental Care)	Twice a year	Staining of soft tissues and margins of restorations, discoloration of tooth after application to carious lesion
	5% NaF varnish	22,600	Duraflor Halo (Medicom) Colgate Duraphat (Colgate-Palmolive) Flor-Opal (Ultradent) NUPRO White (Dentsply) Vanish (3M ESPE) DuraShield (Sultan Healthcare)	Two to four times per year depending on caries risk	Nausea with extensive application in patients with sensitive stomachs
Prescription home use	1.1% NaF gel or toothpaste	5000	Colgate PreviDent (Colgate-Palmolive) Oral-B NeutraCare (Procter & Gamble) DentiCare Gel (Medicom) Fluoridex (Philips Oral Healthcare) Topex Take Home Care (Sultan Healthcare)	Daily	Not for children younger than age 6 years

Continued

Table 18.2 Common In-Office and Home-Use Fluoride Products—cont'd

USE	PRODUCT	FLUORIDE CONTENT (PPM)	COMMON BRANDS	FREQUENCY OF USE	PRECAUTIONS
	0.4% SnF_2 gel	900	Colgate Gel-Kam (Colgate-Palmolive) Oral-B Stop (Procter & Gamble) DentiCare Gel (Medicom) Perio Plus (Oral Dent Pharma) Topex (Sultan Healthcare)	Daily	May cause surface staining of teeth; not for children younger than age 6 years
	0.2% NaF rinse	900	Oral-B Fluorinse (Procter & Gamble) Colgate PreviDent Dental Rinse (Colgate-Palmolive) NUPRO Fluoride Rinse (Dentsply)	Weekly	Not for children younger than age 6 years
Over-the-counter home use	0.05% NaF	250	ACT (Chattem) Colgate FluoriGard (Colgate-Palmolive)	Daily	Not for children younger than age 6 years
	0.02% NaF	100	Listerine Smart Rinse (Johnson & Johnson) Crest Pro-Health (Procter & Gamble)	Daily	Not for children younger than age 6 years
	Toothpaste 0.24% NaF	1100	Numerous brands and manufacturers	Daily	Not for children younger than age 6 years
	Toothpaste 0.8% MFP	1000	Numerous brands and manufacturers	Daily	Use pea-sized amount with children younger than age 6 years

APF, Acidulated phosphate fluoride; *SDF*, silver diamine fluoride; *MFP*, sodium monofluorophosphate; *NaF*, sodium fluoride; SnF_2, stannous fluoride.

Do You Recall?

Why are fluoride-containing toothpastes not recommended for children younger than 6 years old?

KEY POINTS: Benefits of Fluoride Use

1. Lower dental caries risk
2. Contributes to remineralization
3. Protection against erosion
4. Interferes with essential enzyme activity of bacteria
5. Can reduce dentin hypersensitivity

Caution

Parents with children under the age of 6 years should be advised to carefully supervise their children when brushing with fluoride-containing toothpaste. Children at this age tend to swallow the paste and over time could consume enough fluoride to cause mild fluorosis. Only a pea-sized portion of paste should be used.

PIT AND FISSURE SEALANTS

PURPOSE

Sealants are unfilled or lightly filled resins (see Chapter 8) that are used to seal the noncarious pits and fissures of deciduous and permanent teeth. The sealant is a preventive measure to reduce or eliminate dental caries in the pits and fissures. The widespread use of fluoride has caused a significant reduction in dental caries in children who receive regular dental care, but not necessarily in low-income populations. Although the overall caries rate has dropped, the greatest benefit from fluorides has been seen on smooth enamel surfaces. Most caries (about 88%) in children are found in pits and fissures. The nature of the shape of the pits and fissures makes them vulnerable to dental caries. Pits and fissures are:

- Vulnerable to dental caries due to the shape
- Often deep, narrow channels in the enamel surface that can extend close to the dentinoenamel junction (Fig. 18.16)

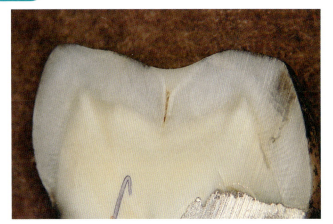

Fig. 18.16 Section of tooth showing a long, narrow fissure containing debris. A sealant is present and covers the opening of the fissure. (Courtesy Steve Eakle, University of California, San Francisco, San Francisco, California.)

- Collect bacteria and food debris that cannot be removed by toothbrushing, so dental caries can occur readily in these locations.

Sealants are not as widely used as they should be. Sealants have been shown in numerous studies to be an effective and conservative means of preventing caries in pits and fissures by blocking bacteria and food products from entering them. The American Dental Association encourages sealant application because sealants have been shown to effectively reduce caries. Caries is often difficult to detect in its early stages in pits and fissures. For this reason, some dentists are reluctant to use sealants for fear of sealing undetected caries. There is ample evidence in the dental literature to indicate if the caries is inadvertently sealed in the pits and fissures, the caries process stops because bacteria are cut off from their nutrients. Only incipient enamel caries should be considered for the sealant procedure. If a sealant leaks because it is not properly placed, caries can occur beneath it. More advanced caries should be treated by conservative restorative procedures rather than with sealants.

INDICATIONS

The lack of an accurate means of predicting where caries will occur has complicated the process of selecting which teeth should be sealed and which should not. Because some individuals will remain caries-free throughout their lifetime, it is not indicated to seal all posterior teeth. Dentist should use their clinical judgment based on specific criteria to determine which teeth should be sealed. Consideration should be given to the patient's:

- Age
- Oral hygiene
- Caries risk
- Diet

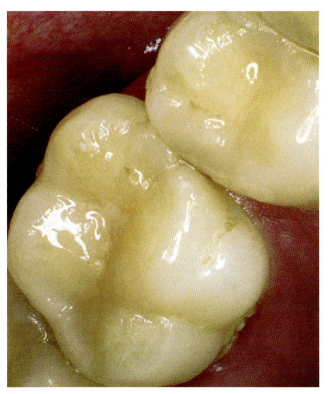

Fig. 18.17 Enamel without significant fissures (well coalesced). (Courtesy Steve Eakle, University of California, San Francisco, San Francisco, California.)

- Fluoride history
- Tooth type
- Tooth morphology

Although the main thrust of sealant therapy is aimed at permanent teeth, primary molars may also be sealed to reduce the caries rate and prevent premature tooth loss. Approximately 44% of caries in primary teeth occurs in the pits and fissures of the molars. Although the occlusal morphology of primary molars is flatter and less fissured than that of permanent molars, sealants are still indicated if deep or stained fissures are found and if the child has a high incidence of caries or high caries risk.

Permanent teeth should be sealed if there is/was evidence of caries susceptibility in the primary dentition or the patient has a high caries risk. Teeth with steep cuspal inclines and deep, sticky fissures are more likely candidates for sealants than teeth with shallow cusps and highly coalesced (fused together) pits and fissures (Fig. 18.17). Molars decay three to four times more frequently than premolars, undoubtedly as a result of the more complex occlusal morphology. Premolars are not generally high-risk teeth, and sealants should be applied selectively when specific indications are present. On occasion, maxillary central and lateral incisors have deep lingual pits that require sealing. However, emphasis is placed on sealing first and second molars as a priority.

Table 18.3 Filler Content and Color of Commercial Sealants

FILLER CONTENT, % BY WEIGHT	BRAND NAME (MANUFACTURER)	COLOR
No filler	Conseal Clear (SDI)	Clear
	Delton (Dentsply Sirona)	Clear, white, amber
	Helioseal (Ivoclar Vivadent)	Clear, white
Lightly filled (6%–8%)	Clinpro (3 M ESPE)	White when set
	Conseal F (SDI)	White
	Natural Elegance (Henry Schein)	White
	Seal-Rite Low Viscosity (Pulpdent)	Off-white
Heavily filled (30%–180%)	Delton Plus (Dentsply)	White
	Embrace WetBond (Pulpdent)	Off-white, tooth colored
	Guardian Seal (Kerr Dental)	White
	Helioseal F (Ivoclar Vivadent)	White
	Grandio Seal (VOCO)	Pearly white
	Ultraseal XT plus (Ultradent)	White, tooth colors A1, A2, clear

SUSCEPTIBILITY OF TEETH TO FISSURE CARIES

Teeth most susceptible to pit and fissure caries are listed in the order of their risk for decay:
- Lower molars—about 50% of the caries occurs in these teeth
- Upper molars—about 35% to 40%
- Upper and lower second premolars
- Upper laterals and upper first premolars
- Upper centrals and lower first premolars

Taken as a group, caries occurs most often in molars, accounting for 85% to 90% of pit and fissure caries.

COMPOSITION

Sealants are chemically similar to composite resins. Their resin component is based on a dimethacrylate monomer that is either:
- Bisphenol A-glycidyl methacrylate (bis-GMA)
- Urethane dimethacrylate (UDMA)

Polymerization of the resin occurs either solely by:
- Chemical reaction (self-cure)
  - Self-cure is by the conventional peroxide-amine system, which requires the mixing of two components.
- Light activation (light cure) (see Chapter 8)
  - Light-cured sealants are one-component systems that are polymerized by blue light.
  - The vast majority of sealants in use today are light cured.

Many manufacturers add very small filler particles to the sealants to make them more wear resistant. Sealants are not as heavily filled (see Table 18.3 for sealant filler content) as most composites because they would be too viscous to flow into the narrow fissures. Some of the filler particles used in sealants may be radiopaque and may allow the sealants to be seen on x-rays. Many sealants, however, are radiolucent.

In 1996 a study done at the University of Granada (Granada, Spain) called into question the safety of dental sealants because of the presence of bisphenol A (BPA) in the saliva of patients after placement of sealants. Bisphenol A can interfere with estrogen (a hormone that regulates reproduction and development) and may have other adverse health effects. In this study only one sealant was tested, but the resin in that sealant (bisphenol A dimethacrylate) is not representative of the resins used in most sealants (bis-GMA or UDMA). Bis-GMA releases very little bisphenol A and UDMA has none. In 2013 the ADA updated a statement indicating that peer-reviewed evidence shows that dental resin materials leach out only very low levels of BPA and do not constitute a health risk for patients (see Chapter 8 regarding concerns about bisphenol A).

Caution

Do not look or stare directly at the curing light. There is potential for damage to the retina with repeated exposures. An appropriate filter should be used to protect the eyes.

WORKING TIME

Self-cured sealant polymerizes to the final set within approximately 2 minutes from the start of mixing of the two components: the initiator and the accelerator. An experienced operator can apply the material to one or two quadrants of posterior teeth with one mix of material, so it has the advantage of being applied faster than light-cured material on a comparable number of teeth. Light-cured material requires a 20-second application of light on each tooth to polymerize the sealant if a standard halogen light is used. Light-emitting diode and laser curing lights can be much more intense and require less curing time (see Chapter 8). Follow the manufacturer's recommendations for curing times. Light-cured material has the advantages of allowing the operator to place and cure the material when the operatory is ready and not requiring mixing prevents the incorporation of bubbles into the material.

COLOR AND WEAR

Manufacturers provide sealants in a variety of colors. Sealants may be:
- Clear
- Amber
- Tooth colored
- Opaque white

Patients usually prefer the clear or tooth-colored sealants, but it is easier for the dental team to identify the presence of the sealants at the time of placement and at subsequent examination visits if they contrast with the tooth color.

Sealants are subject to wear from the occlusion. Sealants that contain no inorganic filler particles will wear faster than those that have filler particles added. Some clinicians use flowable composites as sealants because they are more heavily filled and therefore more resistant to wear, while at the same time having adequate flow to enter the fissures. Wear does not create much of a problem as long as the fissure remains sealed. If part of the fissure is uncovered, repair is recommended.

Sealants seldom flow to the bottom of long, narrow fissures because of the presence of debris (see Fig. 18.16) and trapped air. Some dentists prefer to open the fissures with a small-diameter carbide or diamond bur to look for decay, remove debris, and allow better penetration of the sealant.

PLACEMENT

The ADA Council on Scientific Affairs does not recommend routine opening of fissures with cutting instruments before sealant placement. The technique of placement of sealants requires attention to detail (see Procedure 18.4). This technique has many steps in common with the placement of other bonded restorations (see Chapters 7 and 8). The surface must first be cleaned with pumice to remove any surface debris that would interfere with acid etching or bonding. Retention of the sealant is obtained by etching the enamel with 35–37 % phosphoric acid to roughen it and to open pores in the enamel for penetration of the resin sealant. After etching, rinsing, and drying of the enamel, isolation of the field is very important. Etching enlarges the size and volume of pores in the enamel and roughens the surface so that the sealant can penetrate and mechanically lock into these spaces. Some clinicians like to use a drying agent after etching and rinsing to remove any remaining water in the fissures held thereby capillary action. Drying agents usually consist of alcohol. They will mix with the water, and when evaporated, they will carry off the excess water with them.

Use of Bonding Agent

Studies have shown that application of an enamel bonding resin before placement of the sealant enhances the retention and seal. Many clinicians do not use bonding agents with sealants, as this is a relatively new finding and an additional step in the process. Bonding resins are low-viscosity resins that can flow readily into the fissures and microscopic porosities created by acid etching (see Chapter 7). Resin-containing sealant will then adhere to the bonding resin by a chemical resin-to-resin bond. The sealant is applied to the pits and fissures and surrounding enamel and is cured.

Do You Recall?

How do sealants prevent decay in pits and fissures?

KEY POINTS: Pit and Fissure Sealants

1. Used to protect teeth from caries due to irregular tooth shape or deep pits and fissures
2. Unfilled or lightly filled resins
   - Self-cured
     - Set in 2 minutes
   - Light cured
     - Set in 20 seconds on application of curing light

Clinical Tip

Application of a resin bonding agent after etching the enamel will increase the retention of sealants!

Caution

Place etchant with care to avoid etching adjacent teeth or restorations. Matrix strips could be placed between adjacent teeth, but careful application will prevent inadvertent etching. Avoid contact with the patient's eyes or skin. Protective eyewear should be used by both patient and clinician.

Oxygen-Inhibited Layer

The cured sealant will have a very thin film of uncured resin on its surface. The surface will appear shiny and will be wet to the touch because the set of the resin at its surface is inhibited by contact with oxygen in the air. This film is called the *oxygen-* or *air-inhibited layer*. It should be wiped off with gauze or a cotton roll because it might have an unpleasant taste for the patient.

Caution

Recap sealant and bonding agent bottles promptly after dispensing to prevent loss of volatile monomers that would create a very viscous liquid that cannot penetrate fissures and etched enamel.

Moisture Contamination

Any moisture on the tooth could result in failure of the sealant. Moisture could come from:
- Saliva
- An air-water syringe that leaks water into the airstream
- Moisture from the patient's breath

Sealant failure may be seen as:
- Immediate loss of the sealant
- Complete or partial loss of the sealant seen at subsequent visits
- Retained sealants that are leaking and could result in dental caries beneath the sealant

Maxillary and mandibular second molars are the teeth that most frequently lose sealants, probably because they are the ones for which it is difficult to maintain isolation when a rubber dam is not used. In addition, moisture from the patient's breath could coat the etched enamel and interfere with the bond of the sealant.

Do You Recall?

How does moisture contamination contribute to the failure of sealants?

Clinical Tip

Maintaining good isolation is critical to the success of sealants. Moisture from saliva or even a patient's breath can affect their retention. The most common sites where sealant is lost in the first 6 months are the maxillary and mandibular second molars, and these are the sites where isolation is most difficult to maintain.

Remineralization of Etched, Unsealed Enamel

One concern raised about etching enamel surfaces for placement of sealants is that if the sealant comes off, the exposed surface is more caries susceptible. Studies have shown that the etched enamel begins remineralization after a 24-hour exposure to saliva by deposition of calcium phosphate salts. In areas where sealants wear away, resin tags remaining in the enamel provide some caries protection.

Etching Precautions

Care should be taken in placement of the acid etchant so that adjacent teeth are not etched and the soft tissues are not exposed to the acid. Mylar matrix strips or metal matrix bands can be placed in the interproximal spaces to prevent etching of adjacent teeth, but careful application of etchant will prevent this from occurring. Care should also be taken to avoid contact of the acid with the eyes and skin of the patient and operator. Both should wear protective eyewear.

Bite Interference by Sealant

If a sealant layer is too thick (often described as "high sealant"), it might cause interference with the bite of the patient. Unfilled sealants that are too high will wear down in a few days or weeks. Sealants with filler particles are much more wear resistant. Ideally, all high sealants should be adjusted to be compatible with the patient's bite at the conclusion of the sealant placement appointment. Otherwise sore teeth or jaws may result. Articulating paper should be used to identify the high spots, and an appropriate carbide or diamond bur can be used to make the appropriate adjustments.

PATIENT RECORD ENTRIES

The sealant procedure should be carefully documented in the patient's chart. Chart entries should include the following:
- The date of placement
- Patient (18 years of age or older) or parental consent as obtained
- Type of isolation
- Teeth and surfaces sealed
- Materials used, including percentage of phosphoric acid (etchant) and brand of sealant used
- Statement that the patient or parent was informed of the need for periodic inspection and maintenance of the sealants
- Any adverse events, such as acid splashed on the oral tissues or face, causing a burn, or difficulty with isolation or patient management that may lead to sealant failure

Sealant Retention Studies have shown that retention rates are better when four-handed techniques are used for the placement of sealants. Having an extra pair of hands to help maintain isolation and place or cure the sealants is a definite bonus. In many states, the dental auxiliary can be licensed or certified to place sealants. State dental practice act guidelines must be followed as to the specific oral healthcare providers permitted to place sealants and adjust the occlusion on a high sealant. The dental hygienist can play an important role in the maintenance of sealants by carefully evaluating them at regular hygiene visits.

Clinical Tip

Avoid placing sealant on adjacent unetched enamel. After the sealant is cured, it will look sound, but leakage will occur under the unetched portion of the sealant. When the patient returns for the periodic oral examination there, will be dark staining under the sealant in those areas and the leakage may lead to the development of caries.

EFFECTIVENESS

Carefully placed sealants are very effective at preventing decay in the pits and fissures. See Table 18.4 for advantages and disadvantages of chemical-cured and light-cured sealants.

Table 18.4 Advantages and Disadvantages of Chemical-Cured and Light-Cured Sealants

CHEMICAL-CURED (SELF-CURED OR AUTOPOLYMERIZING) SEALANTS	
ADVANTAGES	**DISADVANTAGES**
• No need for curing light. • No risk of damage to the retina from the curing light. • Sealants can be applied to several teeth without having to go back and individually cure each one with a light.	• Setting time can vary greatly with variations in room temperature; the warmer the material, the faster the set. • Setting time of 2 minutes may be too long if there is trouble maintaining a dry field or controlling a hyperactive child. • Mixing two liquids together introduces bubbles into the material that could produce voids in the completed sealant. • The viscosity (thickness) of the material increases continuously from the start of mixing. When the material is applied to several teeth, the ability of the material to flow well into tight fissures diminishes with time and a new mix may be needed.
LIGHT-CURED SEALANTS	
ADVANTAGES	**DISADVANTAGES**
• Material sets in a short period of time (typically 20 s). This is particularly useful when one is working on an active child or is trying to control heavy salivary flow. • Time for application is not limited as with chemical-cured sealants. • Mixing is not required, so fewer bubbles are introduced into the material. • Viscosity remains low throughout the application period until light is applied.	• The curing light can cause damage to the retina if protection is not used. • The curing light and filter are added expenses. • Only the material directly under the light tip is completely cured, so that when several teeth are done, the total curing time may be significantly increased and it may be difficult to manipulate the light tip to reach the distal pits of maxillary second molars in small mouths.

TROUBLESHOOTING PROBLEMS WITH SEALANTS

Most sealant failures occur within the first 3 to 6 months, and all or part of the sealant comes off. The worst failure is a sealant that leaks but remains in place. The leak can go undetected and can decay significantly underneath the sealant before it is detected. Placing too much sealant can result in excess material flowing into the embrasure space between adjacent teeth (Fig. 18.18). Once the sealant is cured, the contact area is blocked and the patient would not be able to floss. See Table 18.5 for potential problems, their causes, and ways to solve the problems.

GLASS IONOMER CEMENT AS A SEALANT

Glass ionomer cements have been used as sealants because of their adhesion to enamel and release of fluoride into the surrounding tooth structure. However, the retention rate for glass ionomer sealants is rather low. One rationale for their use is to provide protection from caries by sealing the fissures and providing fluoride to the surface of the enamel while the tooth is going through the eruption process, which can be somewhat slow for molars. Then, after the tooth is fully erupted, a resin sealant could be placed. Current recommendations from the ADA Council on Scientific Affairs after a review of the dental literature indicate that resin-based sealants are the preferred materials for pit and fissure sealants.

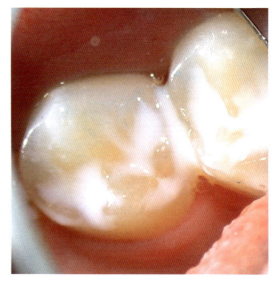

Fig. 18.18 Too much sealant was applied and excess blocks the proximal embrasure. (Courtesy Steve Eakle, University of California, San Francisco, San Francisco, California.)

DESENSITIZING AGENTS

Many patients experience sensitivity in their teeth to a variety of items such as:
• Cold foods or beverages
• Sweets
• Cold air

Table 18.5 Troubleshooting Problems With Sealants

PROBLEM	CAUSE	SOLUTION
Sealant has come off when retention is checked at placement visit	Surface contamination (likely saliva)	Maintain good isolation and reetch and apply the sealant.
Sealant blocks the contact area	Too much sealant was applied Lack of finger rest to control placement	Use just enough sealant to cover fissure and 1 mm beyond. Use good finger rest. Remove excess material before curing it. Remove hardened sealant in contact area with a scaler.
Sealant has holes in surface	Air bubbles in wet sealant Vigorous scrubbing with application brush	Carefully dispense material to avoid bubbles. Gently work sealant into fissures with brush or explorer. Repair by working fresh sealant into holes with explorer tip (reetch first if isolation was lost).
Sealant layer is too high, interfering with bite	Too much sealant was applied	Do not puddle the sealant. Use just enough to cover the fissure and 1 mm beyond

Professionally or OTC materials applied to the teeth by the patient to reduce or eliminate the sensitivity are called **desensitizing agents**. Dental hygienists and assistants may be called on to apply certain types of desensitizing agents or to explain to the patient the causes of the sensitivity.

MECHANISM OF TOOTH SENSITIVITY

Teeth may become sensitive when the gingiva has receded, and dentinal tubules are exposed to the oral cavity. Ordinarily, the root surface has a thin protective coating of cementum. When the cementum is worn away, the dentinal tubules are exposed. Odontoblasts (cells in the pulp that lay down dentin) line the pulp and have extensions within the dentinal tubules that contain nerve endings. When some stimulus causes the fluid within the tubules to move:
- The sensitive nerve endings are deformed.
- Causing them to fire and produce a quick, localized sharp pain (this is the hydrodynamic theory of dentin sensitivity).
- Temperature, usually cold; sugars; and acidic foods are common offenders.

Common Causes of Sensitivity
Common causes of exposed dentin include the following:
- Roots abraded by improper toothbrushing
- Loss of enamel and dentin through the work of dietary or stomach acids (erosion)
- Loss of tooth structure in the cervical part of the tooth by abfraction (grinding of the teeth, which can cause bending of the teeth at the microscopic level with breaking away of enamel and dentin in the cervical area)
- Scaling and root planing procedures

It is estimated that 15% of the population experiences tooth sensitivity. If the dentinal tubules become plugged, the sensitivity stops. Acidic foods and beverages, toothbrushing, or scaling and root planing procedures can remove the plugs and create sensitivity again. Citrus fruits and their juices can readily remove mineral from the surface of the teeth and open plugged dentin tubules. Besides being acidic, they contain citrate that binds and removes calcium from the teeth and saliva, so remineralization is slowed. Desensitizing agents (Fig. 18.19) have been developed to treat tooth sensitivity; however, not all causes of tooth sensitivity respond to desensitizers. Causes of tooth sensitivity such as dental caries, a fracture or crack in the tooth, a high restoration, or a leaking restoration cannot be treated by desensitizers and need corrective measures.

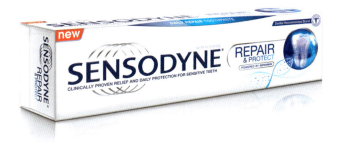
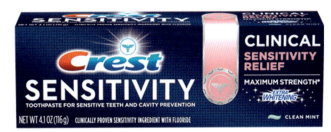

Fig. 18.19 Various desensitizing agents. (Courtesy GlaxoSmithKline, Brentford, United Kingdom; Courtesy Procter & Gamble Co., Cincinnati, Ohio.)

Common Causes of Root Sensitivity
- Root caries
- Toothbrush abrasion
- Erosion by acids
- Abfraction associated with bruxism
- Scaling and root planing
- Leaking restoration on the root

TREATMENT

Treatment for tooth sensitivity is currently centered around two main modalities:
- Occluding (plugging) the open tubules
  - Plugging the open ends of the dentin tubules to reduce fluid movement and stop pressure on the nerve endings
  - Done by a chemical or mechanical blocking process
    - Fluoride compounds in toothpastes, gels, or solutions
    - Ferric or potassium oxalate solutions to precipitate oxalate crystals in the open tubules (Fig. 18.20)
    - Chemical solutions containing resin to block the tubules
  - Dentin bonding agents create a bond with the dentin
  - Amorphous calcium phosphate pastes mineralize the openings of the exposed tubules
- Desensitizing the nerve endings
  - Some desensitizing agents, potassium nitrate in particular, work by passing through the dentinal tubules to the pulp and acting directly on the nerve
    - Potassium depolarizes the nerve so it cannot fire and cause pain
  - Desensitizing agents are used in several different ways
    - At the time of placement of a restoration
    - Prior to or after a prophylaxis or scaling and root planing procedure
    - For teeth with gingival recession and exposed root surfaces that are hypersensitive to touch or temperature

One of the side effects of teeth whitening can be tooth sensitivity during the whitening process. Some whitening products include chemicals, such as potassium nitrate or fluoride, to reduce or eliminate the sensitivity during whitening.

CATEGORIES AND COMPONENTS OF DESENSITIZING AGENTS

Various desensitizing agents are available. They may be categorized as
1. Toothpastes
2. Fluoride gels and varnishes
3. Inorganic salt solutions
4. Resin primers and bonding agents
5. Mineralizing agents
6. Glass ionomer surface sealer (Table 18.6)

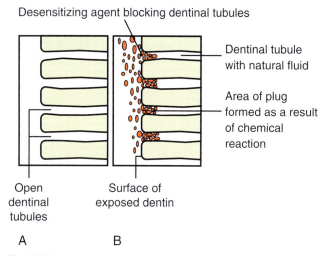

Fig. 18.20 Illustration of **(A)** open dentinal tubules and **(B)** a desensitizing agent that forms a precipitate that occludes the dentinal tubules.

Table 18.6 Desensitizing Agents

PRODUCT CATEGORY	PRODUCT NAME	MANUFACTURER	ACTIVE INGREDIENT
Toothpastes	Sensodyne Deep Clean	GlaxoSmithKline	Potassium nitrate
	Sensodyne True White		Potassium nitrate
	Sensodyne Rapid Relief		Stannous fluoride
	Sensodyne Complete Protection		Stannous fluoride
	Sensodyne Repair and Protect		Stannous fluoride
	Colgate Sensitive	Colgate-Palmolive	Potassium nitrate
	Crest Sensi-Relief Whitening	Procter and Gamble	Potassium nitrate
	Colgate PreviDent 5000	Colgate-Palmolive	1.1% sodium fluoride
	Colgate Duraphat 5000 ppm	Colgate-Palmolive	1.1% sodium fluoride
	Clinpro 5000	3M ESPE	1.1% sodium fluoride
	Colgate Gel-Kam	Colgate-Palmolive	0.4% stannous fluoride
Fluoride varnish	FluoroDose	Centrix	5% sodium fluoride
	Vanish	3M ESPE	5% sodium fluoride
	NUPRO Fluoride Varnish	Dentsply	5% sodium fluoride
	Colgate Duraphat	Colgate-Palmolive	5% sodium fluoride
	Duraflor	Medicom	5% sodium fluoride
	Fluor Protector	Ivoclar Vivadent	Fluorsilane compound

Continued

Table 18.6 Desensitizing Agents—cont'd

PRODUCT CATEGORY	PRODUCT NAME	MANUFACTURER	ACTIVE INGREDIENT
Inorganic salts	D/Sense Crystal	Centrix	Calcium oxalate, potassium nitrate
	BisBlock	BISCO	Oxylates
Potassium nitrate	UltraEZ	Ultradent	3% potassium nitrate plus 0.11% sodium fluoride
	Relief ACP	Philips Oral Healthcare	Potassium nitrate, amorphous calcium phosphate
Resin agents	Gluma Desensitizer	Heraeus Kulzer	5% glutaraldehyde, 35% HEMA
	MicroPrime B	Danville Materials	HEMA, 0.5% sodium fluoride
	HurriSeal	Beutlich	HEMA, 0.5% sodium fluoride
	Pain-Free F	Parkell	4-META resin, fluoride (3000 ppm)
	All-Bond DS	BISCO	NTG-GMA and BPDM primers
	Seal & Protect	Dentsply	Prime and Bond NT with 18% filler
Mineralizing agents	SootheRx	3M ESPE	Calcium sodium phosphosilicate
	Teeth Mate	Kuraray America	Calcium phosphates
	MI Paste	GC America	Amorphous calcium phosphate
Glass ionomer surface sealer	Vanish XT	3M ESPE	Glass ionomer cement

BPDM, Biphenyl dimethacrylate; *HEMA*, 2-hydroxyethyl methacrylate; *4-META*, 4-methacryloxyethyl trimellitate anhydride; *NTG-GMA*, N-(p-tolyl)glycine glycidyl methacrylate.

Desensitizing toothpastes usually require repeated use over several days or weeks to achieve some relief. The relief will only continue while the toothpaste is used. If the patient discontinues the use of the desensitizing toothpaste, the sensitivity will return.

Fluorides may also take a while before results are seen. Some of the inorganic salts that precipitate into the open dentinal tubules and seal their openings will have immediate results; others may take repeated applications.

Resin desensitizing agents will have immediate results if all of the open tubules are sealed. A reduced level of sensitivity may remain if some of the tubules are still open. Desensitizing systems using bonding resins may require etching of the surface first, sometimes creating additional temporary sensitivity, particularly with rinsing and application of air. However, self-etching dentin primers are available that do not require rinsing after etching (see Chapter 7). The duration of relief varies greatly, from a few days to close to 1 year.

None of these agents provides permanent relief. The duration of relief can be prolonged if the original cause of the sensitivity is eliminated. That is, the poor toothbrushing habit, the acidic diet, or the teeth grinding must be curtailed; otherwise, the desensitizing agent will be removed and the tubules reopened. If a patient has a history of sensitivity, the dental hygienist must provide the patient with one of the desensitizing agents after scaling and root planning. Chronically sensitive root surfaces may require restoration with glass ionomers, compomers, or composites to provide definitive relief.

REMINERALIZATION

Remineralization is the process of repairing the surface of tooth structure that has lost mineral because of exposure to:
- Dietary acids
- Environmental acids
- Gastric acids
- Bacterial acids

PRODUCTS

Some of the products used to treat tooth sensitivity can also be used to help remineralize the tooth. As previously discussed, fluorides are helpful in the remineralization process. Because tooth mineral is largely calcium and phosphate, products that contain calcium and phosphate can help replace lost tooth mineral. The main ingredients of these products are amorphous calcium phosphate or calcium sodium phosphosilicate. One product combines fluoride and amorphous calcium phosphate in a varnish (Fig. 18.21). The varnish will prolong the exposure of the covered tooth surfaces to both components. Glass ionomer cements, because they release fluoride, are also helpful.

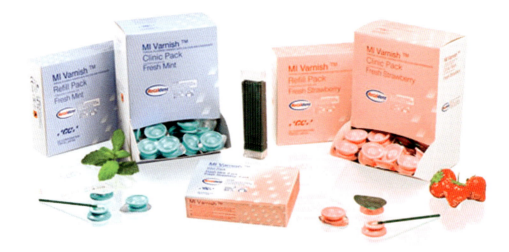

Fig. 18.21 Sample of MI Varnish. (Courtesy GC Corporation.)

RESIN INFILTRATION

A novel approach to halting progression of the early smooth surface white spot carious lesion is to infiltrate the lesion with a low-viscosity resin. As bacterial acids attack the enamel the surface and the body of the developing carious lesion become more porous. The objective for this new approach is to prevent caries progression by blocking the porosity in the enamel with a high-penetration resin.

- First, the right type of lesion is selected.
  - The lesion should be on accessible smooth surfaces of the enamel, with no break or cavitation of the surface of the carious lesion.
  - Interproximal early lesions can be treated but are more difficult technically because they are not readily accessible.
- Next, the area is isolated and the surface of the lesion is cleaned with pumice. Then 15% hydrochloric acid is applied for 2 minutes, extending 2 mm beyond the borders of the lesion. The acid is washed off, the surface is dried, and an ethanol drying agent is applied for 30 seconds followed by air drying.
- Then, the penetrating resin is applied in two applications, totaling 4 minutes, and light cured after each application.
  - Not only does the resin obliterate porosities in the enamel, it makes the white spot lesion much less visible (Fig. 18.22).
  - Although long-term clinical trials have not been done with this technique, the available research supports this conservative approach.

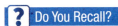 **Do You Recall?**

How does the use of four-handed dentistry during sealant placement contribute to the success of sealants?

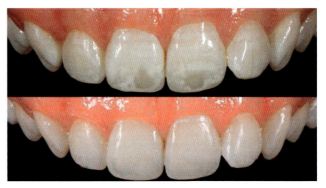

Fig. 18.22 Before and after images of white spot lesions and their improvement after the use of resin infiltration (Icon-infiltrant). (Courtesy DMG America.)

SUMMARY

Conservative dentistry mandates that the dental auxiliary be familiar with the use of the various preventive materials available. By performing caries risk assessment and using topical applications of fluoride, as well as fluoride and antibacterial rinses, early caries can be arrested and tooth structure can often be remineralized. Sealants placed to protect pits and fissures of teeth are recognized as being effective in the prevention of tooth decay. Desensitizing agents are more important now than ever before, because people are retaining their teeth longer, and as a result are subject to the factors that produce root sensitivity. These agents provide relief to patients whose teeth have gingival recession and exposed dentin that subjects them to chronic or episodic pain.

INSTRUCTIONAL VIDEOS

See the Evolve Resources site for a variety of educational videos that reinforce the material covered in this chapter.

Procedure 18.1 Applying Sodium Fluoride Varnish

See Evolve site for Competency Sheet.

EQUIPMENT/SUPPLIES
- Basic examination setup
- Sodium fluoride varnish
- Applicator brush
- 2 × 2 gauze squares
- Air-water syringe tip
- Disposable cup

PROCEDURE STEPS
1. Hand patient cup for use at conclusion of application of varnish.
2. Open fluoride varnish container and mix solution with applicator brush if slight separation has occurred.
   NOTE: Product does expire. The clinician should inspect product and discard if past manufacturer's expiration date.
3. Remove excess fluids from the mouth prior to the application of the varnish.
4. Dry excess saliva from the teeth by wiping dentition with 2 × 2 gauze square or lightly blowing air with air-water syringe.
5. Apply small amount of varnish to each tooth using applicator brush (Fig. 18.23).
   NOTE: Read manufacturer's instructions for recommended application. Some manufacturers recommend painting only one surface of the tooth (i.e., facial or lingual).
6. Once all teeth have been painted, have the patient rub their tongue along all surfaces of the teeth to assist in the distribution of varnish into the interproximal areas.
7. Have the patient expectorate into a disposable cup.

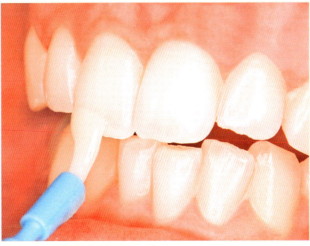

Fig. 18.23 (Courtesy Dentistry Today.)

NOTE: Do not use the saliva ejector or high-volume evacuation to gather excess fluids or varnish from the patient's mouth. The varnish will clog the suction lines over time.

8. Instruct the patient to refrain from eating foods that are extremely hot, crunchy, or contain alcohol as they can remove the varnish from the tooth surface.
9. Instruct the patient to brush their teeth gently after the varnish has remained on the teeth for a period of 6 hours.
   NOTE: Varnish may remain on the teeth for 1 to 3 days if the patient brushes gently.
10. Provide the patient with the home care instructions sheet available from the manufacturer.
    NOTE: Each manufacturer provides home care instruction sheets with their products to be distributed to the patient at the conclusion of treatment.

Procedure 18.2 Applying Topical Fluoride

See Evolve site for Competency Sheet.

EQUIPMENT/SUPPLIES (FIG. 18.24)
- Disposable foam fluoride trays of various sizes
- Topical fluoride foam or gel
- Air-water syringe
- Watch or timer
- Cotton rolls
- Saliva ejector
- High-volume evacuation (HVE) tip

PROCEDURE STEPS
1. Select appropriate disposable foam fluoride tray for the size of the patient's mouth (Fig. 18.4).
2. Examine the patient for the presence of calculus. If present, perform scaling procedure to remove the deposit from the tooth surface before proceeding.
   NOTE: If premanufactured prophylaxis paste during a prophylaxis, the flavoring oils deposited on the surfaces of the teeth may reduce the absorption of fluoride. A slurry of flour of pumice may be used if needed to remove biofilm and prepare the tooth surface for the fluoride application.
3. Seat the patient upright.
   NOTE: This reduces the amount of gel going down the patient's throat.
4. Load trays with a thin strip of fluoride (Fig. 18.25). Do not overfill because that will cause excess fluoride to run into the patient's mouth.

Procedure 18.2   Applying Topical Fluoride—cont'd

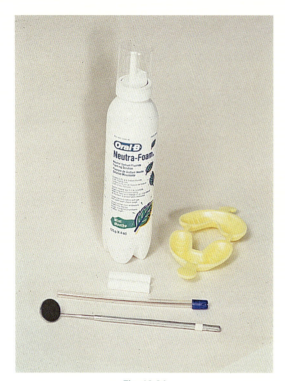

Fig. 18.24

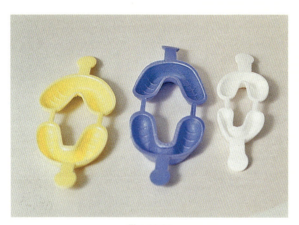

Fig. 18.25

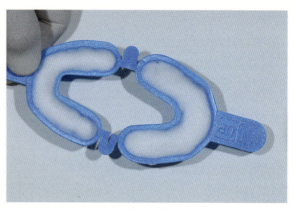

Fig. 18.26

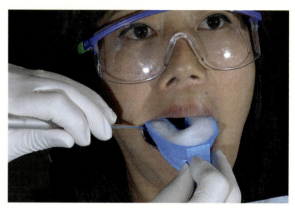

Fig. 18.27

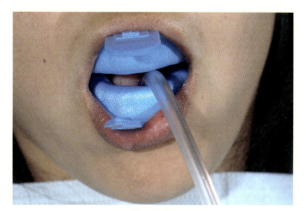

Fig. 18.28

NOTE: Follow appropriate guidelines for the age of the patient.

5. Place trays in the patient's mouth (Fig. 18.27). Place cotton rolls between the trays and have the patient close on the cotton rolls to keep the trays in place.
6. Place the saliva ejector in the mouth on the cheek side or between the trays in the space created by the cotton rolls (Fig. 18.28).

   NOTE: The taste of the gel or foam and the presence of the trays will greatly increase the flow of saliva.
7. Time the fluoride application.
8. Remove the trays after the appropriate time has passed. Remove excess gel/foam and saliva from the patient's mouth by HVE.
9. Instruct the patient not to rinse, eat, or drink for 30 minutes.

   NOTE: Fluoride circulating in the saliva will continue to have a topical effect for a few hours after treatment.

Procedure 18.3 Applying Silver Diamine Fluoride (SDF)

See Evolve Site for Competency Sheet.

EQUIPMENT/SUPPLIES

- Basic examination setup
- Silver diamine fluoride
- Lubricant (Palmer's Cocoa Butter or Vaseline) to prevent staining of tissues
- Plastic Dappen dish
- Microbrush
- Air-water syringe
- Watch or timer
- Cotton rolls, dry angles
- 2 × 2 gauze squares
- Saliva ejector
- High-volume evacuation (HVE) tip
- Super floss
- Bite block

PROCEDURE STEPS

1. Dispense one drop of SDF into plastic Dappen dish.
   NOTE: One drop of solution will treat up to five teeth.
   NOTE: Glass Dappen dish may react with the SDF.
2. Isolate area to be treated with SDF.
   NOTE: Dental dam, cotton rolls, or dry angles can be used to isolate the area being treated.
3. Dry area with 2 × 2 gauze square
   NOTE: Drying area with air-water syringe is not recommended as this may cause the patient sensitivity.
4. Place microbrush into Dappen dish to absorb a small amount of SDF.
5. Apply SDF to the area of caries (see Fig. 18.9).
   NOTE: Keep SDF from touching unwanted areas such as gingival tissues and face as it will stain. If staining of the face occurs, immediately wipe face with hydrogen peroxide. This may reduce the staining that occurs on the face; however, the stain will fade on its own over several days without wiping with peroxide.
6. Keep isolated and allow to dry for 60 seconds.
7. Remove excess material with 2 × 2 gauze square or cotton roll.
   NOTE: Some patients complain of a metallic aftertaste due to the silver content in the solution.
8. Inspect areas of decay to ensure all susceptible areas have absorbed the SDF (see Fig. 18.10).
   NOTE: Glass ionomer can be placed over the tooth treated with SDF to reduce the discoloration that occurs. (See Chapter 9 for benefits of glass ionomer.)

Procedure 18.4 Applying Dental Sealants

See Evolve site for Competency Sheet.

EQUIPMENT/SUPPLIES (FIG. 18.29)

- Basic examination setup
- Prophy setup: slow-speed handpiece with prophy angle, prophy cup, or bristle brush
- High-volume evacuation (HVE), saliva ejector tips, and air-water syringe tip
- Dental dam setup (check for latex allergy); alternative isolation: cotton rolls and holder
- Flour of pumice, pumice preppy, or special prophy paste without oils
- Dappen dish for pumice and mixing well for sealant, if supplied in bulk
- Curing light if using light-cure sealant, and light shield
- Sealant material: Self-cure or light cure
- Etching solution/gel: 35–37% phosphoric acid
- Applicator brush or tips (some sealant materials have an applicator)
- Articulating paper, dental floss
- Bullet-shaped finishing bur or polishing stone

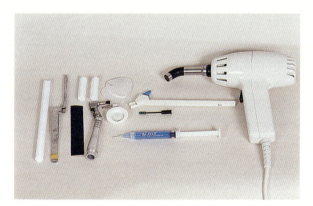

Fig. 18.29

PROCEDURE STEPS

1. Place dental dam or cotton rolls and saliva ejector to isolate teeth to be sealed.
   NOTE: Moisture contamination with saliva or water can cause a loss of or leaking sealant. In this procedure tooth #19 will be sealed.
2. Clean the surfaces of the teeth to be sealed with pumice or oil-free paste (Fig. 18.30).

Procedure 18.4 Applying Dental Sealants—cont'd

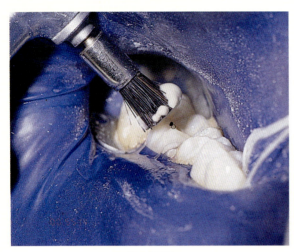

Fig. 18.30

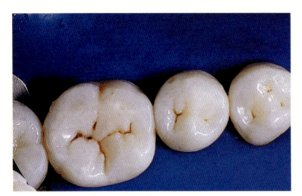

Fig. 18.31

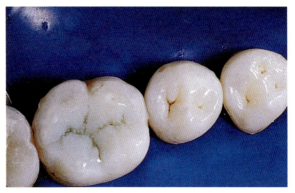

Fig. 18.32

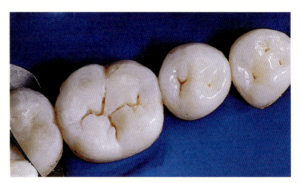

Fig. 18.33

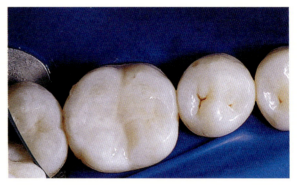

Fig. 18.34

3. Use three-way syringe and HVE to rinse and dry teeth thoroughly. Remove any retained polishing paste (Fig. 18.31).
4. Place etchant on enamel to be sealed for 20 to 30 seconds (Fig. 18.32).
5. Rinse with water for 10 to 15 seconds.
6. If using cotton rolls, carefully replace them or dry them out with the HVE.
   NOTE: Be certain that saliva does not contaminate the freshly etched surfaces or the enamel will need to be reetched for 15 seconds.
7. Dry the teeth thoroughly.
   NOTE: Properly etched enamel should appear frosty (Fig. 18.33). If not adequately etched, reetch for an additional 30 seconds.
8. Apply sealant according to the manufacturer's instructions.

NOTE: Sealant should be gently worked into the pits and fissures to displace trapped air. It should cover the entire fissure but should not overfill the groove pattern because that will probably interfere with the occlusion.

9. Cure appropriately for the required length of time (self-cure or light-cure) (Fig. 18.34).
   NOTE: If light curing, each area under the light probe should be cured for at least 20 seconds. High-powered curing lights may require less time. Follow the manufacturer's recommendations.

Procedure 18.4 Applying Dental Sealants—cont'd

10. Check with an explorer to ensure that all fissures and pits are covered, no holes in the material exist, and sealant is well retained. Apply more material, if needed.
11. Remove dental dam or cotton rolls and thoroughly rinse.
12. Check occlusion with articulating paper and adjust sealant where needed.

    NOTE: Follow the state dental practice act as to which dental professionals are allowed to do adjustments.

13. Check contact areas with floss.

    NOTE: Excess material may have blocked these areas.

14. Check retention at each subsequent visit.

    NOTE: Sealants should be checked for partial or complete loss. Make sure fissures are still covered. With retained sealants, check periphery for staining that may indicate leakage. Extensive decay can occur under leaking sealants if not detected early. Replace lost or leaking sealants.

Review and Discussion

Review Questions

Select the one correct response for each of the following multiple-choice questions.

1. Fluoride helps to protect the teeth from decay by which one of the following?
   a. Neutralizing bacterial acids
   b. Making the enamel more resistant to bacterial acids
   c. Deflecting sugars from the tooth surface
   d. Removing bacterial plaque from the tooth surface
2. When tooth enamel first begins to demineralize, what is one of the corrective measures that can be taken to stimulate remineralization?
   a. Stop eating foods with proteins and amino acids.
   b. Use a daily rinse containing fluoride.
   c. Brush with baking soda and salt.
   d. Check the labels on food packages to determine whether they contain fluoride.
3. What occurs when enamel is remineralized with fluoride?
   a. It is a different color.
   b. The fluoride contains a poison that kills all bacteria associated with dental caries.
   c. The resultant remineralized crystal is more resistant to acids.
   d. All of the calcium is replaced.
4. Fluorosis is always considered to be:
   a. Destructive to the teeth
   b. Very unsightly
   c. A sign that the person has ingested more than the optimal amount of fluoride
   d. A sign that the person will need to have whitening and restorations
5. Nightly home fluoride treatment with 1.1% sodium fluoride as a brush-on gel or in custom trays is indicated for:
   a. Children younger than 6 years of age
   b. Adolescents with one or two pit and fissure caries
   c. Middle-aged females going through menopause
   d. Elderly patients taking medications that cause dry mouth
6. Sealant material is:
   a. Indicated for all permanent molars
   b. Used for protection of smooth surface caries
   c. An unfilled or lightly filled resin
   d. Never in need of replacement once it is placed
7. When a dental sealant is placed, the technique:
   a. Is exactly the same as bonding to dentin
   b. Requires the field to be kept dry
   c. Can be done by dental hygienists and assistants in all states
   d. Always requires the use of a curing light
8. Which one of the following is the best candidate for a sealant?
   a. A newly erupted tooth with numerous deep fissures
   b. A tooth with shallow pits and fissures
   c. A tooth with decay into the dentin
   d. A molar with stained fissures in a 50-year-old patient
9. If caries in a fissure is undetected and is inadvertently covered by a well-placed sealant, what will happen?
   a. Caries will progress rapidly
   b. Caries will progress slowly
   c. Caries will stop progressing
10. Very small filler particles are added to sealant material for which purpose?
    a. To improve the esthetics
    b. To decrease wear of the sealant
    c. To increase adhesion to the enamel
    d. To block the opening of the fissure
11. How is the surface of the tooth prepared before acid etching for sealant placement?
    a. The patient is asked to brush their teeth.
    b. The teeth are wiped with gauze.
    c. A fluoride gel is applied.
    d. The surfaces are cleaned with pumice.
12. Which acid most commonly used to etch the enamel for sealant placement?
    a. Citric acid
    b. Phosphoric acid
    c. Hydrochloric acid
    d. Nitric acid
13. The tip of the light wand of the curing light should be held how close to the sealant?
    a. In contact with the sealant
    b. Very close—about 1 mm away from the surface
    c. About 0.5 inches away
    d. With a good light it does not matter how far away you are
14. After placement of a sealant, which of the following should be checked?
    a. The sealant surface for voids or porosities
    b. The occlusion
    c. The contact areas with adjacent teeth
    d. All of the above
15. Which of the following is the most common reason for loss of a sealant shortly after placement?
    a. Inadequate etching time
    b. Inadequate curing time
    c. The sealant material was bad
    d. Saliva contamination after acid etching
16. How should the surface of the enamel appear after acid etching?
    a. Frosty white
    b. Shiny
    c. Bright gray
    d. Slightly yellow
17. What does acid etching do to the surface of the enamel?
    a. It creates a roughened, irregular surface.
    b. It leaves a smooth, clean surface.
    c. It evenly removes about half the enamel.
    d. None of the above.
18. What is the most important requirement for successfully bonding sealants to enamel?
    a. Good isolation to prevent saliva contamination
    b. A high concentration of acid for etching
    c. Long etching times (60 seconds or longer)
    d. Long drying times (20–40 seconds)

Review and Discussion—cont'd

19. Studies show caries to occur in pits and fissures most often in which group of teeth?
    a. Permanent maxillary incisors
    b. Permanent premolars
    c. Permanent molars
20. How does a sealant adhere to the etched enamel surface?
    a. Micromechanical retention
    b. Chemical bond to the surface
    c. By shrinking; when polymerized it tightly grips the surface
    d. The sealant is very sticky; adheres to the surface like glue
21. The main purpose of most desensitizing agents:
    a. Is to close the openings of the enamel rods to prevent temperature and osmotic changes in the enamel fluids
    b. Is to help the dental hygienist keep the patient comfortable during the dental prophylaxis procedure
    c. Is to plug the openings of the exposed dentinal tubules
    d. When added to toothpaste, is to improve the taste and keep it from burning the gingiva
22. What ingredient in SDF stains the decayed portion of the tooth and anything it comes in contact with?
    a. Fluoride
    b. Ammonia
    c. Silver
    d. Water
23. Application of SDF _____ times per year has shown to arrest caries at 90%.
    a. One
    b. Two
    c. Three
    d. Four

For answers to Review Questions, see the Appendix.

Case-Based Discussion Topics

1. A 14-year-old high school student with no restorations comes to the dental office with poor oral hygiene and early caries in the fissures of the mandibular first molars. An analysis of the diet reveals frequent consumption of sodas and between-meal snacking on sugary foods.
Discuss preventive measures that should be recommended for this patient and the rationale for their use. What diet modifications would you recommend?

2. A 75-year-old retired plumber who takes medication for hypertension comes to the dental office with moderate marginal gingivitis, root caries, and a complaint of dry mouth.
Discuss which of the antibacterial rinses this patient should use. Discuss the type of fluoride regimen that should be used. Explain the rationale for each of these recommendations.

3. A 56-year-old business executive comes to the dental office for an annual examination and cleaning. The patient's chief complaint is that the front teeth are yellowing and thinning on the incisal edges. Sensitivity to cold, sweets, and air on the roots of the maxillary premolars in areas of gingival recession has also been noted. Questioning further reveals a love of lemons, where five lemons are consumed each week and lemon juice is used frequently in cooking and on salads.
Discuss the origin of the patient's complaints and preventive and therapeutic measures that should be recommended.

4. A 3-year-old is brought to the dental office with baby bottle tooth decay on the maxillary anterior teeth. The parent said the child does not complain about the teeth being sore but the parent does not want the child to be in pain if the teeth are left untreated.
Discuss how the teeth can be treated and how the decay can be prevented in the future. Explain how necessary treatment would be described to the parent and what post-op instructions would be provided.

BIBLIOGRAPHY

Aminoshariae A, Kulild JC: Current concepts of dentinal hypersensitivity, *J Endodont* 47(11):1696–1702, 2021.

Azuma Y, Ozasa N, Ueda Y, Takagi N: Pharmacological studies on the anti-inflammatory action of phenolic compounds, *J Dent Res* 65(1):53–56, 1986. https://doi.org/10.1177/00220345860650010901.

Beauchamp J, Caufield PW, Crall JJ, et al., American Dental Association Council on Scientific Affairs: Evidence-based clinical recommendations for the use of pit-and-fissure sealants: a report of the American Dental Association Council on Scientific Affairs, *J Am Dent Assoc* 139(3):257–268, 2008.

Bird DL, Robinson DS: *Modern Dental Assisting*, ed 13, St. Louis, 2021, Elsevier.

Collins FM, Florman M: *Fluoride guide*, 2014, Penwell Continuing Education Course.

Crespin M, Shuman I: *Fluoride and other preventive therapies; maintaining oral health at each stage of life*, 2017, Penwell Continuing Education Course.

Darby M, Walsh M: *Dental Hygiene Theory and Practice*, ed 4, St. Louis, 2015, Elsevier.

Eakle WS, Featherstone JD, Weintraub JA, Shain SG, Gansky SA: Salivary fluoride levels following application of fluoride varnish or fluoride rinse, *Commun Dent Oral Epidemiol* 32(6):462–469, 2004.

Davari A, Ataei E, Assarzadeh H: Dentin hypersensitivity: etiology, diagnosis and treatment; a literature review, *J Dent* 14(3):136–145, 2013.

Doméjean S, Ducamp R, Léger S, Holmgren C: Resin infiltration of non-cavitated caries lesions: a systematic review, *Med Princip Pract: Int J Kuwait Univ Health Sci Centre* 24(3):216–221, 2015.

Featherstone JD: Prevention and reversal of dental caries: role of low level fluoride, *Commun Dent Oral Epidemiol* 27(1):31–40, 1999.

Griffin SO, Jones K, Gray SK, Malvitz DM, Gooch BF: Exploring four-handed delivery and retention of resin-based sealants, *J Am Dent Assoc* 139(3):281–358, 2008.

Handelman SL, Leverett DH, Espeland MA, Curzon JA: Clinical radiographic evaluation of sealed carious and sound tooth surfaces, *J Am Dent Assoc* 113(5):751–754, 1986.

Li Y: Dentin hypersensitivity: diagnosis and strategic approaches, *Inside Dent*, 2018.

Loskill P, Zeitz C, Grandthyll S, Thewes N, Müller F, Bischoff M, Herrmann M, Jacobs K: Reduced adhesion of oral bacteria on hydroxyapatite by fluoride treatment, *Am J Dent* 29(18), 2013.

Mandel ID: Chemotherapeutic agents for controlling plaque and gingivitis, *J Clin Periodontol* 15(8):488–498, 1988.

Oong EM, Griffin SO, Kohn WG, Gooch BF, Caufield PW: The effect of dental sealants on bacteria levels in caries lesions: a review of the evidence, *J Am Dent Assoc* 139(3):271–358, 2008.

Simonsen RJ: Retention and effectiveness of dental sealant after 15 years, *J Am Dent Assoc* 122(10):34–42, 1991.

Uzel I, Gurlek C, Kuter B, Ertugrul F, Eden E: Caries-preventive effect and retention of glass-ionomer and resin-based sealants: a randomized clinical comparative evaluation, *BioMed Res Int* 2022:1–7, 2022.

Teeth Whitening Materials and Procedures

19

http://evolve.elsevier.com/Eakle/materials/

Chapter Objectives

On completion of this chapter, the student should be able to:
1. Describe how whitening materials penetrate the tooth.
2. Compare and contrast the various whitening materials available for in-office, take home, and over-the-counter home use.
3. Describe the necessary precautions to take to protect the oral tissues when applying in-office power whitening products.
4. List the steps in the procedures for in-office power whitening.
5. Identify the potential side effects associated with in-office power whitening, and home whitening products.
6. Describe the methods to whiten nonvital teeth.
7. Discuss the relative effectiveness of whitening products and whitening toothpastes in removing stains from teeth.
8. Demonstrate proper fabrication of home whitening trays.
9. Explain to the patient how various whitening products are used.
10. Identify clinical situations in which enamel microabrasion might be used.
11. Explain how enamel microabrasion works.

KEY TERMS

Whitening a cosmetic process that uses chemicals to lighten or remove discolorations from teeth
Extrinsic Stains stains occurring on the tooth surface
Intrinsic Stains stains that are incorporated into the tooth structure, usually during the tooth's development
Vital Tooth has a living pulp, which produces response to temperature change or electrical stimuli
Power Whitening in-office whitening procedure that uses strong whitening agents and may use a high-intensity light source to accelerate the whitening process

Nonvital Tooth no longer has a living pulp and ceases to give response to electrical stimuli or temperature changes
Walking Bleach Technique whitening technique for nonvital teeth in which whitening materials are sealed inside the tooth crown for a few days and the patient "walks" around with the whitening material in place
Enamel Microabrasion a process that uses hydrochloric acid and an abrasive such as pumice to remove shallow discolorations of the enamel

---

Teeth darken as part of the aging process, although some teeth are discolored from medications or chemicals incorporated into the developing enamel and dentin. In a society where many strive to maintain their youthful appearance, patients desire to regain their brighter, whiter smiles. This has caused an explosion in the demand for cosmetic dental services. The use of whitening products is a fairly inexpensive method to achieve a youthful appearance and has become a significant part of many dental practices. Whitening can be done as an in-office procedure or as a home procedure supervised by the dentist. The dental auxiliary, depending on the state dental practice act, can perform many of the procedures associated with the whitening process, such as making impressions and custom trays, delivering and demonstrating use of the home whitening materials to the patient, providing home use instructions and precautions, and helping with various steps in the in-office whitening procedure. A properly educated auxiliary can answer questions patients have about whitening. This team effort can help in the growth of the practice as pleased patients tell their friends and relatives about the excellent services they have received from a knowledgeable, caring staff.

TEETH WHITENING (BLEACHING)

Evidence-based research indicates that **whitening** with peroxide products is safe and effective. Many stains and discolorations of the teeth can be removed or lightened by whitening procedures. However, some stains are more difficult to remove than others.

TYPES OF STAINS

Teeth may be discolored by:
- **Extrinsic Stains** on the tooth surface
- **Intrinsic Stains** incorporated internally into the tooth structure (often when the tooth is developing)
- A combination of both (Table 19.1)
  - Long-standing extrinsic stains can penetrate the enamel to become intrinsic stains, which makes the removal of the stain more difficult.

Extrinsic Stains

Some common foods or drinks that are known to contribute to extrinsic staining of the teeth include:
- Coffee
- Tea
- Red wine
- Colored cola drinks
- Grape juice
- Various berries

Poor oral hygiene accompanied by pigment-producing bacteria and food stains can also produce extrinsic stains of varying colors (Fig.19.1). Tobacco products and betel leaf chewing also contribute to staining of the teeth (Fig. 19.2).

Antimicrobial mouth rinses, such as chlorhexidine, can contribute to surface staining (Fig. 19.3). Some extrinsic stains limited to the surface can be removed, in part, by:
- Toothbrushing
- Whitening dentifrices
- Whitening mouth rinses

The dental hygienist can remove other stains by:
- Hand or ultrasonic scaling
- Coronal polishing
- Air polishing
  - Using a spray of sodium bicarbonate or aluminum trihydroxide under air pressure

Table 19.1 Causes and Colors of Extrinsic and Intrinsic Discoloration

CAUSE	COLOR
Extrinsic Stain	
Poor oral hygiene	Yellow, brown, green, black
Coffee, tea, red wine, colored cola drinks, foods	Brown to black
Tobacco products and betel leaf chewing	Yellow-brown to black
Antimicrobial rinse (chlorhexidine)	Brown
Intrinsic Stain	
Medications During Tooth Development	
Tetracycline	Brown, gray, black bands
Fluoride	White, brown spots or bands
Medications After Tooth Development	
Minocycline (tetracycline-type drug)	Brown, gray
Diseases/Conditions During Tooth Development	
Conditions such as purpura (a blood disorder)	Red, brown, purple
Trauma	Blue, black, brown
Pulpal Changes	
Pulp canal obliteration	Yellow
Pulp necrosis with hemorrhage	Gray, black
Pulp necrosis without hemorrhage	Yellow, gray-brown
Other Causes in Nonvital Teeth	
Trauma during pulp extirpation	Gray, black
Tissue remnants in the pulp chamber	Brown, gray, black
Restorative dental materials	Brown, gray, black
Endodontic materials (not currently in use in USA)	Gray, black
Combination Intrinsic/Extrinsic Stains	
Aging	Yellow

Adapted with permission from Hayward VB. Current status and recommendations of dentist-prescribed, at home tooth whitening. *Contemp Esthet Rest Pract.* 1999;3(suppl):2–9.

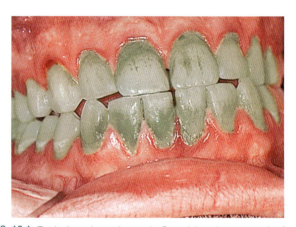

FIG. 19.1 Extrinsic stain on the teeth. Greenish stain as a result of accumulation of plaque, pellicle, food debris, and pigment-producing bacteria. (Courtesy Dr. Steve Eakle, University of California, San Francisco, California.)

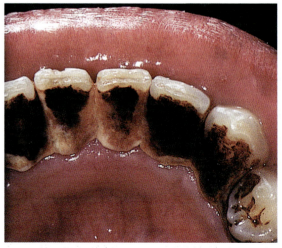

FIG. 19.2 Extrinsic stains on the teeth. Dark brown stains are the result of poor oral hygiene and frequent smoking. (Courtesy Dr. Steve Eakle, University of California, San Francisco, California.)

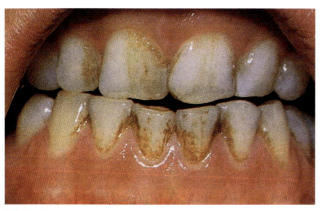

FIG. 19.3 Extrinsic stains on the teeth. Light brown stains on the teeth are a result of chlorhexidine antimicrobial mouthrinse. (From teethandmouth.blogspot.com. Courtesy Asanka.)

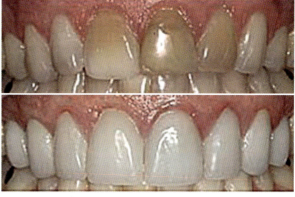

FIG. 19.4 Discolored teeth restored with porcelain veneers. (Courtesy Huefner Sensational Smiles.)

More stubborn stains that have penetrated the enamel surface cannot be polished or scaled away. These may require whitening products (peroxides) to remove them.

Intrinsic Stains

Intrinsic stains are internal and may be a result of developmental disturbances of the teeth during:
- Development
- Hereditary conditions
- Aging

Developmental disturbances can result from:
- Trauma to the developing teeth
- Illness with high fever
- Excessive intake of fluoride
- Certain medications

Intrinsic stains, such as age-related discolorations that are yellow or light brown, are easier to whiten than blue-gray and black stains. Blue-gray, gray-black, and yellow-brown stains are often caused during tooth development by chemicals or drugs, such as tetracycline or doxycycline (see Fig. 19.11). As a consequence, they are incorporated deep within the dentin and are also found in the enamel. Externally applied, vital whitening usually takes much longer to lighten tetracycline stains and achieve an acceptable result. Whitening may make white spots from mild fluorosis less apparent by making the whole tooth whiter.

A single dark tooth should be radiographed and tested for vitality: even if the tooth is symptom free, the pulp may have died. Stains associated with endodontically treated teeth may require internal whitening. Some internal stains, such as those caused by amalgam or dental caries, are resistant to whitening. For stains that cannot be removed by whitening, tooth-colored restorations such as veneers, crowns, or composites must be used to hide the discoloration (Fig. 19.4).

HISTORY OF PEROXIDE WHITENING

In the mid-1960s, some periodontists began applying peroxide in strips to aid in healing of gingival tissues following periodontal treatment. Soon after, an orthodontist began having his patients apply a 10% carbamide peroxide solution to the interior of their orthodontic positioners to reduce gingival inflammation. By accident he discovered that their teeth were also whiter. This discovery was largely ignored until the 1980s when general dentist John Munro also noticed whiter teeth when he had his patients use a 10% carbamide peroxide solution to reduce gingival inflammation. He began using vacuum-formed plastic trays to contain the peroxide solution. He collaborated with a manufacturer to market the first commercial whitening preparation in 1988. Heymann and Haywood in 1989 introduced the technique of "night guard bleaching" using a much more viscous solution to which Carbopol, a thickening agent, was added to allow the whitening agent to remain in the tray longer and increase the whitening time. Soon after, another product with a very thick whitening gel of carbamide peroxide was introduced, and the use of night guard whitening became wildly popular.

HOW WHITENING WORKS

The enamel of the tooth crown is composed almost entirely of mineral (97% by weight) with microscopic spaces between the enamel rods that contain water and organic material (Fig. 19.5). Stains accumulate within these small spaces in the enamel over time and may also penetrate to the dentin. Whitening occurs when a type of peroxide or other whitening material passes through the spaces in the enamel and reaches the dentin, where it releases oxygenfree radicals that oxidize the stains and subsequently lighten the color of the dentin. This process can be accelerated by the use of low-intensity heat or high-intensity light, such as a conventional composite curing light, a laser, high-intensity plasma arc, or light-emitting diode (LED) light. Open carious lesions and leaking restorations can allow the whitening agents to penetrate too deeply into the tooth, resulting in pulpal irritation.

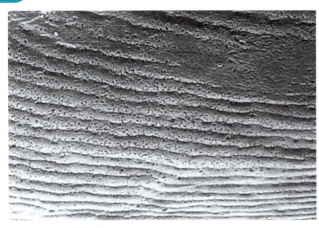 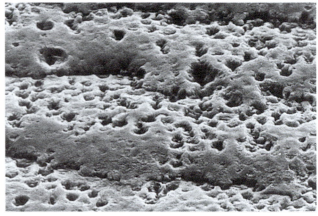

FIG. 19.5 The porosity of the enamel surface may be seen by scanning electron microscopy. An enlargement of the same image is seen on the *right*. (Courtesy Dr. Ole Fejerskov, Aarhus University, Denmark.)

Whitening Materials

Depending on the manufacturer, current whitening products are based on either hydrogen peroxide or carbamide peroxide. Some products also contain additives to help reduce posttreatment sensitivity.

Hydrogen Peroxide. Hydrogen peroxide products range in concentration from 5% to 40% and are available as:
- Liquid
  - liquids can more readily seep under a rubber dam and cause tissue burns
- Varnish
  - Varnishes typically remain in place for a specific period of time due to a clear protective coating placed over them
- Gel
  - Gels usually stay put the best due to viscosity.

Personal protective equipment (PPE) should be worn by operators and auxiliaries when performing in-office hydrogen peroxide whitening procedures, while patients should wear protective eyewear and a cover for their clothing.

Carbamide Peroxide. Carbamide peroxide products are popular for home whitening and range in concentrations from 10% to 44%. They are supplied as:
- Liquids
- Gels

Carbamide peroxide is a weaker oxidizing agent than hydrogen peroxide. A 10% carbamide peroxide gel breaks down into 3.35% hydrogen peroxide and 6.65% urea. The urea further breaks down into ammonia and water and increases the pH value of the solution, subsequently providing beneficial side effects of slowing demineralization by bacterial acids as part of the caries process. Carbamide products also contain either a carbopol or glycerin base, which slows the release of hydrogen peroxide, making it work for a longer period of time.

> **Do You Recall?**
>
> Why are thickening agents added to whitening solutions to make products used in trays?

WHITENING

PRETREATMENT EVALUATION

Prior to starting the whitening process, a thorough evaluation must be done that includes radiographs and a clinical examination to determine the following:
- Cause of the stains
- Other treatments needed before whitening
  - Dental caries, cracked teeth, leaking restorations, abscessed teeth, and root resorption should all be addressed before starting the whitening process
- Alternatives to whitening
- The ideal whitening procedures for the specific patient's problem

If gingival recession has occurred and root surfaces are exposed, the patient should be informed that it is more difficult to whiten the root surface and whitening may not be successful on these surfaces. White spots, such as mild fluorosis, will not be removed by whitening but may be less noticeable when the surrounding tooth surfaces are whitened.

TREATMENT METHODS

There are three main treatment options for patients who wish to whiten their teeth. Treatment may be done as follows:
1. In the dental office, by the dentist and staff
2. At home, with the dentist prescribing and dispensing whitening materials for the patient to use and supervising the course of treatment
3. At home, with the patient purchasing over-the-counter (OTC) whitening products and using them without professional supervision

In-Office Whitening of Vital Teeth

In-office whitening is ideal for patients who want results quickly. Advantages of treatment in the dental office include:
- Direct supervision by the dentist and the staff
- Elimination of patient compliance issues
- Control over the whitening process
- Ability to discontinue treatment if a problem arises

Whitening is done in the dental office for both vital and nonvital teeth. A **vital tooth** has a living pulp, which produces response to temperature change or electrical stimuli.

For years whitening was done by means of a liquid consisting of 35% hydrogen peroxide and the application of a heating lamp. While this method can be effective for single-tooth whitening, it is a time-consuming process and technique sensitive. If any of the liquid contacts the soft tissues:
- It can cause a chemical burn that will turn the affected tissue white
- Cause sloughing of the tissue and may be painful (Fig. 19.6)
- If gingival tissue is affected, vitamin E oil (obtained by breaking open a vitamin E capsule) should be applied to the site as soon as it is discovered
  - Many manufacturers of in-office whitening provide vitamin E oil as part of the kit

A high-concentration gel of 35% (or 45%) carbamide peroxide is more controllable than liquid hydrogen peroxide. All of these high-concentration products require the use of isolation consisting of a dental dam and gingival protection with petroleum jelly, or paint-on light-cured dental dam materials (such as OpalDam; Ultradent Products) (Fig. 19.7).

Prior to completing a whitening procedure, it is best to record the starting shade of the patient's teeth via a Classic Vita shade guide (Fig. 19.8). Intraoral before and after photos should be taken for in-office and take-home whitening procedures (Procedure 19.1). Vita also has a guide for bleaching purposes—see image below the classic guide. Also, the classic guide can be arranged by value so that shades go from light to dark to make comparisons easier.

TYPES OF IN-OFFICE TREATMENTS

Power Whitening - Light_Aided

In-office **"power whitening"** (use of strong whitening agents which may be activated by high-intensity light) has become a popular procedure, because it can be completed in one visit, and there is no need to rely on patient compliance as with home-use systems. Many patients simply do not want to spend the time to whiten their teeth at home for several hours a day over

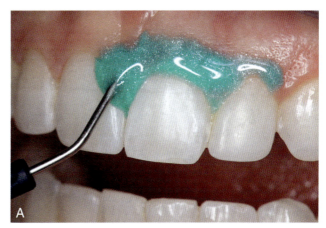

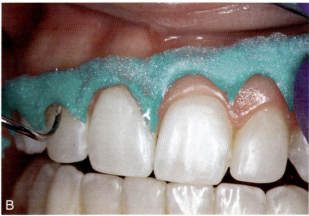

FIG. 19.7 Resin dam material (OpalDam; Ultradent Products) to protect gingiva from whitening agent: **(A)** Material applied from the syringe with a needle cannula, then light cured. **(B)** Material peels right off after use. (Courtesy Ultradent Products, Inc., South Jordan, Utah.)

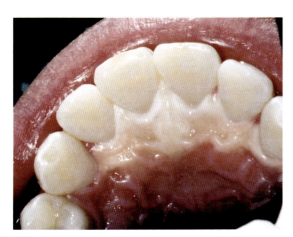

FIG. 19.6 Chemical burn of gingiva from contact with high-concentration hydrogen peroxide. (Courtesy Dr. Steve Eakle, University of California, San Francisco, California.)

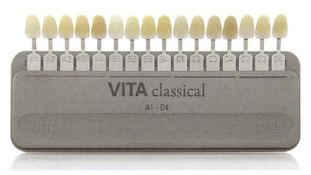

FIG. 19.8 Classic Vita Shade Guide. (Courtesy Vita.)

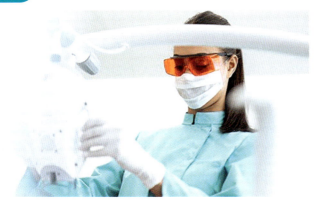

FIG. 19.9 In-office "power" whitening. Patient has protective barriers for oral tissues and eyes. High-intensity light (Zoom, Philips Oral Healthcare) is used to speed whitening. (Courtesy Philips Oral Healthcare, Stamford, Connecticut.)

a period of 2 or more weeks. The treatment time for power whitening is usually 45 to 60 minutes.

Special curing lights, LED light, plasma arc light, or argon laser light may be used with the power whitening in-office systems (Fig. 19.9). Some older systems utilized ultraviolet (UV) lights, and the clinician must be aware if this type of light is being utilized as there are additional precautions to take to protect the patient's lips and nose. It would be best to have the patient provide a sunscreen of choice to limit allergies or breakouts.

Power Whitening—Nonlight Aided

Research shows that the use of high-intensity light is not necessary for whitening to occur and at best, it may accelerate the process. The important factors are the concentration of the whitening material and the contact time with the tooth surface. Since high-intensity light is not essential to successful whitening, products have been developed with strong whitening agents that do not use high-intensity light. It is recommended to store whitening materials in the refrigerator to prolong their limited shelf life.

Electrical-Aided Whitening

Some whitening systems are available that utilize an electrical current to activate the whitening gel or accelerate the whitening process. A special mouthpiece is required to deliver the electrical current without light or heat. Hydrogen peroxide gels utilized in dental whitening systems must be maintained at a lower pH (5.5) to stabilize the materials and increase their shelf life. The systems that use the electrical current to activate the whitening gel and increase the whitening process work by increasing the pH (10.8) of the hydrogen peroxide whitening gel with the electrical current produced in the whitening tray, thus allowing the whitening gel to lighten stains in the teeth more quickly. As with other in-office whitening systems, the tissues must be protected from the peroxide gel as a chemical burn can occur. The paint-on light-cured dental dam materials are the most user-friendly with the design of the mouthpiece used to deliver the electrical current.

Whitening Varnish

As with in-office power whitening, whitening varnish has become a popular procedure. It can be completed in one visit, is not as technique sensitive as power whitening, and only remains on the teeth for 30 minutes rather than an hour like the power whitening. The teeth are isolated and the gingiva is protected with a resin liquid-dam material (see Fig. 19.7). After isolation, the teeth are painted with a 20% hydrogen peroxide whitening varnish. Once all the teeth on the maxillary and mandibular arches have been painted with the varnish, a sealant layer is painted over the varnish to keep it in place. After 30 minutes, the teeth can be brushed or the varnish can be wiped off. Teeth whitening can be continued at home with whitening gel used in custom trays. The whitening varnish is considered a jump-start to home whitening procedures or may be used as a touch-up.

Additional Treatment

Some patients may need a longer whitening time or additional visits, depending on the type of discoloration they present with. Patients who desire maximum whitening may need additional treatments or home whitening to achieve the desired shade. However, every patient has limits as to how white their teeth can become with whitening. Most systems recommend home tray whitening to complement in-office treatment. Power whitening systems have a recommended number of applications per visit, which is established by the manufacturer and usually fall into a range of two to three applications. Applications may need to be repeated until the desired level of whitening has been achieved; however, the maximum number of applications should not be exceeded in one visit as the patient will likely develop sensitivity.

> **Caution**
> High-intensity whitening lights and lasers may generate heat that can irritate the pulp and contribute to posttreatment sensitivity.

In-Office Power Whitening Process

- Isolate teeth with a rubber dam or liquid-dam
- Retract the lips and use a dental napkin to protect skin around the mouth
- Provide the patient with protective eyewear, ideally tinted when a light source is used and with side shields
- Deliver the peroxide whitening gel to the teeth
- Spread the gel over the facial surfaces of the teeth with an applicator brush as recommended by the manufacturer
- Activate the whitening gel with the recommended light source

Continued

- After 20 to 30 minutes, remove the gel with suction and apply a new coating of whitening gel
- Repeat this process for a total of two to three times
- Once the process is complete, thoroughly remove all gel, remove barriers, inspect tissues, and apply vitamin E oil as needed
- Apply desensitizing agents supplied with the whitening kit
- Provide the patient with posttreatment instructions

> **Caution**
>
> The teeth must not be anesthetized during whitening procedures in order for the patient to provide feedback to the clinician pertaining to sensitivity. If the teeth are anesthetized, the patient cannot feel pain produced by heat or the peroxide solution, and permanent pulp damage may result.

> **Caution**
>
> With the use of high-concentration whitening materials, the patient and chairside personnel should all wear PPE and avoid splashes to the eyes or skin that could cause burns.

WHITENING OF NONVITAL TEETH

A **nonvital tooth** no longer has a living pulp and ceases to give response to electrical stimuli or temperature changes. When the pulp of a tooth dies, the necrotic breakdown products of the pulpal tissue or hemoglobin from blood in the pulp escapes into the surrounding dentinal tubules. Chemicals from these tissues (e.g., iron sulfide from hemoglobin) cause intrinsic staining of the dentin, which can turn the tooth dark (Fig. 19.10). Whitening of nonvital teeth in the dental office typically involves teeth that have undergone root canal therapy. Whitening of nonvital teeth requires:
- Removing the restoration from the endodontic access cavity (the hole through which the root canal therapy was performed).
- Whitening internally through this access.

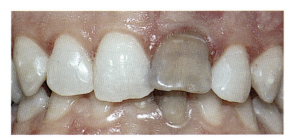

FIG. 19.10 Intrinsic stain in a maxillary central incisor as a result of trauma leading to pulpal death. Staining is due to blood products entering the dentinal tubules. (Courtesy Dr. Steve Eakle, University of California, San Francisco, California.)

- The tooth is isolated with a rubber dam to prevent whitening solutions from contacting and burning soft tissues.
- A 30% to 35% hydrogen peroxide solution or gel is placed in the pulp chamber on a saturated cotton pellet.
- A hot instrument is plunged into the cotton several times to activate the peroxide.

An alternative approach is the "**walking bleach**" technique, in which:
- A commercially prepared bleaching (whitening) gel or paste is made in the office from sodium perborate monohydrate and 30% hydrogen peroxide.
  - Both the sodium perborate monohydrate and hydrogen peroxide products release oxygen that helps whiten the tooth.
- The whitening gel sealed into the pulp chamber with a temporary restoration.
- When the patient returns in 2 to 7 days, the whitening material is removed.
- A composite or amalgam restoration is placed in the endodontic access cavity.

Risk of Root Resorption

All internal whitening procedures require that a seal be established at the base of the endodontic access preparation just coronal to the level of gingival attachment to the tooth. This is done to prevent whitening material from leaking out through open dentinal tubules or accessory canals into the periodontal ligament. There have been cases of external root resorption that occurred when the whitening agent activated an inflammatory reaction in the periodontal tissues. External root resorption is an attack on the root surface by cells and enzymes in the periodontal tissues. It can actually eat a hole through the root, and the patient may lose the tooth.

HOME WHITENING (PRESCRIBED BY THE DENTIST)

Home whitening is a popular and cost-effective method of whitening the teeth, but the treatment interval is much longer compared with in-office treatment (Procedure 19.2). The chemical used in home whitening systems is either:
- 10% to 45% carbamide peroxide
  - Carbamide peroxide products break down into two active ingredients: hydrogen peroxide and urea (an aqueous solution)
- 6% to 15% hydrogen peroxide
  - Hydrogen peroxide breaks down into oxygen and water

Some whitening products have potassium nitrate added to reduce tooth sensitivity. Amorphous calcium phosphate may be added to home whitening to increase tooth whitening efficacy and decrease dentinal hypersensitivity. Nonperoxide gels are also available and claim not to cause tooth sensitivity or gingival irritation, as peroxide products may do with some patients.

Home Whitening Process

The gel is placed in a custom-formed soft, thin plastic tray and is worn by the patient for periods as short as 15 minutes twice daily or as long as overnight. The higher the concentration of the whitening material, application time is decreased. Trays may or may not have spaces, called *reservoirs*, built into them to hold the whitening material. Many offices use reservoirs, but some studies suggest that reservoirs may not be needed. Trays should be trimmed to follow the contour of the gingival crest on the facial aspect of the dentition to avoid contact of the gel with the gingiva because gingival irritation may result (Procedure 19.3). Trimming the tray to follow the contour of the gingival crest on the lingual is not necessary, as the whitening gel will not be placed in the tray to whiten the lingual aspect of the teeth.

The home whitening process is as effective as the in-office process; however, it takes much longer and is sometimes used as a follow-up to the in-office procedure.

Home whitening trays are recommended to be worn daily to achieve optimum results. Hydrogen peroxide solutions oxidize stain more quickly, reducing tray wear time to 15 minutes to 1 hour according to the percentage of solution. Carbamide peroxide solutions oxidize stain slower increasing tray wear time to 30 minutes to 19 hours according to the percentage of solution. The whitening gels used in custom trays are most effective during the first 2 to 4 hours of use and gradually diminish in effectiveness as wear time progresses.

Follow-Up Visits. The recommended time for follow-up visits during treatment is every 2 to 3 weeks, when the procedure is performed under the supervision of the dentist. At the follow-up appointment, the auxiliary will ensure the custom whitening trays still fit appropriately, no gingival burning has occurred, and take a new shade to verify progress.

Length of Treatment. The length of treatment varies for each patient, depending on their discoloration and sensitivity. Yellow and light brown stains caused by aging or foods can usually be whitened more easily in about 2 to 4 weeks. Brown or orange stains caused by systemic or developmental disturbances are more difficult to whiten, resulting in a 1- to 3-month whitening time period. The dark gray, brown, or bluish stains of tetracycline are the most resistant to whitening and may take as long as 6 months to whiten (Fig. 19.11). Intrinsic stains in bands or striations may not whiten evenly or at the same rate. Sometimes, this difference will make the defect more apparent.

Informed Consent. Whether whitening procedures are performed in the office or prescribed for home use, it is essential that the patient be informed of the risks and benefits of treatment and the alternatives to whitening, such as restorative procedures. Standardized informed consent forms can be used or the dentist can fabricate their own. The patient should sign the informed consent only after potential detrimental side effects and limitations of treatment have been presented and all the patient's questions have been answered. The signature of the patient should be witnessed and then the consent should be signed by the dentist or staff member. A copy should be given to the patient, and one copy should be entered into the patient's record.

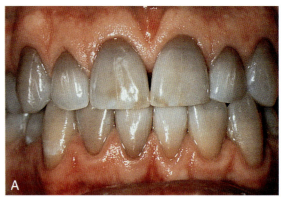
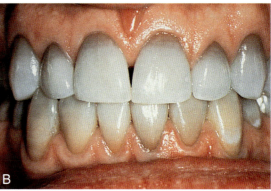

FIG. 19.11 Intrinsic stains. Teeth with tetracycline stains: **(A)** before home whitening; **(B)** after home whitening. (Courtesy Ultradent Products, Inc., South Jordan, Utah.)

> ⚠️ **Caution**
>
> Side effects from home whitening include irritation of oral tissues and throat from contact with the gel, hypersensitive teeth, and sore muscles and jaw joints if trays are worn overnight.

Indications for Whitening

- Discolored teeth
- Surface staining
- Isolated white or brown discoloration, which is shallow or in the surface of the enamel

Contraindications for Whitening

Not everyone is a candidate for whitening procedures. Here are some reasons why:
- Allergy to the products
- Pregnant or nursing
- Open carious lesions
- Cracked enamel
- Excessive dental work on front teeth unless patient is prepared to replace restorations that will no longer match the whitened teeth
- Actively leaking restorations
- Sensitive teeth
- Use of medications causing photosensitivity (light-activated systems could not be used)
- Inability to follow directions
- Unrealistic expectations
- Under the age of 15
- Inability to provide informed consent

OVER-THE-COUNTER PRODUCTS

Over-the-counter (OTC) teeth whitening products are of five basic types:
1. Whitening strips
2. Paint-on whitening pastes
3. Whitening gels applied in stock trays
4. Whitening rinses
5. Whitening toothpastes

With the use of OTC products, professional supervision is not provided during whitening. In addition, no professional evaluation is done before whitening to ensure that decay and leaking restorations are repaired. Individuals with preexisting sensitive teeth could worsen their condition.

Whitening Strips

Whitening strips from various manufacturers have become very popular and are the most widely used OTC whitening products (Fig. 19.12).
- Whitening strips do not require the construction of whitening trays.
- The product typically consists of clear, flexible strips containing 10% peroxide gel and special polymers that help them adhere to the teeth.
- They are placed over the teeth and worn for 30 minutes at a time, once or twice daily.
- The shorter treatment time may be beneficial for patients who have developed sensitivity with longer treatment times when using trays.
- The strips are thin and do not interfere with speech.

Research indicates that OTC whitening strips are just as effective as whitening with carbamide peroxide in custom trays, at a considerable reduction in cost.

Paint-On Whitening Materials

Paint-on materials are viscous liquids applied directly to the enamel surface of the tooth with an applicator such as a brush. The application process is as follows:
- The first step is to dry the teeth with air, a towel, tissue, or gauze.
- Second the solution is painted onto the teeth and in 30 seconds to 1 minute, the liquid solidifies.
- Third the patient needs to keep the mouth open until the material dries.

Some products are applied during the day and should be left on for at least 30 minutes. It is recommended that these materials be applied twice a day to achieve maximum benefit. Because the material is directly exposed to saliva (unlike the gel in strips or trays), the whitening material may be diluted or may come off. Although paint-on products work, they are not known to be as effective as tray-applied whitening products or whitening strips.

Over-the-Counter Tray Whitening Systems

Several tray whitening systems are sold directly to the public by manufacturers. The trays in these systems are preformed stock trays or thermoplastic trays that are heated in boiling water and adapted to the teeth, much like "boil and bite" sports guards (see Chapter 20). These trays are often poorly fitted and are not properly trimmed to prevent excess material from contacting the gingiva. Ill-fitting trays can irritate the gingiva. The whitening agent in these OTC systems is usually 10% to 22% carbamide peroxide gel.

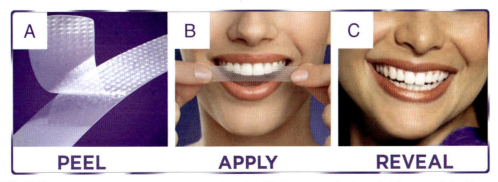

FIG. 19.12 (A) Removal of whitestrip from plastic backing. (B) Placement of strip on facial aspect of dentition. (C) Appearance of teeth on removal of strip. (Courtesy Proctor & Gamble.)

Tooth Whitening Toothpastes

Most of the toothpastes on the market that claim to whiten teeth do so by removing surface stains with abrasives such as hydrated silica or calcium carbonate rather than penetrating the enamel to reach the dentin and whitening the teeth. In addition to mild abrasives, some manufacturers add peroxides to their dentifrices to help with the whitening effect.

Tooth Whitening Rinses

Mouthrinses on the market with whitening properties contain hydrogen peroxide as the active ingredient. The use of the product on a long-term basis is intended to remove surface stains.

NONDENTAL OPTIONS

Whitening has become so popular that it is now offered in retail settings, such as mall kiosks, salons, and spas. These venues have come under scrutiny by the dental community in several states, resulting in actions to limit delivery of whitening services by licensed dental healthcare providers. The rationale for limiting these nondental professionals from providing whitening services is due to the fact that they are not educated in disease screening, infection control, or emergency procedures.

Do You Recall?

How do whitening toothpastes or whitening rinses work to remove surface stains from the tooth structure?

Caution

The US Food and Drug Administration does not require testing for OTC bleaching and whitening products. Manufacturers are not regulated for these products.

KEY POINTS—Vital Teeth Whitening Options

1. Intrinsic stains are more difficult to remove than extrinsic stains
2. Pre-whitening needs should be addressed: caries, leaking restorations, cracked teeth, etc.
3. Main whitening agent is a form of peroxide: hydrogen peroxide or carbamide peroxide
4. In-Office Whitening with high concentration peroxide products—supervised by dentist
   - Power whitening—light aided
   - Power whitening—nonlight aided
   - Electrical-aided whitening
   - Whitening varnish
5. Home Whitening
   - Prescribed and supervised by the dentist
     - Fabricated in the dental office
   - OTC
     - Whitening strips
     - Paint-on whitening materials
     - Prefabricated trays
     - Whitening toothpaste
     - Whitening rinses
6. Most frequent side effect of whitening is tooth sensitivity, followed by gingival irritation

ROLE OF THE DENTAL AUXILIARY

The dental auxiliary can play an important role in the delivery of whitening services to patients. In addition to chairside assistance for in-office whitening, the auxiliary can be active oral health providers for home whitening by:

- Assessing the patient for oral conditions that would contraindicate whitening procedures.
- Performing several important clinical procedures, such as obtaining a pre-whitening shade and taking intra-oral images.
- As permitted by state dental practice acts, provide whitening services in the office.
- Discusing home care remedies for tooth hypersensitivity and advise the patient on foods and beverages that cause staining.

It is important that the patient be fully informed of the pros and cons of whitening. The auxiliary can provide this information to the patient before the dentist completes the informed consent. In addition, the auxiliary can provide the patient with instructions for proper use of the whitening agent and care of the trays.

POTENTIAL SIDE EFFECTS OF TEETH WHITENING

Sensitivity

Tooth sensitivity from the whitening process is usually short term. The sensitivity can be managed by shortening the whitening time each day, alternating days of application, using a lower concentration of whitening agent, or by stopping the whitening process for a few weeks. The sensitivity is likely caused by whitening agent penetrating through the enamel to the dentinal tubules or by passing through open dentinal tubules on exposed root surfaces and into the pulp, causing irritation. Studies have shown that peroxides can penetrate enamel and dentin and reach the pulp within a matter of minutes. Reversible pulpitis may occur with whitening procedures; however, the pain associated with the inflamed pulp will subside as whitening procedures are discontinued. Hydrogen peroxide can be damaging to cells with prolonged exposure or high concentrations.

Foods and beverages such as citrus fruits and their juices, sodas, vinegar, and other acidic foods should be avoided as long as the teeth are sensitive. Acids tend to open dentinal tubules in exposed root surfaces by dissolving plugs of salivary mucins and debris.

Desensitizing products can be useful to reduce symptoms such as:
- Fluoride
- Potassium nitrate
- Amorphous calcium phosphate (ACP)
- Casein phosphopeptide-ACP
- Calcium sodium phosphosilicate
- Arginine calcium carbonate

- Tricalcium phosphate
- Other desensitizing agents, as previously described (see Chapter 18).

In some cases, brushing with desensitizing toothpaste for 2 weeks before whitening is started will reduce sensitivity.

Other Side Effects

Possible side effects caused by excess material coming out of the tray include irritation of the:
- Gingiva
  - Gingival irritation can occur if the trays are not trimmed appropriately and the trays rub the tissues
- Mucosa
- Throat

If patients wear the whitening trays overnight, they may experience some soreness of the muscles of mastication and temporomandibular joints if the trays cause them to clench or grind or slightly displace the condyles (heads of the mandible) from the joints.

 Do You Recall?

What steps can the dental auxiliary recommend for a patient experiencing sensitivity associated with the use of home whitening products?

Home Whitening Instructions Given in the Dental Office

AT THE WHITENING SESSIONS
1. Brush and floss prior to whitening.
2. Place a small amount of whitening gel in the front of each tooth section of the tray. Too much gel in the tray will be displaced by the teeth and may irritate oral tissues and throat.
3. Place the tray over the teeth and seat it gently. Remove excess gel with a toothbrush or paper towel.
4. Wear the tray for the time prescribed by the dentist.
5. At the end of the whitening session, remove the tray, rinse the mouth with water, and use a toothbrush to remove residual gel.
6. Clean the tray under running water with a toothbrush. Liquid soap may be used. Shake off water. Place the tray in a storage container with the lid open to allow the tray to air-dry. Keep out of the reach of children and pets.

ADDITIONAL INFORMATION
1. Store whitening gel in a cool, dry location, out of direct sunlight, or in the refrigerator to prolong shelf life.
2. Whitening is not recommended while pregnant or nursing.
3. Avoid coffee, tea, red wine, colored cola drinks, berries, and tobacco because they can cause staining of teeth.
4. Whitening results usually last 1 to 3 years. Gradual restaining may necessitate occasional rewhitening.
5. Keep the whitening trays for future use or touch-ups; it should only be necessary to buy additional whitening agent for rewhitening.
6. If tooth sensitivity or other problems develop, call the office for guidance.

RESTORATIVE CONSIDERATIONS

Before the whitening process is started, decay should be treated and leaking restorations replaced to prevent excessive penetration of whitening agent through the dentinal tubules, which might irritate the pulp and cause sensitivity. Whitening may be done as a prerestorative procedure to whiten the teeth before composite bonding procedures, veneers, or porcelain crowns. However, bonding procedures, including the placement of composite restorations, should not be attempted on newly whitened teeth, as residual whitening materials may still be present in the tooth structure, which can prevent proper bonding. Additionally, teeth dehydrate when isolated for a period of time. The teeth will appear whiter than they will be after several hours when they have rehydrated. It typically takes at least 2 weeks for the new shade to stabilize. So, if a patient is to have cosmetic restorative treatment after whitening procedures, waiting a minimum of 2 weeks before matching the shade of whitened teeth is recommended.

Prior to whitening procedures, patients need to be informed that the color of existing restorations will not lighten with the whitening of the teeth. If they have tooth-colored restorations in visible areas of the mouth that match the teeth before whitening, the restorations will appear darker after whitening the teeth because the surrounding tooth structure will be lighter. Some patients have whitened their teeth so much that the shades found in regular composite kits may not be light enough to match the color of the whitened teeth. Several manufacturers have now developed whitening shades for composite materials.

During the whitening process, patients should be advised to limit their intake of foods and beverages that can stain the teeth, including coffee, tea, red wine, colored cola drinks, and berries or berry juices. Smoking can also contribute to staining of the teeth.

 Do You Recall?

Why it is important to wait 2 weeks after whitening before picking a shade for a final restoration?

 Clinical Tip

A period of at least 2 weeks is needed after whitening to allow the color of the teeth to stabilize before esthetic restorations are placed. Also, the bond to newly whitened surfaces is weaker than when the teeth are allowed to stabilize.

Contraindications: Whitening Is Not for Everyone

The following people should not attempt to whiten their teeth:
- People allergic to whitening or tray materials
- Pregnant or nursing individuals
- People with open carious lesions, leaking restorations, or cracked teeth
- People with hypersensitive teeth
- People with many tooth-colored restorations who do not want to replace them when whitening of the teeth make them look darker
- People taking medications that make them photosensitive should not have light-activated whitening as they may get skin irritation or burns
- People with unrealistic expectations about what whitening can do
- Adolescents under 15 years of age with recently erupted permanent teeth whose enamel is still porous would allow too much penetration of whitening material, causing sensitivity
- People who have taken sedative medications or are mentally incapable of giving informed consent

RETREATMENT

Both in-office and home whitening will fade with time. One study found a relapse of approximately 40% at 1 year with in-office whitening. Another study evaluating at-home tray whitening found a 26% relapse at 119 months. Some offices provide home whitening kits to their patients who have undergone in-office whitening in anticipation that they will want to rewhiten or touch-up their teeth over time, as retreatment may be required to maintain the lightness of the teeth. Typically, patients may find that in 1 to 3 years they will want to do some additional whitening. With in-office whitening, this often means that patients will have to pay the full bleaching fee again. With home tray whitening, patients only need to purchase additional whitening solution if they keep their custom whitening trays.

ENAMEL MICROABRASION

A variety of noncarious discolorations can occur in the enamel. They may be caused by mild fluorosis, hypermineralized spots that occurred during enamel development, or previous carious white spot lesions that have remineralized but are still whiter than the surrounding enamel. When these discolorations are of concern to the patient, one conservative approach to their removal is called *enamel microabrasion*.

The procedure includes the following steps:

- Determine that the lesion is shallow enough to leave an adequate thickness of enamel after discoloration removal.
- Clean the surface of the lesion with pumice.
- Apply an acid slurry made of flour of pumice and 6% hydrochloric acid (diluted from muriatic acid purchased at a hardware store or a commercial preparation such as PREMA [Premier] or Opalustre [Ultradent]) to the discoloration for 1 minute.
- Agitate the slurry with a ribbed rubber cup (prophy angle) revolving slowly (about 500 rpm) for an additional 1 minute.
- Rinse acid slurry off the tooth.
- Repeat the process if the spot is not gone.
- Do not repeat more than three times as too much enamel will be removed.
- If the spot still remains, another approach, such as covering the spot with composite, might be needed (Fig. 19.13).

ADVERSE OUTCOMES

Care must be taken when performing microabrasion to prevent burns to the soft tissues from the acid. If treatment is too aggressive or prolonged, so much enamel will be removed that the yellow dentin will show through the thinned enamel, and the teeth will look much yellower than before treatment was initiated. The pulp may be irritated by penetration of acid, or by heat generated if the rubber cup is used with too much pressure and speed. As with any dental procedure, the established treatment protocol must be followed as recommended to avoid adverse outcomes.

SUMMARY

Whitening of teeth for cosmetic reasons is a popular aspect of cosmetic dentistry. To be effective in providing whitening services and advice to patients, dental professionals must be knowledgeable about in-office, prescribed home whitening, and OTC products, including their indications and contraindications and potential side effects. Staining of the teeth caused by tetracycline or blood products from nonvital teeth can be the most difficult to remove. Patients need to be advised of potential limitations of treatment and other pros and cons before providing their informed consent to treatment. Dental auxiliaries are important team members in providing these popular cosmetic procedures.

INSTRUCTIONAL VIDEOS

See the Evolve Resources site for a variety of educational videos that reinforce the material covered in this chapter.

Teeth Whitening Materials and Procedures CHAPTER 19

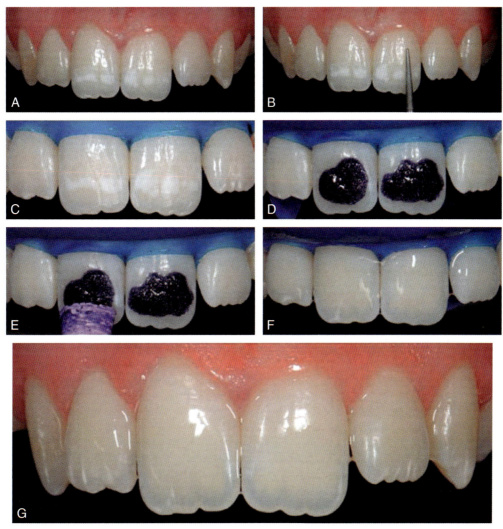

FIG. 19.13 Microabrasion. **(A)** Before treatment: white enamel discoloration. **(B)** Preparation (roughening) of tooth with bur. **(C)** Isolation of teeth with dental dam. **(D)** Application of microabrasion compound. **(E)** Application of microabrasion at slow speed. **(F)** Removal of microabrasion compound. **(G)** After treatment: staining is considerably reduced. After microabrasion, a course of home whitening can further reduce the staining. (From *J Appl Oral Sci.* 2014;22(4):347–354.)

Procedure 19.1 In-Office Whitening

See Evolve site for Competency Sheet.

EQUIPMENT/SUPPLIES (FIG. 19.14)
- Basic examination setup
- Prophy setup: Low-speed handpiece with prophy angle, prophy cup, flour of pumice
- Tooth shade guide
- Dental dam setup (check for latex allergy) or paint on light cured dental dam (liquid-dam material)
- Tissue-protective material (petroleum jelly or manufacturer's coating or foam)
- High-strength whitening material (percentage of solution varies with manufacturer)

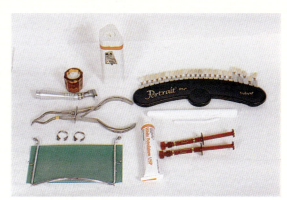

FIG. 19.14

Continued

Procedure 19.1 In-Office Whitening—cont'd

- High-intensity light, curing light, laser, or heat source (depending on whitening material type)
- Appropriately tinted safety lenses or light shield
- Timer or watch
- Three-way syringe and high-volume evacuation with disposable tips
- Waxed dental floss, 2 × 2 gauze
- Optional: Extraoral or intraoral camera for taking photographs

PROCEDURE STEPS

1. Obtain informed consent: One copy for the patient and one for the chart.
2. Clean the teeth with flour of pumice or non-fluoride/oil polishing paste.
3. Determine the starting shade and record. A photograph may also be taken, if desired.
4. Place tissue protection on the gingiva and interdental papillae according to the manufacturer's directions.
   NOTE: The gingiva may be coated with petroleum jelly or other protective layer under the dental dam in case the dam leaks.
5. Place the dental dam, isolating the teeth to be whitened (Fig. 19.15).
   NOTE: Holes in the dental dam must be of appropriate size and spacing to prevent leakage. Invert the edge of the dam around each tooth to form a seal, so that whitening material will not contact the gingiva.
6. Use waxed floss to help tuck in the dam interproximally. Use a hand instrument to invert the dam around each tooth.
7. Place high-strength whitening material as provided by the manufacturer (usually 35% hydrogen peroxide) and follow specific directions for time and light/heat source application (Figs. 19.16 and 19.17). Be aware of developing tooth or gum sensitivity during the procedure. Respond accordingly.

NOTE: Tooth sensitivity may be due to overheating of the tooth, previously exposed root areas, or penetration of strong whitener into vital dentin. Gum sensitivity may be caused by a chemical burn from the whitening agent. Mild sensitivity usually goes away in a few days. Severe burns to the gingiva or mucosa can be painful and cause tissue necrosis that may take weeks to heal. Mild burns with surface whitening of the gingiva heal quickly.

8. Rinse off the whitening material, wipe clean with 2 × 2 gauze, and examine for shade. Repeat the application of whitening solution as needed to achieve the desired shade.
   NOTE: Teeth appear whiter with the dental dam in place because of the contrast in color and the dehydration of the teeth that occurs. The true color appears after the teeth are rehydrated with saliva. Color stability is achieved 2 weeks after whitening.
9. Additional appointments may be needed to achieve the tooth whitening goal.
   NOTE: Desired results cannot always be achieved. Some stains are more resistant to whitening and every patient has a limit as to how white their teeth can get.

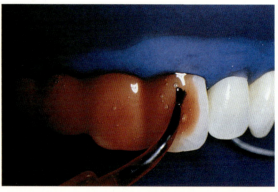

FIG. 19.16

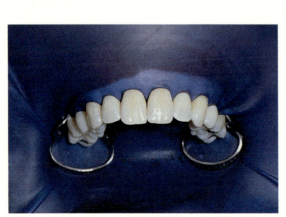

FIG. 19.15

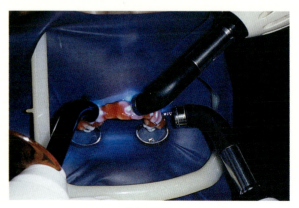

FIG. 19.17

Procedure 19.2 Clinical Procedures for Home Whitening

See Evolve site for Competency Sheet.

EQUIPMENT/SUPPLIES (FIG. 19.18)
- Basic setup for examination
- Rubber mixing bowl and spatula
- Alginate, measures for water and powder
- Alginate impression trays
- Dental plaster or stone
- Dental vibrator
- Tooth shade guide and camera (optional)
- Home whitening kit and instructions

PROCEDURE STEPS

First Appointment

1. Dentist examines the oral cavity and teeth for type of discoloration and oral conditions that might influence the success of whitening. Potential areas of concern are treated or planned for correction.
   NOTE: Dental caries, sensitive teeth, and leaking restorations may need correction before whitening to prevent further sensitivity or pulpal problems.
2. Discuss the pros and cons of whitening with the patient. Obtain informed consent.
   NOTE: A signed informed consent form signifies that the patient fully understands what is involved, has had their questions answered, and agrees to the treatment.
3. Record the patient's tooth shade (Fig. 19.19). Take photographs with a shade tab next to the teeth, if desired.
   NOTE: Many manufacturers include a shade card that can be used to match the initial shade and later to compare it with the whitened shade at future visits.
4. Select impression trays of the correct size and make alginate impressions.
5. Rinse the impressions, spray with disinfectant or immerse in suitable disinfectant for 10 minutes, wrap in moist paper towel, and seal in zippered plastic bag.
6. Pour impressions with dental stone using a vibrator to minimize bubbles. (Block out the tongue and palatal area with a wet paper towel to make trimming the casts easier when making trays.) Trays are fabricated in the office (see Procedure 19.3) or sent to a commercial laboratory.

Second Appointment

7. Insert trays for fit and comfort.
8. Demonstrate loading of trays with gel, tray insertion, and removal of excess gel (Figs. 19.20 through 19.22).

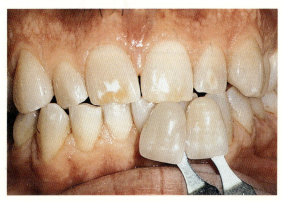

FIG. 19.19 (Courtesy Ultradent Products, Inc., South Jordan, Utah.)

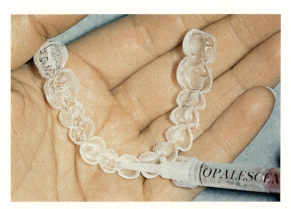

FIG. 19.20 (Courtesy Ultradent Products, Inc., South Jordan, Utah.)

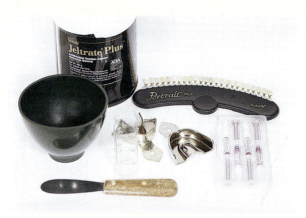

FIG. 19.18

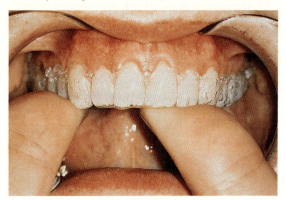

FIG. 19.21 (Courtesy Ultradent Products, Inc., South Jordan, Utah.)

Continued

Procedure 19.2 Clinical Procedures for Home Whitening—cont'd

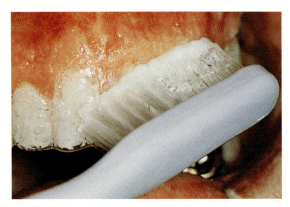

FIG. 19.22 (Courtesy Ultradent Products, Inc., South Jordan, Utah.)

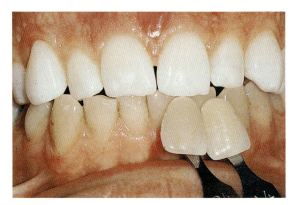

FIG. 19.23 (Courtesy Ultradent Products, Inc., South Jordan, Utah.)

9. Demonstrate cleaning of trays after a whitening session.
10. Give the patient verbal and written instructions to take home after the visit.. Review possible side effects. Dispense home whitening kit.
    NOTE: Written instructions are important because patients sometimes forget what they have been told.
11. Schedule a follow-up appointment in 2 to 3 weeks after initial delivery. Determine and record tooth shade at each subsequent visit (Fig. 19.23). The procedure should be continued until the desired shade is achieved.

NOTE: Whitening will not change the color of existing tooth-colored restorations (composite, glass ionomer, compomer, or ceramic). The patient must understand that these restorations will appear darker than the surrounding whitened teeth and may need to be replaced to achieve the desired cosmetic result. Not all stains respond to whitening, and patients may not achieve the desired results. Cosmetic restorative procedures are done after whitening has stabilized for a period of 2 weeks or longer.

Procedure 19.3 Fabrication of Custom Whitening Trays

See Evolve site for Competency Sheet.

EQUIPMENT/SUPPLIES (FIG. 19.24)

1. Casts (models) of patient's dentition
2. Whitening reservoir material: Light-cured block-out resin
3. Vacuum former
4. Two sheets of 6 × 6-inch by 0.02- or 0.035-inch-thick thermoplastic vinyl tray material
5. Fine-tipped scissors for trimming the trays

PROCEDURE STEPS

1. Trim casts to eliminate much of the facial peripheral border. If the maxillary cast has a palatal area, drill a hole in the deepest part of the palate or grind away most of the palatal area (Fig. 19.25).
   NOTE: Ledges or concave areas on the casts that trap air when the molten tray material is lowered over the casts will prevent good adaptation of the tray to the cast and result in a poorly fitting tray that leaks

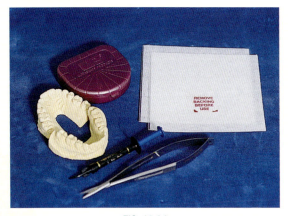

FIG. 19.24

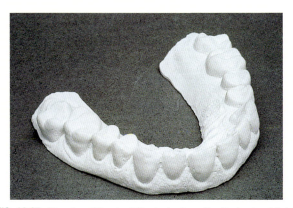

FIG. 19.25 (Courtesy Ultradent Products, Inc., South Jordan, Utah.)

Procedure 19.3 Fabrication of Custom Whitening Trays—cont'd

whitening gel into the patient's mouth. Before pouring stone into the alginate impressions, a wet paper towel should be used to block out the tongue and palate areas. This will save time trimming stone away from these areas later.

2. Allow the casts to dry, and then apply reservoir material (e.g., LC Block-out Resin, Ultradent Products) to the facial surfaces of the teeth (on the cast) to be whitened.
3. Light-cured block-out resin is applied to the facial surfaces of the teeth to be whitened in a thin layer about 1 mm thick. It should extend 1 mm short of the gingival crest and the interproximal embrasures (Fig. 19.26).
4. Resin on each tooth should be cured for 10 seconds with a curing light.

    NOTE: The reservoir is left short of the gingival crest so the tray will seal in that area and prevent the whitening agent from contacting the gingiva.

5. Clamp a sheet of thermoplastic vinyl tray material in the frame of the vacuum-forming unit (Fig. 19.27). Raise the frame until it is just below the heating element. Turn on the heating element.
6. Place one cast in the center of the platform (it contains many holes) of the vacuum former.
7. When the vinyl material has heated and sagged an inch or more (Fig. 19.28), lower the frame to the platform and turn on the vacuum. The molten material will be pulled tightly over the cast.

    NOTE: If a pocket of air is trapped under the vinyl, push it out by adapting the tray to the cast by hand with a damp paper towel while the material is still soft and the vacuum is on.

8. Allow the tray material to cool for at least 1 minute before removing it from the frame. Place it under cold running water to cool thoroughly.
9. Trim excess material away from the cast with scissors. Remove the cast from the tray.
10. Use fine scissors to trim the tray so that it extends over the teeth just to the gingival crest (Fig. 19.29). It should have a scalloped appearance as it traces the outline of the gingival crest (Fig. 19.30).

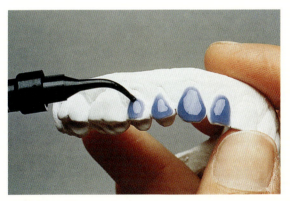

FIG. 19.26 (Courtesy Ultradent Products, Inc., South Jordan, Utah.)

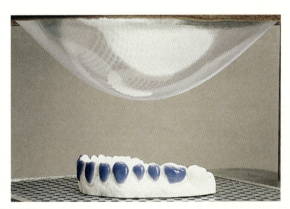

FIG. 19.28 (Courtesy Ultradent Products, Inc., South Jordan, Utah.)

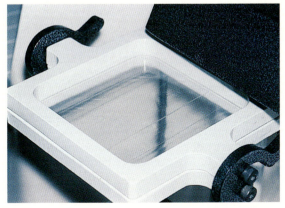

FIG. 19.27 (Courtesy Ultradent Products, Inc., South Jordan, Utah.)

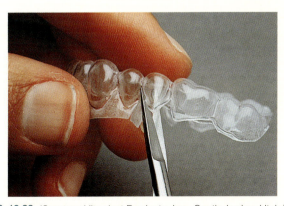

FIG. 19.29 (Courtesy Ultradent Products, Inc., South Jordan, Utah.)

Continued

Procedure 19.3   Fabrication of Custom Whitening Trays—cont'd

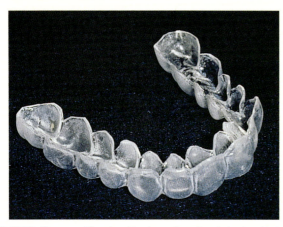

FIG. 19.30 (Courtesy Ultradent Products, Inc., South Jordan, Utah.)

NOTE: If the tray extends over the gingiva on the facial surfaces, a whitening agent can contact the gingiva and cause irritation.

11. Repeat the process for the other cast.
12. Wash the trays with soap and water. Spray the trays with surface disinfectant and store until delivery in a zippered plastic bag marked with the patient's name.

Review and Discussion

Review Questions

Select the one correct response for each of the following multiple-choice questions.

1. What type of whitening solution is painted on the tooth structure and held in place for 30 minutes with a sealer?
   a. Power whitening
   b. Home whitening
   c. Whitening varnish
   d. Whitestrips
2. Whitening of teeth works by:
   a. Removing surface stains
   b. Penetrating both enamel and dentin and oxidizing the stain
   c. Sealing surface porosities so that stain cannot enter the tooth surface
   d. Creating a white coating on the surface of the enamel
3. In-office whitening:
   a. Is superior in results to home whitening
   b. Produces equivalent results to home whitening in a shorter period of time
   c. Does not cause tooth sensitivity
   d. Has no effect if the whitening agent contacts the gingiva
4. The active ingredient in most in-office and OTC whitening products is:
   a. Sodium bicarbonate
   b. Ammonia
   c. Phosphoric acid
   d. Peroxide
5. Which one of the following can remove intrinsic stains?
   a. Prophy cup with polishing paste
   b. Hydrogen peroxide
   c. Air polishing with sodium bicarbonate powder
   d. Ultrasonic scaling
6. Whitening procedures should be avoided if the patient has any of the following *except* one. Which one is the *exception*?
   a. Open carious lesions
   b. Gingivitis
   c. Hypersensitive teeth
   d. Inability to give informed consent
7. Undesirable outcomes from home whitening include all of the following *except* one. Which one is the *exception*?
   a. Soft tissue irritation
   b. Root abrasion
   c. Sore muscles of mastication or temporomandibular joints
   d. Temperature sensitivity
8. The most difficult stains to remove are:
   a. Coffee stains
   b. Chlorhexidine stains
   c. Red wine stains
   d. Tetracycline stains
9. After whitening, how much time should the patient wait until a shade is selected for permanent restorations?
   a. 1 week
   b. 2 weeks
   c. 3 weeks
10. Which one of the following statements about whitening strips is true?
    a. Strips are less effective than paint-on whitening products.
    b. Strips are typically worn for 4 to 6 hours at a time.
    c. Strips interfere with speech.
    d. Strips are just as effective as home tray whitening with 10% to 15% carbamide peroxide.

For answers to Review Questions, see the Appendix.

Continued

Review and Discussion—cont'd

Case-Based Discussion Topics

1. A 35-year-old teacher has been using an OTC whitening system with trays adapted to the teeth after the material is boiled in water. The trays are worn while sleeping. The teacher comes to the dental office complaining of sensitive teeth, inflamed and painful gingiva, and sore jaw muscles.

Discuss possible causes for each complaint and make recommendations to treat the problems and prevent their recurrence.

2. A 16-year-old high school student has just become a cheerleader and wishes to have a brighter smile for public appearances.

Which whitening systems would be appropriate?
What are the potential side effects on patients this young?
What measures can be employed to minimize the side effects?

3. A 45-year-old plumber has high caries activity because of snacking on Snickers bars while out on house calls. The plumber also has dull teeth and wants to whiten them for socializing with friends.

What things should be considered before starting whitening procedures? If anterior composites are placed to restore carious teeth, should they be done before or after whitening? Why?

BIBLIOGRAPHY

American Dental Association (ADA): *Council on scientific affairs: statement on the safety and effectiveness of tooth whitening products.* 2022. Available at: https://www.ada.org/en/about-the-ada/ada-positions-policies-and-statements/tooth-whitening-safety-and-effectiveness.

Bird DL, Robinson DS: *Tooth Whitening.* In *Modern Dental Assisting,* ed 13, St. Louis, 2021, Elsevier.

Darby ML, Walsh MM: *Dental Hygiene Theory and Practice,* St. Louis, 2015, Elsevier.

Epple M, Meyer F, Enax J: A critical review of modern concepts for teeth whitening, *Dent J* 7(3):79, 2019.

Irusa K, Alrahaem IA, Ngoc CN, Donovan T: Tooth whitening procedures: a narrative review, *Dent Rev* 2(3), 2022.

Kugel G, Perry RD, Hoang E, Scherer W: Effective tooth bleaching in 5 days: using a combined in-office and at-home bleaching system, *Compendium Continuing Educ Dent* 18(4):378–383, 1997.

Kwon SR: Innovation in tooth whitening, *Dimens Dent Hyg* 16(01):1821–1823, 2018.

Magid KS: In-office power bleaching with a plasma arc curing light, *Contemporary Esthet Restorat Pract* 9:14–20, 1999.

Robinson DS: *Essentials of Dental Assisting,* ed 7, St. Louis, 2023, Elsevier.

20 Preventive and Corrective Oral Appliances

http://evolve.elsevier.com/Eakle/materials/

Chapter Objectives

On completion of this chapter, the student should be able to:

1. Describe the uses of mouth guards.
2. List the materials for the fabrication of mouth guards.
3. Explain to a patient how to care for a mouth guard.
4. Describe the steps to fabricate a sports mouth guard.
5. Define obstructive sleep apnea.
6. Describe the use of oral appliances to prevent snoring or obstructive sleep apnea.
7. Explain how preventive orthodontics prevent or eliminate the need for full orthodontics.
8. Identify how interceptive orthodontics correct malalignments of the dentition.
9. Describe how thermoplastic orthodontic aligners perform.
10. Identify how 3D printing is being utilized in dentistry.

KEY TERMS

Mouth Guard an appliance made of hard or pliable material that protects teeth from trauma during sports activities or from grinding of the teeth

Custom-Fit made specifically to fit one individual

Obstructive Sleep Apnea a sleep disorder caused when the muscles that support the soft palate, uvula, and tongue relax and the airway narrows or closes

Space Maintainer a fixed or removable appliance used to prevent adjacent teeth from drifting into the space created when a tooth is lost

Thumb Sucking Device a fixed or removable appliance used to discourage tongue thrusting and thumb sucking

Palatal Expansion Device a fixed appliance used to expand the maxillary arch, forcing the maxillary plates apart very slowly while the maxilla is still in development

Crossbite Corrector a fixed or removable appliance used to correct teeth in malalignment, where the maxillary teeth are positioned lingual or facial to the mandibular teeth

Orthodontic Tooth Aligners removable appliances that are designed to gently move teeth into predetermined positions

---

A number of oral appliances are available to prevent damage to the teeth, to keep teeth from shifting, to prevent sleep apnea and snoring, and to orthodontically move teeth. This chapter provides basic knowledge about these appliances. Many of these appliances can be fabricated in the dental office by trained staff or sent to a commercial dental laboratory. The dental auxiliary may be called on to fabricate these appliances or to instruct patients in their use and home care.

PREVENTIVE AND CORRECTIVE ORAL APPLIANCES

SPORTS MOUTH GUARDS

The purpose of sports guards is to protect the teeth and supporting structures (gingival tissues and bone). The widespread use of **mouth guards** in school sports prevents thousands of injuries each year. According to the American Dental Association (ADA), the risk of orofacial injury was 1.6 to 1.9 times higher in players who did not use mouth guards (Fig. 20.1A). The National Youth Sports Foundation estimates that approximately 5 million teeth will be knocked out in sporting activities in a single year. Dental injuries are the most common type of orofacial injury sustained during sports. The Centers for Disease Control and Prevention (CDC) recommend, and most states mandate that participants in school contact sports wear sports guards (also called *mouth protectors* or *mouth guards*) (see Fig. 20.1B).

Most professional and amateur adult athletes also wear sports guards. The protective benefits of sports mouth guards have been well documented.

The three basic types of mouth guards for sports are as follows:
- Stock guards
- Boil-and-bite guards
- Custom-fit guards

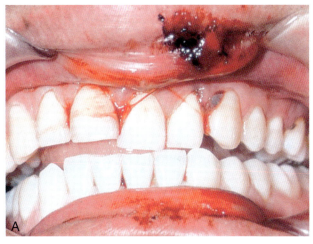
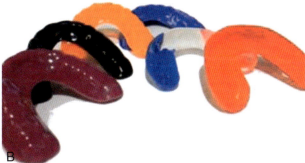

FIG. 20.1 Prevention of sports injuries: **(A)** Injury to the lip and teeth that could be avoided with a sports guard. **(B)** Multilayer sports guard. (Courtesy Acacia Dental Group.)

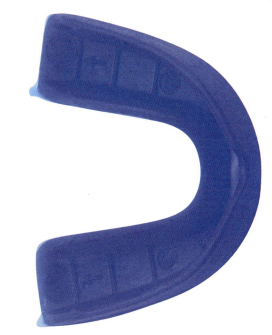

FIG. 20.2 Stock guard. (Courtesy of Athletic Specialties.)

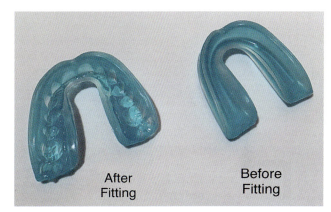

FIG. 20.3 Boil-and-bite guard prior to and after fitting.

Stock Guards

Stock guards (Fig. 20.2) can be purchased over the counter:
- In sporting goods stores
- In some retail stores
- Online

They usually cost less than $25 and come in sizes ranging from small, medium, and large. Along with being the least expensive, stock guards generally have:
- The poorest fit
- May be uncomfortable to wear
- Provide the least amount of protection
- They are not adapted to the patient's bite

Boil-and-Bite Guards

Similar to the stock guards, boil-and-bite guards (Fig. 20.3) can be found:
- In sporting goods stores
- In retail stores
- Online

They typically cost less than $50 and are constructed of a horseshoe-shaped, flexible thermoplastic material that softens when heated.

The material is softened and fitted to the athlete by:
- Boiling water
- Placed in the mouth while still moldable
- Adapted to the teeth and arch by fingers, lips, and tongue
- Then adapted to the bite by closing the teeth into the guard
- Cut away excess material with heavy-duty scissors

This type of guard is often difficult for inexperienced individuals to adapt properly and may have a poor fit interfering with breathing and speaking ability, but the fit is usually better than stock guards. Boil-and-bite guards can provide false protection as they can become very thin when an athlete bites too far into them in a softened state.

Custom-Fit Guards

Professionally made guards are **custom-fit** to casts of the patient's mouth (Fig. 20.4). Because of the added steps, materials, and time involved in their fabrication, custom guards may cost several times more than stock and boil-and-bite guards.

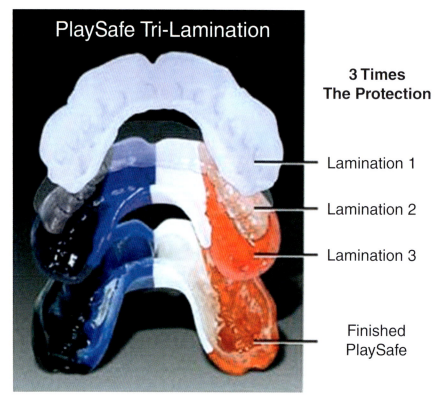

FIG. 20.4 PlaySafe Tri-lamination custom-fit sports guards. (Photo courtesy Glidewell Laboratories Copyright © 2020.)

Custom-fit guards can be made from:
- A single layer of material fabricated in the dental office or commercial laboratory
- Pressure-laminated material in a commercial dental laboratory

The single-layer guard is a sheet of thermoplastic material heated in a vacuum-forming machine and vacuum adapted to the cast (Procedure 20.1). The material may be clear or a variety of colors (Fig. 20.1B). A strap may be attached for sports such as football, where the athlete wears a helmet and wants to attach it to the facemask for easy access. Because the fit is excellent and the bite is comfortable, the athlete is more likely to wear the guard in comparison to the other types.

Pressure-laminated sports guards fabricated in a commercial dental laboratory are highly recommended for contact sports such as hockey, basketball, and football. The thermoplastic material consists of two or three sheets that are heat-fused together. These guards are thicker than single-layer guards, provide more cushion, and are more durable.

Protection

Sports guards can absorb about 80% of the energy from a traumatic hit to the mouth. Sports guards usually extend just short of the height of the vestibule and cover the upper teeth, gingiva, and alveolar bone. On occasion, they are made to cover both arches simultaneously. The guard can protect the teeth and jaws from fracture by a direct blow or cushion the upper and lower teeth when an athlete's jaws are forced together by a blow to the lower jaw. Because these guards provide cushioning to the jaws during collision with another athlete or the ground, some concussions can be mitigated or prevented. The guard can prevent lacerations to lips for athletes with orthodontic braces or brackets and protect dental work such as bridges, anterior veneers, or crowns. Athletes should be directed to leave removable prostheses such as orthodontic retainers out when playing sports because they could become dislodged and enter the throat.

Sports guards need a certain thickness and stiffness to maximize their protective qualities. The heavier the contact in the sport, the thicker the guard should be to provide maximal protection. For heavy-contact sports, where injuries are more likely, a thickness of about 5 mm is desirable. For less physical sports, 2 mm of thickness may suffice.

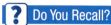 **Do You Recall?**

What types of sports should encourage the use of a sports guard?

NIGHT GUARDS (BRUXISM MOUTH GUARDS)

Many patients who grind (brux) their teeth do so during sleep. They may not even be aware of their grinding until the dental professional points out the wear evident on the teeth.

Common signs of chronic bruxing include:
- Wear facets (flattened tooth surfaces that used to be convex)
- Chipping and wear of incisal edges
- Stress cracks in teeth
- Fractured cusps
- Cracked teeth
- Mobility of teeth
- Enlarged masseters
- Sore muscles of mastication

Guards are recommended for patients who are bruxers. The guard does not stop the grinding habit, but it protects the teeth from wear, chipping, and even fracture of cusps. Guards to protect the teeth from grinding and clenching are also called *occlusal guards, bite splints,* or *night guards*.

Dental offices can provide valuable preventive measures for their patients by offering guards. Dental auxiliaries can play an active role in recommending night guards, making impressions for their fabrication, and even fabricating the guard in the office laboratory.

Patients undergoing treatment for dysfunction of the temporomandibular joint (commonly called *TMD*) are often given devices (called *TMJ splints*) to wear that can serve three functions:
1. Keeping the teeth separated
2. Taking stress off the joints
3. Protecting the teeth

These splints can also be made from hard acrylic or soft thermoplastic material.

Home Care Instructions for Soft Sports or Bruxism Guards

- Wash the guard with room temperature water and brush with a toothbrush and liquid soap after each use.
- Do not soak a soft guard in a commercial denture cleaner or an alcohol-containing mouthwash, as these products will degrade the soft material over time.
- Allow the guard to air-dry. Do not enclose it in an airtight container because mold and bacteria will grow. If storing it in a container, use one with perforations where air can circulate.
- Do not leave the guard in a closed automobile in the sun or expose it to hot water as this will cause warping.
- Do not chew on the guard when in use, as it may tear or distort.
- Do not leave the guard where the family dog might reach it. They have been known to chew them up.
- Sports guards eventually wear out, so when it no longer fits well or has tears and holes in it, it is time to replace it.

Types of Materials

Three types of material are used in the making of night guards:
- *Hard:* Acrylic (methyl methacrylate resin and monomer)
- *Soft:* Thermoplastic sheets of poly(vinyl acetate)-polyethylene material
- *Hard and soft:* Laminates of hard and soft thermoplastic materials

Hard Acrylic Guard. Patients who grind their teeth heavily and frequently should have a hard acrylic guard, due to it being more durable than a soft guard. Hard acrylic guards are usually fabricated in the dental laboratory (Fig. 20.5). The hard guard typically requires more chair-time for adjustment, because the acrylic, like other resins, shrinks when it is cured. They also feel tight on the patient's teeth when first tried on.

Soft Guard. Soft guards are better suited for patients who do not grind their teeth heavily or regularly (daily). Some patients who have had hard guards find the soft guards more comfortable and easier to get used to. These guards are made from soft thermoplastic sheets and may be fabricated in the commercial dental laboratory or the dental office. The auxiliary is often responsible for fabricating the guard in the dental office. Soft guards require much less time to adjust than hard guards. Often chairside adjustment can be made by heating the outside biting surface of the guard with an alcohol torch and, while it is still warm, placing it in the patient's mouth and having them bite into the materials. This process equalizes the bite. Care must be taken to avoid placing the guard in the mouth too hot and should be checked with the gloved hand first. A technique for using upper and lower casts mounted on a simple hinge articulator to adjust the bite at the time the guard is made is described in Procedure 20.1. Adjusting the bite on mounted casts can save chair-time. The poly(vinyl acetate)-polyethylene sheets used to make soft guards come in a variety of thicknesses, and the thinner sheets can also be used as whitening and fluoride trays.

Hard and Soft Laminate Guard. Patients who need the durability of a hard occlusal surface but like the feel of the soft material may prefer a dual hard and soft laminate guards. Guards made from this material are hard on the biting surface and soft internally, allowing them to adapt readily to the teeth while being gentle on the soft tissues. The material comes in sheets that have a firm thermoplastic material laminated with a soft material. A sheet of the material is softened in a vacuum machine similar to the soft guard material and vacuum adapted to the cast.

Design of the Guard

Most night guards and TMD splints cover the maxillary teeth, but some dentists cover the mandibular teeth. Some guards or TMD treatment splints may only cover a few of the anterior teeth (e.g., NTI splints; NTI-Chairside Splints), but some experts contend that guards limited to anterior coverage may actually create a fulcrum that displaces the condyles from their ideal position in the joints, resulting in more damage to the TMJ. Some guards may cover both the lingual and occlusal surfaces

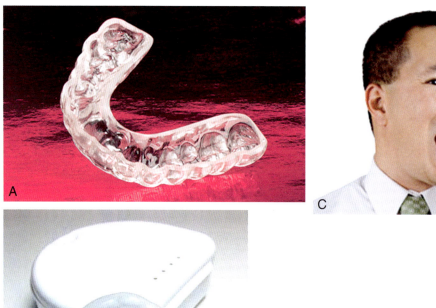
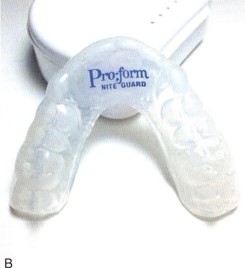

FIG. 20.5 Bruxism guard: **(A)** Laboratory-processed hard acrylic occlusal guard. **(B)** Soft guard made from thermoplastic material. **(C)** Patient aligns the guard with the teeth and presses it in place. (**(A)** Photo courtesy Glidewell Laboratories Copyright © 2020 and **(B)** Courtesy Keystone Industries.)

of the teeth and just lap over cusps of the posterior teeth and the incisal edges of the anterior teeth. Others cover all of the anterior and posterior teeth.

Maintenance

The dental auxiliary should instruct the patient in proper home care of the guard. The following protocols should be shared with the patient:
- Cleaning the guard daily is essential.
- When removed from the mouth, the guard should be rinsed thoroughly to remove saliva.
- Then it should be brushed with a toothbrush or denture brush and liquid soap.
- After the final rinse, excess water should be shaken off.
- Lastly the guard should be stored in a rigid container that is left open to allow the guard to air-dry.
- If the guard is sealed in a container while it is still damp, the growth of bacteria and mold will likely occur.

A rigid storage container prevents the guard from being distorted by other articles inadvertently placed on top of it. Staining is common with all types of guards. Contact with amalgam restorations will cause a dark gray stain over time in the area of contact. Solutions containing alcohol, such as mouthwash, and bleach should not be used because they will degrade the material. Commercially available soaks for orthodontic retainers or dentures are useful to freshen the hard guards but can degrade the soft poly(vinyl acetate)-polyethylene guards over time.

> **KEY POINTS—Preventive Oral Appliances**
>
> 1. Sports Mouth guards—protect teeth and oral structures from sports-type injuries
>   - Variation of guards
>   - Stock guards
>   - Purchased over the counter
>   - Boil-and-bite guards
>   - Purchased over the counter
>   - Custom-fit guards
>   - Made in the dental office or lab fabricated
> 2. Night Guards—protect teeth and oral structures from parafunctional habits such as bruxism
>   - Variation of guards
>   - Hard
>   - Soft
>   - Dual hard and soft
>   - All guards are made in the dental office or lab fabricated

 Caution

Patients should be advised not to immerse their sport guards or night guards in hot water because it can cause distortion of the guard.

ORAL APPLIANCES TO TREAT SNORING AND OBSTRUCTIVE SLEEP APNEA

While snoring may only be considered an annoyance, **obstructive sleep apnea (OSA)** can lead to serious health issues if not treated.

The most serious potential problems include:
- Hypertension
- Heart attack
- Heart failure
- Stroke

Snoring and OSA are often caused by relaxation of the muscles that support the soft palate, uvula, and tongue, causing a narrowing or closing of the airway. Breathing becomes inadequate or stops for a few seconds, causing the blood oxygen level to drop. This alerts the brain to wake the individual up just enough to reopen the airway. Often short, gasping breaths are taken until the oxygen level is restored. Someone with a serious problem may wake up 10 to 20 times an hour. They wake up in the morning feeling exhausted or, surprisingly, they may not notice the lack of sleep.

Risk Factors for Obstructive Sleep Apnea

Risk factors for OSA include:
- A large neck
- Obesity
- Chronic nasal congestion
- High blood pressure
- Diabetes
- Smoking
- Alcohol use
- A narrow airway

Males are twice as likely to have OSA compared to females. It is more common in people who are middle aged or older. To arrive at the proper diagnosis and plan of treatment, those afflicted may be sent to a sleep specialist at a sleep center for evaluation, where sleep patterns may be monitored overnight.

Treatment of Obstructive Sleep Apnea

Treatment for mild OSA may include:
- Weight loss
- Exercise
- Reduced alcohol intake
- Smoking cessation
- Sleeping on one side
- Use of nasal decongestants

Treatment for more severe OSA may involve the use of continuous positive airway pressure (CPAP). With CPAP a mask is worn on the face or nose cannula while sleeping and a device attached to it delivers a continuous positive flow of air to keep the airway open (Fig. 20.6).

Many people find the CPAP mask uncomfortable and have trouble adjusting to it. A more invasive approach to OSA is surgery to reduce the soft palate and uvula (uvulopalatopharyngoplasty) to open the airway. Many patients are willing to try oral appliances as a conservative alternative treatment.

Function of Appliances

Most appliances do one of three things:
- Lift the soft palate
- Hold the tongue in a more forward position
- Reposition the mandible forward to bring the tongue away from the airway

There are at least 80 different designs for oral appliances. Oral appliances do not work for everyone and show the most success for individuals with mild to moderate OSA (Fig. 20.7).

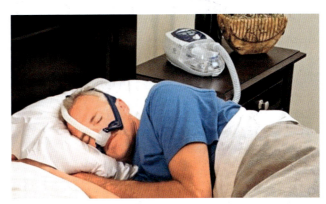

FIG. 20.6 Continuous positive airway pressure (CPAP) device for obstructive sleep apnea. (Courtesy CPAP Global)

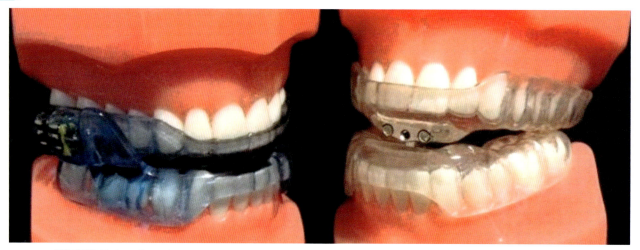

FIG. 20.7 Oral appliance for obstructive sleep apnea positions the lower jaw forward to prevent the tongue and soft tissues of the throat from obstructing the airway. (Courtesy Dental Sleep Apnea Clinic)

> **KEY POINTS—Obstructive Sleep Apnea (OSA)**
> 1. Risk factors for OSA include:
>   - Large neck
>   - Obesity
>   - Chronic nasal congestion
>   - High blood pressure
>   - Diabetes
>   - Smoking
>   - Alcohol use
>   - Narrow airway
> 2. Treatment of OSA:
>   - Weight loss
>   - Exercise
>   - Discontinuing the use of tobacco and alcohol
>   - Side sleeping
>   - Use of nasal decongestants
>   - Use of positive airway pressure (CPAP)
>   - Continuous positive air flow keeps the airway open
>   - Use of oral appliances to reposition oral structures
>   - Lift the soft palate
>   - Hold the tongue more forward
>   - Reposition the mandible forward

PREVENTIVE ORTHODONTICS

Preventive orthodontics are intended to prevent or eliminate malpositions and irregularities in the developing dentition and orofacial region. Preventive orthodontics are intended to eliminate the need for full orthodontics due to their application occurring while the dentition and face are still developing.

SPACE MAINTAINERS

Space maintainers are most frequently used in pediatric dentistry when a tooth is lost too soon. They prevent adjacent teeth from drifting and closing the space created by the missing tooth. Maintaining the space is important to allow the permanent tooth to erupt properly. Sometimes space maintainers are used in adults to hold the space from a lost tooth until a more permanent restoration, such as an implant, bridge, or removable partial denture, can be placed.

Types of Space Maintainers

Space maintainers can be removable or fixed. A removable space maintainer can be in the form of a stayplate or a retainer with a denture tooth or acrylic block attached. Fixed-space maintainers are cemented in place and may have a wire loop attached to a stainless-steel crown or an orthodontic band. The wire loop extends from the crowned or banded tooth to contact the tooth on the opposite side of the open space (Fig. 12.15, Chapter 12).

INTERCEPTIVE ORTHODONTICS

Interceptive orthodontics (corrective appliances) correct problems in the orofacial region as they develop in an attempt to prevent the need for full orthodontics or, at a minimum, decrease the amount of time orthodontics are required. The appliance intervention is necessary to prevent malocclusion.

THUMB SUCKING APPLIANCE

Thumb sucking and tongue thrusting are two main oral habits that interceptive orthodontics or corrective appliances are utilized to treat. The **thumb sucking device** consists of metal protrusions, which resemble spikes or a rake. When the patient places the tongue or the thumb on the device, discomfort will occur. This discomfort is anticipated to break the tongue thrusting or thumb sucking habit (Fig. 20.8).

PALATAL EXPANSION APPLIANCES

Palatal expansion devices are utilized to expand the maxillary arch when it is too narrow in comparison to the mandibular arch. Expansion of the maxillary arch

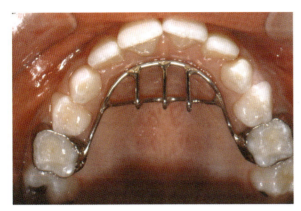

FIG. 20.8 Thumb sucking device. (Courtesy Dr. Frank Hodges.)

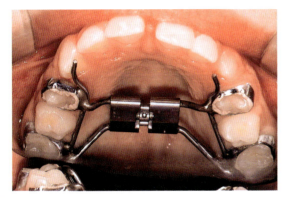

FIG. 20.9 Palatal expansion appliance. (Courtesy Dr. Frank Hodges.)

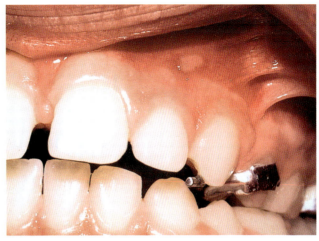

FIG. 20.10 Crossbite correcting device. (Courtesy Dr. Frank Hodges.)

reestablishes the balance between the width of the maxillary and mandibular jaws. Without expansion an abnormal relationship between dental arches would exist. The problems associated with a narrow palate could include airway obstruction due to a narrow nasal cavity and crowding of the maxillary teeth (Fig. 20.9).

CROSSBITE CORRECTOR

A **crossbite corrector** corrects the area where the maxillary teeth are positioned lingually or too far facially to the mandibular teeth. The crossbite is corrected by the use of a fixed or removable device. The device can be a band with an extension that guides the tooth into the appropriate place (Fig. 20.10).

Do You Recall?

Why are preventive orthodontics utilized?

ORTHODONTIC TOOTH ALIGNERS

Many types of minor tooth movement can be achieved with removable appliances that direct forces on the teeth to move them into proper alignment. Traditional removable appliances usually consist of an acrylic base with embedded stainless-steel wires (see Chapter 12) bent into springs or bows (Fig. 20.11) and/or expansion screws. A more recent approach uses a series of clear thermoplastic aligners to gradually move the teeth into the desired position. Because these **orthodontic tooth aligners** are made from a clear thermoplastic material, the clear aligners are used more with adults than children. They are popular because they are more esthetic than conventional retainers, braces, and brackets. However, complex malocclusions will require conventional orthodontic treatment with brackets, bands, and wires.

How Clear Aligners Are Made

Design software creates a 3D model from a digital scan of the teeth or a cast of the teeth. Next, technicians digitally move the individual teeth into the final desired position, using design software. Then, the software is used to simulate moving the teeth in gradual stages, and aligners (made of polyurethane) are fabricated for each stage of movement (Fig. 20.12).

Treatment

The patient wears the clear aligners approximately 20 hours a day. Wearing the aligners for a shorter period of time each day will extend the total treatment time. The aligners are removed only to eat, drink, or clean the teeth. Small nobs made of composite material (called *buttons*) are bonded to the teeth to help the aligners grip well and to facilitate tooth movement (Fig. 20.13). Elastic may be needed to help rotate teeth or to intrude or extrude them.

A new aligner in the series is used every 2 to 4 weeks. This is repeated until the malocclusion or misalignment is corrected. The last and final step is to make a retainer to keep the teeth from shifting. It is usually made from the same clear material as the aligners.

3D PRINTING

The use of 3D printing is becoming increasingly popular in the field of dentistry. A common application of 3D printing is with the use of a desktop 3D printer to fabricate (print) clear orthodontic aligners or implant guides.

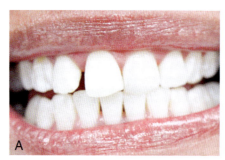
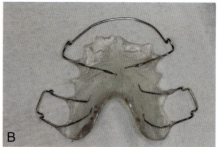
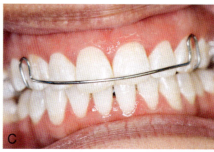

FIG. 20.11 Removable tooth movement appliance (Hawley appliance): **(A)** Protruding right maxillary central incisor. **(B)** Hawley appliance with a labial bow that will be activated by tightening the loops. The pressure created on the incisor will move it lingually. The bow is reactivated as the tooth moves. **(C)** Maxillary incisor has been repositioned with the Hawley appliance, and the appliance will now serve as a retainer. (Courtesy Dr. Scott Rooker, Redmond, OR.)

The aligners can be utilized for the movement of teeth similar to the aligners shown in (see Fig. 20.12) or as a retainer to maintain the position of the dentition after orthodontic treatment has been concluded. The 3D printers utilize a resin-type material to print the appliances.

3D printing is not new to the medical field; however, its use in dentistry is becoming more prevalent. It should be noted that 3D printing is not limited to orthodontic applications. Other applications for 3D printing include the following: prosthodontics, oral surgery, periodontics, and general dentistry.

KEY POINTS—Obstructive Sleep Apnea

Can cause serious medical problems:
- chronic fatigue
- hypertension
- heart failure and heart attack
- stroke

Orthodontic Appliances
Preventive
Fixed and removable space maintainers
Interceptive
Fixed appliances:
- Thumb sucking
- Palatal expansion
- Crossbite corrector

Removable appliances:
- Tooth aligners
- Tooth movement

Do You Recall?

Why do clear aligners need to be changed every 2 to 4 weeks?

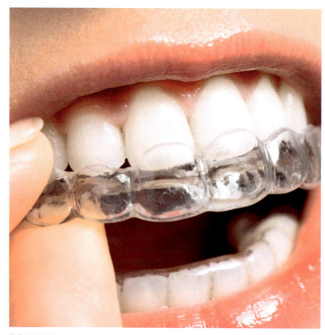

FIG. 20.12 Removable clear tooth aligner Invisalign. (Courtesy Align Technology, San Jose, California.)

KEY POINTS—Preventive Orthodontics

1. Space maintainers
   - Prevent adjacent teeth from drifting and closing the space created by a lost tooth
2. Interceptive orthodontics
   - Correct problems in the orofacial region during development to prevent the need for full orthodontics or decrease time orthodontics are required
3. Thumb sucking appliance
   - Causes discomfort during thumb sucking and tongue thrusting to prevent habit
4. Palatal expansion appliance
   - Expands the maxillary arch when too narrow to re-establish the correct balance between maxillary and mandibular jaws.
5. Crossbite corrector
   - Corrects malposition of a single tooth
6. Orthodontic tooth aligners
   - Removable appliance that directs forces on teeth to move them into proper alignment

SUMMARY

Sports guards prevent many oral injuries each year. The use of mouth guards not only helps those patients with TMJ disorders but is also effective in the prevention of excessive tooth wear and fracture from bruxism. Space maintainers prevent loss of space by drifting of adjacent teeth when teeth are lost prematurely. Treatment of sleep apnea is a growing segment of modern dental practice. More adults are requesting orthodontic treatment to correct misaligned teeth, and they demand "invisible" braces when possible. A dental auxiliary must be able to answer questions about the procedures and materials used. They must also be able to provide home care instructions for the appliances.

INSTRUCTIONAL VIDEOS

See the Evolve Resources site for a variety of educational videos that reinforce the material covered in this chapter.

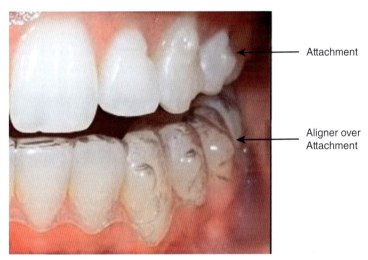

FIG. 20.13 Aligner buttons bonded to teeth. Spaces are created in an aligner over the facial surfaces of selected teeth. Composite resin is packed into these spaces. The teeth are prepared for bonding of the composite buttons. The aligner is positioned over the teeth and the composite buttons are bonded to the teeth. These buttons aid in tooth movement.

PROCEDURE 20.1 Fabrication of a Sports Mouth Guard (Protector)

See Evolve site for Competency Sheet.

Consider the following with this procedure: safety glasses are recommended for the patient, personal protective equipment is required for the clinician, ensure appropriate safety protocols are followed, and check your local state guidelines before performing this procedure.

EQUIPMENT/SUPPLIES (FIG. 20.14)
- Trimmed casts (study models)
- Mouth guard material: One sheet 6 × 6 in, 0.15 in thick
- Vacuum former unit
- Heavy-duty scissors
- Straight-line hinge articulator
- Petroleum jelly
- Alcohol torch
- Disinfectant spray and zippered plastic bag

PROCEDURE STEPS

1. Inspect casts (study models) and remove any blebs of dental stone on the teeth.
   NOTE: These blebs (bumps) of stone represent trapped air bubbles in the impression. Painting alginate on the occlusal surfaces of the teeth and in the palate just before inserting the loaded tray will help minimize trapped air in the impression.
2. Trim casts in a horseshoe shape so that the central portion representing the tongue and palate areas is mostly removed.
   NOTE: To save time trimming the casts, these areas can be blocked out with a piece of wet, crumpled paper towel once the impressions are poured.
3. Insert a sheet of mouth guard material in the frame of the vacuum former and clamp it in place. Lift the clamping frame up to a heating element and turn on the heat to soften the material.
   NOTE: The guard material comes in sheets in a variety of colors that are appealing to young athletes, or they can be clear.
4. Place the maxillary cast on the platform and center it under the sheet of guard material.
5. Lower the frame when the sheet of material has softened and sags an inch or more. Turn on the vacuum when the molten guard material covers the cast. Leave the vacuum on for at least 30 seconds to allow the molten material to adapt to the cast (Fig. 20.15).
   NOTE: With some machines, the vacuum activates automatically when the frame is lowered. If air is trapped between the cast and the guard material, use a wet paper towel to quickly press the guard material against the cast while the vacuum is still on in order to force the air out and closely adapt it to the cast.
6. Remove the guard material and the cast from the clamping frame and allow it to cool.
   NOTE: Hold it under cold water to cool it rapidly.
7. Trim excess material from the cast. Carefully remove the cast from the guard material.
   NOTE: Removing excess guard material at the sides of the cast will help free the cast more easily.
8. Place the maxillary and mandibular casts together in their proper bite relationship (centric occlusion) and mount them on the articulator, using fast-set plaster (Fig. 20.16).
   NOTE: For patients whose bite relationship is not clear, a separate bite registration should be taken when the alginate impressions are made.
9. Trim excess guard material away, using heavy-duty scissors, until the guard extends about 1/4 inch onto the palatal and facial gingiva of the cast.
   NOTE: The guard is extended over the gingiva to give added protection, but is kept short of the depth of the vestibule so that it will not irritate the tissues when the athlete bites on the guard.

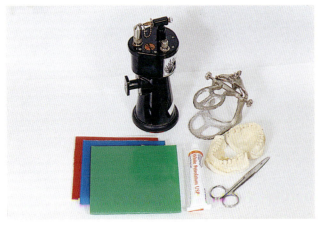

FIG. 20.14

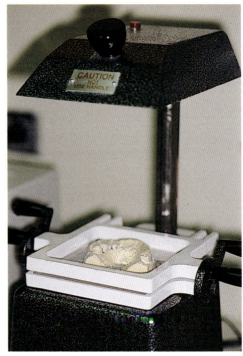

FIG. 20.15

Procedure 20.1 Fabrication of a Sports Mouth Guard (Protector)—cont'd

10. Place the guard on the maxillary cast and check to see that the guard material is not too thick in the molar area (Fig. 20.17). The mandibular cast should close evenly onto the guard and not prop the bite open.
11. Correct the bite. If the guard hits the mandibular molars first, apply a thin coat of petroleum jelly to the occlusal surfaces of the mandibular cast, soften the guard in both right and left molar areas with an alcohol torch, and close the casts together into the softened guard material (Fig. 20.18). Repeat this process by heating the guard in the molar, premolar, and cuspid areas until the mandibular teeth touch the guard evenly in the posterior and anterior.

    NOTE: A guard corrected in this manner will allow the athlete to close comfortably and not be in a strained jaw position.

12. Round out, using an acrylic bur in the laboratory handpiece, the indentations in the guard caused by the mandibular cast. The borders extending in the vestibule may also be rounded with an acrylic bur in the laboratory handpiece. Next, smooth the occlusal surface and borders altered by the acrylic bur and by flaming with an alcohol torch to soften the material, then lightly rubbing the surface of the guard with a gloved finger coated with petroleum jelly.

    NOTE: Be careful not to overheat the guard. Just soften the surface by lightly flaming it. If it is too hot, it could cause a burn to the finger. Overheating the guard can also cause it to burn.

13. A commercially purchased strap can be added to the anterior part of the guard for those sports in which a face guard is used. The strap allows the athlete to remove the guard from the mouth while not in activity and have it attached to the face guard and ready to reinsert when needed. While still on the cast, heat the guard on the facial surface and heat the back surface of the strap attachment base with an alcohol torch and press the two soft surfaces together. Allow it to cool. Insert the face guard strap into the slot on the strap attachment base (Figs. 20.19 and 20.20).
14. Wash the guard with liquid soap and water. Rinse thoroughly and spray it with a disinfectant. Store it until the delivery appointment in a zippered plastic bag marked with the patient's name.

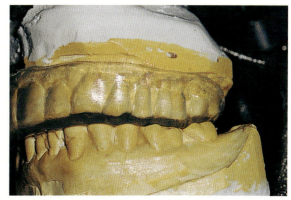

FIG. 20.18

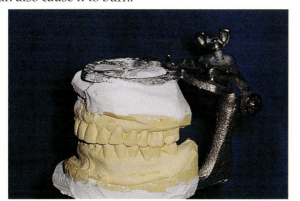

FIG. 20.16

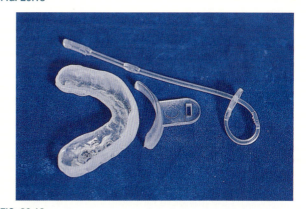

FIG. 20.19

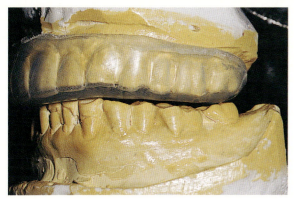

FIG. 20.17

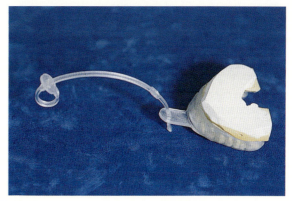

FIG. 20.20

Review and Discussion

Review Questions

Select the one correct response for each of the following multiple-choice questions.

1. When a soft mouth guard is prescribed by the dentist, fabrication can be done by:
   a. The dental assistant
   b. The dental hygienist
   c. The laboratory technician
   d. All of the above
2. What appliance is utilized to correct a malocclusion where the maxillary teeth are positioned lingually to the mandibular teeth?
   a. Thumb sucking device
   b. Palatal expander
   c. Crossbite corrector
   d. Space maintainer
3. What is the main purpose of a sports mouth guard?
   a. To help protect the teeth and supporting structures during contact sports
   b. To keep the airway open
   c. To keep the tongue out of the way
   d. To keep teeth in alignment after orthodontic treatment
4. Custom-made mouth guards and splints may be made of:
   a. A plastic material softened by boiling
   b. Thermoplastic resilient plastic or hard processed acrylic resin
   c. Composite resin
   d. Tray acrylic
5. A palatal expander is a fixed appliance used to expand the:
   a. Mandibular arch
   b. Maxillary arch
   c. Both maxillary and mandibular arches
   d. Neither maxillary nor mandibular arches
6. Obstructive sleep apnea can lead to:
   a. Chronic fatigue
   b. High blood pressure
   c. Heart problems
   d. All of the above
7. Oral appliances used for obstructive sleep apnea work by:
   a. Holding the tongue forward
   b. Holding the mandible forward
   c. Supporting the tissue of the soft palate
   d. Any one or more of the above
8. The treatment objectives of oral appliances for sleep apnea include all of the following *except* one. Which one?
   a. Lift the soft palate
   b. Hold the tongue in a more forward position
   c. Open the nasal passages
   d. Reposition the mandible forward to bring the tongue away from the airway
9. Which one of the following statements about space maintainers is *true*?
   a. They are always cemented into place.
   b. They are used only when primary teeth are lost.
   c. They prevent teeth adjacent to the space from drifting into the space.
   d. Denture teeth are never used in conjunction with space maintainers.
10. With Invisalign orthodontic treatment, the removable aligners are changed about every:
    a. 2 to 4 weeks
    b. 5 to 8 weeks
    c. 9 to 12 weeks
    d. 13 to 15 weeks
11. Which one of the following statements about removable orthodontic aligners is *true*?
    a. All malocclusions can be treated with aligners.
    b. Aligners are made for each stage of tooth movement simulated by design software.
    c. Aligners are made from processed acrylic resin.
    d. Treatment with aligners takes much longer than conventional treatment because a series of aligners must be used.
12. Boil-and-bite sports guards may appear to be protective but may not be. This is due to the material becoming very thin when athletes bite into it in a softened state.
    a. The first statement is true, and the second is false.
    b. The first statement is false, and the second is true.
    c. The first and second statements are true.
    d. The first and second statements are false.

For answers to Review Questions, see the Appendix.

Case-Based Discussion Topics

1. On examination, a 37-year-old truck driver is found to have chipped and worn incisal edges on the anterior teeth and flattened occlusal surfaces on the first and second molars. The enamel is almost worn through. The teeth are not mobile, periodontal health is good, and no caries are present. The patient suspects clenching and grinding the teeth while driving in heavy traffic. The spouse has reported observations of the patient grinding during sleep.
Is this patient a candidate for an occlusal guard? If so, what type of guard material would best be suited for this condition? Should the guard be worn at night, during the day, or both? Why?
2. A 16-year-old will be playing left tackle for the high school football team. The patient is 6 ft 2 in, weighs 190 lb, and is very strong.
Should the football player wear a sports guard? If so, is a single-layer guard appropriate? What types of injuries can a sports guard prevent?

BIBLIOGRAPHY

American Academy of Dental Sleep Medicine: *Oral appliances*. Available at: http://www.aadsm.org/obstructive_sleep_apnea.php, 2024.

American Dental Association (ADA) Science and Research Institute 2021. Available at:https://www.ada.org/en/resources/research/science-and-research-institute/oral-health-topics/athletic-mouth-protectors-mouthguards, 2021

Academy for Sports Dentistry: *Frequently asked questions*. Available at: http://www.academyforsportsdentistry.org/faq-s. 2021.

Bird DL, Robinson DS: *Modern Dental Assisting,* ed 13, St. Louis, 2021, Elsevier.

Darby ML, Walsh MM: *Dental Hygiene: Theory and Practice*, St. Louis, 2015, Saunders/Elsevier.

Powers JM, Wataha JC: *Dental Materials: Foundations and Applications,* ed 11, St. Louis, 2017, Elsevier.

Robinson DS: *Essentials of Dental Assisting,* ed 7, St. Louis, 2023, Elsevier.

University of Washington: Classification of space maintainers. In: *Atlas of Pediatric Dentistry [web-based textbook]*. Atlas maintained by the Department of Pediatric Dentistry, University of Washington, Seattle, Washington. Available at: http://depts.washington.edu/peddent/AtlasDemo/space009.html.

Appendix A

Answers to Review Questions

Chapter 2
1. c
2. d
3. b
4. c
5. d
6. b
7. c
8. b
9. b
10. a
11. d
12. c
13. c
14. c
15. d
16. c
17. d
18. a
19. b
20. e

Chapter 3
1. a
2. b
3. c
4. c
5. d
6. b
7. a
8. b
9. c
10. c

Chapter 4
1. d
2. d
3. d
4. c
5. c
6. d
7. c

Chapter 5
1. b
2. a
3. c
4. d
5. c
6. d
7. d
8. a
9. b
10. a
11. c
12. d
13. b
14. c
15. a
16. b
17. b
18. d
19. d
20. b
21. b
22. a
23. d
24. a
25. d
26. c
27. b

Chapter 6
1. b
2. c
3. c
4. c
5. a
6. c
7. a
8. a
9. d
10. a
11. d
12. c

13. d
14. a
15. d

Chapter 7
1. d
2. a
3. d
4. c
5. b
6. a
7. b
8. c
9. c
10. a

Chapter 8
1. a
2. d
3. d
4. a
5. c
6. c
7. b
8. c
9. d
10. b
11. c
12. d
13. a
14. c
15. d
16. a
17. b
18. a
19. d
20. b
21. a

Chapter 9
1. d
2. c

3. d
4. a
5. b
6. d
7. b
8. c
9. a
10. a

Chapter 10
1. a
2. c
3. a
4. a
5. d
6. d
7. d
8. b
9. d
10. c
11. b
12. b
13. c
14. b
15. c
16. c
17. b
18. a
19. d
20. b
21. c
22. c

Chapter 11
1. c
2. c
3. c
4. d
5. c
6. c
7. a
8. d

9. d
10. c
11. a
12. b
13. d
14. a
15. c
16. d
17. a
18. a

Chapter 12
1. b
2. a
3. c
4. a
5. d
6. b
7. a
8. d
9. d
10. c
11. c
12. d
13. a
14. a
15. d
16. d
17. a

Chapter 13
1. d
2. b
3. b
4. c
5. e
6. b
7. d
8. b
9. d
10. a
11. a
12. d

13. c
14. a
15. d
16. a
17. b
18. c
19. b

Chapter 14
1. c
2. a
3. d
4. a
5. b
6. d
7. c
8. a
9. d
10. d
11. d
12. c
13. d
14. d
15. c
16. c
17. d
18. a
19. d
20. b
21. d
22. a
23. b

Chapter 15
1. c
2. b
3. d
4. d
5. c
6. d
7. b
8. d
9. b

10. a
11. c
12. c

Chapter 16
1. b
2. b
3. d
4. c
5. b
6. c
7. a
8. d
9. d
10. d
11. a
12. d
13. d
14. b
15. d
16. a
17. a

Chapter 17
1. d
2. c
3. d
4. b
5. b
6. c
7. c
8. b
9. a
10. a

Chapter 18
1. b
2. b
3. c
4. c
5. d
6. c
7. b

8. a
9. c
10. b
11. d
12. b
13. b
14. d
15. d
16. a
17. a
18. a
19. c
20. a
21. a
22. c
23. b

Chapter 19
1. c
2. b
3. b
4. d
5. b
6. b
7. b
8. d
9. b
10. d

Chapter 20
1. d
2. c
3. a
4. b
5. b
6. d
7. d
8. c
9. c
10. a
11. b
12. c

Glossary

Abrasive: A material that comprises particles of sufficient hardness and sharpness to cut or scratch a softer material when drawn across its surface.

Accuracy: Ability of a material to adapt to and flow over the surfaces of the oral structures to record fine detail.

Addition Polymerization: Common form of polymerization for dental materials; monomer molecules are added one to another sequentially as the reactive group on one molecule initiates bonding with an adjacent monomer molecule and frees another reactive group (free radical) to repeat the process.

Addition Silicone: A silicone rubber impression that also sets by linking of molecules in long chains but produces no by-product. The most commonly used addition silicones are the polyvinyl siloxanes.

Adhesion: The act of sticking two things together. In dentistry, it is used to describe the bonding or cementation process. The attractive forces of atoms or molecules that join two surfaces together. Chemical adhesion occurs when atoms or molecules of dissimilar substances bond together and differs from cohesion in which attraction among atoms and molecules of like (similar) materials holds them together.

Adhesive: An intermediate material that causes two materials to stick together.

Adverse Response: An unintended, unexpected, and harmful or unwelcomed response of an individual to dental treatment or biomaterial.

Agar: A powder derived from seaweed that is a major component of reversible hydrocolloid.

Air Polishing: The process of polishing or finishing using fine particles with air pressure to remove biofilm and stain for enamel surfaces and in pits and fissures; an alternative to prophy pastes. Air polishing uses soft particles (Mohs ranking of 3) and an air pressure of approximately 40 to 60 pounds per square inch (psi).

Air Abrasion: Like air polishing but using greater air pressure (40–160 psi) and harder particles (aluminum oxide; Mohs harness ranking of 9). Used to cleanse cast appliances before cementation, repair porcelain and composite restorations, prepare tooth surfaces before bonding, and cut tooth structure for restorative preparations.

Alginate: A versatile, irreversible hydrocolloid impression material that is used most often in the dental office; however, it lacks the accuracy and fine surface detail needed for impressions for crown and bridge procedures.

All-Ceramic Restoration: Ceramic restorations with no metal core.

Allograft: Tissue taken from a donor (usually deceased) for grafting in another human.

Alloplast: Synthetic graft material.

Alloy: A mixture of two or more metals; a solid compound made up of two or more elements of which at least one is a metal.

Alloy, Admixed: A mixture of lathe-cut and spherical alloys for amalgam.

Alloy, Base Metal: An alloy that comprises nonnoble metals which corrode more readily.

Alloy, High Noble: An alloy that contains at least 60% noble metals, 40% of which must be gold.

Alloy, Lathe-Cut: Irregularly shaped particles formed by shaving fine particles from an alloy ingot for amalgam.

Alloy, Noble: An alloy that comprises metals that do not corrode readily; at least 25% must be noble metals.

Alloy, Porcelain Bonding: Special casting alloy manufactured for its compatibility with porcelain that has been bonded to it at high temperature.

Alloy, Spherical: Alloy particles produced as small spheres for amalgam.

Alloy, Wrought Metal: An alloy that has been mechanically changed into another form to improve its properties.

Amalgam, Dental: Restorative material that comprises silver-based alloy mixed with mercury.

Amalgamation: A reaction that occurs when silver-based alloy is mixed with mercury.

Amalgam Separator: A device that collects amalgam particles and mercury from evacuation systems that might otherwise escape into the wastewater and therefore enter the environment.

Anneal: To modify physical properties of a metal by heating it.

Annealing Controlled heating of a cast metal to modify physical properties.

Antibacterial Mouth Rinse: A liquid used to rinse the oral cavity to reduce or suppress bacteria associated with dental caries or periodontal disease.

Antimicrobial Mouth Rinse: Liquid used t o rinse the oral cavity to reduce or suppress bacteria, fungi, and viruses associated with dental caries or periodontal disease.

Archwire: A curved, flexible wire that approximates the general shape of the dental arches and when slightly bent and attached to orthodontic brackets or bands tries to regain its original form creating forces that move the teeth.

Astringent: A chemical used in tissue management during gingival retraction to control bleeding and constrict tissues.

Autograft: Graft tissue harvested from the patient's own body.

Auxiliary Materials: Materials used to fabricate and maintain restorations, directly or indirectly.

Barrier Membrane: Protective membrane that prevents the in-growth of fibrous connective tissue into a graft site and also holds the graft material in place.

Base: A thick layer of cement used in a cavity preparation to protect the pulp from chemical insult or to act as a thermal insulator and to support restorations in deep cavity preparations.

Base-Metal Alloy: Alloy composed of nonnoble metals which corrode more readily.

Bioactive Dental Materials: Materials that interact with living tissue and are used to remineralize and repair dentin.

Bio-Aerosol: A cloud-like mist that contains, tooth dust, materials dust, and bacteria, fungi, and viruses.

Biocompatible: The property of a material that allows it not to impede or adversely affect living tissue.

Biofilm: A complex community of oral microorganisms living on surfaces within the mouth. When these colonies are found on teeth or restorations, they are commonly called dental plaque.

Biointegration: A total integration of the implant fixture with the bone (without a microscopic space) that occurs with ceramic implant materials.

Bite Registration: An impression of the occlusal relationship of opposing teeth in centric occlusion (patient's normal bite).

Bleaching: A cosmetic process that uses chemicals to remove discolorations from teeth or to lighten them.

Bond or Bonding: To connect or fasten; to bind (*Webster's New World Dictionary*). Basically, items are joined together at the surface in two ways: by mechanical adhesion (physical interlocking) and chemical adhesion.

Bonding Agent: A low-viscosity resin that penetrates porosities and irregularities in the surface of the tooth or restoration created by acid etching, for the purpose of facilitating bonding.

Bonding Resin: A low-viscosity resin that penetrates porosities and irregularities in the surface of the tooth or restoration created by acid etching for the purpose of facilitating bonding. Also called bonding agent.

Brittle: Hard materials that break easily when stress is applied. They break suddenly with little plastic deformation, for example, glass.

Brittleness: Property of a material to break when stressed without deforming.

Buildup: A thick layer of restorative material such as amalgam, composite resin, or glass ionomer cement that is used to replace missing tooth structure in a badly broken-down tooth and to act as support for a restoration such as a crown.

Bulk-Fill Composites: Composites with greater depth of cure that permit placement in large increments up to 4 mm thick instead of the standard 2 mm; their use speeds up the filling process.

Burnishing: After the amalgam mix is placed an instrument is used to further condense and smooth the amalgam surface.

CAD/CAM: Computer-assisted design/computer-assisted machining technology that uses a scanning device to capture an image of the preparation and integrates the image with computer software to design then cut restorations from blocks of dental materials.

Calcium Hydroxide: Used as a low-strength liner and a direct pulp-capping material to stimulate secondary dentin formation.

Cariogenic: Substances or microorganisms that promote dental caries.

Casts: Replicas of hard and soft tissue of the patient's oral cavity made from gypsum products. They are also referred to as *models*.

Cavity Varnish: A thin layer of resinous material placed on the floor and walls of the preparation to seal the tubules and minimize microleakage.

Ceramics: Materials composed of inorganic metal oxide compounds, including porcelain and similar ceramic materials that require baking at high temperature to fuse small particles together to form the restoration, or a preformed ceramic block from which the restoration is milled using CAD/CAM techniques.

Chemical-Set Materials: Materials that set through a timed chemical reaction with the combination of a catalyst and base.

Chroma: The intensity or strength of a color (e.g., a bold yellow has more chroma than a pastel yellow).

Cleaning: The removal of soft deposits from the surface of restorations and tooth structure. Polishing and cleaning are done to remove surface stains and soft deposits from the clinical crowns and exposed root surfaces of teeth after all hard deposits are removed. Aside from abrasives, there are also chemical cleaning products that are used primarily for removable prostheses.

Closed-Tray Impression: Impression for implant that removes the impression with the impression abutment still attached to the implant fixture; the abutment is later removed and placed in the impression.

Coefficient of Thermal Expansion (CTE): The measurement of change of volume or length in relationship to change in temperature.

Colloid: Glue-like material composed of two or more substances in which one substance does not go into solution but is suspended within another substance. It has at least two phases a liquid phase called a sol and a semisolid phase called a gel.

Compomer: A composite resin that has polyacid, fluoride-releasing groups added.

Composite, Dual-Cured: Composite that contains components of light-cured and self-cured composites. When the two parts are mixed together, it polymerizes by a chemical reaction that can be accelerated with blue light activation.

Composite, Flowable: A light-cured, low-viscosity composite resin that contains fewer filler particles.

Composite, Hybrid: Composite that contains both macrofiller and microfiller particles to obtain the strength of a macrofill and the polishability of a microfill.

Composite, Light-Cured: Composite that polymerizes when a chemical is activated by light in the blue wave range.

Composite, Macrofilled: An early generation of composite that contained filler particles ranging from 10 to 100 μm.

Composite, Microfilled: Composite that contains very small filler particles averaging 0.04 μm in diameter.

Composite, Packable: A light-cured, highly viscous, heavily filled composite resin for dentists who use a placement technique with composite that is similar to that of amalgam.

Composite Resins: Direct-placement, tooth-colored materials that comprises an organic resin matrix and inorganic filler particles.

Composite, Self-Cured: Composite that polymerizes by a chemical reaction when two resins are mixed together.

Compressive Force: Force applied to compress an object.

Condensation: The act of pressing amalgam mix into a cavity preparation with instruments to produce a dense mass.

Cone Beam Computed Tomography (CBCT): Type of digital tomographic radiography used to produce three-dimensional images of the jaws; useful for analyzing the structures before surgery.

Condensation Silicone: A silicone rubber impression material that sets by linking of molecules in long chains but produces a liquid by-product through condensation.

Conditioning: The process of preparing the surface of a tooth or a restoration for bonding. The most common etching material (etchant) used is phosphoric acid. (Also see "Etching.")

Contamination: Contact with a substance that changes the chemical or mechanical properties (e.g., contamination of the etched surface of the tooth with saliva before bonding).

Coping: A thin covering like a thimble that serves as a substructure for a porcelain-bonded-to-metal crown (in this case, the coping is metal).

Corrosion: Deterioration of a metal caused by a chemical attack or electrochemical reaction with dissimilar metals in the presence of a solution containing electrolytes (such as saliva).

Corrosive: Usually an acid or strong base that can cause damage to skin, clothing, metals, and equipment, a gradual chemical destruction of metallic materials, as the rusting of metal instruments.

Cover Screw: Component placed in the top of the implant fixture to prevent tissue from growing into the screw hole when the fixture is covered with the flap in a two-stage surgical procedure.

Creep: Gradual change in the shape of a restoration caused by compression from occlusion or adjacent teeth and can cause amalgam to bulge out of the cavity preparation.

Crossbite Corrector: A fixed or removable appliance used to correct teeth in mal-alignment where the maxillary teeth are positioned lingual to the mandibular teeth.

Cross-Linked Polymers: Adjacent long-chain polymers joined by the bonding of short chains along their sides to enhance the properties of the polymer.

Crown: An indirect restoration that covers all or part of the coronal tooth structure (extracoronal) and is composed of metal, ceramic or a combination of the two.

Cure or Polymerize: A reaction that links low molecular weight resin molecules (monomers) together into high molecular weight chains (polymers) that harden or set. The reaction can be initiated by strictly a chemical reaction (self-cured), by light in the blue wave range (light-cured), by a combination of the two (dual-cured), or by heat.

Custom-Fit/Custom-Made: Made specifically to fit one individual.

Delayed Expansion: Expansion of amalgam containing zinc when it is contaminated with moisture (e.g., saliva) during condensation. Inside the amalgam hydrogen gas develops from the interaction of water and zinc, and it creates an outward pressure that causes creep to occur.

Demineralization: The action usually caused by acids that remove minerals from the tooth.

Density: The measure of the weight of a material compared with its volume.

Dental Amalgam: Restorative material composed of silver-based alloy mixed with mercury.

Dental Caries: A process whereby bacteria in plaque metabolize carbohydrates and produce acids that remove minerals from teeth and permit bacteria to invade.

Dental Stone: A stronger, less porous form of gypsum product used in dentistry.

Depth of Cure: The depth to which light from a curing unit can penetrate and cure composite resin.

Desensitizing Agent: A chemical that seals open dentinal tubules to reduce tooth sensitivity to air, sweets, and temperature changes.

Diagnostic Casts: Casts generally made from dental plaster or stone and used for patient education, treatment planning, and tracking the progress of treatment, as with orthodontic models; these casts are also known as *study models*; positive replicas of the teeth and surrounding oral tissues and structures produced from impressions that create a negative representation of the teeth.

Dies: Replicas of the prepared teeth that are generally removable from the working cast.

Die Stone: The densest form of gypsum product used in dentistry.

Digital Impression: Detailed digital images of the preparation, surrounding and opposing teeth, and tissues taken by a digital scanner for the purpose of making a restoration.

Dimensional Change: A change in the size of matter. For dental materials, this usually manifests as expansion caused by heating and contraction caused by cooling.

Dimensional Stability: Ability of a material to maintain its size and shape over a period of time.

Direct Fabrication: Provisional restorations made directly inside the patient's mouth on the prepared tooth/teeth.

Direct-Placement Esthetic Materials: Tooth-colored materials that can be placed directly into the cavity preparation without being constructed outside of the mouth first.

Direct Restorative Materials: Restorations placed directly into cavity preparations.

Dual-Set Materials: Materials that polymerize by a chemical reaction that occurs when the material is mixed with a catalyst or that is initiated by exposure to blue light (or by a combination of chemical or light reaction).

Dual-Cured Composite: Composite that contains components of light-cured and self-cured composites. When the two parts are mixed together, it polymerizes by a chemical reaction that can be accelerated by blue light activation.

Ductility: The ability of an object to be pulled or stretched under tension without rupture.

Durability: The ability of a material to withstand damage due to pressure or wear.

Edge Strength: The ability of a material to withstand fracture at a thin edge such as at the margins of a restoration.

Elastic Deformation: Deformation of a material that recovers its original shape and size when the force is removed.

Elasticity: The ability of a material to recover its shape completely after deformation from an applied force.

Elastic Limit: The greatest stress a structure can withstand without permanent deformation.

Elastic Modulus (also called Young's Modulus): A measure of the stiffness of a material; the higher the elastic modulus the stiffer the material and a low modulus a more flexible one.

Elastomers: Highly accurate elastic impression materials that have qualities similar to rubber. They are used extensively in indirect restorative techniques, such as crown and bridge procedures.

Enamel Microabrasion: A process that uses hydrochloric acid and an abrasive such as pumice to remove shallow discolorations of the enamel.

Endodontic Post: A metal or nonmetal dowel placed within the root canal to retain a core buildup for a crown.

Erosion: The loss of tooth mineral caused by dietary or gastric acids, not by bacterial metabolism (caries process).

Esthetic Materials, Direct Placement: Tooth-colored materials that can be placed directly into the cavity preparation without being constructed outside of the mouth first.

Esthetic Materials, Indirect Placement: Tooth-colored materials that are used to construct restorations outside of the mouth on replicas of the prepared teeth in the dental laboratory or at chairside. Later, they are cemented to the teeth.

Etch-and-Rinse (also called Total-Etch) Technique: A clinical technique that includes etching of both enamel and dentin, then rinsing the etchant off as a separate step from the application of bonding agents. Products that use this technique are called Etch-and-Rinse Bonding Systems.

Etching: The process of preparing the surface of a tooth or restoration with an acid for bonding. The most commonly used acid is phosphoric acid. (Also see "Conditioning.")

Excess Residue: A wax film that remains on an object after the wax is removed.

Exothermic Reaction: The production of heat resulting from the reactions of the components of some materials when they are mixed.

Extracoronal Restoration: A restoration that covers all or part of the external surface of the clinical crown of the tooth and may extend over the cusp tips on facial or lingual surfaces, such as onlays, three-fourth crown, full crowns, and veneers.

Extrinsic Stains: Stains that occur on the tooth surface.

Fatigue Failure: A fracture that results from repeated stresses that produce microscopic flaws that grow.

Film Thickness: The minimum thickness obtainable by a layer of a material. It is particularly important to dental cements.

Final Impression: A detailed impression of oral structures used to make an accurate cast from which restorations or prostheses are made.

Final Set Time: The time needed for the reaction that begins when the material is mixed to go to completion, and the material hardens to its permanent state.

Finish Line: The continuous edge that borders the preparation to which the restoration is fit or finished; it is also called the *margin*.

Finishing: A procedure used to reduce excess restorative material to develop appropriate occlusion, contour, and functional form. This usually is done with rotary cutting instruments. Finishing removes surface blemishes and produces a smooth surface.

Fixed Bridge: A dental prosthesis that replaces one or more missing teeth and is cemented to adjacent natural teeth or implants. It is composed of the same materials as crowns.

Firing: A process of heating porcelain at high temperature until it fuses.

Flash: Feather-like excesses of material that extends beyond the cavity margins, present at the margins of a restoration typically on occlusal and proximal surfaces.

Flash Point: The lowest temperature at which the vapor of a volatile substance will ignite with a flash. A low flash point means that a substance can catch fire very easily.

Flexural Strength: The ability to withstand bending forces without fracturing.

Flexural Stress: The maximum stress a material can be subjected to before it bends or breaks.

Flow: The movement of the wax as it approaches the melting range.

Flowable Composite: A light-cured, low-viscosity composite resin that contains fewer filler particles.

Fluorapatite: A tooth mineral that results when fluoride is incorporated into hydroxyapatite.

Fluoride: A naturally occurring chemical that helps to protect tooth structure from dental caries.

Fluorosis: Enamel abnormality caused by consumption of excessive levels of fluoride.

Fracture Toughness: Material's ability to resist fracture from crack propagation.

Free Radical: A reactive group on one end of a monomer that initiates the joining of adjacent monomer molecules to form a polymer; an atom with one unpaired electron in its outer shell making it highly reactive.

Galvanism: An electrical current transmitted between two dissimilar metals in contact and in a solution containing electrolytes, such as saliva.

Gamma-2 Phase: A chemical reaction between tin in the silver-based alloy and mercury that causes corrosion in the amalgam.

Gauge: A measure of the thickness of a wire. For example, an 8-gauge wire is thicker than a 16-gauge wire.

Gel: A semisolid state in which colloidal particles form a framework that traps liquid (e.g., Jell-O).

Glass-Based Ceramics: Ceramic materials with a silica (glass) matrix with or without fillers such as leucite or lithium disilicate.

Glass Ionomer: A self-cured, tooth-colored, fluoride-releasing restorative material that bonds to tooth structure without an additional bonding agent.

Glass Ionomer Cement: One of the most versatile cements; used as a permanent luting agent and restorative material, and for low- and high-strength base and core buildups; a tooth-colored, self-adhesive, fluoride-releasing material used mainly for fillings or cementing crowns and bridges.

Glazing: Firing porcelain at high temperature to achieve a smooth, shiny surface.

Grit: The particle size of the abrasive, typically classified as coarse, medium, fine, and superfine.

Gypsum: A material found in nature and composed of the dihydrate of calcium sulfate; used to make dental casts and dies.

Hardness: The resistance of a solid to penetration, the ability of a material to resist abrasion.

Hard Liner: A rigid reline material used inside a denture to improve the fit and stability.

Hazardous Chemical: A chemical that can cause burns to the skin, eyes, lungs, etc. It can be poisonous or flammable.

Heat-Pressing: Pressing molten ceramic material into a mold at high temperature and pressure.

Healing Abutment: A component placed temporarily on the implant fixture during the healing phase to allow the gingiva to adapt to it and form a cuff that will function around the implant.

Hue: The color of the tooth or restoration. It may include a mixture of colors, such as yellow-brown.

Hybrid Composites: Composite that contains both fine fill (2–4 µm) and microfill (0.04–0.2 µm) particles to obtain the strength of a macrofill and the polishability of a microfill.

Hybrid (resin-modified) Glass Ionomer: A glass ionomer to which resin has been added to improve its physical properties.

Hybrid Layer: A resin/dentin layer formed by the penetration of the dentin bonding resin through collagen fibrils exposed by acid etching and into the etched dentin surface. It serves as an excellent resin-rich layer onto which the restorative material, such as composite resin, can be bonded.

Hydrocolloid: Glue-like material that comprises two or more substances in which one substance does not go into solution but is suspended within another substance. It has at least two phases: (1) a liquid phase called a sol and (2) a semisolid phase called a gel.

Hydrocolloid, Irreversible: An impression material that is mixed to a sol state, and as it sets, it is converted to a gel by a chemical reaction that irreversibly changes its nature.

Hydrocolloid, Reversible: An impression material that can be heated to change a gel into a fluid sol state that can flow around the teeth, then cooled to gel again to make an impression of the shapes of the oral structures.

Hydrodynamic Theory of Tooth Sensitivity: Pain caused by movement of pulpal fluid in open (unsealed) dentinal tubules. Actions that cause a change in pressure on the fluid within the dentinal tubules stimulate nerve fibers in the processes of odontoblasts in the pulp to send out a pain response.

Hydrophilic: An attribute that allows a material to tolerate the presence of moisture.

Hydrophobic: An attribute that does not allow a material to tolerate or perform well in the presence of moisture.

Hysteresis: The property of a material to have two different temperatures for melting and solidifying, unlike water, which has one temperature for both.

Ignitable: A material or chemical that can erupt into fire easily.

Imbibition: The act of absorbing moisture.

Implant, Abutment: Metal or ceramic component that connects the implant crown to the implant fixture.

Implant, Analog: A substitute for the implant fixture used during the laboratory fabrication of the implant crown.

Implant, Fixture: Metal or ceramic component placed into bone to support a crown or prosthesis.

Implant, Endosseous (endosteal): Implant placed into the bone.

Implant, Subperiosteal: Implant placed on top of the bone and under the periosteum.

Implant, Transosteal: Implant that penetrates entirely through the bone.

Impression Abutment: Component used in the implant impression to align the implant analog in the same way as the implant fixture was in the mouth.

Impression Compound: An impression material that comprises resin and wax with fillers added to make it stronger and more stable than wax.

Impression Plaster: An impression material that comprises a gypsum product similar to plaster of paris.

Incremental Placement: A technique for composites that places and cures small increments individually to reduce the overall polymerization shrinkage and shrinkage stress in the restoration and permit curing throughout the increment.

Indirect Fabrication: Construction of provisional or final restorations on a cast outside the patient's mouth; provisional restorations made on a cast or milled in a computer-aided design/computer-aided milling machine outside the patient's mouth before delivery.

Indirect Restorative Materials: Materials used to fabricate restorations outside the mouth that are subsequently placed into the mouth.

Indirect-Placement Esthetic Materials: Tooth-colored materials that are used to construct restorations outside of the mouth in the dental laboratory or at chairside on replicas of the prepared teeth. They are later cemented to the teeth.
Initial Set Time: The time at which the material can no longer be manipulated within the mouth and coincides with the end of working time.
Inlay: An indirect restoration composed of ceramic, composite resin, or metal that is fitted to a cavity preparation that is within the crown of a tooth (intracoronal).
Inorganic Filler Particles: Fine particles of quartz, silica, or glass that give strength and wear resistance to the material.
Insulators: Materials that have low thermal conductivity.
Interface: The boundary between the walls of the preparation and the restoration.
Intermediate: Referring to materials expected to last from a few weeks to a year.
Intermediate Restorations: Restorations expected to last several weeks to months.
Intracoronal Restoration: A restoration within the crown of the tooth, such as an inlay.
Intraoral Scanner: A type of camera that takes digital images (typically in continuous video form) of oral structures for CAD/CAM procedures, such as crown preparations.
Intrinsic Stains: Stains that are incorporated into the tooth structure, usually during the tooth's development.
Irreversible Hydrocolloid: An alginate impression material that is mixed to a sol state and as it sets converts to a gel by a chemical reaction that irreversibly changes its nature.
Light-Activated Materials: Materials that require light in the blue wave range to initiate a reaction.
Light-Cured Composite: Composite that polymerizes when a catalyst is activated by light in the blue wave range.
Liner: A thin layer of material placed to protect the pulp from the chemical components of dental materials and microleakage, from oral fluids and microorganisms associated with microleakage, to stimulate reparative dentin, or to act as a pulp capping.
Lithium Disilicate Ceramics: glass-based ceramics with lithium disilicate fillers to enhance physical and mechanical properties, especially flexural strength.
Lost Wax Technique: A technique for fabricating a metal restoration by encasing the wax pattern in stone then vaporizing the wax under high temperatures to leave an empty impression space (pattern) once occupied by the wax; molten metal is then cast into the space and takes the shape of the pattern.
Luting: Cementing two components together such as an indirect restoration cemented on or in a tooth (e.g., inlays, crowns, bridges, veneers, orthodontic bracket and bands, posts and pins).
Macrofilled Composite: An early generation of composite that contained filler particles ranging from 10 to 100 microns (μm).
Malleability: The ability to be compressed and formed into a thin sheet without rupture.
Margination: A procedure for removal of excessive restorative material from margins of restorations.
Safety Data Sheet (SDS): Printed product report from the manufacturer that contains important information about the chemicals, hazards, cleanup, and special PPE related to a product.
Melting Range: A range of melting points of the individual components of wax that starts when the first part begins to liquefy and finishes when the wax is completed melted.
Microfilled Composite: Composite that contains very small filler particles averaging 0.04 μm in diameter.
Microhybrids: Hybrid composites that contain fillers that are smaller fine-particle (0.04–1 μm) and microsized fillers.

Microleakage: Leakage of fluid and bacteria caused by microscopic gaps that occur at the interface of the tooth and the restoration margins.
Mini-Implant: A very small–diameter implant that can be placed with minimal surgery involved.
Mixing Time: The amount of time allotted to bring the components of a material together into a homogeneous mix.
Model Plaster: The weakest, most porous form of gypsum product used in dentistry. Often used for study models.
Mohs Hardness: A measure of hardness on a scale of 1 to 10 where 1 is a very soft material and 10 is the hardest material.
Monomers: Small, low organic molecules that are joined in long chains to form polymers. As used in dentistry, monomers are usually liquids.
Mouth Guard: A hard or pliable resin that protects teeth from trauma during sports activities or from teeth grinding.
Nanocomposites: Composites that contain all nanosized fillers to enhance physical properties.
Nanohybrids: Microhybrids to which nanosized fillers (less than 100 nm) have been added.
Nitinol: An alloy of nickel and titanium often used for orthodontic wires.
Non–Glass-Based Ceramics: Crystalline-based ceramics without a glass matrix.
Nonvital Tooth: No longer has a living pulp and ceases to give response to electrical stimuli or temperature changes.
Obstructive Sleep Apnea: A sleep disorder caused when the muscles that support the soft palate, uvula, and tongue relax and the airway narrows or closes.
Onlay: Restoration that is similar to an inlay but covers or replaces one or more cusps.
Opaque: Optical property in which light is completely absorbed by an object.
Open-Tray Impression: Impression for implants that uses a tray with a hole over the impression abutments to be able to remove the abutments with the impression.
Organic Resin (polymer) Matrix: Thick liquids made up of two or more types of organic molecules (polymers) that form a matrix around filler particles.
Orthodontic Tooth Aligners: Removable appliances that are designed to gently move teeth into predetermined positions.
Osseointegration: Bone growth in intimate contact with an implant.
Overhang: Excessive restorative material present at the cervical cavosurface margin.
Over-the-Counter (OTC): Available in retail or drug stores without a doctor's prescription.
Oxygen-Inhibited Layer: (Also called *air-inhibited layer*) a layer of unset resin on the surface of a polymerized resin that is prevented from curing by contact with oxygen in the air.
Packable Composite: A light-cured, highly viscous, heavily filled composite resin for dentists who use a placement technique with a composite that is similar to that of amalgam.
Palatal Expander/Palatal Expansion Device: A fixed appliance used to expand the maxillary arch forcing the maxillary plates apart very slowly while the maxilla is still in development.
Particulate Matter: Very small particles (e.g., dust from dental plaster or stone).
Percolation: Movement of fluid within the microscopic gap of the restoration margin as a result of differences in the expansion and contraction rates of the tooth and the restoration with temperature changes associated with ingestion of cold or hot fluids or foods.
Peri-Implantitis: an infection around an implant that can cause gingival inflammation and loss of bone around the implant
Permanent: Lasting indefinitely.
Permanent Restorations: Restorations expected to be long-lasting.

Personal Protective Equipment (PPE): Gloves, masks, gowns, eyewear, and other protective equipment for the employee.

Pigments: Coloring agents that give composites their color.

Plastic Deformation: Deformation of a material causing permanent changes in size or shape due to an applied force.

Plasticizer: Liquid added to acrylic resin to soften it and make it more pliable.

Primer: A low-viscosity resin applied as the first layer to penetrate etched surfaces to enhance bonding.

Provisional Coverage: A restoration that temporarily holds the place of a permanent restoration, typically for up to 2 to 4 weeks. In the case of implant, complex prosthodontic and periodontal treatments, provisional restorations may be required to last for extended periods of time and are called interim restorations.

Polishing: A procedure that produces a shiny, smooth surface by eliminating fine scratches, minor surface imperfections, and surface stains using mild abrasives frequently found in the form of pastes or compounds. Polishing produces little change in the surface.

Poly(methyl methacrylate): A polymer that comprises numerous methyl methacrylate monomers linked together into a long chain.

Polyether: A rubber impression material with ether functional groups. It has high accuracy and is popular for crown and bridge procedures.

Polymer: A long-chain, high molecular weight molecule produced by the linking of many low molecular weight monomer molecules.

Polymerization: The act of forming polymers by chemically linking monomers into long chains; the process can be activated by chemicals, heat, or light.

Polymerization, Addition: A common form of polymerization of dental materials. Monomer molecules are added to one another sequentially as the reactive group on one molecule initiates bonding with an adjacent monomer molecule and frees another reactive group to repeat the process.

Polymers, Cross-Linked: Adjacent long-chain polymers by bonding of short chains along their sides to enhance the properties of the polymer.

Polysulfide: A rubber impression material that has sulfur-containing (mercaptan) functional groups.

Poly(Methyl Methacrylate) (PMMA): A polymer composed of numerous methyl methacrylate monomers linked together into a long chain. Methyl methacrylate is commonly used in denture fabrication.

Polyvinyl Siloxane (also referred to as Vinyl Polysiloxane): Very accurate addition silicone elastomer impression material. It is used extensively for crown and bridge procedures because of its accuracy, dimensional stability, and ease of use.

Porcelain: A tooth-colored ceramic material that comprises crystals of feldspar, alumina, and silica that are fused together at high temperatures to form a hard, uniform, glass-like material.

Porcelain Bonding Alloys: Special casting alloys manufactured for their compatibility with porcelain that is bonded to them at high temperature.

Porcelain-Fused-To-Metal Restoration: Restoration that has a metal core over which porcelain is fused at high temperature. Also called porcelain-bonded-to-metal.

Porcelain-Metal Restorations: Restorations that have a metal core over which porcelain is fused at high temperature.

Porosity: Numerous microscopic holes or voids within a material often caused during polymerization of resins when a monomer vaporizes and is lost; can also be caused by entrapping of air during mixing of powder and liquid or two pastes.

Post: A metal or nonmetal dowel placed within the root canal to retain a core buildup.

Post, Active: A post that engages the root canal surface like a screw.

Post, Custom: A post cast to fit precisely within the root canal space; it usually has the core attached.

Post, Passive: A post that sits within the prepared canal space but does not engage the root surface.

Post, Pre-formed: A factory-made post supplied in several sizes.

Pouring: *Pouring the cast* refers to the process of vibrating the flowable gypsum product into the impression; this process must produce a cast that is the exact replica of the structures captured in the impression.

Power Whitening: In-office whitening procedure that uses strong whitening agents and may use a high-intensity light source to accelerate the whitening process.

Precious Metal: The classification of metal based upon its high cost.

Preliminary Impression: An impression of the dentition or edentulous arch and surrounding tissues taken as a precursor to other treatment; often used to make casts (models) of oral structures for planning, and to construct custom trays or provisional restorations.

Prevention/Preventive Aids: Chemicals, devices, or procedures that reduce or eliminate disease or tooth destruction in the oral cavity.

Primary Bonds: The strongest bonds that hold atoms together because they involve the exchanging or sharing of electrons.

Primary Consistency: Less-viscous, easily flowing state of a material which can be drawn to a 1-inch string with a spatula lifted from the center of its mass, and is suitable for luting.

Proportional Limit: The greatest stress a structure can withstand without permanent deformation.

Prosthesis: A device used for the replacement of missing teeth and/or soft tissues. It can serve both cosmetic and functional roles.

Provisional Coverage: A restoration that temporarily occupies the place of a permanent restoration, typically for up to 2 to 3 weeks. In the case of implant and complex prosthodontic and periodontally involved cases, provisional restorations may be used to last for extended periods of time. These restorations are also commonly referred to as temporaries.

Reactive: Ability of a substance to take part in a chemical reaction, resulting in a different end product; the reaction of opposing chemical substances that creates a different end product.

Remineralization: Process that replaces mineral lost from the tooth by an acid attack.

Resilience: The resistance of a material to permanent deformation.

Resin-Based Cement: Modified composite used to bond ceramic indirect restorations, conventional crowns and bridges, and orthodontic brackets.

Resin-Modified (or Hybrid) Glass Ionomer: A glass ionomer to which resin has been added to improve its physical properties.

Restorative Agents: Materials used to reconstruct tooth structure.

Retention: A material's ability to maintain its position without displacement under stress.

Sealant: A protective coating usually composed of resin that is bonded to enamel to protect pits and fissures from dental caries.

Secondary Bonds: The weaker bond that holds atoms together. Unlike with primary bonds, there is no transfer or sharing of electrons.

Secondary Consistency: Thick, putty-like, condensable physical state of material which can be rolled into a ball or rope and is suitable for use as a base.

Sedative: To soothe or act in a sedative manner; to relieve pain.

Selective Etching: Technique where enamel is etched first with phosphoric acid prior to the application of self-etch acidic primers that lack sufficient acidity to produce a good etch of the enamel.

Self-Cured Composite: Composite that polymerizes by a chemical reaction when two resins are mixed together.

Self-Etch Bonding System: A bonding system that does not use a separate etching procedure with phosphoric acid. The acid is contained in the resin primer and no rinsing is needed.

Shearing Force: Force applied when two surfaces slide against each other or in a twisting or rotating motion.

Shelf Life: The useful life of a material before it deteriorates or changes in quality.

Silane Coupling Agent: A chemical that helps to bind the filler particles to the organic matrix.

Silicone, Addition: A silicone rubber impression material that sets by linking of molecules in long chains but produces no by-product. It is commonly known as polyvinyl siloxane and is the most popular material for crown and bridge procedures because of its accuracy, dimensional stability, and ease of use.

Silicone, Condensation: A silicone rubber impression material that sets by linking of molecules in long chains but produces a liquid by-product through condensation.

Sintering: Fusion of ceramic particles at their borders by heating them to the point that they just start to melt.

Sinus Lift: A surgical procedure that lifts up the floor of the maxillary sinus to allow placement of a bone graft. It is used to provide adequate bone for an implant when there was not enough available over the maxillary sinus.

Slip-Casting: Process whereby ceramic powder is mixed with a water-based liquid to form a mass or slip. The slip is pressed into a form and is baked at high temperature.

Smear Layer: A tenacious layer of debris on the enamel or dentin surface resulting from cutting the tooth during cavity preparation. It comprises fine particles of cut tooth structure, bacteria, and salivary components.

Soft Liner, Long-term: A soft material that lines a denture for use in patients who have problems with hard-acrylic denture bases. It is expected to last 1 to 3 years.

Soft Liner, Short-term: A soft provisional (temporary) material that lines a denture for a short period of time to improve tissue health. It is also called a *tissue conditioner*, and it typically lasts from a few days to a few weeks.

Sol: A liquid state in which colloidal particles are suspended. Through cooling or by chemical reaction, it can change into a gel.

Solder: An alloy used to join two metals together or to repair cast metal restorations.

Solubility: Susceptible to being dissolved.

Space Maintainer: A fixed or removable appliance used to prevent adjacent teeth from drifting into the space created when a tooth is lost.

Splatter: Small particles that may contain blood, saliva, oral particulate matter, water, and microbes.

Stiffness: A material's resistance to deformation.

Strain: Distortion or deformation that occurs when an object cannot resist a stress.

Stress: The internal force, which resists the applied force.

Subperiosteal Implant: Implant placed on top of the bone and under the periosteum.

Substantivity: Property of a material to have a prolonged therapeutic effect after its initial use.

Subgingival Air Polishing: The process of polishing the anatomical crown and clinical root surface using fine, soft particles under air pressure to remove biofilm subgingivally.

Supragingival Air Polishing: The process of polishing or finishing the clinical crown using fine, soft particles under air pressure to remove biofilm and stain from enamel surfaces and in pits and fissures; an alternative to prophy pastes.

Surface Energy: The electrical charge that attracts atoms to a surface.

Surfactant: A chemical that lowers the surface tension of a substance so it is more readily wetted. For example, oil beads on the surface of water, but soap acts as a surfactant to allow the oil to spread over the surface.

Sutures: Natural or synthetic material with the appearance of thread used to hold tissues together or to reposition tissues after trauma or surgical procedures. They can be absorbable (sutures broken down naturally by the body's enzymes and absorbed) or nonabsorbable (sutures made of materials that are not broken down by the body and require removal by a dental professional).

Sutures, Absorbable: Sutures broken down naturally by the body's enzymes and absorbed.

Sutures, Nonabsorbable: Sutures made of materials that are not broken down by the body and require removal by a dental professional.

Syneresis: A characteristic of gels to contract and squeeze out some liquid, which then accumulates on the surface.

Tarnish: Discoloration that results from oxidation of a thin layer of metal at its surface. It is not as destructive as corrosion. Oxidation affecting a thin layer of a metal at its surface that does not change the metal's mechanical properties.

Tear Resistance: Ability to avoid tearing when the material is in thin sections.

Temporary Anchor Devices (TADs): Small, tack-like mini-implants used on a temporary basis as anchors for orthodontic tooth movement.

Temporary/Provisional: Referring to materials expected to last from a few days to a few weeks.

Temporary Restorations: Restorations expected to last several days or weeks.

Tensile Force: Force applied in opposite directions to stretch an object.

Therapeutic Agents: Materials used to treat disease.

Therapeutic Materials: Materials used to treat disease.

Thermal Conductivity: The rate at which heat flows through a material.

Thixotropic: Having a viscosity that flows more readily under mechanical force such as mixing, stirring, or shaking.

Thixotropy: A characteristic of some gels and liquids that they will flow more readily under mechanical force such as mixing, stirring, or shaking.

Thumb Sucking Device: A fixed or removable appliance used to discourage tongue thrusting and thumb sucking.

Total-etch (also called Etch and Rinse) System: A bonding system that includes etching of both enamel and dentin as a separate step from the application of bonding agents.

Toughness: The ability of a material to resist fracture.

Toxicity: The quality of a material to cause damage to the body; the degree to which a product or a chemical can cause damage to the body.

Translucency: Varying degrees of light passing through and being absorbed by an object.

Transosteal Implant: Implant that penetrates entirely through the bone.

Transparent: Light passing directly through an object.

Trimming: The process of removing excess hardened gypsum from the cast for ease in working with the cast and for appearance in presentation.

Triturator (amalgamator): A mechanical device used to mix silver-based alloy particles with mercury to produce amalgam.

Ultimate Strength: The maximum amount of stress a material can withstand without breaking.

Universal Bonding System: A bonding system capable of bonding to tooth structure as well as most restorative dental materials.

Universal Composites: Composites that have physical and mechanical properties such as strength and polishability that allows them to be used in both the anterior and posterior parts of the mouth.

Value: How light or dark a color is. A low value is darker and a high value is brighter.

Varnish: A thin layer placed on the floor and walls of the cavity preparation to seal the dentinal tubules and minimize microleakage.

Veneers: Thin layer of ceramic or composite resin material that is bonded to the fronts of teeth to improve their appearance. It can also be a sticky material that allows delivery of fluoride to the enamel surface.

Viscosity: The thickness of a liquid; describes its resistance to flow.

Vital tooth: Has a living pulp, which produces response to temperature change or electrical stimuli.

Vitality: A life-like quality.

Walking Bleach Technique: Whitening technique for nonvital teeth in which whitening materials are sealed inside the tooth crown for a few days and the patient "walks" around with the whitening material in place.

Water Sorption: The ability to absorb moisture.

Wax Pattern: A duplicate of the restoration carved in wax.

Whitening: A cosmetic process that uses chemicals to lighten or remove discolorations from teeth.

Wet Dentin Bonding: Bonding to dentin that is kept moist after acid etching to facilitate penetration of bonding resins into etched dentin.

Wetting: The ability of a liquid to wet or intimately contact a solid surface. Water beading on a waxed car is an example of poor wetting.

Wire: A wrought metal alloy that can be soft and easily bent or can be heat-treated to be hard and resist bending. It has numerous applications in dentistry.

Working Casts: Casts generally made from one of the dental stones and strong enough to resist the stresses of fabricating an indirect restoration or prosthesis; these casts are also known as *master casts or working models*.

Working Time: The lapse of time from the start of mixing the material until it begins to harden and is no longer workable because it has reached its initial set.

Wrought Metal Alloy: An alloy that has been mechanically changed into another form to improve its properties (including ductility and malleability).

Xenograft: Graft tissue taken from an animal (usually bovine) for use in a human.

Yield Strength: The amount of stress at which a substance deforms.

Yield Stress: The stress at which a material deforms permanently; also called yield point on a stress-strain curve.

Young's Modulus or Elastic Modulus: Measures the resistance of a material to being deformed or its stiffness.

Zinc Oxide Eugenol: A hard and brittle impression material used in complete denture procedures. A variation of this material is used as a provisional filling material.

Zinc Oxide Eugenol Cement: A cement generally used as a provisional material or to temporarily cement provisional coverage.

Zinc Phosphate Cement: The oldest of the cements; used primarily for permanent luting.

Zinc Polycarboxylate Cement: The first cement developed with adhesive bonds; used primarily for permanent luting.

Zirconia: a nonglass polycrystalline ceramic that is the strongest ceramic used in dentistry.

Index

Page numbers followed by *f* indicate figures, *t* indicate tables, and *b* indicate boxes.

A

Abrasion, 369–393
  factors affecting, 371–373
  materials used in, 374–379
    aluminum oxide, 375*t*
    calcium carbonate, 375*t*
    dentifrice (toothpaste), 378, 378*b*
    denture cleansers, 378–379
    diamond, 375*t*, 376*f*
    glycine, 375*t*, 377*f*
    potassium and sodium, 375*t*
    prophylaxis (prophy) paste, 374–377, 378*t*
    pumice, 375*t*
    rouge, 375*t*
    sand, 375*t*
    silicon carbide, 375*t*
    silicon dioxide, 375*t*
    sodium bicarbonate, 375*t*, 377*f*
    tin oxide, 375*t*, 376*f*
    tungsten carbide finishing burs, 375*t*
  mode of delivery of, 373–374, 373*f*
    bonded abrasives, 373, 373*f*
    coated abrasives, 373–374, 374*f*
    loose abrasives, 374
    paste abrasives, 374
    three-body, 374
    two-body (direct contact), 373
  particles
    number of with contact on surface, 372
    size irregularity and hardness of, 371–372, 371*b*, 371*t*
  patient education in, 387
  resistance, of gypsum, 96–97
  safety/infection control, 387, 387*b*
  speed and pressure, 372–373, 373*b*
Abrasive particles, 268, 269*f*
Abrasives, 369, 371
  microparticles, 374
  three-body, 374
    loose, 374
    paste, 374
  two-body, 373
    bonded, 373, 373*f*
    coated, 373–374, 374*f*
Absorbable sutures, 246, 269, 269*f*
Absorption, directly through breaks in skin, 38
Accelerators, gypsum setting time and, 102–103
Accuracy, 51–52, 54
Acetone, 127
Acid etchant, 123, 123*f*
Acid etching, 121, 122*f*
Acid reflux, 396
Acidic primers, 130
  pH of, 130
Acids
  chemical spills, control of, 40
  in layer of skin, 38
Acrylic, staining of, 12
Acrylic denture bases, polishing of, 382–383, 382*f*
Acrylic provisional materials, 314–315, 314*f*, 315*b*
  properties of, 316*t*
Acrylic resins (plastics), 276
  allergic reaction to, 278, 278*b*
  for denture bases, 278, 279*f*
  dentures, care of, 298–300
  injection molding of, 282
  light-cured, 283
  microwave processing of, 282
  modifiers of, 277
  polymerization reaction of, 278–280, 279*b*, 280*f*, 280*t*
  properties of, 277
    chemical-cured, 277
    dimensional change as, 277
    heat-cured, 277, 278*t*
    polymerization shrinkage as, 277
    porosity as, 278, 278*b*, 278*f*
    strength as, 277
    thermal conductivity as, 277
  teeth, 290–292
  uses of, 276–277, 277*f*
Activator, 132
Active posts, 239
Acute chemical toxicity, 38
ADA. *See* American Dental Association
ADA Seal of Acceptance, 251
ADA's Council on Scientific Affairs, 3–4
Addition polymerization, 276
  definition of, 275
Addition silicone, 64
  definition of, 51–52
  features of, 68*t*
Adhesion
  definition of, 7–8, 14, 120–121, 333
  of dental cement, 341–342, 341*b*, 342*f*
Adhesive, use of, 62–63, 63*f*
Adhesive cements, 339, 348–349, 349*b*
Adhesive resins, 126
Admixed alloy, 204, 204*f*, 205*t*
  definition of, 203
  example of, 204*f*
Admixed amalgam, 206*t*
Adverse response, definition of, 7–8, 10
Aerosols, 387
Agar, 51–52, 55–56. *See also* Reversible hydrocolloid
Air, restorations, 21
Air abrasion, 369, 374, 384–386, 386*b*, 386*f*
Air polishing, 267–268, 269*f*, 369, 374, 377*f*, 384–386, 384*t*, 385*b*
  contraindications for, 268–269
Alginate. *See also* Irreversible hydrocolloid
  definition of, 51–52, 56
  substitutes of, 67
Alginate impressions, 61, 63*f*
  criteria for acceptable, 61*t*
  dispensing of, 58, 58*b*, 59*f*
  mixing of, 58–59, 59*f*
  procedure for making, 80*b*–82*b*, 80*f*, 81*f*, 82*f*
  troubleshooting for, 62*t*
Alginate system, two-phase of, 61–62, 63*f*, 65*f*
All-ceramic restorations
  advantages and disadvantages of, 181
  CAD/CAM for, 185–188, 186*f*
  cementation of, 191–192, 192*b*
  definition of, 180
  finishing and polishing, 191
    principles of, 191, 191*b*
  heat-pressing and, 185
  introduction of, 181
  layers in, 194*f*
  maintenance of, 192–193
  shade matching for, 197
  shade selection for, dental assistant/hygienist and, 195, 195*f*
  shade taking, 195–198
    device, 197–198, 197*f*, 198*f*

All-ceramic restorations *(Continued)*
    sintering, 182*f*, 185
    slip-casting and, 185
Allergy, to nickel, 232
Allied oral health practitioner, role of, 1–2
Allografts, 246, 261, 261*f*
Alloplasts, 246, 261, 262*f*
Alloys, 226–227
    composition of, 204, 205*t*
    definition of, 203
    dispensing of, 213
    particle shapes, 205*t*
    stainless steel, 235–236
    structure of, 227–229
    titanium and, 231–232
    used in dental amalgam, 204
Alumina, 183
    glass-infiltrated
        flexural strength of, 183*t*
        indications and contraindications to, 189*t*
Aluminum oxide, for polishing composite restorations, 383
Aluminum shell crowns, 310*f*, 311
Aluminum trihydroxide powders, in air polishing, 384
Amalgam, 203–225
    advantages and disadvantages of, 215*b*
    allergy to, 217
    alloy used in, 204
    ANSI/ADA standard No.1 for, 205–206, 206*t*
    applications for, 207
    bonding of, 217
    class II, placing and carving of, 209*b*, 220*b*–223*b*, 220*f*, 221*f*, 222*f*, 223*f*
    composition of, 204, 205*t*
    corrosion of, 207, 207*f*
    creep in, 206
    definition of, 203
    delayed expansion of, 206, 206*f*
    dimensional change of, 206
    expansion and contraction of, 206
    failure of, 216*b*
    finishing of, 215
    longevity of, 216–217
    manipulation of, 213
    matrix bands and, 207–213, 208*f*, 209*b*, 209*f*, 210*f*, 211*f*, 212*f*, 213*f*, 214*f*
    mercury and
        health concerns for, 217–218
        setting reactions of, 205, 205*t*
        setting transformation of, 204–205
    placement and condensation of, 215, 215*b*
    polishing of, 12–13, 215, 215*b*
    practices for waste of, 218*t*
    repair of, 217
    restrictions on use of, 218–219
    safety procedures for, 217–219
    separator, 203

Amalgam *(Continued)*
    strength of, 206
    tarnish of, 206–207
    thermal conductivity of, 207
    trituration of, 213–214, 214*b*, 215*f*
    use of, 204
    working and setting times, 214–215
Amalgam restorations
    finishing of, 370*f*, 381, 381*f*
        procedure for, 388*b*–389*b*, 388*f*, 389*f*
    polishing of, 383
Amalgam War, 3*t*
Amalgamation, 203–205
    definition of, 203–204
Amalgamator (triturator), 203, 213–214
American Dental Association (ADA)
    evidence-based dentistry, 2
    Seal of Acceptance, 3–5
        example of, 4*f*
        for toothpaste, 378, 378*t*
    stance on dental amalgam safety, 217
    standards in dentistry and, 3–5, 4*f*
American National Standards Institute (ANSI), 5
American National Standards Institute/American Dental Association (ANSI/ADA), Standard No.1
    for amalgam, 205–206, 206*t*
American Society of Dental Surgeons, 3*t*
Amorphous solid, 26
Annealing, 226, 229
Anorexia nervosa, 396
ANSI. *See* American National Standards Institute
Antibacterial agents, for implant home care, 265–266
Antibacterial mouth rinse
    chlorhexidine gluconate as, 396
        side effects of, 397
    definition of, 396
    Listerine as, 397
Antimicrobial mouthrinse, 394
Appearance, gold teeth and, 3
Application, materials classified by, 29
Archwire, in orthodontics, 226, 236–237, 236*t*
    arch forms, 236–237, 237*f*
    ligation, 237
    materials, 236
    shapes in cross-section, 237
    size, 237
Astringent, definition of, 51–52
Astringents/hemostatic agents, 69–70, 70*b*, 70*f*
Atom, 25, 25*f*
Atraumatic restorative treatment, for glass ionomer cements, 173
Attrition, 373
Atypical wedge placement, 211–212, 211*b*, 212*f*

Autografts, 246, 260–261
Automixing dental cement, advantages and disadvantages of, 354*t*
Auxiliary materials, 9
    definition of, 7–8

B

Balsa wood triangular sticks, for implant home care, 265
Bands
    matrix, 156
    orthodontic, 237, 238*f*
        cement for, 336–337
Base, 141–142, 335–336, 336*b*
    definition of, 333
    high-strength, 335
    line drawing of, 335*f*
    low-strength, 335
Base-metal alloy, 226, 229
    orthodontic wires as, 236
    removable partial dentures, 231, 231*f*
Base-metal dental casting alloys, 230–231
Baseplate wax, 108, 108*f*
Beryllium, 232, 232*b*
Bioactive cements, 353
Bioactive dental materials, 170, 177–178, 177*b*
    definition of, 170
    physical properties, 177
    uses for, 177
Bio-aerosol
    definition, 34
    dental, 35–36
    in dental setting, 35–36, 36*f*
    management of, 36*b*
Biocompatibility, 134, 134*b*, 231–232, 232*f*
    of base metals, 231–232
    of ceramics, 184–185
    of composite resin, 143
    of dental cement, 341, 341*b*
    of glass ionomer cements, 171
Biocompatible, 2
    definition of, 7–9
    dental materials and, 9–10, 10*f*
Biofilm, definition of, 7–8, 12
Biointegration, 246, 250
Biological contaminants, exposure to, 35, 35*f*
Biological seal, 263
Biomechanics, 10
Bis-acrylic composite provisional material, 315
    properties of, 316*t*
Bis-acrylic urethane, 149
Bis-GMA, 140–141
Bisphenol A (BPA), 143, 143*b*
    exposure to, 38
Bisphosphonates, as contraindication to dental implants, 248

Bite registration, 51–53
  procedure for making, with elastomeric material, 85b–87b, 85f, 86f
Bite registration materials, 54
  addition silicone as, 66
  application of, 66f
Bite registration trays, 54
Bite registration wax, 109
  procedure for, 115b–117b, 115f, 116f, 117f
Biting force, 10–11
Bleaching, 421–424. See also Whitening
  contraindications to, 429b
  dental auxiliary in, role of, 430
  at home
    clinical procedures for, 435b–436b
    over-the-counter products for, 429–430
  in-office
    of nonvital teeth, 427, 427f
    procedure for, 433b–434b, 433f, 434f
    varnish, 426
    of vital teeth, 425–427, 425f, 430b
  non-dental options of, 430, 430b
  potential side effects of, 430–431
  restorative considerations before, 431–432, 431b
  retreatment for, 432
  rinses, 430
  tooth sensitivity from, 430–431
  toothpastes for, 430
Body and incisal porcelains, 193–194
Boil-and-bite guards, 441, 441f
Bond strength, 125–126
  of glass ionomer cements, 171
Bonded abrasives, 373, 373f
Bonding, 347
  of amalgam, 217
  clinical applications of, 132–134
  components, 127
  definition of, 7–8, 15–16, 120–121
  dentin for, 126–127
  principles of, 120–138
  retention and, 14
  self-etch, 129t, 130–134, 131f
  surface wetting and, 121, 122f
  systems, 126–128, 131
  "wet" dentin, 124–125
Bonding agents, 127, 127b
  definition of, 120–121
  universal, 131–132, 132b, 133f
  use of, 406, 406b
Bonding resins, 126f, 127b
  components of, 121
  definition, 120–121
  dentin, 126–127
  enamel, 126, 126f
Bonding restorations, benefits of, 127b
Bonding systems, 129t, 134b
  classification of, 129–135
  components of, 126–127
  etch-and-rinse, 129–130

Bonding systems (Continued)
  history of development of, 127–128
  main steps of, 135b
  one-bottle self-etch, 131
  packaging, 131
  refrigeration, 131
  self-etch, 130–134
  time line of development of, 127b
  total-etch, 128
  two-bottle self-etch, 130–131, 131f
  universal, 131–132, 132b, 133f
Bone grafting, 259–261
  purpose of, 259
  types of, 259–261
Border molding, 287–288
Boxing method, for casts, 103f, 104
Boxing wax, 108
BPA. See Bisphenol A
Brackets, orthodontic, 237, 238f
  cement for, 336–337, 337f
Brazing, soldering and, 234
Bridge
  fixed, 191
  procedures, components of impression making for, 69–73
  restorations/endodontic procedures, 1–2
Brittleness, 24–25, 27–28, 28f
Brushes, for implant home care, 264–265, 265f
Bruxism, 10–11
Bruxism guard, mouth, 442–445
  design of, 443–444
  home care instructions for, 443b
  maintenance of, 444–445, 445b
  types of materials for, 443, 444f
Buccal mucosa, inflammatory response of, 217f
Buildup, 333, 336, 336f
Bulimia, 396
Bulk-fill composites, 147–148
  definition of, 139–140
Buonocore, Michael, 121
Burlew wheels, 382
Burnishing
  definition of, 203
  matrix band, 209f
Burns, chemicals, causing, 38

C

CAD/CAM
  for all-ceramic restorations, 185–189, 186f
  basic components of, 185, 186f
  for ceramic inlays, onlays, and fixed bridges, 191, 191b
  ceramic materials in, 185–188
    firing the blocks, 187, 188f
    glass-based, 187
    milling the blocks, 187, 188f
    nonglass, 187, 187f
    polishing, restoration, 188
    resin hybrid, 188, 188f

CAD/CAM (Continued)
    stains and glazes, 187–188
  definition of, 180
  restorations, 185–188
CAD/CAM provisional (temporary) materials, 319–320, 319f, 320b
Calcination, 95
Calcium carbonate, in abrasion, 385
Calcium hydroxide
  alkaline pH of, 335
  cavity liner, 216f, 335b
  as low-strength base/liner, 335
Calcium sodium phosphosilicate powder, in air polishing, 384
Calcium sulfate hemihydrate, 95
Canadian Centre for Occupational Health (CCOH) Bloodborne Pathogens Standard, 35
Candida albicans in silicone liners, 287
Carbamide peroxide, 424
Cariogenic bacteria
  definition of, 394
  fluoride preventing, 395
Cast, 94f
  construction of, 3t
  definition of, 93
  disinfection of, 79, 105
  pouring procedure for
    anatomic portion, 112b–113b, 112f, 113f
    art portion, 114b, 114f
  separating impression from, 105
  procedure for, 115b, 115f
Casting alloys
  classification of, 228
  color of, 229
  metal, 228
  noble metals for, 228–229
  nongold noble metals, 230, 230t
  properties of, 229–232, 234b
  removable partial dentures, 231, 231f
Casting metal
  biocompatibility, 231–232
  IdentAlloy program, 234
  resistance to tarnish and corrosion, 229–230
  restorations, 228, 228f
Casting wax, 108
Catalyst, 30, 141–142
Cavity sealer, 215–216, 216f
Cavity varnish, 333
CBCT. See Cone beam computed tomography
CDC. See Centers for Disease Control and Prevention
Celluloid crown, 313, 313b, 313f
Cement
  for crown, 336f
  line drawing of, 335f
  primary consistency of, 333
  properties of, 340t
    viscosity and film thickness of, 340–341

Cement *(Continued)*
  secondary consistency of, 337
Cement-retained implant crowns, 258, 258*b*, 259*f*
Cementation, 334–339
  of all-ceramic restorations, 191–192, 192*b*
    preparation of, 192
    tooth preparation in, 192
    try-in of, 192
  cleanup, disinfection, and sterilization after, 356
  loading crown for, 355*b*, 355*f*
  luting agent for, 339*b*
  preparation for, 350–351
  removal of excess, 192
  of zirconia, 183
Centers for Disease Control and Prevention (CDC), 35
  mouth guard, use of, 440
Ceramic inlays/onlays, 191
Ceramic restorations
  finishing of, 382–383, 382*b*
  polishing of, 385
Ceramics, 180–202
  classification of, 181
  clinical applications of, 189–195
  coatings, 251
  definition of, 180
  as dental implant coating, 250
  history of, 181
  processing techniques of, 185
  properties of
    optical, 184, 184*f*
    physical and mechanical, 183–185
    thermal, 184
  selection of, rationale for, 189
  shade guides for, 195
CEREC system, 181
Cermets, 172
Cervical matrices, in matrix systems, of composite resin, 158, 159*f*
Chairside Economical Restoration of Esthetic Ceramic (CEREC) system, 181
Chairside reline, for dentures, 287–289, 289*b*
Checkups, dental, dentures and, 298
Chemical
  disposal of, 41–42
    empty containers, 41–42
    hazardous waste disposal, 41*b*–42*b*, 42
  toxicity, acute and chronic, 38–39
Chemical cleaning products, 371
Chemical containers, labeling of, 44, 44*b*, 45*f*
Chemical cure, of composite resin, 141–142
Chemical-cured acrylic resin, 277, 282
  for custom impression tray and record base material, 295–297
  for denture repair, 294–295, 295*b*

Chemical-cured acrylic resin *(Continued)*
  polymerization of, 280
  pour technique for, 282
Chemical-cured resins, 347, 350*b*
Chemical-cured sealant, 408*t*
Chemical inventory, hazard communication program, 43
Chemical properties, 28
Chemical-resistant glove, 39
Chemical retention, 14–15
Chemical safety, in dental office, 36–38, 36*b*
Chemical set materials, 24–25, 30
Chemical spills, 40–41
  acids, 40
  eyewash, 40, 40*t*, 41*f*
  flammable liquids, 40
  mercury, 40, 40*f*
  ventilation, 40–41
Chlorhexidine, 253
Chlorhexidine gluconate, 396–397, 396*f*, 397*f*
  side effects of, 397
Chroma, 139–140, 150
  definition of, 7–8, 16
Chronic chemical toxicity, 38–39
Circumferential matrix systems, of composite resin, 157–158
Class II composite resin restoration, placement of, 165*b*–167*b*, 165*f*, 166*f*, 167*f*
Clay retraction material, 72*f*
Cleaning, 369
Cleanup, of gypsum, 105, 105*b*
Closed-bite trays. *See* Triple trays
Closed-tray impression, 246, 255, 257*f*
Coated abrasives, 373–374, 374*f*
Coefficient of thermal expansion (CTE)
  of ceramics, 184
  definition of, 7–8, 13
Coffee, staining from, 12
Colloid, 51–52, 54–55
Color
  components of, 16–17
  of glass ionomer cements, 171
  optical properties, 17
  sensing, 16
  viewing, 17
Coloring resins, 141
Community of microorganisms, 17
Community water fluoridation program, 3, 3*t*
Compatibility
  of provisional material, 309
  resins, 134–135
Compomer cements, 351
Compomers, 170–179, 176*f*
  bonding, 176
  definition of, 170
  fluoride release, 176
  packaging, 176, 176*f*
  placement and finishing, 176

Compomers *(Continued)*
  properties of, 176, 177*t*
  restorative material, 176*f*
  setting reaction in, 176
  uses for, 176
Composite resin, 141–163
  classification by filler size, 145–147
  classification methods for, 148*t*
  clinical handling of, 150–153
  comparison of properties of, 149*t*
  compomers, 176
  components of, 141
    coupling agent, 141
    filler particles as, 141
    matrix, 141
    pigments, 141
  contaminants of, 153–154
  cross-contamination of, 155–156, 155*b*
  definition of, 139–140
  dental assistant/hygienist involvement, 151
  dispensing of, 155–156, 155*b*, 156*f*
  failure of, 163
  finishing and polishing of, 163, 163*b*
  history of development of, 140
  incremental placement of, 144*b*, 144*f*
  indirect-placement of, 163–164, 164*f*
  introduction of, 181
  layering (stratification) of, 154–155
  light-curing of, 160–163
  matrix systems of, 156–160
  modes of cure of, 141–142
  polymerization and, 141–142
  posterior, advantages and disadvantages of, 150*t*
  repair of, 163
  resin-to-resin bonding, 153, 154*f*
  selection of materials for, 150
  shade guides for, 152–153, 152*f*, 153*b*
  shade matching for, 151–152, 152*b*, 153*b*
  uses of, 150
Composite resin provisional materials, 315–316, 315*f*, 316*b*
Composite resin teeth, 292
Composite restorations
  finishing of, 381–382, 381*b*, 381*f*
  polishing of
    during oral prophylaxis, 383–386
    procedure for, 389*b*–390*b*, 390*f*, 391*f*
Composites, 139–169
  kits, 147
  physical and mechanical properties of, 142–145, 144*b*
    biocompatibility, 143
    coefficient of thermal expansion and, 144
    elastic modulus and, 144
    polymerization shrinkage, 143–144
    radiopacity of, 144–145

Composites (Continued)
    shelf life of, 155
    strength, 143
        thermal conductivity of, 144
        water sorption of, 144
        wear, 143
    properties, 147b
    provisional (temporary) restorative, 149–150
    viscosities, 149b
Composition
    of material, 29–30
    and reaction, 29–30
    of waxes, 106
Compression molding technique, 280–282, 281f
Compressive force
    definition of, 7–8
    oral environment and, 11
Compressive strength
    amalgam and, 206
    of glass ionomer cements, 171
Condensation
    definition of, 203, 215
    final evaluation of matrix bands before, 212–213, 212f
Condensation polymerization, 276
Condensation silicone, 51–52, 63–64
Cone beam computed tomography (CBCT), 246, 251, 252f
Containers, labeling, exemptions to, 44–46
Contaminants
    biological, exposure to, 35, 35f
    bonding site, 135
    of composite resin, 153–154
    dental impressions as, 78
Contamination
    definition of, 120–121
    moisture, 407
Contraction
    of alloy, 214
    of amalgam, 206
    effects of, 13–14
Conventional feldspathic porcelain, 182
Copal resin varnish, 215, 216f
Copal varnish, 335
Coping, 226, 233
Copolymers, formation of, 276
Copper
    as composition of amalgam alloy, 205t
    primary molars, T-band for, 214f
Cord packing instruments, 69, 70b, 70f
Cord placement, evaluation of, 70–71
Cordless impression device, 74–75
Core buildup composites, 148–149, 149b, 149f
Corrective impression wax, 109
Corrosion, 28
    in alloy, 214, 229
    of amalgam, 207, 207f

Corrosion (Continued)
    definition of, 7–8, 12–13, 203
    oral environment and, 12–13
    resistance to, 229–230
Corrosive, 34, 41b–42b
Covalent bonds, 25
Cover screw, 246, 249, 253, 254f
Creep, 206
    in alloy, 214
    definition of, 203
Crossbite corrector, 447, 447f
    definition of, 440
Cross-linked polymers
    definition of, 275
    formation of, 276
Crown
    cement-retained implant, 258, 258b, 259f
    components of impression making for, 69–73
    definition of, 180–181
    designs of, 233–234, 233f
    double-bite impression for, 83b–85b, 83f, 84f, 85f
    film thickness and, 15
    implant, 248–249
    loading for cementation, 355, 355b, 355f
    provisional, 236, 308f
    screw-retained, 255–258, 258f
    seating and cementing for, 336f, 355b
Crystal formation, 229
Crystalline structure
    density and, 26, 26f
    solids and, 26
CTE. See Coefficient of thermal expansion
Cure, definition of, 120–121
Curing
    methods, 276
        by restoration type, 350b
    modes of, 128–129
Custom abutment, 248
Custom-fit, definition of, 440
Custom-fit guards, 441–442, 442f
Custom impression trays, 295–298
    chemical-cured, 295–297, 301b–303b, 301f, 302f
    fabrication of, 295
    light-cured, 297
Custom post, 241
Custom trays, 54, 56f
Custom whitening trays, fabrication of, procedure for, 436b–438b
Customized provisional crowns, 313–314, 314f

D

Deformation, 27
Delayed expansion, 203, 206, 206f
Demineralization
    definition of, 394
    dental caries and, 395

Density, 27, 27f
    of alloys, 229
    definition of, 24–25
    of solids, 27
Dental amalgam, 203. See also Amalgam
Dental assistant, esthetic materials, handling of, 181
Dental auxiliary, role of, 1–2, 2b
    in bleaching, 430
Dental bio-aerosol, 35–36, 36b
Dental caries
    antibacterial rinses for, 396–398, 396f
    classification of, 146t
    definition of, 394–395
    teeth susceptibility to, 403–404
Dental casting alloys, 228
Dental cement, 333–368
    classification of, 334
    delivery system for, 354t
    loading crown for, 355f
    manipulation of, 353
        considerations for, 354b
        mixing of, 352f, 353–354, 354b
        storage of, 353
        working and setting times of, 354–355
    properties of, 339–342
        biocompatibility and anticariogenic properties, 341
        esthetics, 342
        radiopacity, 342
        retention and adhesion, 341–342, 341b
        solubility of, 340
        strength of, 340, 340b
        viscosity and film thickness, 340–341
    radiopaque, 345f
    removal of excess, 350–351, 350b, 355–356, 355b–356b
    resin-based cements (adhesive and self-adhesive resin), 347–351
        advantages and disadvantages of, 351b
        composition of, 347
        procedure for, 363b–364b, 364f
        properties of, 347
    uses of, 334–339, 334t
        cavity varnish, 335
        pulpal protection, 334–336
    zinc oxide eugenol as, 351–353
        advantages and disadvantages of, 352b
        composition of, 351–352
        manipulation of, 352–353
        primary and secondary consistency of, 359b, 359f, 360f
        properties of, 352
    zinc phosphate as, 343–344
        advantages and disadvantages of, 343b
        composition of, 343

Dental cement (Continued)
  manipulation of, 344
  primary consistency of, 360b–361b, 360f, 361f
  properties of, 343–344
  zinc polycarboxylate as, 344–345
    advantages and disadvantages of, 344b
    composition of, 344
    manipulation of, 345, 345b
    primary consistency of, 361b–362b, 361f, 362f
    properties of, 344–345
Dental ceramics, 181–182
Dental environment, material hazards in, 34–35, 35b
Dental fluorosis, severe, 4f
Dental hygienist
  intraoral tasks, 1
  role of, in bleaching, 430
Dental implants, 246–274
  benefits of, 248
  components of, 248–249, 249f
  contraindications for, 248
  designs, 250–251, 250f
  dimensions of, 250–251
  home care of, 263–266
  hygiene visit after, 266–269
  indications for, 247–248
  longevity, 261–263
  materials for, 249–250
  mechanical properties of, 250t
  surface treatment of, 251
  types of, 247f
    endosseous, 247–251, 248f
    subperiosteal, 247
    transosteal, 247
Dental impression compound, 77–78
  uses for, 77–78, 77f
Dental laboratory infection control, 42–43, 42b, 43f
Dental materials, 1–6
  allied oral health practitioners, 1–2
  biocompatibility of, 9–10
  biofilm on, 18
  biomechanics, 10
  classification of, 9
  developments in, 5
  esthetics and color and, 16–17
  exothermic reaction, 14b
  force, stress and strain, 10–12
  handling and safety of, 34–50
  historical development of, 3, 3t
  materials of, 9
  oral biofilm and, 17–19, 19b
  physical and mechanical properties of, 24–33
  precautions for storing and disposing chemicals, 41, 41b
  retention, 14–16, 15f
  study of, 2b
Dental office
  mercury and, 219b

Dental office (Continued)
  other waxes utilized in, 109
Dental personnel, microorganisms exposure to, 35
Dental stone, 96
  for casts, 95f
  definition of, 93
  high-strength, 96f
  high-strength/low-expansion
    type III, 99
    type IV, 99
    type V, 99
  properties of, 98t
Dental waxes
  classification of, 107–109, 107f, 108t
  composition and properties of, 106–107
  lost wax technique for, 109–111, 110f
  manipulation of, 109–111
Dentifrice, abrasion
  before, 378, 378b, 378f, 378t
  factors contributing to, 378b
Dentin
  bonding agent, 124–125
  hardness of, 371–372
  smear layer in, 123
Dentin bonding resins, 126–127
Dentin etching, 123–125
  smear layer in, 123, 123f
Dentin matrix, 123–124
Dentistry, evidence-based, 2–3, 2f
Denture cleansers, before abrasion, 378–379, 378b, 379f
Denture liners, 285–290
  hard relining materials for, 287–289, 287b
    chairside reline, 287–289, 289b
    laboratory reline, 289
  infection control procedures for, 297–298, 298b
  over-the-counter, 289
  soft relining materials for, 286–287
Denture repair, 294–295
Denture sores
  cause of, 289, 289b
  detection and management of, 289
  home care for, 290
  signs and symptoms of, 289, 290f
  treatment for, 289–290
    use of dye transfer method, 290, 292f, 293f
    use of pressure indicating paste, 290, 290f, 291f
Denture stomatitis, 18
Dentures
  bases, acrylic resin for, 278, 279f
  care of acrylic resin, 298–300
  characterization of, 292, 295f
  components of, 282b
  digital, 284–285, 284f, 285f
    advantages of, 285b
  fabrication of, steps in, 279b
  of George Washington, 4f

Dentures (Continued)
  hard relining materials for, 287–289, 287b
    chairside reline, 287–289, 289b
    laboratory reline, 289
  home care of, 299, 299f
  in-office care of, 299–300, 300f
  soft relining materials for, 286–287
  spring closed, 4f
  stabilize, 259
  storage of, 300, 300b
  teeth, 290–292
  wearers of, instructions for, 298
Depth of cure, 142, 147–148
  definition of, 139–140
Dermatitis, 38
Desensitizing agents, 408–411, 409b, 409f, 410t–411t
  bleaching and, 430–431
  categories/components of, 410–411
  definition of, 394, 409
  tooth sensitivity, causes of, 409–410
  treatment for, 410, 410f
Desensitizing system, 411
Diagnostic casts, 94f
  definition of, 93–94
  fabricating and trimming of, 103–104, 103f
    boxing method in, 103f, 104
    double-pour method in, 104
    single-step method in, 104
    poured, criteria for evaluation of, 104b
    trimming of, 103–104, 106b, 115b–117b, 115f, 116f, 117f
    procedure for, 115b–117b, 115f, 116f, 117f
  uses of, 94, 99b
Diamond, in abrasion, 372, 376f
Diamond polishing paste, 382f
Diastema, 9f
Die stone, 95b, 96, 96f, 99
  definition of, 93
  resin-reinforced, 99
Dies
  definition of, 93–94
  metal-plated and epoxy, 99
Digital impressions, 73–77, 255, 258f
  advantages of, 76, 76b
  definition of, 51–52
  disadvantages of, 76, 76b
  expanded use of, 77, 77f
  learning curve, 73–74
  scanning devices of, 74–76, 75f, 76t
  soft tissue management of, 76–77
Digital photography, 196
Dimensional change
  of acrylic resins, 277
  of amalgam, 206
  definition of, 7–8, 13
Dimensional stability, definition of, 51–52, 54, 57
Direct fabrication, 306

Direct-placement esthetic materials, 140
   definition of, 139–140
Direct restorations, 9
Direct restorative material, 29
   definition of, 24–25
Direct technique, for provisional coverage, 316–319, 317f, 318b
Disclosing agents, for implant home care, 264–266
Disinfecting solutions, selecting, 79
Disinfection
   after cementation, 356
   of casts, 79
   of impressions, 78–79, 78b, 79b, 79t
Double-bite impression, 53f
   procedure for making, for crown, 83b–85b, 83f, 84f, 85f
Double-pour method, for casts, 104
Dough stage, of polymerization, 280
Doxycycline, teeth staining from, 423
Dual-cure process, 128
Dual-cured composites, 142
   definition of, 139–140
Dual-cured resins, 348, 350b
Dual set material, 24–25, 30
Ductility, 24–25, 27–28, 27f
Durability, 24–25, 28
   of bond, 125–126
Dusts, inhalation of, 38
Dye transfer method, use of, 290, 292f, 293f

E

Eating, dentures and, 298
EBDM. *See* Evidence-based decision-making
Eco-conscience green practices, 46–47, 46b
Edge strength, 24–25, 27–28
Elastic deformation, 24–25, 27
Elastic impression materials
   elastomers as, 62–68
   features of, 68t
   hydrocolloids as, 54–62
   polyethers as, 67–68
Elastic limit, 24–25, 27
Elastic modulus, 24–25, 27, 144, 226, 229
   definition of, 139–140
Elastic recovery, 63
Elasticity, 24–25, 27
Elastomers, 62–68
   bite registration with, 85b–87b, 85f, 86f
   definition of, 51–52
   polysulfides as, 63
Electrical conductivity, of alloys, 229
Electrical-aided whitening, 426
Electrons, of primary bonds, 25, 27
Electroplating dies, 99
Employee training, 45b

Empty containers, disposal of chemical, 41–42
Enamel
   composition of, 423–424, 424f
   erosion from stomach acid, 396f
   hardness and, 27
   remineralization of etched, unsealed, 407
Enamel bonding resins, 126, 126f
Enamel etching
   acid, 122f
   composition of, 121–123
Enamel microabrasion, 432, 433f
   adverse outcomes of, 432
   definition of, 421
Endodontic files and reamers, 239, 240f
Endodontic posts, 226, 239–242
   classification of, 226, 241t
   custom, 241
   preformed, 241–242, 241f, 242f
   purpose of, 226
Endosseous implant, 246–251, 248f
   components of, 248–249, 249f
   immediate loading, 254–255
   immediate-placement surgical procedure, 254
   one-stage surgical procedure, 253–254, 254f
   two-stage surgical procedure, 253
      first stage, 253, 254f
      second stage, 253
End-tuft brushes, 264–265, 265f
Environment, safety for, mercury and, 218
Epithelial seal, 251
Epoxy dies, 99
Erosion
   definition of, 394
   protection against, 396
   from stomach acid, enamel, 396f
Esthetic dentistry, 16
Esthetic material
   ceramics as, 181
   dental assistant handling of, 181
   direct-placement, 140
Esthetic resin cements, 348
Esthetics
   of dental cement, 342, 348b
   provisional coverage for, 309, 309b
   of provisional material, 309–310
   of zirconia, improvement of, 183
Etch-and-rinse systems, 129–130
Etch-and-rinse (also called total-etch) technique
   definition of, 120–121
   procedure of, 136b–137b, 136f, 137f
Etching
   definition of, 120–121
   of dentin, 123–125
      smear layer, 123, 123f
   enamel, 121–123, 122b, 122f
   times, 122–123
Etching sclerotic dentin, 124

Ethanol, 127
Ethyl methacrylate provisional materials, 315, 315b
Evidence-based decision-making (EBDM), 2
Excess residue
   definition of, 93
   of dental waxes, 107
Exothermic reaction, 95
   definition of, 7–8, 14
Expansion
   of alloy, 214
   cause of, 125–126
   delayed, 203
      of amalgam, 206f
      definition of, 203, 206
   effects of, 13–14
Extracoronal restoration, 306
Extrinsic stains
   causes and colors of, 422–423, 422f, 422t, 423f
   definition of, 421
   example of, 422f
Eye protection, 39
   for light-curing, 162
Eyes, chemicals absorbed in, 38
Eyewash, availability of, 40, 40t, 41f

F

Facemask, 40
Fast-set alginates
   setting time for, 57
   working time for, 56
Fatigue, 28, 29f
Fatigue failure
   definition of, 7–8
   oral environment and, 12
Feldspathic porcelain, 182, 182b, 182f
   flexural strength of, 183t
   indications and contraindications to, 189t
Felt cones, 386, 387f
Files
   breakage, 239
   endodontic, 239
Filler particles, 132
   composite resin and, 141
Film thickness
   definition of, 7–8, 15
   of dental cement, 340–341, 340b
   of zinc phosphate, 343
Final impression, 51–53
Final set time, 24–25, 30, 30f
Finish line, 306
Finishing, 18, 369, 380b
   of amalgam restorations, 370f, 381, 381f
      procedure for, 388b–389b, 388f, 389f
   benefits of, 379–380
   of ceramics, 382–383, 382b
   of composite restorations, 381–382, 381b, 381f

Finishing (Continued)
  flash, margination and removal of, 380–381, 380b, 380f
  of gold alloy, 382
  in laboratory, 386, 386f
  patient education in, 387
  of restoration, characteristics of, 382b
  safety/infection control, 387, 387b
Fissure sealants, 147
  glass ionomer cements as, 173
Fit, of dentures, 298
Fixed bridge, 180–181
Flammable liquids, in control of chemical spills, 40
Flash, 369
  definition of, 51–52, 72
  margination and removal of, 380–381, 380b, 380f
Flash point, 34, 40
  dental materials solvent, 40
Flexural strength, 182–183
Flexural stress, 7–8, 11
Flosses, for implant home care, 265, 266f
Flow
  definition of, 93
  of dental waxes, 107
Flowable composites, 147, 148f
  definition of, 139–140
Fluorapatite, 395
  definition of, 394
Fluoride, 132, 395–403, 398f
  antibacterial rinses for the control of dental caries, 396–398, 396f
  bacterial inhibition and, 396
  definition of, 394
  home-use in, 402t–403t
  in-office in, 402t–403t
  methods of delivery of, 398–402
    dietary supplements as, 398
    in-office application (topical) as, 398–400
    over-the-counter rinses, 401, 401f
    prophylaxis paste, 401–402
    self-applied topical gels and pastes as, 400, 401f
    toothpaste as, 401
  protection against erosion, 396
  safety in, 402–403, 403b
  topical, applying, 413b–414b, 414f
  topical and systemic effects of, 395–396
Fluoride-containing prophylaxis pastes, 401–402
Fluoride release, of glass ionomer cements, 171
Fluoride varnish, as desensitizing agent, 410t–411t
Fluorosis, 395
  definition of, 394
  example of, 395f
Flux, 235

Foams, in fluoride applications, 399–400, 400f
Follow-up visits, in teeth whitening, 428
Food and Drug Administration, 5
Force
  compressive, 7–8, 11
  shearing, 11
  tensile, 11
  types of, 11
Fracture toughness, 7–8, 11
  definition of, 180, 183
Free radical, definition of, 275
Function, provisional coverage for, 308f

G

Galvanic reaction, 207
Galvanic shock, 13
Galvanism
  definition of, 7–8, 13, 13f
  effects of, 207b
  electric current and, 13
Gamma phase, 205t
Gamma-1 phase, 205t
Gamma-2 phase, 205t
Gas
  characteristics of, 26
  inhalation of, 38
Gauge, 226
  of wire, 237
Gel, 51–52, 55–56, 72
  etchant, 123, 123f
  in fluoride applications, 399–400, 400f
GICs. See Glass ionomer cements
Gingival retraction, 69–72
Giomers, 176–177
Glass-based ceramics, 182–183, 185b
  bonding restorations, surface treatment for, 198b–199b, 199f
  definition of, 180–181
  preparation of, 192
Glass ionomer cements (GICs), 170, 175b–176b, 345
  advantages and disadvantages of, 173b
  atraumatic restorative treatment for, 173
  bond to enamel and dentin, 171, 173b
  caries control, 173
  cermets for, 172
  clinical application of, 172f, 174–176
  conventional, 170–173
  definition of, 170
  delivery systems, 172f
  encapsulated preferred, 172
  finishing and polishing, 175–176
  as fissure sealant, 173
  hybrid, 346–347
    advantages and disadvantages of, 347b

Glass ionomer cements (GICs) (Continued)
  lamination or "sandwich" technique for, 173, 173f
  liners and bases for, 172–173
  luting cements for, 171
  mixing of, 174–175
  packaging of, 174–175
  pediatric dentistry, 172
  physical and mechanical properties of, 171
  placement and manipulation, 175
  predosed capsule, procedure for, 362b–363b, 362f, 363f
  properties of, comparison of, 177t
  proximal surface caries, 172
  resin-modified, 346–347
  restorative materials for, 171–173, 172f
  root abrasion/erosion, 171–172
  root caries, 171
  traditional
    advantages and disadvantages of, 346b
    composition of, 345
    manipulation of, 346, 346f
    mixing of, 346b
    properties of, 345–346
  uses for, 171–173
Glass ionomer surface sealer, as desensitizing agent, 410t–411t
Glass ionomers, 170–179
Glazing, 194, 195f
Gloves, chemical-resistant, 39
Glycine, for abrasion, 377f, 384
Gold
  solders, 234–235
  tooth restoration for, 4f
Gold alloy
  finishing of, 382
  polishing of, during oral prophylaxis, 383, 384f
Goodyear brothers, 3t
Grains, 227, 229
Grit, 369, 372, 372f
  as three-body abrasive, 374
Gypsum products, 93–119
  behaviors of, 95–98
  classification of, 98–100, 100b
  cleanup of, 105, 105b
  desirable qualities of, 94–95
  dimensional accuracy of, 97
  fabricating diagnostic/working casts in, 103–104, 103f
  final setting time of, 101–102, 102b
  formation of, 95
  infection control and safety issues in, 105
  manipulation of, 100–106
    factors in, 103t
    material selection in, 100, 100f
    mixing in, 100–101, 101f

Gypsum products (Continued)
    proportioning (water-to-powder ratio) in, 100, 100b, 101t
    metal-plated and epoxy dies and resin-reinforced die stone in, 99
    mixing procedure for, 111b–112b, 112f
        equipment/supplies for, 112f
    physical properties of, 96–98
    production of, 95–96
    properties of, 98t
    qualities of, 94–95
    reproduction of detail of, 97, 97f
    separating impression from cast in, 105
    setting time in, 101, 102f
        accelerators and retarders in, 102–103
        altering W/P ratio in, 102
        control of, 102–103
        spatulation in, 102
        temperature in, 102
        using clean equipment and impressions, 103, 103t
    solubility of, 97–98, 98b, 98t
    storage of, 104–105, 104b
    trimming of, 103f, 105–106, 106b, 106f
    type IV and V, 99
    uses of, 94, 100b

H

Halogen, 161, 161b
Hand mixing dental cement, advantages and disadvantages of, 354t
Hand protection, 39, 39f
Hand spatulation, of gypsum materials, 101
Hard acrylic guard, for mouth, 443
Hard laminate guard, for mouth, 443
Hard liner, definition of, 275
Hard relining materials, for dentures, 287–289, 287b
    chairside reline, 287–289, 289b
    laboratory reline, 289
Hardness, 27
    abrasion and, 369, 371–372
    of alloys, 229
    definition of, 24–25
    of gypsum, 96–97
    of provisional material, 309
    of solids, 27
Hazard communication program, 43–44, 43b, 45f
    chemical inventory, 43
    containers, labeling of, 44, 45f, 46b
        exemptions to, 44–46
    safety data sheets, 43–44, 44b
    written, 43
Hazardous chemical, 34, 36–38, 37f
Hazardous waste disposal, of chemical, 41b–42b, 42
Healing abutment, 246, 253, 254f
Healing screw, 254f

Heat-cured acrylic resin, 277, 278t
    polymerization of, 278–280
Heat-pressing, 180, 185
High-copper alloy
    admix and spherical, 206t, 214t
    common, 216t
    compressive strength of, 205
    creep and, 206
High-noble alloy, 226, 228–229
High-strength base/liners, 335
High-strength stone, properties of, 96, 98t
Home care
    for acrylic resin dentures, 299
    for denture sores, 290
    for soft liners, 287
Home care, for implant, 263–266
    antibacterial agents, 265–266
    brushes, 264–265, 265f, 266f
    disclosing agents, 264–266
    flosses, 265, 266f
    wooden plaque removers, 265
Home whitening, 427, 428b
    chemical used in, 427
    clinical procedures for, 435b–436b, 435f, 436f
    instructions for, 431b
    over-the-counter products for, 429–430
    process, 428–429
Hue, 139–140, 150
    definition of, 7–8, 16
Humidity, in manipulation of materials, 31
Hybrid composites, 145–146
    definition of, 139–140
Hybrid glass ionomer cements, 346–347
    advantages and disadvantages of, 347b
    manipulation of, 347, 347b
Hybrid (resin-modified) ionomers, 173–176
    curing modes, 174
    definition of, 170
    pediatric dentistry, 174
    properties of, comparison of, 173–174, 177t
    uses for, 174
Hybrid layer
    definition of, 120–121
    formation of, 127, 128f
Hydrocolloid. See also Irreversible hydrocolloid; Reversible hydrocolloid
    definition of, 51–52
Hydrofluoric acid, 132b
Hydrogen bonds, 26
Hydrogen peroxide, 424
Hydrophilic, 120–121, 128
Hydrophobic, 127
    definition of, 120–121
Hydroxyapatite crystals, 123–124

Hygiene visit, for implant home care, 266–269
Hypersensitivity
    from bleaching, 427
    cause of, 9

I

Identalloy program, 234, 234f
Ignitable, 34, 41b–42b
Illumination, 21
Imbibition, 51–52, 62
Immediate-placement surgical procedure, for endosseous implant, 254
Implant
    abutment, 246, 248
    analog, 255
    fixture, 246, 248
    longevity, 261–263
        adverse outcomes from, 262b
        implant failure, 262–263
        long-term success, 261
    maintenance, 263, 264f
        home care, 263–266
        hygiene visit, 266–269
    placement and restoration, 252–255, 263b
        immediate loading, 254–255
        immediate-placement surgical procedure, 254
        informed consent, 252
        one-stage surgical procedure, 253–254, 254f
        patient, preparation of, 253
        postsurgical instructions, 253
        surgical risks, 252
        two-stage surgical procedure, 253
    planning, image-guided, 251–252, 252f
        advantages of, 251–252
        software for, 251
    polishing of, 384
Implant abutment, 246
Implant analog, 246, 255
Implant maintenance
    home care
        aids for, 266b
        antibacterial agents, 265–266
        brushes, 264–265, 265f, 266f
        disclosing agents, 264–266
        flosses, 265, 266f
        wooden plaque removers, 265
    hygiene visit
        implant surface, cleaning of, 267–269, 267f, 268f
        mobility, 267
        probing, 267, 267f
        radiographic assessment, 266–269
        visual assessment, 266–267
Implant planning, 252f
Impression, 62b
    abutment, 246, 255
    accurate, obtaining, 73b

Impression (Continued)
  as contaminated, 78
  criteria for clinically acceptable, 61, 61f, 61t
  disinfection of, 78–79, 78b, 79b, 79t, 105
    procedure for, 89b
  double-bite, 53f
    for crown, 83b–85b, 83f, 84f, 85f
  handling of, 60–61
  optical scanners and, 185
  troubleshooting for, 62t
  types of, 53
Impression making
  components of, for crown and bridge procedures, 69–73
  criteria for successful, 72, 72b
  evaluation of, 72–73, 73b, 77f
  objective for, 57–58
  tray selection for, 58–61, 58f
Impression materials, 51–92
  key properties of, 53–54
  types of, 53
Impression plaster, 78, 98
Impression tray, 54, 295–298
  chemical-cured, 295–297, 301b–303b, 301f, 302f
  example of, 55f
  fabrication of, 295
  light-cured, 297
  loading, 59
  removing of, 60
  seating, 59–60, 60b, 60f
  selection of, 58–61, 58f
  sterilization of, 79
Impression wax, 78
Improper handling, consequences of, 214
Incremental placement, of composites, 144b, 144f
  definition of, 139–140
Indirect fabrication, 306
Indirect restorations, 9
Indirect restorative material, 29
  definition of, 24–25
Indirect technique, for provisional coverage, 318–319, 318b
Indirect-direct technique, for provisional coverage, 319, 319b
Indirect-placement esthetic materials, 163–164
  definition of, 139–140
Inelastic impression materials
  dental impression compound, uses for, 77–78, 77f
  impression plaster as, 78
  wax as, 78
Infection control
  in gypsum products, 105
  for light-curing, 162–163
Infectious disease, personal chemical protection, 39

Informed consent, in teeth whitening, 428–429
Ingestion, of chemicals, 38
Inhalation, of chemicals, 38
Inhalation protection, 39–40
Inhibitors, 141–142
Initial set time, 24–25, 30
Initiation, of free radicals, 276
Inlay, definition of, 180–181
Inlay wax, 107–108, 107f
In-office fluoride treatment, 402t–403t
In-office tartar and stain remover, 379f
In-office whitening
  of nonvital teeth, 427, 427f
  procedure for, 433b–434b, 433f, 434f
  of vital teeth, 425–427, 425f, 430b
Inorganic filler particles, 139–140
Inorganic salts, as desensitizing agent, 410t–411t
Insulators, 7–8, 14
Interceptive orthodontics, 446
Interface, 7–8, 16
Intermediate, 333
Intermediate restoration, 24–25, 29
  cement consistency for, 337
International Organization for Standardization (ISO), 5
Interproximal brushes, 264, 265f
Intracoronal cement provisionals, 321, 321b, 321f
  procedure for, 328b–330b, 329f, 330f
Intracoronal restoration, definition of, 306, 310
Intraoral scanner, 73
  definition of, 51–52
Intrinsic stains
  causes and colors of, 422t, 423, 423f
  definition of, 421
  example of, from tetracycline, 428f
Investment materials, 99–100
Ionic bonds, 25
Irreversible hydrocolloid (alginate), 51–52, 56–57
  composition of, 56, 56t
  dimensional stability of, 57
  disinfection of, 79t
  impression making, 57–61
  permanent deformation of, 57
  setting reaction of, 56
  setting time for, 57, 57b
  tear strength of, 57
  working time for, 56–57
ISO. See International Organization for Standardization
Ivory, as denture material, 4f

K
Knoop hardness test, 371, 371t

L
Labeling, exemptions, 44–46
Laboratory reline, for dentures, 289

Lathe-cut alloy, 203, 205t
Lattice structure, 227, 227f
Length of treatment, in teeth whitening, 428
Leucite-reinforced ceramics
  glass, flexural strength of, 183t
  indications and contraindications to, 189t
Light aided power whitening, 425–426
Light-activated materials, 24–25, 30, 31f
Light-cured cements, 354b
Light-cured composites, 142, 160–163, 162b
  definition of, 139–140
  factors affecting, 160, 160b, 160f
  guidelines for, 162b
  infection control methods, 162–163, 162b
  matching of, 161–162, 162b
  position of, 160–163
  in proximal box, 161
  rapid, 161
  types of, 161
Light-cured resins, 128, 283
  for denture repair, 295
Light-cured sealant, 408t
Light-curing, 347–348, 350b
Light-emitting diode (LED), 161, 161f
Liner, 335
  definition of, 333
  high-strength, 335
  line drawing of, 335f
  low-strength, 335
Lingual retainer, 237–238, 238f
Liquids
  characteristics of, 26
  etchant, 123
  flammable, in control of chemical spills, 40
Liquidus, 229
Listerine, 397, 397f
Lithium disilicate ceramics, 182–183
  definition of, 180
  flexural strength of, 183t
  indications and contraindications to, 189t
Long-term soft liners, 286, 286f
  definition of, 275
Longevity, of materials, 29
Loose abrasives, 374
Looseness, of dentures, 298
Lost wax technique, 109–111, 110f
  definition of, 93
Low-copper alloy, compressive strength of, 205
Low-fusing porcelain, 193
Low-strength base/liner, 335, 336b
Luting, 333, 336
Luting cements, 171
  classification of, 342–353
  functions of, 343b
  loading crown for, 355, 355b

M

Macrofilled composites, 145
  definition of, 139–140
Magnification, 21
Malleability, 24–25, 27–28, 28f
Mandibular impressions, criteria for acceptable, 61t
Manipulation
  considerations for, 354b
  of dental cement, mixing of, 352f, 353–354, 360b–361b
  of gypsum products, 100–106
    factors in, 103t
    material selection in, 100, 100f
    mixing in, 100–101, 101f
    proportioning (water-to-powder ratio) in, 100, 100b, 101t
  of material, 31
    variables for, 31
Margin, breakdown, 27–28, 28f
Margin configuration, 233, 233f
Margination, 369, 380–381, 380b
  indications for, 380b
Margins, care on, 356–357
Mastication, stress during, 12
Masticatory force, 10–11
Materials, classification of, 28–29, 29b
Matrix bands, 207–213, 208f, 209b, 209f, 210f, 211f, 212f, 213f, 214f
Matrix system, 207–216, 210f
  of composite resin, 156–160
    bands in, 156, 157f, 158f
    cervical matrices, 158, 159f
    circumferential, 157–158
    sectional, 158, 159f
    wedges in, 158–160, 160f
Matter, three states of, 26
Maxillary impressions, criteria for acceptable, 61t
Maxillofacial prostheses, plastics for, 293, 296f
Mechanical properties, of dental materials, 27–28
Mechanical retention, 14–15
Melting range, 229
  definition of, 93
  of dental waxes, 106–107
Mercury, 215f
  alloy and
    setting reactions of, 205, 205t
    setting transformation of, 204–205
  dispensing of, 213
  exposure to, 38
  handling of spills of, 219b
  health concerns for, 217–218
  office staff exposure to, 219b
  vapor reduction, methods for, 219b
Mercury spill kits, 40, 40f
Mercury vapor
  reduction of, 219b
  release of, 217–218
Metal casting alloys, 228

Metal matrix band, posterior, types of, 208f
Metal-plated dies, 99
Metallic bonds, 25
Metals
  moisture and acid levels in, 12–13
  in orthodontics, 236–239
  structure of, 227–232, 227b
Metamerism, 17, 17f, 151
Methyl methacrylate provisional materials, 314–315, 314f, 315b
Microabrasion, 369, 385–386, 386b, 386f
  enamel, 432, 433f
    adverse outcomes of, 432
Microfilled composites, 145, 146t, 177t
  definition of, 139–140
Microhybrids, 146
  composite, 177t
  definition of, 139–140
Microleakage, 16f, 135, 135f
  definition of, 7–8, 16
  effects of, 16
  of glass ionomer cements, 171
Microorganism, 35
  community of, 17
Microparticle abrasives, 374
Microwave processing, of acrylic resin, 282
Milling, all-ceramic restorations, 185, 187f
Mineral (hydroxyapatite), 121
Mineralizing agents, as desensitizing agent, 410t–411t
Mini-implants, 246, 250–251, 258–259
  uses for, 259, 260f, 261f
Mixing, in manipulation of materials, 31, 31f
Mixing time, 24–25, 30
Model plaster
  definition of, 93, 95
  formation of, 95b
  properties of, 98t
  use of, 98–99, 99b
Modulus of elasticity, of glass ionomer cements, 171
Mohs scale of hardness, 369–371, 371t
Moist dentin, for bonding, 124–125, 124f
Moisture contamination, 30, 407
Monomers, 141
  definition of, 139–140, 275
Mouth guards
  definition of, 440
  sports, 440–442, 441f
    boil-and-bite guards and, 441, 441f
    custom-fit guards and, 441–442, 442f
    fabrication of, 450b–451b, 450f, 451f
    protection by, 442
    stock guards and, 441, 441f
  use of, 440–442, 441f

N

Nanocomposites
  of composite resin, 146–147, 147f
  definition of, 139–140
Nanohybrids, 146
  definition of, 139–140
Nano-ionomers, 174
  definition of, 170
National Fire Protection Association labels, 44–46
National Institute of Occupational Safety and Health (NIOSH)-approved dust and mist respirator facemask, 40
National Institutes of Health (NIH), amalgam safety, 217
Neoprene apron, 39
Nickel, allergy to, 232
Night guards, 442–445
  design of, 443–444
  home care instructions for, 443b
  maintenance of, 444–445, 445b
  types of materials for, 443
NIH. *See* National Institutes of Health
Nitinol, 239
Noble alloy, 226, 229
Noble metal casting alloys, 228–229
Noble metals, biocompatibility of, 231–232
Non-absorbable sutures, 246, 269, 270f
Non-adhesive cements, 339
Non-glass-based ceramics, 183, 185b
  definition of, 180, 182
  preparation of, 192
Non-vital tooth, definition of, 421
Nonlight aided power whitening, 426

O

Obstructive sleep apnea
  definition of, 440
  function of appliance, 445, 446f
  oral appliances for prevention of, 445–446
  risk factors for, 445
  treatment of, 445, 445f
Occlusal surface configuration, 233
Occupational Safety and Health Administration (OSHA), 35
  Hazard Communication Standard, 43
  mercury exposure, 218
Odontoblasts, 124
  hypersensitivity and, 409
Office staff, safety for, mercury and, 218
Oil-based luting cements, 351–353
One-bottle adhesive systems, 129–130
One-bottle self-etch bonding systems, 131, 131b, 131f
One-stage surgical procedure, for endosseous implant, 253–254, 254f
Onlay, definition of, 180–181

Opacity, of ceramics, 184, 196
Opaque, 7–8, 17
Open-tray impression, 246, 255–258, 255b, 256f
Optical reader, 197, 197f, 198f
Optical scanner, 185
Oral appliances, preventive and corrective, 440–449, 445b, 450b–451b
Oral disease, biofilm and, 18
Oral environment
 esthetics and, 16–17
 moisture and acid levels, 12–13, 12f
 patient concerns, 8
 and patient considerations, 7–23
 preventive/therapeutic materials, 9
 temperature of, 13–14
Oral prophylaxis, polishing in, 383–386
Organic resin matrix, 141
 definition of, 139–140
Orthodontic band, 237, 238f
 cement for, 336–337
Orthodontic bracket, 237
 bonding, 121
 cement for, 336–337, 337f
Orthodontic plaster, 99b
Orthodontic tooth aligners, 447–449, 448f
 creating, 447, 448f
 definition of, 440
 treatment for, 447, 449f
Orthodontic wax, 109
Orthodontics, metals used in, 236–239
 archwires, 236–237, 236t
 brackets and bands, 237, 238f
 endodontic files and reamers, 239, 240f
 retainers, removable orthodontic appliances and, 237–238, 238f, 239f
 space maintainers, 238
OSHA. See Occupational Safety and Health Administration
Osseointegration, 246, 249, 250f, 254
OTC. See Over-the-counter
Overhang, 369, 380, 380f
Over-the-counter (OTC), 394, 397f
 fluoride rinses, 401, 401f
Over-the-counter (OTC) liners, 289
Oxidation, tarnish and, 12–13
Oxides, 251
Oxygen-inhibited layer, 129
 definition of, 120–121
 of sealant, 406–407, 406b

P

Packable composites, 148
Packaging, 131
Paint-on whitening materials, 429
Palatal expansion appliances, 446–447, 447f
Palatal expansion device, definition of, 440

Palladium, 230
Particulate matter, 34–35
 exposure to, 34–35
Passive post, 239
Paste abrasives, 374
Patient education, restoration and, 321–322, 387
Patient safety, 47–48, 47f
 mercury and, 218
Pattern waxes, 107–108
PBM restorations. See Porcelain-bonded-to-metal restorations
Percolation, definition of, 7–8, 14
Peri-implant disease, cement-associated, 356, 356b, 356f
Peri-implantitis, 246, 259f, 263
Permanent, 333, 337
Permanent dipoles, 25
Permanent restoration, 24–25, 29
Peroxide whitening, history of, 423
Personal chemical protection, 39–40
 eye protection, 39
 hand protection, 39, 39f
 inhalation protection, 39–40
 protective clothing, 39
Personal protective equipment (PPE), 34–35
PFM restorations. See Porcelain-fused-to-metal restorations
pH
 of acidic primers, 130
 of saliva, 12–13
Phosphoric acid etching, dentin and, 123–125, 124f, 125b
Physical properties, of dental materials, 26–27
Physical structure, of materials, 25–26, 26b
Pigments, 141
 composite resin and, 141
 definition of, 139–140
PIP. See Pressure indicating paste
Pit and fissure sealants, 147, 403–408
 application of, 413f
 bite interference by, 407
 chemical-cured and light-cured, advantages and disadvantages of, 408t
 color and wear of, 406
 composition of, 405, 405b
 effectiveness of, 407
 etched, unsealed enamel, remineralization of, 407
 etching precautions of, 407
 filler content/color of, 405t
 glass ionomer cement as a sealant, 408
 indications for, 404, 404f
 oxygen-inhibited layer of, 406–407, 406b
 patient record entries of, 407, 407b
 placement of, 406–407, 406b
 purpose of, 403–404, 404f

Pit and fissure sealants (Continued)
 susceptibility of teeth to fissure caries, 405
 troubleshooting problems with, 408, 408f, 409t
 working time for, 405
Plaque removers, for implant home care, 265
Plastic deformation, 24–25, 27
Plasticizer
 aromatic esters as, 277
 definition of, 275
Platinum, 230
Pneumatic press, 280
Polishing, 369–393, 374b
 in laboratory, 386, 386f
 during oral prophylaxis, 383–386
  air abrasion, 384–386, 386b, 386f
  air polishing, 384–386, 384t, 385b
  of amalgams, 383
  of composite, 383, 389b–390b, 390f, 391f
  of gold alloys and ceramics, 383
  of implants, 384
  of resin/cement interface, 384
 patient education in, 387
 safety/infection control, 387, 387b
Poly(methyl methacrylate), 275
Polycarbonate crown, 312–313, 313b
 procedure for, 324b–326b, 325f, 326f
Polyether, 67–68
 block out undercuts, 67–68, 68f
 consistency and setting reaction of, 67
 definition of, 51–52
 disinfection of, 79t
 features of, 68t
 hydrophilic nature, 68
 mixing and dispensing of, 67, 67f
 properties of, 67, 67f
 working and setting times of, 68
Polymer chains, cross-linking of, 141, 142f
Polymerization, 141–142
 addition, 276
 of chemical-cured resins, 282
 condensation, 276
 definition of, 120–121, 139–140, 275
 formation of, 276–284
 of heat-cured resins, 280
 methods of, 276
 physical stages of, 280
 reactions, 276
 of resin-based cements, 347–348
Polymerization shrinkage, 143–144, 148
 of acrylic resins, 277
 clinical consequences of, 143–144
 reducing the effects of, 144b
Polymers, 141
 definition of, 275
 formation of, 276–284
  review of, 276–284

Polymers *(Continued)*
    for prosthetic dentistry, 275–305
Polysulfides, 63, 63*b*
    definition of, 51–52
Polyvinyl siloxane (PVS), 64–68
    bite registration, 66
    definition of, 51–52
    disinfection of, 79*t*
    dispensing system of, 64–65, 64*b*, 65*f*
    features of, 68*t*
    hydrophobic nature of, 64
    putty/wash techniques, 65–67
    surface detail of, 64
    viscosities of, 64
    working and setting time of, 65
Porcelain, 19–20
    alumina, 182
    body and incisal, 193–194
    composition of, 182
    definition of, 180, 182–183
    failure, 194–195
    feldspathic, 182, 182*b*, 182*f*
    fusing temperatures of, 182
    hardness of, 27, 371
    high fusing, 182
    low fusing, 182
    medium fusing, 182
    metal oxides and, 194–195
    reinforced, 182
    surface preparation, 190
    uses of, 182
Porcelain application, metal coping, 233
Porcelain bonding alloys, 226, 232–234, 232*f*
Porcelain teeth, 3*t*, 292, 294*f*
Porcelain veneers, 189–190
    example of, 190*f*
Porcelain-bonded-to-metal (PBM) restorations, 193, 233–234
    layers of, 194*f*
Porcelain-fused-to-metal (PFM) restorations, 180, 193–195
    advantage of, 193
    coefficient of thermal expansion of, 194–195
    color modification in, 194
    color selection in, 193
    glazing and, 194, 195*f*
    metal oxides and, 194–195
    porcelain failure of, 193*f*
    sintering and, 193
    soldering of, 233
Porosity
    of acrylic resins, 278, 278*b*, 278*f*
    definition of, 275
Postoperative sensitivity, 9, 16, 130
Potassium nitrate, as desensitizing agent, 410*t*–411*t*
Pour technique, for chemical-cured resins, 282
Pouring
    of cast, procedure for

Pouring *(Continued)*
    anatomic portion, 112*b*–113*b*, 112*f*, 113*f*
    art portion, 114*b*, 114*f*
    definition of, 93
    of gypsum in casts, 94*f*, 101
Power whitening
    definition of, 421
    in-office, 425–426, 426*b*, 426*b*–427*b*, 426*f*
    light aided, 425–426
    nonlight aided, 426
PPE. *See* Personal protective equipment
Pre-cementation check, 353
Precious metals, 226, 230
Predose package, 30*b*
Predosed capsules, advantages and disadvantages of, 354*t*
Preformed abutment, 248
Preformed post, 241–242, 241*f*, 242*f*
Preformed/prefabricated crowns, 310–311, 310*b*, 310*f*
Preliminary impression, definition of, 51–53
Pressure indicating paste (PIP), use of, 290, 290*f*, 291*f*
Prevention/preventive aids, 394
Preventive dentistry, fluoride and, 3
Preventive material, 29
Primary bond, 24–25, 26*b*
    types of, 25
Primary consistency, 340
    definition, 333
    zinc oxide eugenol procedure for, 359*b*, 359*f*, 360*f*
    zinc phosphate procedure for, 360*b*–361*b*, 360*f*, 361*f*
    zinc polycarboxylate procedure for, 361*b*–362*b*, 361*f*, 362*f*
Primer, 120–121
    acidic, 130
Probiotics, biofilm and, 18
Processing waxes, 107–109
Propagation, of free radicals, 276
Properties of waxes, 106
Prophylactic polishing paste, 372, 372*f*
    before abrasion, 374–377, 374*b*
Prophylaxis pastes, for implants, 267
Prosthesis, 248–249
    definition of, 275
    maxillofacial, plastics for, 293, 296*f*
Protective clothing, 39
Protective measures, 232
Provisional coverage
    advanced techniques for, 319–320
    criteria for, 307
        esthetics and speech, 309, 309*b*
        exposed tooth surfaces, 307–309, 308*b*
        function, 308, 308*f*
        gingival tissues, 308, 308*b*, 308*f*
        retention, 309, 309*b*

Provisional coverage *(Continued)*
        tooth position, 307
    custom, direct technique for, 327*b*–328*b*, 327*f*, 328*f*
    definition of, 306
    dental procedures requiring, 307, 307*t*
    direct technique for, 316–319, 317*f*, 318*b*
    indirect technique for, 318–319, 318*b*
    indirect-direct technique for, 319, 319*b*
    intracoronal cement provisionals for, 321, 321*b*, 321*f*
    patient education for, 321–322, 322*b*
    vacuum former acetate technique for, 316
Provisional crown, 308*f*
    cementing of, 320, 320*b*
    materials for, 310
    procedure for
        metal, 322*b*–324*b*, 322*f*, 323*f*, 324*f*
        polycarbonate, 324*b*–326*b*, 325*f*, 326*f*
Provisional materials
    acrylic, 314–315, 314*f*, 315*b*
    aluminum shell crowns, 310*f*, 311
    bis-acrylic composite, 315, 316*t*
    composite resin, 315–316, 315*f*, 316*b*
    customized, 313–314, 314*f*
    ethyl methacrylate, 315, 315*b*
    fitting the crown, 311–312, 312*f*, 313*b*
    manipulation of, 316, 316*b*, 316*t*
        methods of fabrication, 316
        type and uses of templates, 316, 317*f*
    methyl methacrylate, 314–315, 314*f*, 315*b*
    polycarbonate crown forms, 312–313, 313*b*
    preformed/prefabricated crowns as, 310–311, 310*b*, 310*f*
    properties of, 309–314
        esthetics, 309–310, 310*b*
        hardness, 309
        strength, 309
        tissue compatibility, 309
    stainless-steel crowns as, 311, 311*f*
Provisional resin cements, 351, 351*f*
Provisional restorations, 306–322, 322*b*–324*b*, 324*b*–326*b*, 327*b*–328*b*, 328*b*–330*b*
    cement consistency for, 337
    removal of, 320–321, 320*f*, 321*b*
Provisional/temporary, 337
Pulp-capping agent, 335
Pumice, 372, 372*f*
    in abrasion, 374
Pure metals, 227, 227*b*
Putty/wash techniques, 65–67
    one-step technique, 65, 65*bd*
    potential distortions of, 66, 66*b*
    removing of set impression, 66

Putty/wash techniques (Continued)
two-step technique, 65–66, 65b
PVS. See Polyvinyl siloxane

R

Radiographs, restorations, 21, 21f
Radiopacity
of composite resin, 144–145, 145f
of dental cement, 342
of glass ionomer cements, 171
Rag wheel, 376f, 386
Ratios, in manipulation of materials, 31
Reaction
exothermic, definition of, 7–8, 14, 14b
of material, 30–31, 30f
Reactive, 34, 41b–42b
Reamers, 239
Record bases, 295–298
chemical-cured, 295–297
fabrication of, 296
light-cured, 297
Reflectance, of ceramics, 184
Regular-set alginates
setting time for, 57
working time for, 56
Reline, for dentures, 285–290
Reline jig, 289
Remineralization, 395, 411–412
definition of, 394
products of, 411, 412f
resin infiltration, 412, 412b, 412f
Removable partial denture (RPD), processing of, 283–284, 283b, 283f, 284f
Removable prosthesis, procedure for cleaning of, 379b
Removable retainer, 238
Resilience, 7–8, 11, 24–25, 27
Resin agents, as desensitizing agent, 410t–411t
Resin-based cements (adhesive and self-adhesive resin), 347–351, 348b, 349f
advantages and disadvantages of, 347b
categories of, 348–350
composition of, 347
procedure for, 363b–364b, 364f
properties of, 347
Resin bonding agent, 121, 122f, 128–129
Resin/cement interface, polishing of, 384
Resin cement systems, 192
Resin-modified glass ionomer cements (RMGIC), 346–347
Resin-modified ionomer, 177t
Resin-reinforced die stone, 99
Resin tags, 121, 126
Resin-to-resin bonding, 153, 154f
Resins, staining of, 12
Restoration
bleaching and, 431–432
bonding of, 135

Restoration (Continued)
cement consistency for, 340
conditions for assessing, 21b
curing methods for, 350b
loading of, 355
mechanisms, tooth structure, 121
permanent, intermediate, and temporary/provisional, 337
try-in of, 350
Restorative materials, 8–9
allied oral health practitioners, 16
definition of, 7–8
detection of, 19–21, 20f
identification methods, 19–21
thermal properties of tooth and, 14t
Restorative phase, 255–258
implant impression and laboratory components, 255
impression procedures, 255–258
removable prosthesis, retention of, 258, 260f
retention of implant crown, 255
Retainer
lingual, 237–238, 238f
in matrix bands, 208, 210f
placement of band in, 208
removable, 237–238, 238f
Retainerless matrix systems, 213, 213f, 214f
Retarders, gypsum setting time and, 102–103
Retention
definition of, 7–8, 14
of dental cement, 341–342, 341b
provisional coverage for, 309, 309b
restorative materials and, 14–16
Retentive undercuts, 15f
Retraction cord, 69f
checklist of, 71, 71f
evaluation of, 71, 71f
methods of, 69
Retraction paste, 72
Reversible hydrocolloid (agar), 55–56
definition of, 51–52
Rim-lock trays, 54
RMGIC. See Resin-modified glass ionomer cements
Root canal sealers, 337
Root canal therapy, 239
Root resorption, risk of, in teeth whitening, 427
Rotary brushes, 265
Rotary files, 239, 240f
Rotary instruments, 239
Rouge, in abrasion, 376f, 382
Roughening, surface implants, 251
RPD. See Removable partial denture
Rubber base, 63
Rubber stage, of polymerization, 280

S

Safety
fluoride and, 402–403, 403b

Safety (Continued)
issues, in gypsum products, 105
measures, 105
Safety data sheets (SDS), 34, 36–38, 43–44, 44b
Saliva
abrasion and, 372
excess, dentures and, 298
pH of, 12–13
"Sandwich" technique, for glass ionomer cements, 173, 173f
Sandy stage, of polymerization, 280
Screw-retained crowns, 255–258, 258f
SDS. See Safety data sheets
Sealants
bite interference by, 407
color and wear of, 406
composition of, 405, 405b
definition of, 394
dental, application of, 415b–417b
effectiveness of, 407
glass ionomer cement as, 408
indications for, 404
oxygen-inhibited layer of, 406–407, 406b
patient record entries of, 407, 407b
pit and fissure, 403–408
placement of, 406–407, 406b
troubleshooting problems with, 408, 409t
working time for, 405
Secondary bonds, 24–25, 26b
of materials, 25–26
Secondary consistency, 333, 335
for temporary/provisional and intermediate restorations, 335
zinc oxide eugenol procedure for, 359b, 359f, 360f
Sectional matrix systems, 213
of composite resin, 158, 159f
Sedative, 333, 337
zinc oxide eugenol as, 352
Sedative provisional restoration, 337
Selective etching, definition of, 120–121, 130
Self-adhesive resin cements, 349–350, 349f, 350b
Self-adhesive technique, for indirect restorations, 365b–366b, 365f, 366f
Self-applied topical gels and pastes, 400, 401f
Self-cured composites, 141–142
definition of, 139–140
Self-curing process, 128, 347, 350b
Self-etch bonding systems, 129t, 130–134
definition of, 120–121, 130
Self-etch cements, 348
Self-etch systems, 128, 132f, 133b, 134–135
Separating medium, 280
Separator, amalgam, 203, 218

Shade guides
　for ceramics, 195
　example of, 197f
Shade mapping, 196
Shade matching
　for all-ceramic restorations, 197
　custom, 196–197
Shade taking
　for ceramic restorations, 195–198
　　dental assistant/hygienist in, 195, 196f
　　characterizing, 196–197
　　device, 197–198, 197f, 198f
　　example of, 197f
　　involving dental assistant/hygienist and patient in, 195, 195f
　　lighting for, 196
　　matching of, 196
Shear, amalgam and, 206
Shearing force, 7–8, 11
Shelf life
　definition of, 24–25
　of material, 31–32
Short-term soft liners, 286–287, 287f, 288f
　application of, 287
　definition of, 275
Shrinkage, of glass ionomer cements, 171
Silane, 132
Silane coupling agent
　composite resin and, 141
　definition of, 139–140
Silica particles, 387
Silicone, 72
　addition, 64
　condensation, 63–64
Silicone die technique, 67
Silicone rubber impression materials
　addition, 64
　condensation, 63–64
　types of, 63
Silver, 204
　as component of amalgam alloy, 205t
Silver alloy phase, 205t
Silver-based amalgam alloys, classification of, 204
Silver diamine fluoride, 398, 398f, 399t
　application of, 398–399, 399f, 415b, 415b–417b, 415f, 416f
Silver paste, 3t
Single-step method, for casts, 104
Sintering, 182, 182f, 185
　definition of, 180
Sinus lift, 246, 261, 263f
Skin, chemicals absorbed in, 38
Slip-casting, 180, 185
Smear layer, 123, 123f
　definition of, 120–121
Snoring, oral appliances for prevention of, 445–446
Sodium bicarbonate, in abrasion, 377f
Soft guard, for mouth, 443

Soft laminate guard, for mouth, 443
Soft relining materials, for dentures, 286–287
Sol
　definition of, 51–52
　gelling of, 55–56
Solders, 226, 234
　gold, 234–235
　silver, 235, 235f
Solids, characteristics of, 26, 26f
Solidus, 229
Solubility
　definition of, 7–8
　of dental cement, 340
　dental materials and, 12
　of glass ionomer cements, 171
　of gypsum, 97–98, 98b, 98t
　of zinc phosphate, 343
Solvents, type of, 126–127
Soreness, from dentures, 298
Space maintainers, 446
　definition of, 440
　types of, 446
Spatulation of gypsum, 101f, 102
Speaking, dentures and, 298
Spectrophotometer, 197, 197f
Spherical alloy, 205t
　definition of, 203
Splatter, 34–35
Sports mouth guards, 440–442, 441f
　boil-and-bite guards and, 441, 441f
　custom-fit guards and, 441–442, 442f
　fabrication of, 450b–451b, 450f, 451f
　protection by, 442
　stock guards and, 441, 441f
　types of, 440–441
Spring closed denture, 4f
Staining, 12
　of restorations, 387
Stainless-steel alloy, 235–236
Stainless-steel crowns, 311, 311f
Stains, on teeth
　causes and colors of, 422t
　types of, 422–423
Standards in dentistry, American Dental Association (ADA) and, 3–5, 4f
Sticky wax, 108–109
Stiffness, 24–25, 27
Stock guards, 441, 441f
Stock trays, 54
　sectional, 54
Storage, of gypsum products, 104–105, 104b
Storing chemicals, precautions for, 41, 41b, 41f
Strain
　definition of, 7–8, 11
　example of, 11f
Strength
　of acrylic resins, 277
　of alloys, 229
　of amalgam, 206

Strength (Continued)
　of dental cement, 340, 340b
　of gypsum, 96–97, 97b
　of provisional material, 309
　of zinc oxide, 351
　of zinc phosphate, 343
Stress, 27, 27f
　definition of, 7–8, 10
　dental materials and, 11, 11f
　during mastication, 12
Stringy stage, of polymerization, 280
Sub-gingival air polishing, 369, 377f, 385, 385f
Subperiosteal implants, 247
Substantivity, 394
Sulcus, prepacking of, 69, 70f
Supra-gingival air polishing, 369, 377f, 384–385
Surface characteristics, 15–16
Surface energy, definition of, 7–8, 16
Surface luster and texture, 196
Surfactant, 51–52, 68
　in impression materials, 97, 97f
Surgical dressings
　cement for, 337, 338f, 339b
　materials and supplies for mixing, 338f
　placement of, 338f
　well-placed, criteria for, 339b
Sutures, 246, 269–270
　characteristics of, 269
　needles for, 269–270, 270f
　removal, 270, 271b–272b, 271f, 272f
　techniques for, 270, 270f
　types of, 269–270
Systemic diseases, biofilm and, 18

T
Tactile evaluation, 19–20
TADs. See Temporary anchor devices
Tarnish
　causes of, 206–207, 207f
　definition of, 7–8, 12–13, 203
　and oxidation, 12–13
　resistance to, 229–230
Tea, staining from, 12
Tear resistance, definition of, 51–52, 54
Tear strength, of irreversible hydrocolloid, 57
Teeth whitening
　contraindications for, 429b
　materials for, 424
　procedures, 421–439
Temperature
　gypsum setting time and, 102
　hypersensitivity and, 409
　in manipulation of materials, 31
　of oral environment, 13–14
Temporary anchor devices (TADs), 246, 259, 261f
Temporary dipoles, 26
Temporary/provisional, 333, 337
Temporary restorations, 24–25

Tensile force
　definition of, 7–8
　oral environment and, 11
Tensile strength, of glass ionomer cements, 171
Tension, amalgam and, 206
Termination, of free radicals, 276
Tetracycline, teeth staining from, 423
Therapeutic materials, 8–9, 29
　definition of, 7–8
Thermal conductivity
　of acrylic resins, 277
　of alloys, 229
　of composite resin, 144
　conductor for, 14
　definition of, 7–8, 14
Thermal expansion
　and contraction, of glass ionomer cements, 171
　of dental waxes, 107
　of metals, 229
Thermal protection, of glass ionomer cements, 171
Thixotropy, 24–26
Three-body abrasives, 374
　loose, 374
　paste, 374
Thumb sucking appliance, 446, 447f
Thumb sucking device, definition of, 440
Tin, 205
　as component of amalgam alloy, 205t
Tin oxide
　in abrasion, 374, 376f
　for implants, 267
Tissue conditioners, 286–287, 287f, 288f
Tissue management, 263
Titanium
　in alloy, 231–232
　alloy screws, 249–250
　oxides of, 249
Tofflemire-type retainer, 208
　use of, 208f, 210f
Tongue, surface changes and, 373
Tooth
　characteristics, 196
　dental caries susceptibility, 405
　placement of band in, 208–210, 210f
　sensitivity of, mechanism of, 409–410, 409b
Tooth restoration, gold for, 4f
Tooth structure, 123f
　bond to, of glass ionomer cements, 171
Tooth whitening rinses, 430
Toothpaste, 378
　abrasion from, 378f
　as desensitizing agent, 410t–411t
　fluoride-containing, 401
　tooth whitening, 430
Torque wrench, 249, 255–258
Torsion/torque, 7–8, 11, 11f
Total-etch cements, 348

Toughness, 24–25, 27
　fracture, 7–8, 11
Toxicity, 34, 38–39
Traditional glass ionomer cements
　advantages and disadvantages of, 346b
　composition of, 345
　manipulation of, 346
　properties of, 345–346
Transillumination, 21
Translucency, 7–8
　of ceramics, 184, 196
Transosteal implant, 247
Transparency, of ceramics, 184, 184f
Transparent, 7–8, 17
Tray whitening systems, over-the-counter, 429
Trimming, 105–106, 106b, 106f
　definition of, 93
　of diagnostic casts, 103–104, 103f
　　procedure for, 115b–117b, 115f, 116f, 117f
Triple trays (closed-bite trays), 54
Trituration, 213–214, 214b, 215f
　alloy and, 213–214
Triturator (amalgamator), 203, 213–214
Two-body abrasives, 373
Two-bottle adhesive systems, 129–130, 130f
Two-cord retraction technique, 70
Two-stage surgical procedure, for endosseous implant, 253
　first stage, 253, 254f
　second stage, 253

U

UDMA. *See* Urethane dimethacrylate
Ultimate strength, 7–8, 11, 27
　definition of, 24–25
Ultrasonic implant tips, 267–269, 268f
Undercut, retention and, 14, 15f
Universal bonding adhesive, clinical application of, 132–134, 133b, 133f
Universal bonding system, definition of, 120–121
Universal composites, 146
　definition of, 139–140
Urethane dimethacrylate (UDMA), 141
Utility wax, 108, 109f

V

Vacuum former acetate technique, for provisional coverage, 316
Value, 139–140, 151
　definition of, 7–8, 16
Van der Waals forces, 25–26
Vapor, inhalation of, 38
Varnish, 335
　sodium fluoride, applications, 399, 400f, 413b, 413f
Veneer, 181, 189–191, 190b
　crown, cross-section of, 184f

Veneer *(Continued)*
　definition of, 180
　materials used for, 189
　porcelain, 189–190
Ventilation, type of chemical, 40–41
Vinyl polyether silicone hybrid, 68
Vinyl polysiloxane (VPS), 64–68
Viscosity, 24–26
　of cement, 340–341
　definition of, 7–8, 15
　of dental cement, 340–341, 340b
　of zinc oxide, 352
VITA Lumin system, 195
Vital tooth, definition of, 421
Vitality, 7–8, 17
　of ceramics, 184
Vitapan classical shade, 17f
Vomiting, tooth erosion and, 396
VPS. *See* Vinyl polysiloxane

W

"Walking bleach" technique, 427
　definition of, 421
Washington, George, 4f
Water
　abrasion and, 372
　air polishing and, 385
　as solvent, 130
Water-based luting cements, 343–347
Water sorption
　definition of, 7–8
　dental materials and, 12
Wax bite, 66, 67f
　registration, 87b–88b, 87f, 88f
Wax pattern, definition of, 93
Wear resistance, of glass ionomer cements, 171
Wedge, 210–211, 211f
　in matrix systems, of composite resin, 158–160, 159b, 160f
Welding, 234
"Wet" dentin bonding, 124–125
　definition of, 120–121
Wettability, 63, 63b
Wetting
　characteristics, 15f
　definition of, 7–8, 15, 120–121
　of gypsum materials, 97
　liquid adhesive and, 15
Wheels, 386, 387f
Whitening
　contraindications of, 429b
　definition of, 421
　indications for, 428b
　materials, 424
　pretreatment evaluation of, 424
　treatment methods, 424–432
Whitening strips, 429, 429f
Wire
　gauge of, 237
　in orthodontics, 226, 229, 236
Wooden plaque removers, for implant home care, 265

Working casts, 94, 95f
  definition of, 93
  fabricating and trimming of, 103–104, 103f
    boxing method in, 103f, 104
    double-pour method in, 104
    single-step method in, 104
Working time, 24–25, 30
Written hazard communication program, 43
Wrought metal alloys, 226, 235–236, 235f, 241b–242b

X

Xenografts, 246, 261, 262f

Y

Yield strength, 226, 229, 231
Yield stress, 24–25, 27
Young's Modulus, 24–25, 27, 144

Z

Zinc, as component of amalgam alloy, 205t
Zinc oxide, as base material, 335–336, 336b
Zinc oxide eugenol (ZOE), 351–353
  advantages and disadvantages of, 352b
  composition of, 351–352
  impression material, 78
  manipulation of, 352–353
  primary and secondary consistency of, 359b, 359f, 360f
  properties of, 352
Zinc phosphate, 343–344
  advantages and disadvantages of, 343b
  composition of, 343
  manipulation of, 344
  primary consistency of, 360b–361b, 360f, 361f
  properties of, 343–344
Zinc polycarboxylate, 344–345
  advantages and disadvantages of, 344b
  composition of, 344
  manipulation of, 345, 345b
  primary consistency of, 361b–362b, 361f, 362f
  properties of, 344–345
Zirconia, 183
  definition of, 180
  in dental implants, 250
  esthetics of, improvement of, 183
  flexural strength of, 183t
  glass-infiltrated, indications and contraindications to, 189t
  with or without veneering, indications and contraindications to, 189t
ZOE. See Zinc oxide eugenol